Canine and Feline Behavior for Veterinary Technicians and Nurses

Canine and Feline Behavior for Veterinary Technicians and Nurses

SECOND EDITION

EDITED BY

Debbie Martin

LVT, CPDT-KA, KPA CTP, VTS (Behavior)
TEAM Education in Animal Behavior, LLC
Veterinary Behavior Consultations, LLC
Texas, USA.

Julie K. Shaw

RVT, KPA CTP, VTS (Behavior)
Julie Shaw Consulting
Indiana, USA.

WILEY Blackwell

Edition history
First edition © 2015 by John Wiley & Sons

Published by John Wiley & Sons, Inc., Hoboken, New Jersey.
Published simultaneously in Canada.

Library of Congress Cataloging-in-Publication Data
Names: Martin, Debbie, 1970– editor. | Shaw, Julie K., 1963– editor.
Title: Canine and feline behavior for veterinary technicians and nurses / edited by Deborah Ann Martin, Julie Kay Shaw.
Description: Second edition. | Hoboken, NJ : Wiley-Blackwell, 2023. | Includes bibliographical references and index.
Identifiers: LCCN 2023004393 (print) | LCCN 2023004394 (ebook) | ISBN 9781119765400 (paperback) | ISBN 9781119765578 (adobe pdf) | ISBN 9781119765592 (epub) | ISBN 9781119765585 (obook)
Subjects: MESH: Dogs–psychology | Behavior, Animal | Cats–psychology | Veterinary Medicine–methods | Animal Technicians
Classification: LCC SF433 (print) | LCC SF433 (ebook) | NLM SF 433 | DDC 636.7/0887–dc23/eng/20230215
LC record available at https://lccn.loc.gov/2023004393
LC ebook record available at https://lccn.loc.gov/2023004394

Cover Design: Wiley
Cover Image(s): Courtesy of Debbie Martin

Set in 8.5/11pt MeridienLTStd by Straive, Pondicherry, India

SKY10069152_030824

Dedication

This text is dedicated to Dr. Andrew Luescher, DVM, Ph.D, DACVB. Dr. Luescher envisioned the role of a veterinary technician in animal behavior in 1998 and then developed and defined that role over the years. He believed pet owners were best served with a team approach to the treatment of behavior issues and he saw the importance of veterinary technicians on that team. He is our mentor, teacher, and friend and without him, it is unlikely this text would have ever come to fruition. Thank you Dr. Luescher for all you have done to promote, protect, and support the human–animal bond and veterinary technicians over the years. We hope we have made your proud.

Julie and Debbie

Contents

Appendix Section 1: Forms and Questionnaires

Appendix Section 2: Training Exercises

Appendix Section 3: Samples and Letters

Contributors

Lindsey M. Fourez, BS, RVT
Purdue Comparative Oncology Program, Purdue University, West Lafayette, IN, USA

Lindsey grew up in a small rural town in Illinois. After high school she attended Purdue University where she studied animal science and veterinary technology. In 2004 she graduated with her Associate in Science degree in veterinary technology, and then in 2005 with a BS in veterinary technology. Currently Lindsey works in the Purdue Comparative Oncology Program.

Sarah Lahrman, RVT
Purdue Comparative Oncology Program, Purdue University, West Lafayette, IN, USA

Sarah Lahrman is a graduate of Purdue University and obtained her Associate degree in veterinary technology in 1998. Following graduation she began work at a small animal practice in Fort Wayne, Indiana and later moved to another small animal practice in Columbia City, IN. In 2007, her family relocated to Lafayette, IN and Sarah was inspired to work at Purdue University's Small Animal Teaching Hospital. She currently works in the Purdue Comparative Oncology Program.

Rachel M. Lees, LVMT, KPA CTP, Elite FFCP (Veterinary), LSHC – Silver, VTS (Behavior)
The University of Tennessee College of Veterinary Medicine, Knoxville, TN, USA

Rachel Lees is proud to be a veterinary nurse and member of the Academy of Veterinary Behavior Technicians. She is also delighted to be a Certified Training Partner through the Karen Pryor Academy Dog Trainer Professional program.

Rachel graduated from Cuyahoga Community College in May 2009 with her Associate degree in veterinary technology. Immediately after graduation, Rachel was employed at a multi-doctor practice in a suburb near Cleveland, Ohio. She became the behavior advocate of her veterinary hospital introducing the need for happy visits and performing behavior modification with behavior cases in the practice. In June 2013, Rachel left her position in general practice to accept a position at The Behavior Clinic in Olmsted Falls, OH. In April 2014, she graduated and became a Certified Training Partner with the Karen Pryor Academy. After an eight-year adventure with The Behavior Clinic, in May 2021 Rachel uprooted herself and took a position at The University of Tennessee College of Veterinary Medicine with Dr. Julia Albright, DACVB.

Rachel has a special interest in teaching cooperative care techniques for veterinary protocols to small animals and has even worked with some exotic species. Rachel is an Elite Fear Free Certified Professional, is on the Fear Free Speakers Bureau, and an active member of the Fear Free Advisory Panel. Rachel is the current CVTS liaison for the Academy of Veterinary Behavior Technicians and is an active instructor and member of VIN/VSPN, NAVTA (National Association of Veterinary Technicians of America), and TVTA (Tennessee Veterinary Technician Association).

Debbie Martin, LVT, Elite FFCP (Veterinary), CPDT-KA, KPA CTP, FFCP (Trainer), VTS (Behavior)
TEAM Education in Animal Behavior, LLC, Spicewood, TX, USA
Veterinary Behavior Consultations, LLC, Spicewood, TX, USA

Debbie is a licensed veterinary technician and a Veterinary Technician Specialist (VTS) in Behavior (2010). She is a Certified Professional Dog Trainer (Knowledge Assessed) and Karen Pryor Academy Certified Training Partner and Faculty Emeritus. She has a Bachelor of Science degree from The Ohio State University in human ecology, and an Associate of Applied Science degree in veterinary technology from Columbus State Community College. She has been working as a registered/licensed veterinary technician since graduation in 1996 and has been actively involved in the field of animal behavior. Debbie was president of the Academy of Veterinary Behavior Technicians (AVBT) from 2012 to 2014 and is the treasurer. She is an active member and the previous recording secretary for the Society of Veterinary Behavior Technicians (SVBT). She is co-author of the book *Puppy Start Right: Foundation Training for the Companion Dog* and the Puppy Start Right for Instructors Course. Debbie is an Elite Fear Free Certified Professional-Veterinary and Fear Free Certified Professional-Trainer and is a subject matter expert for Fear Free Pets and Fear Free Happy Homes. She presents seminars and presentations internationally regarding animal behavior and training.

Kenneth M. Martin, DVM, Elite FFCP (Veterinary), DACVB
TEAM Education in Animal Behavior, LLC, Spicewood, TX, USA
Veterinary Behavior Consultations, LLC, Spicewood, TX, USA

Dr. Martin completed a clinical behavioral medicine residency at Purdue University's Animal Behavior Clinic in 2004. He graduated from Louisiana State University – School of Veterinary Medicine in 1999. He is a licensed veterinarian in Texas. He practiced companion animal and exotic animal medicine and surgery, and emergency medicine and critical care prior to completing his behavioral medicine residency. His professional interests include conflict-induced (owner-directed) aggression, compulsive disorders, behavioral development, psychopharmacology, and alternative medicine. Dr. Martin is co-author of the book *Puppy Start Right: Foundation Training for the Companion Dog* and Puppy Start Right for Instructors Course. He is a member of the American Veterinary Medical Association, the American Veterinary Society of Animal Behavior and the previous recording secretary. Dr. Martin is an Elite Fear Free Certified Professional-Veterinary and is a subject matter expert for Fear Free Pets and Fear Free Happy Homes. Veterinary Behavior Consultations in Spicewood, TX was the first behavior-only veterinary speciality hospital to earn Fear Free Hospital certification (2019).

Virginia L. Price, MS, CVT, VTS (Behavior)
St. Petersburg College, St. Petersburg, FL, USA

Ginny Price is a professor at St. Petersburg College where she teaches small animal behavior (in the AS and BAS programs) and lectures in animal nursing. Between 2009 and 2011 she was the Critical Thinking Champion for the AS College of Veterinary Technology. From 2012 to 2013, Ginny served as the Center of Excellence for Teaching and Learning representative for the SPC College of Veterinary Technology. From 2009 through 2011 she was privileged to serve on the board of directors for the Western Veterinary Conference as their Technician Director. She graduated from St. Petersburg College Veterinary Technology in 1981. She is certified in the state of Florida with the Florida Veterinary Technician Association. She has a Master's degree in psychology earned in 2007 from Walden University. She is a founding member of the Society of Veterinary Behavior Technicians and the Academy of Veterinary Behavior Technicians. At this time, 2022, Ginny serves at the pleasure of the AVBT President as the Parliamentarian. She also serves on the Clinical Animal Behavior Conference Speaker Committee. She earned her Veterinary Technician Specialist in Behavior in 2010. She earned her Fear Free level 3 in 2021.

Lisa Radosta DVM, DACVB
Florida Veterinary Behavior Service, West Palm Beach, FL, USA

Dr. Radosta is a board-certified veterinary behaviorist and owner of Florida Veterinary Behavior Service. She has spoken from Miami to Moscow, penned books, including *Behavior Problems of the Dog and Cat, 4th edition* and *From Fearful to Fear Free*. She has served on the Fear Free Executive Council and the AAHA Behavior Management Task Force. She is frequently interviewed for print, radio, podcast, and television media. She strives to help veterinary team members understand that behavior is medicine and help pet parents understand their companion's behavior.

Julie K. Shaw, KPA CTP, RVT, VTS (Behavior)
Julie Shaw Consulting, Lafayette, IN, USA

Julie Shaw became a registered veterinary technician in 1983. After working in general veterinary practice for 17 years and starting her own successful dog training business. She became the Senior Animal Behavior Technologist at the Purdue Animal Behavior Clinic working with veterinary animal behaviorist, Dr. Andrew Luescher, PhD, DVM, DACVB. While at Purdue, Julie saw referral behavior cases with Dr. Luescher, organized and co-taught the acclaimed five-day DOGS! Behavior Modification course, taught many classes to veterinary and veterinary technician students, and instructed continuing education seminars for veterinary technicians, veterinarians, and trainers.

Julie is a charter member of the Society of Veterinary Behavior Technicians and the Academy of Veterinary Behavior Technicians. She is also a faculty emeritus for the Dog Trainer Professional Program through the Karen Pryor Academy for Animal Training and Behavior.

Julie has received many awards including the North American Veterinary Conference Veterinary Technician Speaker of the Year Award and the Western Veterinary Conference speaker of the year, and was named the 2007 NAVC Mara Memorial Lecturer of the year for her accomplishments and leadership in the veterinary technician profession.

Julie currently sees referral behavior cases and is active in animal-assisted interventions.

Thank you to the following contributors of content for the first edition of the book. Although they were not involved in the revisions of the chapters noted for the second edition, much of their organization and content remain in the updated chapters. Their original contributions were invaluable.

Chapter 2: Andrew U. Luescher, DVM, PhD, DACVB, ECAWBM (BM)

Chapter 7: Linda M. Campbell, RVT, CPDT-KA, VTS (Behavior), Marcia R. Ritchie, LVT, CPDT-KA, VTS (Behavior)

Chapter 9 (1e chapter 8): Julie K. Shaw, KPA CTP, RVT, VTS (Behavior)

Chapter 10 (1e chapter 9): Carissa D. Sparks, BS, RVT, VTS (Neurology), Sara L. Bennett, DVM, MS, DACVB

Preface

The human–animal bond is a powerful and fragile union. Pets, dogs specifically, have evolved from being primarily for utilitarian purposes to taking on the role of a human companion and family member. Consequently, pet owners' expectations have changed and are continuing to change. As the stigma of human mental and emotional health begins to be shattered, so is the stigma of treating animals with behavioral issues. Pet owners are beginning to recognize their pet's emotional and mental needs and are reaching out to veterinary professionals for assistance.

We believe it takes a mental healthcare team that includes a veterinarian, veterinary technician, and a qualified trainer to most successfully prevent and treat behavior issues in companion animals.

The veterinary technician is in a unique position to be a pivotal and key component in that mental healthcare team. Technicians interact and educate pet owners on a daily basis about preventive and intervention medical treatments. Through behavioral preventive services and assisting the veterinarian with behavioral intervention, communicating and working closely with the qualified trainer, veterinary technicians can become the "case manager" of the team, in turn saving lives and enhancing the human–animal bond.

Many books have been published geared toward the role of the veterinarian in behavioral medicine. The purpose of this text is to provide the veterinary technician with a solid foundation in feline and canine behavioral medicine. All veterinary technicians must have a basic understanding of their patient's behavioral, mental, and emotional needs. Companion animal behavior in this regard is not a specialty but the foundation for better understanding and treatment of our patients. General companion animal behavior healthcare should no longer be an "elective" in veterinary and veterinary technician curriculums but rather a core part of our education. How can we best administer quality healthcare if we do not understand our patient's psychological needs?

The reader will learn about the roles of animal behavior professionals, normal development of dogs and cats, and be provided with an in-depth and dynamic look at the human–animal bond with a new perspective that includes correlations from human mental healthcare. Learning theory, preventive behavioral services, husbandry and veterinary care, standardized behavior modification terms and techniques, and veterinary behavior pharmacology are also included.

There is vibrant change occurring in the world of animal behavior professionals. It is as though a snowball that took some work to get started has begun rolling and growing on its own. People like you are propelling that snowball forward and improving the lives of animals and the people who love them.

After the first moment you open this book we hope it becomes outdated – because you will continue to push the snowball forward with new ideas and techniques.

Thank you for improving the lives of animals.

Julie K. Shaw and Debbie Martin

Acknowledgments

Debbie Martin

I would like to thank Julie Shaw, a wonderful teacher, mentor, and friend. It was her passion for educating others and initiative that brought this book to fruition. I was honored to have been invited to co-edit the book with her for the first edition and equally honored she trusted me to be the primary editor for the second edition.

I would also like to acknowledge my husband, Kenneth Martin, DVM, DACVB, for his patience, guidance, and understanding as I spent countless hours, days, weeks, and months on this project. His insights and feedback provided much needed support and assistance throughout the process.

Julie K. Shaw

Thank you to Ginny Price, MS, CVT, VTS (Behavior), Danielle Bolm, RVT, LVT, KPA CTP, VTS (Behavior), and Dr. Liam Clay, Ph.D, B. App. Sc. (Vet tech) VTS (Behavior) B. App. Sc.(Hons) for their research assistance.

I would like to thank my friend Debbie Martin for making my life better and making this book possible.

About the companion website

This book is accompanied by a companion website:

www.wiley.com/go/martin/behavior

The website includes:

- Powerpoints of all figures from the book for downloading
- Appendices from the book for downloading
- Self-assessment quizzes
- Videos cited in the chapters

1 The role of the veterinary technician in animal behavior

Kenneth M. Martin[1,2] and Debbie Martin[1,2]
[1]*TEAM Education in Animal Behavior, LLC, Spicewood, TX, USA*
[2]*Veterinary Behavior Consultations, LLC, Spicewood, TX, USA*

CHAPTER MENU

The veterinary staff plays a significant role in preventing, identifying, and treating behavioral disorders of pets. Inquiring about behavior at each veterinary visit, as well as creating client awareness about behavior disorders and training problems, strengthens the client–hospital bond, the human–animal bond, and prevents pet relinquishment. The veterinary technician can excel and be fully utilized in the behavior technician role. The responsibilities of the veterinary technician in animal behavior begin with educating and building awareness regarding the normal behavior of animals. The veterinarian–veterinary technician partnership allows for prevention and treatment of behavioral disorders and training problems. Distinguishing and identifying behavior disorders, medical disorders, lack of training issues, and being able to provide prevention and early intervention allows for the maintenance and enhancement of the human–animal bond. Clearly defining the roles and responsibilities of the veterinary behavior team facilitates harmony within the team without misrepresentation. The veterinary technician's role as part of the behavior team is often that of "case manager"; the technician triages and guides the client to the appropriate resources for assistance. Before delving into the extensive role

Canine and Feline Behavior for Veterinary Technicians and Nurses, Second Edition. Edited by Debbie Martin and Julie K. Shaw.

Companion website: www.wiley.com/go/martin/behavior

of the veterinary technician in the behavior team, the roles of the veterinarian and the animal trainer will be explored. By understanding these roles first, the pivotal role of the technician will become evident.

- The veterinary technician's role as part of the behavior team is often that of "case manager"; the technician triages and guides the client to the appropriate resources for assistance.

Veterinarian's roles and responsibilities

The veterinarian is responsible for the clinical assessment of all patients presented to the veterinary hospital. The veterinarian's role in behavior includes

1. setting the hospital's policy and procedures,
2. determining which behavioral services are offered,
3. developing the format of the behavior consultation history form for medical documentation,
4. establishing a behavioral diagnosis and list of differentials, as well as medical differentials,
5. providing the prognosis,
6. developing a treatment plan and making any changes to the plan,
7. prescribing medication and changing medication type or dosage, and
8. outlining the procedure and protocols for follow-up care.

- The veterinarian is responsible for the clinical assessment of all patients presented to the veterinary hospital.

Only a licensed veterinarian can practice veterinary medicine. The practice of veterinary medicine means to diagnose, treat, correct, change, relieve, or prevent any animal disease, deformity, defect, injury, or other physical or mental conditions, including the prescribing of any drug or medicine (Modified from: Title 37 Professions and occupations Chapter 18. Veterinarians Louisiana Practice Act [La. R.S. 37: 1511–1558]). The mental welfare of animals and the treatment of mental illness are included in many states' veterinary practice acts. Only by evaluating the patient's physical and neurological health and obtaining and reviewing the medical and behavioral history, can the veterinarian establish a diagnosis and prescribe appropriate treatment. When dealing with the behavior of animals, it must be determined whether the behavior is normal, abnormal, the manifestation of a medical condition, an inappropriately conditioned behavior, or simply related to a lack of training.

The veterinarian, by establishing a diagnosis and prescribing behavioral treatment, is practicing veterinary behavioral medicine comparable to a medical doctor practicing human psychiatry, this medical specialty deals with the prevention, assessment, diagnosis, treatment, and rehabilitation of mental illness in humans. The goal of human psychiatry is the relief of mental suffering associated with behavioral disorder and the improvement of mental well-being. The focus of veterinary behavior is to improve the welfare of pets and consequently enhance the well-being of clients. This strengthens the human–animal bond. When addressing the behavior of animals, the mental well-being of the patient should be evaluated in direct relation to the patient's medical health. In this manner, the veterinarian is using a complete or holistic approach and treating the entire patient. This may be accomplished only by a visit to the veterinarian (Figure 1.1).

The veterinarian or veterinary technician should obtain behavioral information during every hospital visit. Many behavioral issues are overlooked in general veterinary practice without direct solicitation.

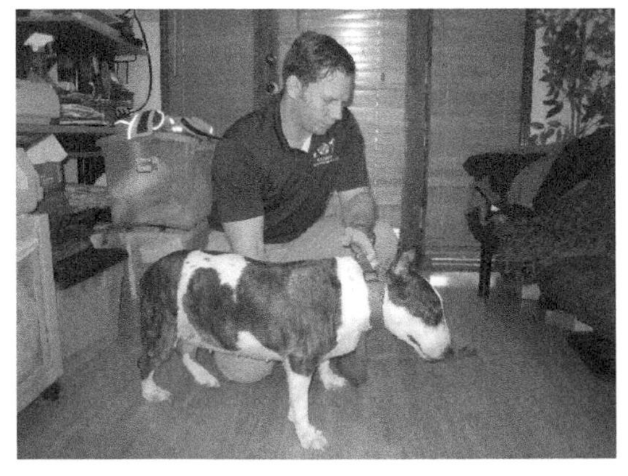

Figure 1.1 Veterinarian performing a physical examination of the patient at home.

Current pet management information regarding feeding, housing, exercising, training, and training aids should be documented in the medical record. Behavioral topics for puppy visits should include socialization, body language, house training, play biting, husbandry care, and methodology for basic training and problem solving. Behavioral topics for kitten visits should include play biting and scratching, litter-box training and management, husbandry care, and carrier training. All senior patients should be screened annually for cognitive dysfunction syndrome. Only through questioning clients regarding their pet's behavior will potential behavioral disorders or training problems be identified. The veterinary staff may then recommend suitable behavior services to address the specific issues. This may prompt scheduling an appointment with the appropriate staff member: the veterinarian, veterinary behavior technician, or a qualified professional trainer.

- Many behavioral issues are overlooked in general veterinary practice without direct solicitation.

When a behavioral disorder is suspected, interviewing the client and obtaining a thorough behavioral history is essential for the veterinarian to make a behavioral diagnosis. The behavioral history should include the signalment, the patient's early history, management, household dynamics and human interaction schedule, previous training, and a temperament profile. The temperament profile determines the pet's individual response to specific social and environmental stimuli. Triggers of the undesirable behaviors should be identified. Pet owners should describe the typical behavioral response of the pet. In addition, the chronological development of the behavior, including the age of onset, the historical progression, and whether the behavior has worsened, improved, or remained the same, must be documented. Discussing a minimum of three specific incidents detailing the pet's body language before, during, and after the behavior, as well as the human response, is necessary. The medical record should document previous treatments including training, medical intervention, and drug therapy. Changes in the household or management should be questioned. Inducing the behavioral response or observing the behavior on previously recorded video may be necessary. However, caution should be used in regard to observing the behavior. Often the behavioral history provides sufficient information for a diagnosis. If the description of the behavior does not provide sufficient information, then observation of the patient's *first* response to a controlled exposure to the stimulus may be required. Safety factors should be in place to prevent injury to the patient or others. This should only be used as a last resort as it allows the patient to practice the undesirable behavior and carries risk. (For an example of behavior history forms, see Appendices 1–5.)

The veterinarian and veterinary staff are instrumental in recognizing behavior issues when a pet is presented for an underlying medical problem. All medical diseases result in behavior changes and most behavioral disorders have medical differentials. A behavior disorder may lead to the clinical presentation of a surgical or medical disease. Surgical repair of wounds inflicted by a dog bite may prompt the veterinarian to recommend behavior treatment for inter-dog aggression. A cat or dog presenting with self-inflicted wounds may indicate a panic disorder or compulsive behavior (Figure 1.2). Dental disease including fractured teeth may prompt the veterinarian to inquire about anxiety-related conditions such as separation anxiety. Frequent enterotomies may indicate pica or some other anxiety-related condition. The astute veterinarian must use a multimodal approach with the integration of behavioral questionnaires and medical testing to determine specific and nonspecific links to

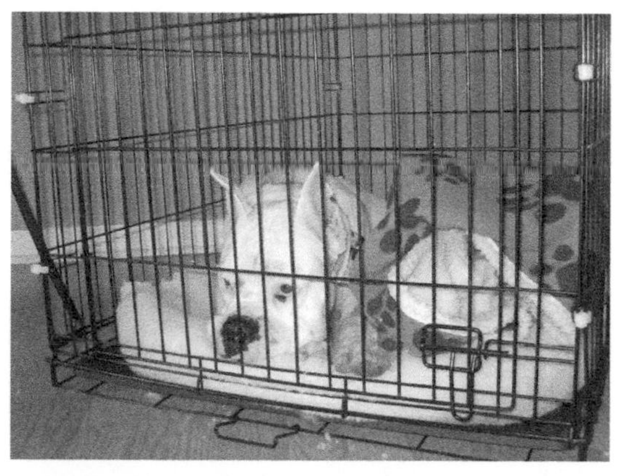

Figure 1.2 Boxer presenting for excoriation of the muzzle due to separation anxiety (barrier frustration) with frequent attempts to escape the crate.

behavioral disorders. Medical disease may cause the development of a behavior disorder. Feline lower urinary tract disease may lead to the continuation of inappropriate elimination even after the inciting cause has been treated. Many behavior disorders require and benefit from concurrent medical and pharmacological treatment.

- All medical diseases result in behavior changes and most behavioral disorders have medical differentials.

- The astute veterinarian must use a multimodal approach with the integration of behavioral questionnaires and medical testing to determine specific and nonspecific links to behavioral disorders.

Medical differentials to behavior disorders

When faced with a behavior problem, the veterinarian must determine if the cause is medical and/or behavioral. The rationale that the problem is only either medical or behavioral is a flawed approach. Neurophysiologically, any medical condition that affects the normal function of the central nervous system can alter behavior. The nonspecific complaint of lethargy or depression may be caused by a multitude of factors including pyrexia, pain, anemia, hypoglycemia, a congenital abnormality such as lissencephaly or hydrocephalus, a central nervous system disorder involving neoplasia, infection, trauma, or lead toxicity, endocrine disorders such as hypothyroidism or hyperadrenocorticism, metabolic disorders such as hepatic or uremic encephalopathy, and cognitive dysfunction or sensory deficits. Behavioral signs are the first presenting signs of any illness.

- Behavioral signs are the first presenting signs of any illness.

As a general rule, veterinarians should do a physical and neurological examination and basic blood analysis for all pets presenting for behavioral changes. The practitioner may decide to perform more specific diagnostic tests based on exam findings. Additional diagnostics will vary on a case-by-case basis.

The existence of a medical condition can be determined only after a thorough physical and neurological examination. Completing a neurological examination is difficult in patients displaying fear and/or aggression with handling. The neurological examination may be basic and limited to the cranial nerves, muscle symmetry and tone, central proprioception, ambulation, and anal tone. Other minimum diagnostic testing should include a complete laboratory analysis (complete blood count [CBC], serum chemistry profile, and urinalysis) and fecal screening. A further look into sensory perception may include an electroretinogram (ERG) or brainstem auditory evoked response (BAER). Thyroid testing (total thyroxine, free thyroxine, triiodothyronine, thyrotropin, and/or antithyroid antibodies) may be indicated based on clinical signs, suspicion, and the class of medication considered for behavioral treatment. Imaging techniques, such as radiographs, ultrasound, magnetic resonance imaging (MRI) or computed axial tomography (CT) may provide invaluable information. The workup for medical conditions and behavioral conditions is not mutually exclusive. However, exhausting every medical rule out may pose financial limitations for the client. After all, diagnosis is inferential behaviorally and medically, and the purpose of establishing a diagnosis is not to categorize but to prescribe treatment.

- After all, diagnosis is inferential behaviorally and medically, and the purpose of establishing a diagnosis is not to categorize but to prescribe treatment.

Behavioral dermatology

A relationship between dermatologic conditions and anxiety-related conditions exists in humans and pets. Environmental and social stress has been shown to increase epidermal permeability and increase the susceptibility to allergens (Garg et al. 2001). A dermatological lesion can be caused behaviorally by a compulsive disorder, a conditioned behavior, separation anxiety, or any conflict behavior. Behavioral dermatologic signs in companion animals may include alopecia, feet or limb biting, licking or chewing, tail chasing, flank sucking, hind end checking, anal licking, nonspecific scratching, hyperesthesia, and self-directed aggression. Medical reasons for tail chasing may include lumbosacral stenosis or cauda equina syndrome, a tail dock neuroma or a paresthesia. Anal licking may be associated with anal sac disease, parasites, or food hypersensitivity. Dermatological conditions may be related to staphylococcal infection, mange, dermatophytosis, allergies, hypothyroidism, trauma, foreign body, neoplasia, osteoarthritis, or neuropathic pain. Diagnostic testing may include screening for ectoparasites, skin scraping, epidermal cytology, dermatophyte test medium (DTM), woods lamp, an insecticide application every three weeks, a food allergy elimination diet (FAED), skin biopsy, intradermal skin testing or enzyme linked immunosorbent assay (ELISA), and a corticosteroid trial. It is important to realize that corticosteroids have psychotropic effects in addition to antipruritic properties. A favorable response to steroids does not rule out behavioral factors. Steroid-treated dogs with pruritus may show increased reactivity to thunderstorms and noises (Klink et al. 2008).

Conversely, behavioral disorders may be maintained even after the dermatological condition has resolved. Dermatological lesions may be linked to behavioral disorders and lesions can facilitate and intensify other behavior problems including aggression. Dogs with dermatological lesions are not necessarily more likely to be aggressive, but dogs with aggression disorders may be more irritable when they have concurrent dermatological lesions. In a study of dogs with atopic dermatitis, pruritus severity was associated with increased frequency of problematic behaviors, such as mounting, chewing, hyperactivity, coprophagia, begging for and stealing food, attention-seeking, excitability, excessive grooming, and reduced trainability (Harvey et al. 2019).

Aggression

The relationship between the viral disease of rabies and aggression is very clear. All cases of aggression should be verified for current rabies vaccination status and/or clients should be advised to maintain current rabies vaccination for their pet to protect from liability. Iatrogenic aggression in canine and feline patients has been induced by the administration of certain drugs such as benzodiazepines, acepromazine, and ketamine.

- All cases of aggression should be verified for current rabies vaccination status and/or clients should be advised to maintain current rabies vaccination for their pet to protect from liability.

The relationship between hyperthyroidism in cats and irritable aggression is very likely present, although not definitively established. The relationship between hypothyroidism and aggression in dogs is inconclusive. Hypothyroidism may lead to structural and functional changes in the brain that can potentially lead to changes in behavior such as aggression, apathy, lethargy or mental dullness, cold intolerance, exercise intolerance, and decreased libido (Camps et al. 2019). Numerous case reports suggesting a link between aggression in dogs and thyroid deficiency have been published in the veterinary literature. The effect of thyroid supplementation on behavior without the benefit of a control group in these case studies offers limited evidence of a causative relationship. In a controlled study of nonaggressive and aggressive dogs no significant differences in thyroid levels were found (Radosta-Huntley et al. 2006). Thyroid hormone supplementation in rats results in elevation of serotonin in the frontal cortex (Gur et al. 1999). Serotonin is a neurotransmitter associated with mood stabilization (see Chapter 10). The possible elevation of serotonin due to thyroid supplementation may result in beneficial behavioral changes in dogs that display aggression. In a small study of dogs with spontaneous hypothyroidism, thyroid supplementation produced no significant difference in circulating serum concentrations of serotonin at six weeks and six months when compared to baseline (Hrovat et al. 2018). Spontaneous resolution of aggression with thyroid supplementation is probably overstated and hypothyroidism is unlikely the cause of aggression. While malaise can lead to irritability, many dogs that have hypothyroidism do not show aggression.

The presence of sensory deficits may contribute to aggressive behavior and anxiety. This is particularly important when assessing the behavior of senior patients with concurrent medical disorders. Age-related behavioral changes in the brain can lead to the presentation of clinical signs consistent with cognitive dysfunction syndrome. These signs may include disorientation, interaction changes with the owner, changes in the sleep–wake cycle, and house soiling. Activity level may be decreased or increased.

Elimination disorders

Elimination problems in dogs may be related to urinary tract infection, urolithiasis, polyuria/polydipsia, incontinence, prostatic disease, renal disease, constipation/diarrhea, acute or chronic pain, neoplasia, or acute or chronic stress. Elimination problems in cats may be related to idiopathic cystitis, urolithiasis, infection, neoplasia, incontinence, acute or chronic pain, polyuria/polydipsia, constipation/diarrhea, acute or chronic stress, or associated with long hair. Urological diagnostics may include a CBC, chemistry, urinalysis, urine culture, adrenocorticotropic hormone (ACTH) stimulation, water deprivation tests, imaging, cystoscopy, or a urethral pressure profile. Gastrointestinal diagnostics may include a CBC, chemistry, and urinalysis to assess for contributing or concurrent problems that may affect treatment decisions, fecal float/smear/PCR, abdominal-thoracic imaging studies, GI panel (B12/folate/TLI/PLI), baseline cortisol or ACTH stimulation test for Addison's disease, and gastrointestinal endoscopy/laparotomy/biopsy.

When one is uncertain whether it is a behavioral or medical problem, one must do some reasonable fact finding and treat the entire patient, physically and psychologically. When necessary, infer the most likely diagnosis and treat all contributing factors. Medical and psychological factors must be treated concurrently. A treatment plan that includes conventional medical treatment and behavioral intervention is necessary for successful resolution of the inciting problem.

- When one is uncertain whether it is a behavioral or medical problem, one must do some reasonable fact finding and treat the entire patient, physically and psychologically.

Chronic pain conditions

Chronic and undiagnosed pain-related conditions are extremely common in veterinary patients. They can directly contribute to and exacerbate behavioral disorders. The anticipation of pain can change behavior and lead to anxiety. It is imperative that patients, regardless of age and activity level, are routinely evaluated for pain. Pain automatically creates fear, anxiety, and stress in pets. If a behavioral condition is being treated but the patient is experiencing chronic pain, we are not treating the well-being of the entire patient and behavioral therapy might not be as effective.

Through learning, a dog might pair the approach of a person or another animal in the house, while the dog is resting on the couch, with pain. The dog when approached moved or shifted his body and experienced a sharp pain in his back. Now when approached he anticipates pain and might begin to display defensive aggression to inhibit the approach of the person or other animal. Ruling out pain conditions when a pet displays aggression when approached, especially by familiar people, is imperative.

Another example is with food-related aggression. Consider pain-related conditions contributing to difficulty apprehending, chewing, or ingesting food in cases of food-related aggression. Dogs may be hungry and motivated to eat, but frustrated and irritable due to dental or oropharyngeal pain or discomfort with eating. Gastrointestinal upset and discomfort may be associated with aggression around food. Musculoskeletal disease may lower the dog's threshold to display irritable behavior. Rather than rising and moving away with the object, a dog with musculoskeletal pain may be more likely to remain stationery and display aggression.

There has also been a correlation between musculoskeletal pain and noise sensitivities in dogs (Lopes Fagundes et al. 2018). The non-pain and pain groups in the study showed similar behavioral response to loud noises. However, in the pain group the onset of noise sensitivity was later; on average four years later than the non-pain group. Dogs with pain were more likely to generalize and show avoidance of associated environments and other dogs. All dogs (pain or non-pain groups) responded well to treatment but the pain group only once pain was treated.

Behavior disorder versus training problem

Behavioral disorders of animals are emotional disorders that are unrelated to training. Training problems relate to pets that are unruly or do not know or respond to cues or commands. These problems are common in young puppies and adolescent dogs without basic training. These dogs lack manners.

Training involves the learning of human-taught appropriate behaviors that are unrelated to the emotional or mental well-being of the patient. There are many different approaches to training. Some are purely force free or free of aversives (positive reinforcement) and others use aversive methodology (positive punishment and negative reinforcement). Trainers may also be "balanced" or somewhere in the middle regarding methodology, using a combination of pleasant and unpleasant consequences. Depending on the methodology used, positive and negative associations can be made by the dog. Aversive-free methods are less emotionally damaging and can strengthen the human–animal bond. Aversive methods risk creating a negative emotional state and may contribute to the development of a behavioral disorder. Dogs that are behaviorally normal and emotionally stable yet lack basic manners training related to heeling on leash, coming when called, sitting, lying down and staying, fit into the category of a training problem. Yes, some emotionally unstable dogs may, in addition, have training problems, but training problems and behavior disorders are treated independently as separate entities. Dogs with fear- or anxiety-related conditions can benefit from aversive-free training in much the same way as shy children benefit from team sports or other confidence-building activities. Dogs previously trained using aversive methodology often need to be retrained using force-free methods for performing behavioral modification techniques as a result of the negative emotional response caused by the previous aversive training. Many well-trained dogs have behavioral disorders (Figure 1.3).

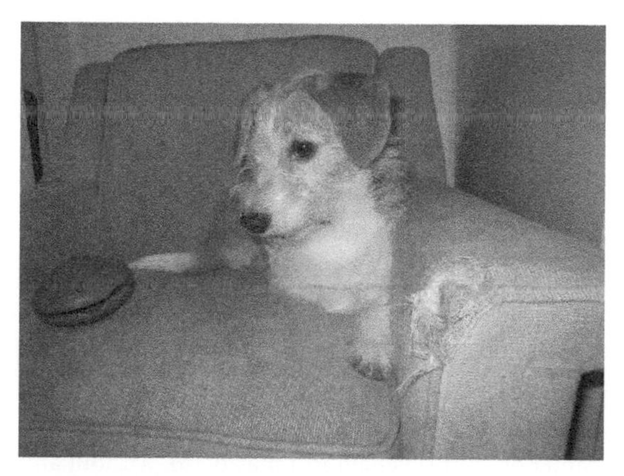

Figure 1.3 Therapy dog who suffers from thunderstorm phobia.

Examples include separation anxiety or human-directed aggression. These disorders occur in spite of the fact that the dog may be very well trained and responsive to the handler. Dog training does not directly treat behavioral disorders and is not considered practicing veterinary behavioral medicine.

- Behavioral disorders of animals are emotional disorders that are unrelated to training.

- Training involves the learning of human-taught appropriate behaviors that are unrelated to the emotional or mental well-being of the patient.

- Some emotionally unstable dogs may, in addition, have training problems, but training problems and behavior disorders are treated independently as separate entities.

It should be noted that there are many benefits to having an aversive-free trainer associated or working within the veterinary practice. Pet owners have been shown to search the internet for information and call their veterinary hospital for their pet's behavioral and training needs (Shore et al. 2008).

Qualified professionals to treat animal behavior disorders

When the pet's behavior is considered abnormal, with an underlying medical or behavioral component, comprising fear, anxiety, or aggression, owners should seek guidance from a trained professional. The veterinarian is the first person who should be contacted when a pet exhibits a problem behavior or the pet's behavior changes. Changes in behavior or behavior problems reflect underlying medical conditions, which must be evaluated by a veterinarian. Many underlying medical problems, including pain, can alter the pet's behavior in ways that are difficult for pet owners to identify. Once medical conditions have been ruled out, behavioral advice should be sought. It is important to understand the qualifications of people who use titles that indicate they are behavior professionals. This is difficult because, unlike the titles veterinarian, psychologist, and psychiatrist, which are state licensed, the title "animal behaviorist" or similar titles can be used by anyone, regardless of their background (modified from www.certifiedanimalbehaviorist.com). Qualified animal behavior professionals include a veterinarian with special interest and training in animal behavior, a Diplomate of the American College of Veterinary Behaviorists (DACVB), or a Certified Applied Animal Behaviorist (CAAB).

- The veterinarian is the first person who should be contacted when a pet exhibits a problem behavior or the pet's behavior changes. Changes in behavior or behavior problems can reflect underlying medical conditions, which must be evaluated by a veterinarian.

- Qualified animal behavior professionals include a veterinarian with special interest and training in animal behavior, a DACVB or a CAAB.

The American Veterinary Society of Animal Behavior (AVSAB) is a group of veterinarians and research professionals who share an interest in understanding the behavior of animals. AVSAB emphasizes that the use of scientifically sound learning principles that apply to all species is the accepted means of training and modifying behavior in pets and is the key to our understanding of how pets learn and how to communicate with our pets. AVSAB (https://avsab.org) is thereby committed to improving the quality of life of all animals and strengthening the human–animal bond.

The American College of Veterinary Behaviorists or ACVB (https://www.dacvb.org) is a professional organization of veterinarians who are board-certified in the specialty of Veterinary Behavior. This veterinary specialty is recognized by the American Board of Veterinary Specialization. Board-certified specialists are known as *diplomates*. Veterinarians who have the honor of calling themselves diplomates may use the designation "DACVB" after their names. The requirements for veterinarians include completing the equivalency of a one-year veterinary internship, completing a conforming approved residency program or a nonconforming training program mentored and approved by ACVB lasting usually three to five years, authoring a scientific paper on behavior research and publishing it in a peer-reviewed journal, writing three peer-reviewed case reports, and successfully completing a comprehensive two-day examination.

The Animal Behavior Society (ABS) is a professional organization in North America for the study of animal behavior. Certification by the ABS (www.animalbehaviorsociety.org) recognizes that, to the best of its knowledge, the certificant meets the educational, experimental, and ethical standards required by the society for professional applied animal behaviorists. Certification does not constitute a guarantee that the applicant meets a specific standard of competence or possesses specific knowledge. Members who meet the specific criteria may use the designation, "CAAB," after their names. CAABs (http://corecaab.org) come from different educational backgrounds and may include a PhD in Animal Behavior or Doctor of Veterinary Medicine. CAABs, who are not veterinarians, usually work directly with veterinarians or through veterinary referral to provide behavioral care.

Trainer's and consultant's roles and responsibilities

The role of the animal trainer in behavior is coaching and teaching of pets and pet owners about basic training and manners. Trainers are teachers. Some trainers function as coaches for competitive dog sports such as obedience, tracking, agility, rally, or protection. Those who work with veterinarians provide an instrumental role in implementing behavior modification as prescribed in a treatment plan.

Comparatively, as it would be inappropriate for a schoolteacher to diagnose or prescribe treatment for a child with a behavioral disorder, dog trainers may not diagnose or prescribe treatment for veterinary behavioral disorders (Luescher et al. 2007). Although the treatment of animal behavior disorders is considered the practice of veterinary medicine, many states have been unwilling to prosecute when treatment is done in the name of animal training.

Animal training is a largely unlicensed and unregulated profession in the United States. As of 2022, anyone who wishes to call himself/herself a dog trainer or animal behaviorist may do so, without any formal education or true understanding of learning theory. The trainer's reasoning for the behavior may vary greatly from the actual motivation and the training methodology may be inhumane, outdated, or inappropriate. For example, some trainers base all dog behavior and training on dominance theory. The assumption that dogs misbehave because they are striving for higher rank often leads trainers to use force or correction to modify undesirable behaviors. This negatively affects the human–animal bond and is a flawed approach (Luescher and Reisner 2008; Landsberg et al. 2008).

When the pet's behavior is considered normal, without an underlying medical or mental disorder, owners may seek guidance from a trained professional. That person may be a Karen Pryor Academy Certified Training Partner (KPA CTP) (www.karenpryoracademy.com; www.greatdogtrainers.com), a Certified Professional Dog Trainer, or a Veterinary Technician Specialist in Behavior (VTS-Behavior).

Choosing an animal trainer can be a difficult decision for the veterinarian, the veterinary staff, and the client. An animal trainer should have all the desirable attributes of a good teacher. They should keep up with current training tools and methods by attending workshops and continuing education conferences; should be calm, patient, open-minded, understand how animals learn, and be able to convey this knowledge to the pet owner in a positive and motivational manner; should describe the behavior being trained, explain why it is important, and be able to demonstrate it. In a group setting, ample time should be allotted to individually assist students and allow time for practice. The AVSAB Position Statement on Punishment states: Trainers who use or advocate physical force (e.g. hitting, alpha rolling, pushing a dog into position, choke chain, or pinch collar correction) or methods/devices that have the potential to harm, as an acceptable way to train should be avoided (Eskeland 2007). Trainers must adapt humane training methods to the individual dog or problem situation. The most outstanding trainers are motivational and avoid aversives in their techniques. Trainers who do not use rewards should be avoided. Motivational trainers use rewards (e.g. food, toys, play, affection) rather than teaching the dog using fear, pain, correction, or punishment as a means to get behavior. In this situation, the dog works for the possibility of a reward, rather than to avoid physical or psychological punishment. Punishment is rarely necessary, does not teach an appropriate desirable behavior, and should only be used as a last resort by a trainer who can fully explain the possible adverse effects. Before referring to a trainer, veterinarians should interview the trainer about vaccination requirements for attending training classes. In addition, the veterinarian or veterinary technician should observe the trainer instructing a class (Box 1.1). Are rewards used liberally? Are the handlers smiling and using upbeat voices? Are the dogs having fun? Do you hear any yelling or scolding? See any harsh physical correction? And if so, how does the instructor handle the situation? See Appendix 6 for a Trainer Assessment Form.

BOX 1.1: ASSESSING AN ANIMAL TRAINER'S COMPETENCE AND ETHICS

- Welcomes potential clients to observe a class prior to making a decision to enroll
- Explains a skill and gives examples of how the skill is useful in everyday life
- Demonstrates the skill
- Utilizes handouts and other instructional guides
- Circulates through the students giving assistance and guidance when needed
- Remains conscious of the emotional state of all animals in the classroom setting and acts appropriately
- Arranges the classroom to optimize the success of each handler and animal
- Does not become focused on one student
- Keeps the class moving at an appropriate pace
- Can adjust the teaching plan as needed for individual student's needs
- Is professional and respectful at all times to owners/handlers
- Is appropriate and liberal with positive reinforcement or rewards to both the owners and animals
- Is familiar with TAGteach (www.tagteach.com) and utilizes it frequently and appropriately to instruct clients (see Chapter 5)
- Uses appropriate management tools to decrease unwanted behaviors while teaching the desired behaviors
- Utilizes only humane training methods that promote and protect the human–animal bond and are not harmful to the handler or animal in any way
- Does not recommend or utilize choke collars, pinch collars, electronic shock collars, or physical or verbal punishments
- Does not coach or advocate the outdated and disproved "dominance hierarchy theory" and the subsequent confrontational training and relationship that follows from it

CHAPTER 1

- Understands and addresses the emotional and motivational state of the animal
- Recommends and utilizes training tools designed not to inflict physical pain
- Understands the value of education and attends continuing education seminars regularly
- Is a certified member of a standardized and policed credentialing program
- Because of variables in dog breeding, temperament, owner commitment, and experience, a trainer cannot and should not guarantee the results of their training, although should ensure client satisfaction
- Builds and maintains a mutually communicative, respectful, and professional relationship with veterinary professionals
- Understands veterinarians are exclusively responsible for diagnosing behavioral disorders, for medical and behavioral differential diagnoses, and for prescribing a treatment plan, which may include pharmacological intervention

Before veterinary professionals refer their client to a trainer, they should be familiar with the trainer's level of education and the methodology and tools used to achieve behavior modification. One should be wary of trainers who guarantee results and refer to themselves as a behaviorist, while lacking credentials. The ideal trainer should collaborate openly with the veterinarian when faced with possible underlying medical and behavior disorders (fear, anxiety, or aggression). In doing so, the veterinarian may diagnose and prescribe behavior modification and/or pharmacological treatment. The trainer then may instruct and assist the pet owner on implementation of the prescribed behavior modification plan. A holistic team approach should be developed between the veterinary team, trainer, and client (Table 1.1).

- Before veterinary professionals refer their client to a trainer, they should be familiar with the trainer's level of education and the methodology and tools used to achieve behavior modification.

Fortunately, the trend is toward the licensing of animal trainers who have some level of education; continuing education is also required. The AVSAB Position Statement on Dominance recommends that veterinarians do not refer clients to trainers or behavior consultants who coach and advocate dominance hierarchy theory and the subsequently confrontational training. Rather, behavior modification and training should focus on reinforcing desirable behaviors, avoiding the reinforcement of undesirable behaviors, and striving to address the underlying emotional state and motivations, including medical and genetic factors that are driving the undesirable behavior.

There are numerous dog trainer schools and organizations that offer online educational correspondence courses. These through-the-internet courses offer to "certify" the participant as a "professional" in the field of dog training and behavior. Many courses are offered by self-proclaimed animal behaviorists and dog trainers to those willing to become "certified" professional dog trainers or certified "canine behavior therapists." The person's or place's reputation, credentials, and qualifications should be determined before accepting any title or degree. Some organizations are "bogus," while others are well known and taught by professional, qualified staff. The best schools and educational programs for trainers offer their students a strong foundation in learning theory with hands-on workshops, seminars, and continuing education. Reputable certifying organizations "police" their members by holding them to a standardized level of ethics and care. If those ethics and care are violated, certification can be revoked. It is beyond the scope of this chapter to identify all reputable professional animal training organizations, but we will mention a few.

The Karen Pryor Academy or KPA (www.karenpryoracademy.com) is an educational organization that offers online education and hands-on workshops in order to certify dog trainers. Graduates of KPA become part of a community of trainers who have achieved and demonstrated a consistent level of excellence and can represent themselves as a KPA CTP. Training partners must teach and train using force-free principles and techniques, are subject to a policed credentialing process, and are expected to demonstrate the highest level of professionalism and ethics. KPA CTPs must demonstrate an ability to communicate clearly, professionally, and positively with associates, veterinary professionals, and pet owners. Veterinarians should seek out KPA CTPs in their area to develop mutually beneficial working relationships.

The Association of Pet Dog Trainers (APDT) is a professional organization of individual dog trainers who are committed to becoming better trainers

Table 1.1 The roles and responsibilities of the veterinary behavior team.

Roles and responsibilities	Veterinarian	Veterinary technician	Dog trainer
Initial client communication	×	×	×
Client education and awareness	×	×	×
Obtaining clinical history	×	×	—
Setting hospital policies	×	—	—
Medical differentials	×	—	—
Behavioral diagnosis	×	—	—
Prognosis	×	—	—
Develops and modifies treatment plans	×	—	—
Prescribes medications	×	—	—
Implementing prescribed treatment plan	—	×	×
Follow-up communication with client	×	×	×
Follow-up communication with veterinarian	—	×	×
Follow-up behavior consultation	×	—	—
Demonstrate training methods	—	×	×
Demonstrate training tools	—	×	×
Assess pet's trainability	—	×	×
Identifying normal versus abnormal behavior	×	×	×
Problem prevention	×	×	×
Teaching puppy and kitten classes	—	×	×
Teaching manners and life skills classes	—	×	×

through education. APDT (www.apdt.com) provides membership networking and sharing of ideas through educational conferences, newsletters, and seminars. Membership is open to any member of the public who is interested in dog training. APDT does not offer trainer certification directly. It encourages its members to make use of "dog-friendly" training methods that use reinforcement and rewards, not punishment, to achieve the desired behavior. There is no policing of training methodology or education requirements to be an APDT member.

The Certification Council for Professional Dog Trainers (CCPDT) was originally created by the APDT in 2001.

The CCPDT (www.ccpdt.org) was the first national certification program for professional pet dog trainers and offers an international testing program. All certified trainers must earn continuing education credits to maintain their designations. They must also agree to adhere to a code of ethics. Candidates who meet the following requirements and pass the written exam earn the title Certified Professional Dog Trainer-Knowledge Assessed and may use the designation, "CPDT-KA," after their name.

CCPDT has recognized the importance of evaluating the hands-on skills of trainers. In 2011, they launched a practical assessment of a trainer's skills. A trainer who is already a CPDT-KA may be evaluated and tested on hands-on skills via video submission. If the candidate passes the hands-on practical assessment, they earn the title of Certified Professional Dog Trainer-Knowledge and Skills Assessed (CPDT-KSA). CCPDT has added another level of certification, CBCC-KA, which stands for Certified Behavior Consultant Canine-Knowledge Assessed. It is their advanced certification for dog trainers who offer canine behavior modification training.

Another animal training/consultant organization that deserves mention is the International Association of Animal Behavior Consultants (IAABC). The goals of IAABC are to standardize and support the practice of animal behavior consulting, to provide quality, evidence-based education and peer and supervising mentoring, and to provide resources for pet owners needing advice (https://m.iaabc.org/about).

Fear Free Pets, LLC also offers a Fear Free Certified Trainer course available to credentialed trainers. This program is designed to familiarize the professional animal trainer with Fear Free® techniques and the importance of working with veterinary and other animal professionals to provide a consistency of care throughout the pet's life (https://fearfreepets.com/fear-free-animal-trainer-certification-program-overview).

The Society of Veterinary Behavior Technicians (SVBT) is a professional organization open to veterinary technicians or nurses, veterinary technician or nursing students, and certified animal trainers. SVBT's mission is to enrich human–animal interactions by promoting scientifically based techniques of training, management, and behavior modification. SVBT (www.svbt.org) provides a forum for discussion and continuing education while working with allied professional organizations to strengthen the veterinary healthcare team. In 2008, the National Association of Veterinary Technicians in America (NAVTA), through the AVBT (www.avbt.net), recognized the specialty for veterinary technicians in animal behavior. The first VTS-Behavior technicians were inducted in 2010. A veterinary technician or nurse wishing to become a VTS-Behavior must complete extensive required tasks over a three-to-five-year period to apply for consideration to take the three-part examination. For details on the requirements and application process, visit www.avbt.net.

The role and responsibilities of a VTS-Behavior are described in Box 1.2.

BOX 1.2: THE ROLE AND RESPONSIBILITIES OF A VTS-BEHAVIOR

- Triage behavior concerns of clients, both in the clinic and on the phone, including determining when to refer to a Veterinary Behaviorist (i.e. prevention vs. intervention).
- Observe and triage behavior of animals in shelters, rescues, zoological parks, laboratories, and similar animal-related facilities, following procedures developed and approved by the veterinarian on record for that facility.
- Give management and safety advice to clients before their appointments.
- Take a history and perform a physical examination.
- Observe or assess behaviors in the context in which they are offered.
- Obtain samples and perform diagnostic testing.
- Discuss diagnostic procedures.
- Dispense prescribed medications.
- Discuss medication effects, side effects, and contraindications.
- Demonstrate a comprehensive understanding of operant and classical conditioning.
- Demonstrate a comprehensive understanding of behavior modification techniques.
- Assist the veterinarian during behavior consultations.
- Rehabilitate animals with problem behaviors in veterinary clinics, shelters, rescues, zoological parks, laboratories, and similar animal-related facilities, implementing procedures developed and prescribed by a veterinarian or veterinary behaviorist.
- Demonstrate good communication, rapport, and teaching ability with owners.
- Demonstrate a high level of expertise and understanding of scientifically based positive reinforcement training methods.
- Create a positive and safe learning experience for the animal and owner.
- Execute hands-on training and behavior modification with the client, animal caretaker, or the animal after the diagnosis and recommended treatment of a behavior problem.
- Assist the client at the hospital or in-home visits to understand and implement the prescribed behavior modification and management techniques.
- Educate clients on products used to manage behavior cases.
- Teach owners to properly fit and condition patients with tools such as head collars and basket muzzles.
- Create criteria for client behavior logs.
- Be proficient in medical, behavioral, training, and research record keeping.
- Perform follow-up telephone calls, email contacts, and home or hospital visits with clients as directed by the veterinarian.
- Implement changes to the treatment plan based on client feedback and consultation with the veterinarian.
- Present at conferences, seminars, and workshops on the role of the veterinary technician in animal behavior, normal behavior and problem prevention strategies to the public, clients, volunteers, staff members, and other veterinary technicians.
- Write professional scientific material for the veterinary public.
- Develop animal-behavior-related handouts for clients.
- Condition animals to handling and husbandry practices common within the veterinary environment to create a more cooperative patient.
- Train veterinary staff in behavior protocols for that hospital, including scheduling, interacting with animal patients, and desensitizing patients to procedures.
- Educate clients about normal behavior and how to train their animal to be more comfortable during veterinary visits.
- Perform pet selection counseling.

- Perform problem prevention counseling.
- Counsel owners on common training techniques.
- Develop and implement programs of preventive behavior medicine. This includes creating, organizing, and updating handouts and staff training.
- Review current literature and behavioral information directed toward veterinary professionals and the general public.
- Evaluate and network with area animal trainers and other pet care professionals who provide supportive services.
- Create and teach puppy and kitten classes.
- Create and teach training classes for adult animals.
- Assist with behavior wellness appointments.
- Perform grief counseling.
- Promote and protect the human–animal bond.
- Be a Fear Free or Low-stress handling advocate for the hospital.

Source: Adapted from Luescher et al., 2007; 2008 Academy of Veterinary Behavior Technician's Petition to the National Association of Veterinary Technicians of America.

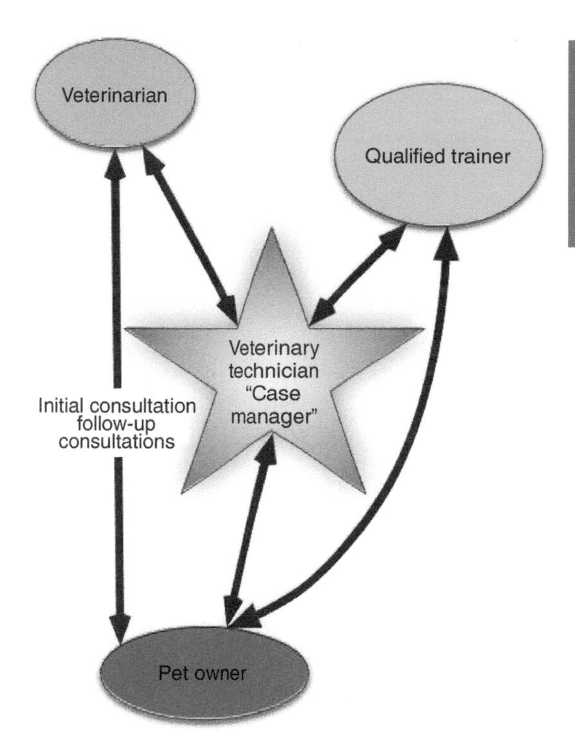

Figure 1.4 The technician's role as the "case manager" in veterinary behavior.

There are a variety of choices when looking for an animal trainer to complement veterinary behavior services. The credentials of an individual should not take the place of first-hand experience and interviewing potential training partners. When referring clientele to a trainer, clients will assume that the trainer's methodology is representative of the hospital. Although we have mentioned a few specific organizations in this chapter, the list is not exhaustive as there are other reputable animal training organizations which have not been mentioned.

- There are a variety of choices when looking for an animal trainer to complement veterinary behavior services. The credentials of an individual should not take the place of first-hand experience and interviewing potential training partners.

The role of the veterinary technician in the veterinary behavior consultation

The veterinary technician will have many roles in the veterinary behavior team. The technician will often first assess the situation and help determine the appropriate type of service needed. Not only will the behavior technician be able to triage the situation, but they will also assist with the clinical behavior consultation and may also act as the trainer for the hospital. Acting as the liaison for the client, trainer, and veterinarian, the veterinary behavior technician could be considered the "case manager," helping facilitate communication between all parties. Figure 1.4 shows a simple schematic of the role of the behavior technician as the "case manager."

Triaging the issues

Clients contacting the veterinary hospital are often unaware of the types of services available and necessary to address their pet's behavior. The veterinary staff or veterinary technician must triage the situation and determine whether a pet may be suffering from a possible medical/behavioral disorder, whether the situation is still in a preventive stage, or has progressed into a situation of behavior problem intervention (Figure 1.5). Medical as well as behavioral conditions may be factors that must be considered and evaluated prior to the appointment being

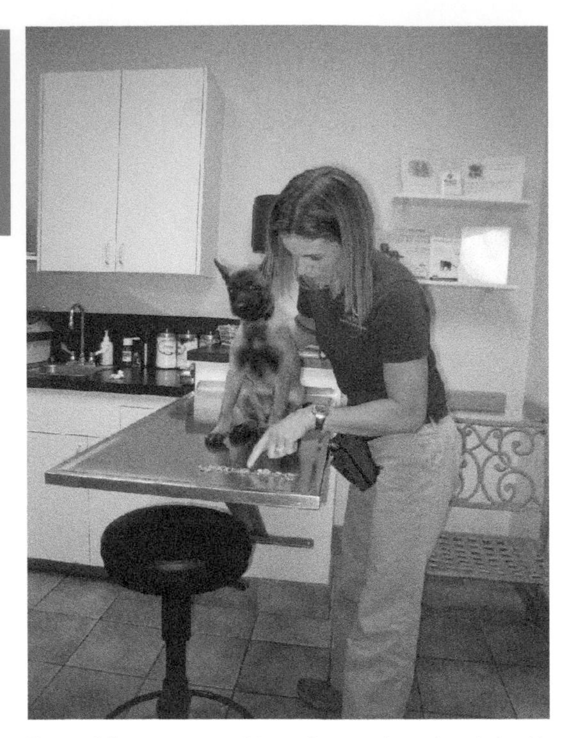

Figure 1.5 First puppy visit to the veterinary hospital. This puppy is exhibiting fear and not taking treats.

scheduled with the appropriate personnel. Clients may contact the veterinary hospital requesting training for their pet, when in reality the pet is suffering from a behavioral disorder.

Determining whether the animal's behavior requires a veterinarian's diagnosis and attention is often a gray area that a veterinary technician must become adept at distinguishing by asking the client appropriate questions.

Generally, conditions will fall into one of two categories.

Medical and/or behavioral disorder (veterinary diagnosis required)

Medical conditions can cause or exacerbate behavioral issues and therefore must be ruled out and/or treated concurrently. Any acute change in behavior should alert the veterinary technician to a primary medical disorder. Physical pain or malaise may increase irritability and contribute to anxiety, aggression, or elimination disorders. Changes in sensory perception will alter the pet's behavioral responses and social interactions. Pets with behavioral disorders in conjunction with medical disorders may present at any age. These cases must be promptly examined and evaluated by the veterinarian.

Case 1 A client calls about their cat, a 13-year-old male neutered orange tabby named Logan, who is urinating outside of the litter box. The problem could be medical, related to diabetes, kidney disease, a urinary tract infection, crystaluria or stones, osteoarthritis, and so on. The problem could be a behavioral disorder and ultimately given a diagnosis of urine marking, litter-box aversion–substrate aversion/preference, or cognitive dysfunction. The patient should be seen by the veterinarian to determine the etiology and make a diagnosis.

Case 2 A client presents with their dog, a 10-month-old male intact Bull Mastiff named Rex, who has shown aggression when the owners have attempted to move him while resting. The comprehensive behavioral history limits aggression to one specific situation, moving him while resting. The dog is slow to rise and reluctant to go for walks off the property. Physical examination reveals pain and aggression with flexing and extending the coxofemoral joint. Radiographs suggest severe hip dysplasia. A veterinary diagnosis of pain-induced aggression is made. Concurrent behavioral and medical treatment is required.

Case 3 Duke is a four-year-old male intact Boxer. The owners report they cannot trim Duke's nails and would like to be able to do so. Upon questioning the owners, the veterinary technician is told the owners have been bitten not only when trimming Duke's nails, but also when they have hugged him. Duke has growled at strangers as well.

Although the client's primary complaint is that they are unable to trim Duke's nails, his preliminary history indicates aggression with nail trimming and concurrent behavioral issues which should be addressed by the veterinarian. Because aggression has been displayed, a diagnosis by a veterinarian is required.

Case 4 Brie is a two-year-old female spayed Dalmatian. The owners would like tranquilizers for the Fourth of July fireworks.

The technician notices Brie is very frightened and trembling next to the owner. Upon questioning the owner, the owner reports this is Brie's usual reaction to leaving the house or toward anything "new." Brie also reportedly stares at the ceiling excessively, which could be an indication of a compulsive disorder. The technician advises that Brie's behavior and welfare could be improved through behavioral therapy with a veterinarian. A veterinary behavior consultation is recommended.

Case 5 Cujo is a three-month-old male Saint Bernard. He presents to the veterinary hospital for his last set of vaccinations. The technician noted that Cujo showed signs of fear and growled when she approached and handled him to get his pulse and respiration rate. The patient's elevated level of fear, anxiety, and stress leads to further behavioral questioning of the dog's behavior outside the veterinary clinic. The technician advises that Cujo's behavior and welfare in hospital could be improved through veterinarian prescribed pre-veterinary visit pharmaceuticals and scheduling formal training sessions with a skilled trainer in the hospital (see Chapters 7 and 8). A veterinary behavior consultation is recommended because abnormal behavior is identified.

Situations in which it is unclear if the behavior is normal or abnormal, or there is a component of fear, anxiety, and/or aggression, require a veterinary diagnosis.

Prevention and training (no veterinary diagnosis required)

Some situations may not have progressed into a behavioral disorder and a veterinary technician may preempt the development of a behavior problem through appropriate preventive and training services. Situations may include prevention, lack of training, or conditioned unwanted behaviors.

Prevention

Prevention of behavior disorders is easier than treatment. Preventive situations most often will be with new puppies or kittens presenting to the veterinary hospital. Normal canine behavior and the prevention of behavioral problems should be discussed in puppy socialization classes and/or during puppy wellness visits (Figure 1.6). Kitten classes may focus on normal feline behavior and management, as well as the prevention of behavior problems.

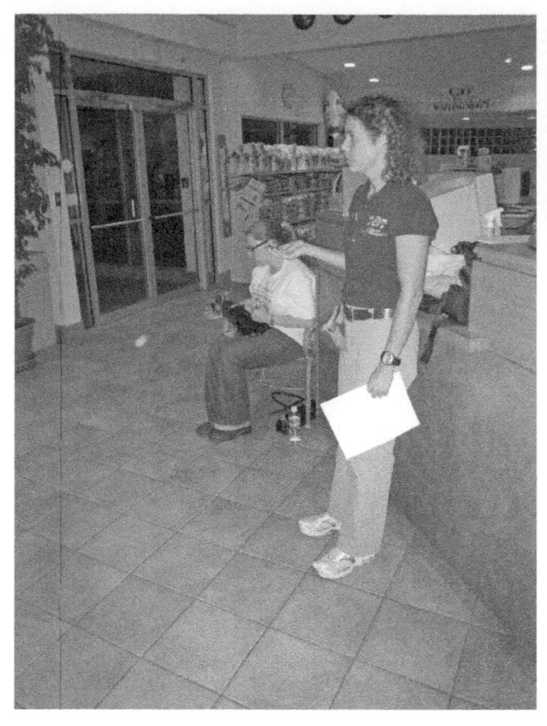

Figure 1.6 A veterinary technician conducting puppy socialization classes at the veterinary hospital.

Case 1 A client calls complaining that their eight-week-old Chinese Lion Dog, better known as the *Shih Tzu*, named Mufasa, is biting the family. Is the behavior normal mouthing and biting that is commonly seen in puppies? Often owners call normal puppy mouthing "biting." The client reports that the puppy is growling and biting. His bites sometimes break the skin. Is this a fearful puppy or a lack of bite inhibition? The pet should be screened as to whether the behavior is normal puppy mouthing or abnormal behavior for a puppy. This may be accomplished through a puppy behavior wellness appointment or an in-hospital puppy socialization class. During puppy class, it can be determined if there are other areas of concern (such as guarding of resources) and a veterinary examination and diagnosis may be required.

Case 2 A six-month-old sheltie named "Cosmo" has attended puppy classes and is currently enrolled in the hospital's clicker-training classes. The owner reports Cosmo occasionally steals and chews household items (socks, paper towels, etc.). The behavior is not associated with owner departure and is not excessive. Cosmo does not show aggression in these contexts. Having Cosmo in both your puppy classes and clicker-training classes, you are familiar with him, and it is obvious Cosmo is a stable and outgoing adolescent with no apparent anxiety issues. The client reports they are thrilled with Cosmo's behavior in all other aspects. Chewing is a normal behavior for adolescent dogs. The technician can recommend management, supervision, supplying a variety of appropriate chew toys, and teaching relinquishment of objects. The technician may also consider recommending a trainer to assist the client.

Lack of training or conditioned unwanted behaviors

Conditioned unwanted behaviors are behaviors that have been inadvertently reinforced by the owners and are problematic or undesirable. The behavior could be considered normal for the breed/species and not be considered excessive to the point of having a fear, aggression, anxiety, or hyperexcitability component. This is an emotionally stable pet that has not been taught cues related to manners or presents for learned unwanted behaviors. One helpful technique is for the veterinary technician to ask the client to describe the pet's personality. This may prompt the client to express a fear or anxiety-related component. Even after elaborate questioning, one may still be unsure of the true etiology of the condition. Many dogs present during adolescence for training problems. A consistent protocol or informational handout should be followed for dealing with the specific problem. These pets may benefit from private, semiprivate, or group training lessons.

Case 1 A client informs you that their dog, a nine-month-old intact male Siberian Husky named Bolt, needs training. Specifically, he runs away and does not come when called. You may be tempted to assume that based on the breed's genetic basis to run, that this is purely a training problem. But you do not have enough information. One must first determine the situation when Bolt runs away. Is he digging out of the yard or jumping the fence? The client reports when she opens the front door, Bolt dashes out running. Next, one must determine Bolt's motivation. Is he roaming because the neighbor's dog is in estrus? Does he want to chase things, such as small animals or children running? Does Bolt have any aggression issues (such as growling or excessive barking) with people at the door or passing the property? The client reports that Bolt is not chasing anything or anyone and has never met a person or dog he has not liked. He is very friendly. Finally, one must determine, what the client does when Bolt runs away. The client reports they chase him. His favorite game is "keep away" – he loves to be chased with a toy in his mouth. Now, after gathering a variety of information, one may assume Bolt's behavior is likely a training problem typical for the breed and related to previous learning experiences. Bolt has likely not been taught to wait at the door. Not coming when called and running away has been inadvertently conditioned by routinely being chased and playing "keep away." Private or group training sessions may be recommended to work on the training concerns.

Case 2 Fang is a six-month-old male neutered medium-sized mixed-breed dog. The owner reports they cannot trim Fang's nails. The veterinary technician asks what Fang does when they attempt to trim his nails and the owner reports he tries to run away. The veterinary technician asks if he growls or attempts to bite the owner in these situations and the owner reports he does not; he "just wiggles." The veterinary technician asks if there are other situations such as brushing, touching body parts, or medicating Fang that are also problematic. The owner reports, "We can do anything, but trim Fang's nails." The veterinary staff has not had difficulty handling Fang for medical treatments.

Because there is no aggression and the fear is mild and considered normal given the context and situation, the veterinary technician does not need a diagnosis from the veterinarian. Most dogs do not enjoy having their nails trimmed and mild fear/anxiety in this

Table 1.2 Triage.

Scenario	Comments	Veterinarian's DX?
The issue is still in "preventive" stages	See preventive definition	No diagnosis required
The behavioral issue is likely a lack of training issue or a conditioned unwanted behavior	Send to a qualified trainer (see definition)	No diagnosis required
The issue is very specific (handling feet) and the only issue. There has been no history of aggression or extreme fear. A mild fear response or avoidance is evident	Rare	No diagnosis required, but with more in-depth assessment, the handling issue may be a symptom of a larger problem – then diagnosis required
There are multiple behavioral issues	Likely a complex situation and issues will need to be prioritized. Issues may be due to general temperament	Diagnosis likely required
Multiple triggers or unknown triggers	Difficult to/impossible to manage	Diagnosis required
Issue is anxiety or fear based	Anxiolytic medication may be needed	Diagnosis required
Any history of aggression (growling, snapping, or biting not in the context of play)	Lack of bite inhibition increases risk	Diagnosis required
Any acute change in behavior	Rule out health issues	Diagnosis required
Geriatric patient with behavior changes	Rule out health issues, including cognitive dysfunction	Diagnosis required
Puppy 8 wk of age showing aggression toward people (growling, snapping, biting not associated with normal puppy play mouthing)	Rule out health issues including neurological conditions, if behavioral usually genetic	Diagnosis required and counseling regarding the severity of the problem.
Behavior is uncharacteristically intense or out of context	Rule out health issues, possible abnormal brain chemistry or arousal issues	Diagnosis required

BOX 1.3: COMMON DEFINITIONS

Behavior problem: The animal's behavior is a problem for the owner. The issue could be lack of training, a conditioned unwanted behavior, a behavior disorder, or a combination of issues.

Behavior disorder: Psychological or behavioral patterns outside the behavioral norms for the species. Often there is an affective (emotional) component.

Behavioral assessment: An informal impression or evaluation of a situation; the first step in triaging a behavior problem or disorder.

Preventive care: Refers to measures taken to prevent the development of behavior problems or disorders, rather than treating the symptoms of an existing problem or disorder. Preventive care is a primary role for veterinary technicians.

Intervention care: Refers to measures taken to improve or alter an existing behavior disorder. Intervention requires a veterinary diagnosis and treatment plan.

Qualified trainer: An animal trainer who is certified from a standardized, positive-based curriculum and is policed by an organization in which certification can be revoked if the trainer acts unprofessionally or outside the organization's code of ethics.

context is normal. The technician can instruct and demonstrate to the owner basic behavior modification techniques for desensitization to trimming nails (see Chapters 7 and 9).

If the dog panicked to the point of losing bladder or bowel control or remains in a heightened state of arousal after being removed from the situation, then the fear and anxiety would be considered excessive, and a veterinary behavior consultation should be recommended.

Table 1.2 summarizes how to determine whether the behavioral issue is associated with lack of training, preventive in nature, or intervention, and requires a veterinary diagnosis.

Box 1.3 provides a quick reference to common terminology and definitions.

Prior to the consultation

The veterinary technician's responsibilities prior to the behavior consultation involve client communication tasks, office tasks including record keeping, and inventory management. Pre-appointment client communications may be the responsibility of the veterinary behavior technician or a trained receptionist. Providing awareness that there are viable treatment options for behavior disorders and educating clients about the difference between a training problem and a behavior disorder may be the first step in client communication. Preliminary information obtained should include the signalment (species, breed, color, sex, and age), medical problems, and behavioral issues. It is necessary to determine what prompted the call and what behavioral services are warranted (see sections **Triaging the issues** and **Qualified professionals to treat animal behavior disorders**). The expectations of the client should also be assessed. If the client makes an ultimatum, "If Fido growls at me one more time, he is out of here," attempting to educate the client briefly on normal canine communication and setting realistic goals for behavior intervention are important for the client's overall satisfaction. A thorough description of the services available and what is involved, as well as the cost of the services should be understood by the client. If the pet owner is expecting the behavior issues to be "cured" in a two-hour consultation, they will be dissatisfied with the service and may be less likely to implement the treatment plan. When the client understands that the assessment will give the appropriate knowledge and tools to address the pet's behavior issues, the client will be more accepting of the information and treatment plan. Informing the client that treatment options are available for their pet's behavioral issues, provides the client with some immediate relief. The client should be informed of any cancelation policies.

When any form of aggression is described by the client, the veterinary technician should advise the client to avoid triggers of aggression until the behavior disorder can be addressed through a behavior consultation. The client should also be advised to avoid punishment and manage the environment to avoid further learning of the undesired behaviors. This may include separating two dogs in the house that are fighting, avoid leaving the separation-anxiety dog alone, or blocking access to soiled areas for feline elimination disorders. The initial contact is usually a 10–15-minute phone conversation. If an appointment is scheduled, requesting video footage of the pet and the problem behaviors, without eliciting aggression or endangering the pet or people, may be suggested to enhance the behavior consultation.

Depending on the business model, a detailed behavioral history might be obtained prior to the consultation with the veterinarian or obtained during the initial consultation. Some clinicians prefer to review the medical and behavioral history prior to meeting with the client and pet, so a diagnosis, prognosis, and treatment recommendations can be provided during the initial visit. However, some clinicians prefer to obtain the behavioral history during the initial consultation via interview with the client and then have the client and pet return for future visits to provide more in-depth treatment recommendations. Both methods have their advantages and disadvantages. Attempting to obtain a detailed behavior history and provide treatment recommendations concurrently would result in a lengthy (likely more than 2.5 hours) consultation.

Since the authors of this chapter obtain and review a detailed behavior history prior to meeting with the client, that model will be outlined here. The behavioral history should include questions regarding general management, current medications (including heartworm and flea preventives), the pet's disposition, and historical information such as the age the pet was obtained and source from which the pet was obtained. The primary undesirable behaviors should be identified and ranked in order of importance to the owner. A brief general description of the behavior should include the antecedent, the behavior, and the consequence or outcome of the behavior. The context of the behavior, including the individuals present, the location, the owner's reaction, and the pet's reaction, should be obtained. A temperament evaluation to screen for other potential behavior concerns that might impede or modify treatment recommendations, provides vital information for safe and individualized guidance to address the pet owner's behavioral concerns.

The history form may be emailed or mailed to the client, but an easy-to-use online form is the preferred method for most clients. Allowing the client to complete the form decreases staff time and may facilitate multiple family members' input. When utilizing online forms, the software should ideally allow the client to save their information and return to it at another time rather than needing to complete the entire form in one session. A detailed behavior history form might take the client an hour to complete, and they might need to reference information they do not have available at the time. To minimize frustration and lost information, use a system that autosaves the information and allows the client to return to the form later. If you would like to see examples of online forms, you may complete a mock form at the links provided in Box 1.4 and Appendix 5.

BOX 1.4: LINKS FOR EXAMPLES OF ONLINE BEHAVIORAL HISTORY FORMS

Feline history form: https://veterinarybehavior.formstack.com/forms/cat_behavior_history_copy
Canine history form: https://veterinarybehavior.formstack.com/forms/dog_behavior_history_copy
Feline follow-up history form: https://veterinarybehavior.formstack.com/forms/cat_follow_up_copy
Canine follow-up history form: https://veterinarybehavior.formstack.com/forms/dog_follow_up_copy

Informing the client of safety precautions for the appointment and client preparation prior to the appointment (video footage, training tools, treats, etc.) are communication tasks performed by the veterinary technician. For home behavior consultations when aggression toward strangers entering the home is identified, the client should be instructed to place the pet in a safe contained area to prevent injury to veterinary staff entering the home. If other pets live in the home, inquire about their reactivity to strangers. This helps to protect the veterinary team. Similarly, with clinic consultations, if reactivity to other animals or people is an issue, the pet should be managed upon arrival at the veterinary hospital to prevent an incident. This may include managing the pet outside the building or in the car until the pet can be safely escorted into the consultation room.

If behaviorally and medically appropriate, the pet should be hungry for the consultation. Advise the client to withhold food for 6–12 hours prior to the appointment or feed a quarter to half the normal meal that morning. The client should bring video footage, training collars or training devices used, the pet's favorite treats and toy, and routine medications to the consultation.

With clinic consultations the veterinarian will not be able to observe the pet in its natural environment; video footage allows evaluation of interactions with household members and other pets (Figure 1.7). Once the appointment has been scheduled, the veterinary technician should impress upon the client the importance of video footage. Resting, feeding, drinking, and exercising areas should be included in the video.

The veterinary technician's responsibilities might also include making sure the patient file and pertinent forms are prepared prior to the appointment.

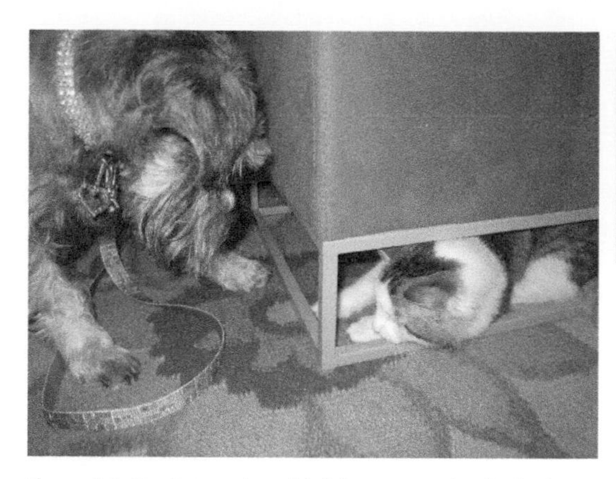

Figure 1.7 Dog interacting with feline companion in the home environment. When not providing in-home consultations, video footage is helpful in assessing the dynamics of the household.

This provides for a smooth and efficient consultation. If the consultation is taking place within the veterinary hospital, training tools, treats, and toys should be readily accessible to the staff but out of reach of the pet. Stocking the room prevents unnecessary interruptions during the behavior appointment. Examples of such items, depending on the case, would be a variety of clickers, toys and treats, appropriate-size head halters, harnesses and basket muzzles, bluetooth speaker for sound desensitization exercises, calming music, non-slip surfaces, leashes, and training books.

Any interruption may be upsetting to the patient and distracting to the client. Team members should be settled in the examination room before the patient enters. Phones and pagers should be turned off prior to entering the consultation room. A sign should be placed on the outside of the consultation door notifying staff that a behavior consultation is in progress, to prevent accidental interruption. The ideal architectural design for a behavior consultation room would allow the client and pet to enter directly into the room from outside of the building. A large room with couches and no visual obstruction between the veterinarian and the clients is ideal (Figure 1.8). The staff would have a separate interior entrance to the room. Safety precautions, such as a secure tether system, should also be implemented in the behavior consultation room (Figure 1.9).

When providing home behavior consultations, the vehicle should be stocked appropriately. Similarly, a

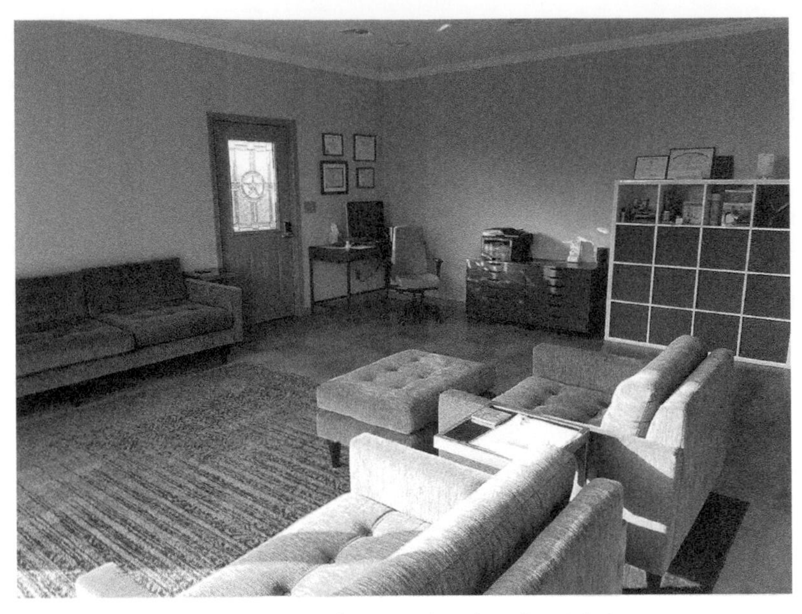

Figure 1.8 Large consultation room with direct entrance from outside and couch and chairs.

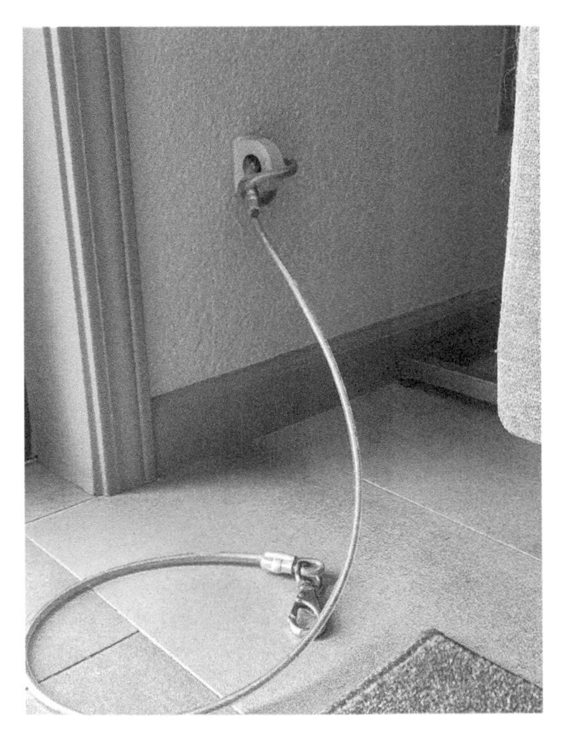

Figure 1.9 Tether system embedded in a stud in the consultation room.

laptop computer, power charger, charged cell phone, directions to the home, the patient file and behavioral and medical history should all be packed into the vehicle. Inventory of behavior training tools should be assessed at least weekly, especially on items that are commonly recommended or size specific (basket muzzles, head halters).

For cats and for dogs that will be uncomfortable in a new environment or around unfamiliar people, consider modifying the consultation format to limit the amount of stress the pet (and consequently, the pet owner) must experience. Many clients can assimilate more information during the consultation when most of it is performed via audiovisual telemedicine. Attending to the pet's emotional and physical needs during an in-clinic or in-home consultation can be distracting for the pet owner. With required modifications to services during the COVID-19 pandemic, the utilization of audiovisual telemedicine consultations has become more practiced and accepted. Although most states require the establishment of a valid veterinarian–client–patient relationship (VCPR) be established with an in-person appointment, once established, telemedicine consultation can be an option. This might entail: (i) a brief visit outside of the clinic, at the pet's home, or in the veterinary building. This is simply to establish a valid VCPR and legally be able to provide care to the pet. (ii) Following the brief visit to establish a VCPR, an approximately 1–1.5-hour video consult would be scheduled to provide the bulk of the behavior consultation and treatment recommendations.

During the consultation

The veterinary technician's responsibilities during the consultation involve working directly with the patient whenever possible, as well as assisting the client with the implementation of the treatment plan as outlined by the veterinarian. During the behavior consultation, ideally the veterinary technician should

1. offer nonthreatening body language and treats while waiting for the pet to approach and become comfortable with veterinary technician interaction,
2. assess the pet's trainability and interest in a variety of rewards (assorted treats and toys),
3. assess the pet's current level of reliability with cued behaviors required for implementation of the treatment plan (sit, stay, come, go to mat, loose leash walking),
4. introduce the pet to training tools needed to implement the treatment plan (Figure 1.10),
5. convey to the veterinarian the pet's responsiveness and reaction to training and the training tools,
6. demonstrate and explain training methods and training tools required for implementing the treatment plan,
7. encourage and give positive feedback to clients regarding their skills while utilizing the training tools (i.e. clicker, head halter) and performing the behavior modification exercises,
8. clarify and problem-solve with the client to integrate the treatment plan into their lifestyle,
9. answer any questions the client may have regarding the diagnosis, prognosis, or treatment plan and refer questions to the veterinarian as needed, and
10. provide the client with resources for recommended training supplies or tools, when applicable.

The veterinarian will complete the history and temperament evaluation, make a diagnosis and prognosis, and outline a treatment plan. While the

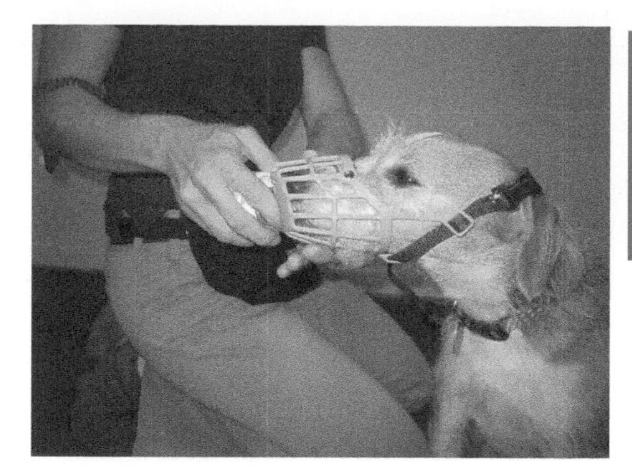

Figure 1.10 Desensitization and conditioning to a basket muzzle, using canned cheese.

veterinarian is interviewing the client, the veterinary technician should interact with the pet in a nonthreatening manner. This includes letting the pet approach on its own, avoiding prolonged eye contact, facing sideways to the pet, and avoid reaching toward the pet. The client and other members involved in the consultation should ignore the pet. This will make the veterinary technician the only person that "pays off." The veterinary technician may toss a variety of small, tasty treats in an underhand manner toward the pet.

- While the veterinarian is interviewing the client, the veterinary technician should interact with the pet in a nonthreatening manner. This includes letting the pet approach on its own, avoiding prolonged eye contact, facing sideways to the pet, and avoid reaching toward the pet.

Once the pet is comfortably interacting with the veterinary technician, the veterinary technician may begin to assess the trainability of the pet. Some pets will warm up immediately and others may never feel comfortable enough to eat a treat throughout the entire consultation. It is important for the veterinary technician to wait until the pet is relaxed with the interactions before prompting or asking the pet to perform a behavior such as sit. Otherwise, the veterinary technician risks making the pet wary. For example, imagine meeting an unfamiliar person for the first time. As long as that person does not immediately ask something of us and is nonthreatening, we are more likely to be comfortable with the interaction.

The pet's comfort level with handling and tendency toward guarding objects and/or food will be assessed in the temperament evaluation. This is important when considering placing a head collar and utilizing treats and toys. Although the pet's body language determines how the veterinary technician will proceed, it is good to know beforehand if the pet has any known triggers, such as a sensitive area, or shows a tendency to guard food or toys. For example, a Golden Retriever presents for destructive behavior when left at home alone. The temperament evaluation reveals previous aggression when touched around the ears. This invaluable information may not be immediately offered by the client because it is not a presenting complaint. The veterinary technician should wait until the temperament evaluation is completed by the veterinarian prior to desensitizing to a head halter, harness, muzzle, or introducing toys. This increases safety with handling of the patient. Toys should be on a rope or tether when introduced to the pet. This provides a nonconfrontational way for the veterinary technician to retrieve the toy.

- Although the pet's body language determines how the veterinary technician will proceed, it is good to know beforehand if the pet has any known triggers, such as a sensitive area, or shows a tendency to guard food or toys.

The veterinary technician may introduce training tools (e.g. clicker, head collar, muzzle) (see Chapter 9) and training cues needed for behavior modification exercises (e.g. sit, stay, go to a mat, loose leash walking) to the pet while the veterinarian describes the diagnosis and treatment plan. On occasion, the veterinary technician may take the canine patient for a walk to assess reactivity to environmental factors and temperament away from the owner. This may determine whether the owner will be capable of walking the dog and if undesirable behaviors have been inadvertently conditioned by the owner. For example, some dogs are only reactive to other dogs while with their owner. The technician may also observe defensive or fearful behaviors that can be reported to the veterinarian. The technician may notice the dog stop taking treats, which is likely a sign of anxiety. The walk also allows the veterinary technician to assess the dog's reaction to a head collar, if applicable. The veterinary technician's insight should be conveyed to the veterinarian during the consultation.

While the veterinarian prepares the written behavior assessment summary and treatment plan, the veterinary technician should explain and demonstrate any training tools or skills required in implementing the treatment plan. This should include how to teach the pet appropriate behavior responses and their importance with regard to the treatment of the behavioral disorder. Clients are more likely to comply with the treatment plan when they understand the significance of the exercises. Specific behavior modification exercises and desensitization to training tools should be demonstrated. The client should be provided an opportunity to practice some of the exercises with assistance and positive feedback from the veterinary technician (Figure 1.11). While observing the client's training skills, the veterinary technician may foresee potential training problems and provide insight to remediate those problems. During this time the veterinary technician should also accompany the client and dog on a walk. Not only will the veterinary technician be able to observe the dog's behavior with the client, but the veterinary technician may also assess the client's leash and handling skills. Behavior modification techniques used on walks should be demonstrated by the behavior technician. Client questions regarding the diagnosis, prognosis, and treatment plan may be answered by the

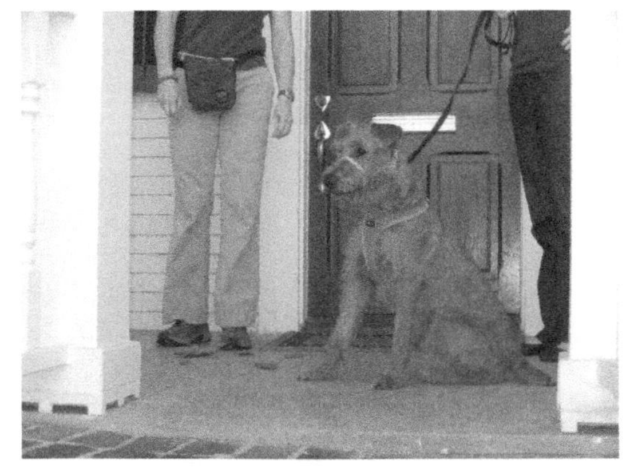

Figure 1.11 Technician coaching a client on behavior modification exercises with a dog that reacts to other dogs.

veterinary technician or referred back to the veterinarian for clarification.

- Clients are more likely to comply with the treatment plan when they understand the significance of the exercises.

The veterinary behavior technician will need to develop communication skills to assist the client without putting the client on the defensive (see Chapter 5). For example, the veterinary technician observes a dog that reluctantly returns to the client when called. If the veterinary technician says, "Fido doesn't look happy when he comes to you, because he thinks you are going to punish him," the client is likely to take the comment personally and feel less competent as a trainer. Instead, the veterinary technician might say, "That is great, that Fido came when you called him. The next step in his training will include. . .". The veterinary technician would suggest a few things to make Fido's recall enjoyable and provide the handler with tips regarding nonthreatening body language. This acknowledges the success of the client's previous training with the dog; the dog did come when called. The client is now in an open frame of mind for the "next step" to teaching the recall.

When the patient is a cat, bird, or a dog showing extreme fear and/or anxiety, the veterinary technician may be more limited with patient interactions. Birds may be wary of new people and are less likely to be amenable to interacting with a stranger. Similarly, some cats will avoid interactions with new people or will lose interest in treats and toys quickly. Some dogs will not be comfortable enough to interact with the veterinary technician even after a sustained period of time. There will also be some canine patients that are too unsafe for the veterinary technician to handle directly. The veterinary technician will need to rely on their ability to explain and demonstrate implementation of the treatment plan without the pet. Coaching the client regarding problem solving and training is an important role of the veterinary technician in these cases.

- When the patient is a cat, bird, or a dog with extreme fear and/or aggression, the veterinary technician may be more limited with patient interactions.

The flow of the behavior consultation is shown in Box 1.5.

BOX 1.5: BEHAVIOR CONSULTATION FLOW CHART (DURING THE CONSULTATION)

- Appropriate safety measures in place prior to appointment or on presentation to the veterinary hospital.
- Introductions and assessment of environment (video or directly)
  - Technician may be offering the pet treats.
- Review of the submitted behavioral and medical history of the pet
  - Veterinarian: summarizes the presenting complaints and the medical and behavioral history asking for verification or further input from the client.
  - Technician: offers nonthreatening body language and observing and noting the pet's body language in the medical record.
- Diagnosis, prognosis, and treatment plan
  - Veterinarian
    - explains the diagnosis (diagnoses), prognosis, and treatment plan, including any supplements or medications.
  - Technician
    - assesses the pet's trainability and interest in a variety of rewards (assorted treats and toys),
    - assesses the pet's current level of reliability with behaviors required for implementation of the treatment plan (sit, stay, come, go to mat, loose leash walking),
    - introduces the pet to training tools needed to facilitate the treatment plan,
    - takes the dog for a walk if safe and appropriate to do so,
    - conveys to the veterinarian the pet's response and reaction to training and the training tools.
- Training plan demonstration and implementation
  - Veterinarian
    - prepares the written behavior assessment summary and treatment plan.
  - Technician
    - demonstrates and explains training methods and training tools required for implementing the treatment plan,
    - encourages the client and offers positive feedback while the client practices using the training tools (e.g. clicker, head halter) and during behavior modification exercises,
    - clarifies and problem-solves implementation of the treatment plan with the client,

- answers any questions the client may have regarding the diagnosis, prognosis, or treatment plan or refers to the veterinarian, and
- provides the client with resources for recommended training supplies or tools, if applicable.

- Conclusion of appointment
  - Veterinarian
    - sends the client the written behavior assessment summary and treatment plan,
    - prescribes medication (when applicable),
    - explains follow-up recommendations (written into the behavior summary), and
    - answers client's questions.
  - Technician
    - conveys any pertinent information revealed during the training exercises that may affect the treatment plan,
    - asks veterinarian's opinion on questions presented by client during training, if applicable,
    - relays to the veterinarian a summary of the training and behavior modification exercises performed,
    - updates the patient's medical record (including the Emotional Medical Record – see Chapter 8),
    - prepares medications and supplements being prescribed by the veterinarian,
    - schedules the next appointment or provides the client with information on how and when to schedule the next appointment.

After the consultation: follow-up care

The role of the veterinary technician regarding follow-up care is to provide continued support for the client and promote fluent communication. Clarification of the treatment plan and evaluation of the human–animal bond should be determined at each contact. The veterinary technician can evaluate through home visits, phone contacts, emails, or video correspondence, the implementation of training and behavior modification exercises. Answering questions regarding the treatment plan, prescribed medications, training, and behavior modification may also be addressed by the veterinary technician.

- The role of the veterinary technician regarding follow-up care is to provide continued support for the client and promote fluent communication.

When the pet shows no signs of improvement, worsening of the behavior, or a new undesirable behavior, the veterinarian should be informed and assess whether changes in the treatment plan are necessary. With the veterinary technician's insight, the veterinarian may make changes to the treatment plan. Only a veterinarian can change the treatment plan, including changing prescribed medications or medication dosages. When improper implementation of the behavior modification is suspected, a behavior modification appointment with the veterinary technician may be suggested. The veterinarian may determine that a follow-up behavior consultation is required to reevaluate the pet.

- Only a veterinarian can change the treatment plan, including changing prescribed medications or medication dosages.

If new problem behaviors, which were not addressed in the consultation, arise, then another behavior consultation with the veterinarian would be necessary. For example, Herman, a five-year-old neutered male Himalayan, was seen for urinating and defecating daily on the floor next to the litter box. The veterinarian diagnosed feline inappropriate elimination with a litter-box aversion. Litter-box factors were changed, and environmental and behavior modifications were implemented. Herman's behavior was significantly improved, and he is found to only eliminate inappropriately when the owner is negligent about cleaning the litter boxes. After several months, the client reports that Herman is having a relapse. Further questioning reveals that Herman is now urinating on the owner's bed, bathroom rug, and the new kitten's bed. It is only urine, never stool. Not only should this warrant a thorough medical workup to evaluate Herman's urinary tract health, but it should also be recognized that this is an entirely different behavior disorder. This warrants another behavior consultation with the veterinarian because the behavior is likely anxiety-related urine marking. Although the initial complaint is the same, the cat is not always using the litter box; the description of the behavior is different.

A set protocol for follow-up care should be determined by the veterinarian and documented in the treatment plan. Follow-ups may be performed by the veterinary behavior technician. The suggested minimum follow-up communication should occur between one and three weeks post the initial behavior consultation. Follow-up may be either by telephone/email/video call or in clinic with or without the pet. The first follow-up communication centers around answering questions regarding the treatment plan. If medication was prescribed, the veterinary technician should ask the client if the pet has been started on the medication. It should not be assumed that the prescribed medication is being administered or given appropriately. Confirm the dosage and frequency of the medication. The client should be questioned regarding side effects of the medication. During the first follow-up communication, determine which parts of the treatment plan the client has begun to implement. Updates should be provided to the veterinarian and the treatment plan modified as directed. When providing in-clinic follow-up, avoid mistaking the follow-up assessment with a behavior modification appointment. If the client requires further assistance with training or behavior modification, an appointment should be scheduled with appropriate personnel. Ideally, this person may be a veterinary behavior technician or an animal trainer who is knowledgeable about implementation of behavior modification techniques.

- It should not be assumed that the prescribed medication is being administered or given appropriately.

Continued follow-up care should be tailored to the case. Any changes to the treatment plan should be reevaluated two to three weeks post implementation. If no changes to the treatment plan are made and the client is satisfied with the pet's progress, reassessment should be rendered in an additional one to two month (approximately two to three months following the initial consultation). The three-month follow-up may be either a phone-, video-, or in-clinic assessment. Follow-up appointments should be required every six months to yearly in order to continue providing behavioral assistance. The majority of veterinary computer software programs support phone and appointment reminder systems. This makes follow-up care easier to implement. Routine follow-up care initiated by the veterinary team provides for continued guidance and support from the veterinary team, thereby facilitating and enhancing the human–animal bond.

The veterinary technician's roles encompass client communication, including education, awareness, and prevention before, during, and after the consultation, as well as assisting the veterinarian with the clinical behavior consultation. Utilization of the veterinary technician provides for a more comprehensive and successful behavior service for the hospital and the client/patient.

- The veterinary technician's roles encompass client communication, including education, awareness, and prevention before, during, and after the consultation, as well as assisting the veterinarian with the clinical behavior consultation.

Summary of the roles of the veterinarian, veterinary technician, and animal trainer in veterinary behavior

Table 1.1 summarizes the roles of the veterinarian, veterinary technician, and animal trainer in the veterinary behavior team. Although many of the tasks may overlap, there are clearly defined roles that are exclusive to the veterinarian because they involve the practice of veterinary medicine.

Home versus clinic behavior consultations

Offering in-home or in-clinic veterinary behavior consultations to clients can be a service added to a general practice or the sole focus of a veterinary practice. Behavior consultations in the home can provide additional insight that may affect the diagnosis and treatment plan. Perhaps a combination of in-clinic and in-home behavioral services could be offered in order to balance the advantages and disadvantages of each service.

Pros and cons of the home behavior consultation versus the clinic behavior consultation

Providing home veterinary behavior consultations has some distinct advantages and disadvantages compared to clinic behavior consultations. With the home consultation, the pet and client are in their natural environment. This increases the likelihood that the pet will exhibit typical characteristic behaviors. It is easier for the entire household to attend the in-home consultation. This may lead to better compliance and will definitely allow for better insight. By observing the home environment, management problems and environmental stressors may be more easily identified. Home consultations also allow the veterinarian and veterinary technician to observe the human social relationships and dynamics within the household. Another distinct advantage to the home consultation is direct application of behavior and environmental modification to the home setting. Home visits increase the perceived value of the service to the client. It adds a personal touch because the veterinarian and veterinary technician have spent time in the home with the client and the pet. During home consultations, the veterinarian is less likely to be interrupted by ancillary hospital staff, yet the client may have personal distractions. Home visits may be less stressful for the client and the pet. If the veterinary service is dedicated solely to treating behavior problems, providing in-home consultations eliminates operating costs associated with a building and additional personnel (Figure 1.12).

The main disadvantage of home behavior consultations is the risk of injury to staff members. It is an unknown environment and therefore safety is a major concern. Often the patient is more offensive, more protective, and has a lengthy learning history in the home environment, making aggression more prone to occur. The veterinary technician may take dogs for brief walks during the consultation. Unfamiliarity with the neighborhood, neighborhood pets, and the dog can be potential safety issues. There is risk of injury to the dog and veterinary technician due to stray dogs. Attempting to implement as many safety precautions and protocols as possible will help prevent dangerous situations. The clinic behavior consultation allows for existing safety measures and familiarity with the setting (Figures 1.13 and 1.14).

Home visits require travel time and may take longer than in-clinic consultations. This may be due to the social nature of the home appointment setting. See Tables 1.3 and 1.4 for average time

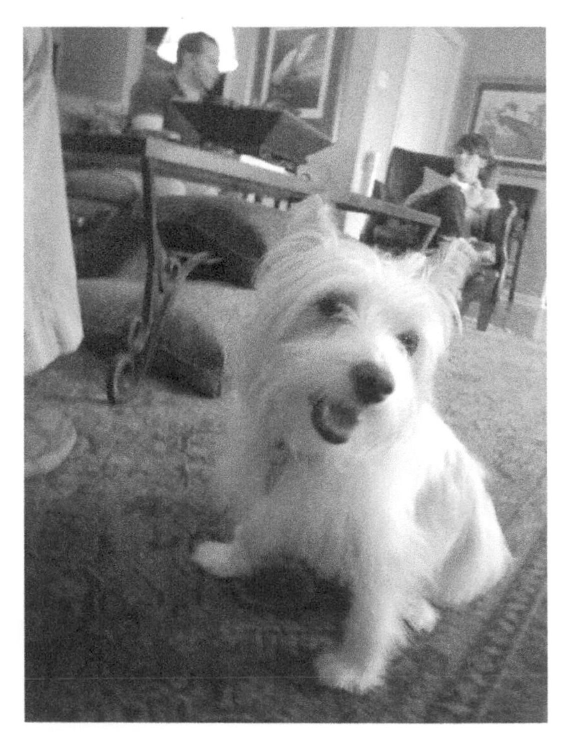

Figure 1.12 Patient evaluated in the home setting for aggression toward family members and strangers entering the home.

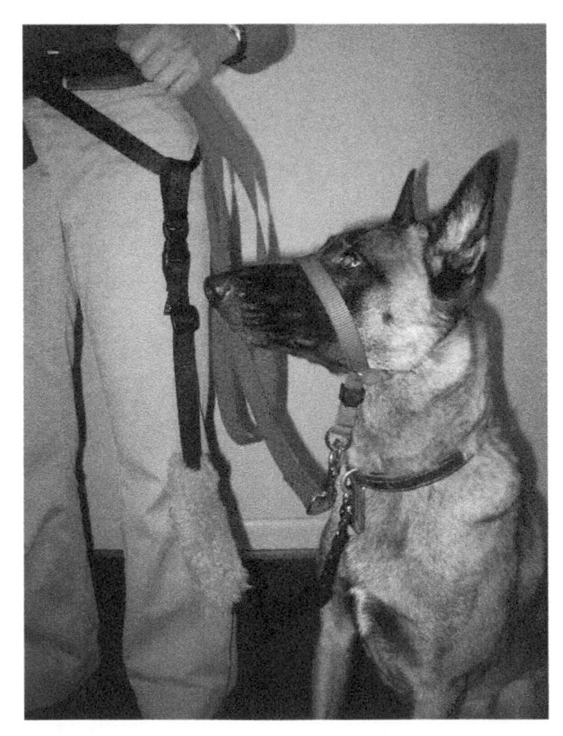

Figure 1.13 Dual leash method, with one leash attached to the head collar and waist leash attached to flat buckle collar. This adds safety and security with dogs, who display reactivity on leash.

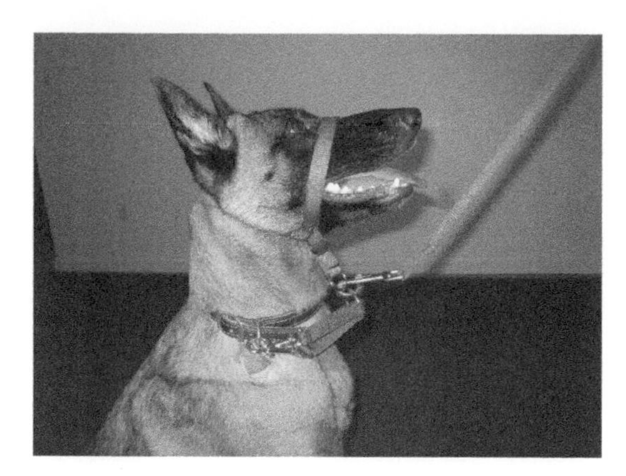

Figure 1.14 Coupler attaching head collar to flat buckle collar. This adds security should one device fail with reactivity.

Table 1.3 Home behavior consultations.

Initial contact phone call	10–15 min
Appointment preparation	15 min
Travel time (varies)	30–60 min
Consultation	2–2.25 h
Fax/Email/Call RDVM[a] (if applicable)	5–15 min
Follow-up contact	30–60 min
Total time	3.5–5 h

[a] Referring DVM.

Table 1.4 Clinic behavior consultations.

Initial call	10–15 min
Appointment preparation	15 min
Appointment	1.5–2 h
Fax/Email/Call RDVM[a] (if applicable)	5–15 min
Follow-up contact	30–60 min
Total time	2.5–3.75 h

[a] Referring DVM.

commitments related to the home versus clinic behavior consultation.

Home behavior consultations typically require follow-up to be facilitated by phone, email, or video conferencing. Ideally, an in-person follow-up would be performed three to four weeks following the initial consultation. This may not be financially feasible due to travel time. Private behavior modification appointments may be recommended for continued follow-up. In-clinic follow-up, training, and behavior modification appointments may be more cost- and time effective for the veterinary staff. A general practice that is offering home behavior consultations may have the capability to perform follow-up appointments and behavior modification appointments in the clinic.

Veterinary-technician-driven behavior services

Besides assisting with behavior consultation, the behavior technician may also provide a variety of other behavior services. Potential veterinary technician-instigated behavior services include behavior modification appointments, puppy socialization classes, kitten classes, pet selection counseling, new puppy/kitten appointments, basic manners/training classes, head-collar fitting, behavior wellness visits, avian classes, and staff and client seminars. Many of these services will be covered in more detail in Chapter 7.

- Besides assisting with behavior consultation, the behavior technician may also provide a variety of other behavior services.

Behavior modification appointments

Behavior modification appointments assist clients with the implementation of the veterinarian-prescribed treatment plan. Behavior modification appointments should last less than one hour. Some pets and owners would benefit from 20- to 30-minute behavior modification appointments. The pet will require scheduled training breaks throughout the appointment; these breaks allow for discussion with the client. Appointments may occur in the hospital setting or at the pet's home. Behavior modification appointments performed in the home allow for further insight and implementation of the treatment plan in the pet's natural environment. This may be beneficial, especially if the initial consultation was performed in the hospital. In contrast, when applying behavior modification for fear at the veterinary hospital, the hospital is the preferred choice unless a non-stressful starting point in the hospital setting is not identified (see Desensitization, Chapter 9).

The same safety and pre-appointment measures implemented during the consultation should be applied to behavior modification appointments. Review the temperament evaluation prior to the appointment to determine if the pet has a history of guarding objects or food from people.

- The same safety and pre-appointment measures implemented during the consultation should be applied to behavior modification appointments.

The first part of the appointment is discussion with the client regarding the status of the pet's progress. What parts of the treatment plan have they implemented? What problems have they encountered? The client should demonstrate the behavior modification exercises with the pet. While the pet is given something enjoyable to do, the veterinary technician can give feedback to the client. Always offer verbal encouragement regarding two or three things the client did well, then discuss alternatives for problem areas. Make it a joint effort, demonstrate for the client, and then allow the client to practice. The conclusion of the appointment should review the major topics covered, present realistic expectations for progression, and set a date for follow-up communication. Detailed notes should be recorded in the patient's file regarding the behavior modification appointment. The veterinarian should be provided with a status update, allowing for any necessary adjustments to the treatment plan.

A specific type of behavior modification appointment is a victory visit. A victory visit is also referred to as a cooperative care training visit, or formal training for veterinary experiences. These sessions are geared toward either preventing handling sensitivities or addressing an already diagnosed handling issue. Victory visits are explored in more detail in Chapters 7 and 8.

Semiprivate behavior modification classes are another option. Dogs that are reactive with other dogs may benefit from "reactive" group dog classes. Careful management and safety are imperative with these classes. Dogs may be required to wear a basket muzzle throughout the class in order to minimize risk associated with handler error. Classes may be formatted in a variety of different ways. One option is to allow only one dog each week to attend the session. All the owners benefit from observing the behavior modification in practice. A volunteer decoy dog or stuffed animal may be used, depending on the dog's reactivity and the clients' ability to safely handle their dog. Pets that demonstrate other behavioral disorders, such as fear and aggression at the veterinary hospital, may also benefit from semiprivate classes at the veterinary hospital focusing on behavior modification techniques. Semiprivate classes may be more cost effective than private lessons. Clients learn by observing implementation of behavior modification with other dogs. Similarly, the client is also provided with a network of people with pets presented for similar behavior disorders.

Because behavior modification appointments require specialized training and knowledge, appropriate charges should apply. An additional fee should be assessed when traveling to the client's home. Travel fees may be a variable or fixed rate, based on mileage or travel time. The travel radius should be predetermined.

- Because behavior modification appointments require specialized training and knowledge, appropriate charges should apply.

Puppy socialization classes

Poor socialization or deprivation of environmental exposure early in life often leads to lifelong deficits and dysfunctional behaviors. Lack of positive exposure is as detrimental as a bad experience. The socialization period is a finite period of development in which the dog is genetically programmed to be more accepting of novelty. Puppy socialization classes help to provide immunity against the development of behavior disorders (Figure 1.15).

The benefits of offering puppy socialization classes in the veterinary hospital include bonding the client to the puppy and veterinary hospital, educating the client on normal canine behavior, addressing common puppy-training issues, and providing a controlled and safe environment for play. Puppy socialization classes also help prevent behavior disorders such as inter-dog aggression, separation anxiety, and fear disorders related to lack of socialization. Teaching puppies to enjoy restraint and handling will make the veterinary staff's job easier. Puppy classes also help identify problem puppies or high-risk puppies for the development of future behavior

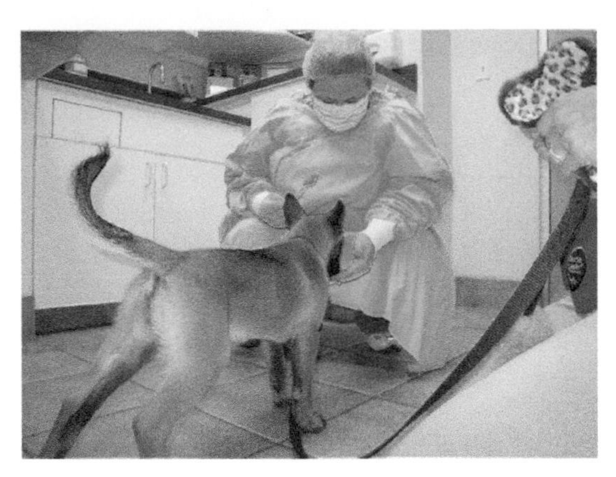

Figure 1.15 Exploration and desensitization to the veterinary hospital and staff using treats during a puppy class.

disorders. They are intended for behaviorally normal puppies and are not designed to address abnormal behaviors. The focus of a puppy class is on education and prevention. Puppy socialization classes are the number one preventive behavior service a veterinary hospital can offer its clients. Puppy classes can be started with minimal work and capital investment. Instructing and assisting puppy socialization classes can be extremely enjoyable and rewarding for the veterinary technician. Puppy socialization classes are discussed in more detail in Chapter 7.

- Puppy socialization classes are the number one preventive behavior service a veterinary hospital can offer its clients.

Kitten classes

Kitten classes are similar to puppy socialization classes, but because most kittens are out of their socialization period (feline socialization period is two to seven weeks of age) by the time they are obtained, there are some distinct differences. Rather than focusing on socialization, kitten classes focus on normal feline behavior and the prevention of behavior disorders. They allow for positive exposure to the veterinary hospital, desensitization to handling, and controlled exploration, thereby bonding the client to the kitten and veterinary hospital. Understanding why cats perform certain behaviors fosters client empathy for the cat. Kitten classes provide the client with the knowledge necessary to modify unwanted behaviors using humane, relationship-building, cat-friendly techniques. Responsible cat ownership with regard to allowing the cat outdoor versus indoor, environmental enrichment, and minimizing stress in multicat households should be addressed. Kitten classes identify and prevent behavior disorders, teach appropriate owner play, address litter-box factors, play biting and scratching, handling, and carrier/kennel training. Often, basic cue training such as sit, come, touch, and place are taught, using positive reinforcement training.

Pet selection counseling

Pet selection counseling is the first defense in the prevention of behavior disorders. The goals of pet selection counseling are to educate the client about normal canine behavior and breed selection (as most pet selection cases are usually regarding obtaining a dog), prepare the client for the new arrival, promote positive reinforcement training, and promote hospital services. If the pet does not meet the client's expectations or is a mismatch to the client's personality or lifestyle, it is unlikely to be retained. Offering pre-purchasing counseling is a way to educate clients prior to their pet's first veterinary visit. This service should be promoted through the hospital website, client mailings, newsletters, email, telephone correspondence, and the hospital bulletin board. Because pet selection counseling is time consuming, hospitals should charge appropriately for technician/staff time. Pet selection counseling appointments can be a valuable service, enhancing the human–animal bond, as well as the client–veterinary–hospital bond.

- Pet selection counseling is the first defense in the prevention of behavior disorders.

New puppy/kitten appointments

The first veterinary hospital visit for puppies and kittens sets the trend for future visits. This can be problematic when the first visit is not enjoyable for the pet. A bad experience potentiates fear or aggression with future visits to the veterinary hospital. Ideally, for all wellness visits, clients should be encouraged to bring a hungry pet and a variety of high-value treats such as string cheese, canned cheese, peanut butter, and small pieces of hotdog. The client should be informed to offer the pet a treat in the parking lot, upon entering the hospital, in the waiting room, and in the exam room. If the puppy/kitten fails to acclimate during the first visit, reschedule the appointment and delay vaccination until the pet is comfortable and taking treats. The goal is for the pet to associate the veterinary hospital with good things (food). Consequently, regardless of the pet's actions, the pet should be offered treats. Scheduling of all new puppy/kitten visits as an extended appointment allows the pet to become acclimatized to the hospital/staff and allows for time to cover specific behavioral topics.

- The first veterinary hospital visit for puppies and kittens sets the trend for future visits.

Veterinary technicians play a critical role in educating clients and staff members about the prevention of behavioral disorders and training problems. Prevention is the most important step in the treatment of behavior. Preventive measures include educating clients about what is normal behavior for the particular breed or species. With each additional wellness visit, specific behavior topics should be covered. Behavioral topics for puppy visits should include socialization, body language, house training, play biting, handling for veterinary and grooming care, jumping, and methodology for basic training and problem solving. Behavioral topics for kitten visits should include play biting and scratching, litter-box training and management, handling for veterinary and grooming care, and carrier training. The importance of veterinary behavioral services such as puppy socialization classes and kitten classes should be stressed to the client. These topics or services may be additionally covered in instructional handouts. Receptionists should be trained to discuss behavioral services regarding preventive medicine over the telephone when scheduling appointments.

- Veterinary technicians play a critical role in educating clients and staff members about the prevention of behavioral disorders and training problems.

Life skills and basic manners training classes

Life skills and basic manners training classes should focus on life skills and foundation behaviors for all young dogs and puppies. Life skills include polite greetings with people and other dogs, cooperative care training for veterinary and grooming care, and building resilience with novelty and sounds. Foundation behaviors may include targeting, attention, position changes (sit, down), settle or go to a place, coming when called, and loose leash walking. Ideally, this class should follow the completion of a puppy socialization class and build on the skills started in that class. Classes may be group, semiprivate, or private, depending on the facility. Training should utilize positive reinforcement and avoid aversive techniques. Offering more advanced classes may also be incorporated. For more information on curriculum development and class formats, see Chapter 7.

- Life skills include polite greetings with people and other dogs, cooperative care training for veterinary and grooming care, and building resilience with novelty and sounds.

Head collar and harness fitting

Many clients and dogs presenting to the veterinary hospital will benefit from the proper fit and usage of head collars or harnesses. When fitted improperly, they are likely to be rejected by the dog and may cause physical abrasion. Head collars and harnesses offer clients control of their dog and facilitate humane leash walking. This increases the likelihood that clients will exercise their pet, benefiting the pet mentally and physically. Head collars are often a necessity for reactive dogs. The behavior veterinary technician should be utilized when offering this service. A specific appointment should be scheduled for a harness or head collar fitting. The hospital should be compensated for the veterinary technician's time and knowledge when educating about these devices (see Chapter 7).

Behavior wellness visits

Although information regarding animal behavior should be solicited during every veterinary visit, pet behavioral wellness appointments are a specific appointment to identify and prevent potential behavioral disorders and training problems. This routine appointment should be scheduled with the veterinary behavior technician. The ideal time to identify behavior and training issues is during the juvenile and adolescence periods. The onset of behavior and training problems is typically prior to social maturity. In dogs, this is prior to two to three years of age.

A behavioral wellness visit should also be scheduled for senior pets. Dogs are typically considered senior by an average of seven years of age, compared to cats between 10 and 12 years of age. Senior pets should be screened for cognitive dysfunction syndrome. The format of the appointment may be conversational and/or a questionnaire.

The longer the duration of the behavioral disorder or learning history for training problems, the more difficult it is to rectify. Behavior wellness visits focus on identifying and preventing problem behaviors and training issues. Veterinary behavioral consultation services or referral to a veterinary behaviorist may be necessary, depending on the disorders or problems identified.

- The longer the duration of the behavioral disorder or learning history for training problems, the more difficult it is to rectify.

Avian classes

In a hospital that provides care to birds, the veterinary behavior technician may consider providing avian classes. Classes may be in a lecture format, discussing management and enrichment recommendations for parrots or hands-on, providing training directly with the birds and clients. Birds should be free of contagious diseases and recently examined by a veterinarian prior to attending classes. Setting specific guidelines for health prerequisites may be determined by the veterinarian-veterinary technician team.

Staff and client seminars

The veterinary behavior team not only has the responsibility of educating the public, but also the veterinary staff, including receptionists, veterinary assistants, kennel assistants, veterinarians, technicians, and the grooming staff. Providing team members with behavior training through staff seminars ensures that the entire veterinary team is providing and promoting consistent behavior information. Contradictory information will confuse the client and may be detrimental to the human–animal as well as the client–hospital bond. New team members should be given immediate education on hospital policies regarding animal behavior. At least biannual seminars to refresh and strengthen the entire team's behavior knowledge are recommended. Information provided should be well documented and not merely based on personal experience.

- Providing staff members with behavior training through staff seminars ensures that the entire veterinary team is providing and promoting consistent behavior information.

Similarly, providing the hospital's clientele with monthly seminars on a variety of behavior topics is an added service the behavior technician may implement. Examples of topics include problem prevention, body language, normal development and behavior, safety with children and pets, husbandry and cooperative care training, and avian management. Charging clients a fee for attendance is appropriate.

Fear Free®/Low Stress Handling® hospital advocate

- The veterinary behavior technician is the optimal team member to be a principal participant of the Fear Free® and/or Low Stress Handling® advocacy committee for the veterinary hospital.

The veterinary behavior technician is the optimal team member to be a principal participant of the Fear Free® and/or Low Stress Handling® advocacy committee for the veterinary hospital. Involvement can include designing team training and hospital policies around creating a culture within the hospital to prevent and alleviate fear, anxiety, and stress for all team members including the pets in our care. We must take our patient's emotional well-being into consideration concurrently with their physical well-being as they are intricately related. As one of the founding members of Johns Hopkins Hospital, William Osler stated, "The good physician treats the disease. The great physician treats the patient who has the disease."

Financial benefits

Behavior services not only generate additional revenue for the hospital with the addition of behavioral services, but they also assist in maintaining and enhancing the human–animal and client–hospital bonds. The direct financial benefits are realized through the income produced by behavioral services. However, indirect financial benefits are equally as profound and are associated with an increase in pet retention, client referrals, veterinary visits, and a decrease in required staff assistance and examination time.

Behavioral issues have been estimated to result in 15% of pets being relinquished, rehomed, or euthanized each year (Patronek and Dodman 1999). Even a 5% loss of a veterinary hospital's patients has a profound impact on revenue.

For example, consider the following:

- A hospital with 2500 active patients.
- An annual loss of 5% results in 125 patients.
- Average estimated annual veterinary expenses for a healthy pet in 2022 is $400–$1200 (biannual to annual exam cost $200–$300, annual lab work $100–$300, and preventive products and care $100–$600).
- Total annual loss $50 000–$150 000 (125 patients).
- A 10% loss would be $100 000–$300 000 (250 patients).
- A 15% loss would be $150 000–$450 000 (375 patients).

Preventive behavior services and early intervention are likely to increase pet retention and decrease financial loss due to unresolved behavioral concerns. When the human–animal bond is weakened due to behavior issues, pet owners are less likely to seek veterinary care and follow veterinary recommendations (Lue et al. 2008).

Through the implementation of compassionate care that integrates low stress and fear free interactions, handling, and restraint, veterinary patients will have a more pleasant experience at the veterinary hospital. Owners, whose pets enjoy coming to the hospital, will visit more often. Similarly, satisfied clients will recommend the hospital to friends and family, thus potentially increasing clientele through referrals.

By offering puppy socialization and kitten classes, participating dogs and cats will have repetitive positive experiences in the hospital and become acclimated to handling and restraint. Consequently, examination time and the need for extra staff assistance with restraint will be decreased.

The veterinary behavior technician can be instrumental in providing direct and indirect financial benefits to the hospital.

Conclusion

At a minimum, the veterinary technician and veterinary staff should be familiar with preventive behavior services and even if not directly involved with the implementation of behavior services, they need to be able to provide clients with appropriate resources that will enhance the human–animal bond.

Should the technician choose, they can play an instrumental role in the success of preventive behavior services. Behavior can be a specialty area in which the veterinary technician can excel. The inspired behavior technician can develop and implement a variety of preventive behavior services and in doing so, increase animal retention, save animals, and improve client satisfaction while simultaneously improving hospital revenue and veterinary technician's job satisfaction.

- The inspired behavior technician can develop and implement a variety of preventive behavior services and in doing so, increase animal retention, save animals, and improve client satisfaction while simultaneously improving hospital revenue and veterinary technician's job satisfaction.

References

Camps, T., Amat, M., and Manteca, X. (2019). A review of medical conditions and behavioral problems in dog and cats. *Animals* 9 (12): 1133. MDPI AG, https://doi.org/10.3390/ani9121133.

Eskeland, G. (2007) Educational methods as risk factors for problem behaviours in dogs. School of Psychology, University of Southampton. Dissertation for the degree of MSc in Companion Animal Behaviour Counselling, p. 127.

Garg, A., Chren, M.M., Sands, L.P. et al. (2001). Psychological stress perturbs epidermal permeability barrier homeostasis: implications for the pathogenesis of stress-associated skin disorders. *Archives of Dermatology* 137 (1): 53–59.

Gur, E., Lerer, B., Newman, M. et al. (1999). Chronic clomipramine and triiodothyronine increase serotonin levels in rat frontal cortex in vivo: relationship to serotonin autoreceptor activity. *Journal of Pharmacology and Experimental Therapeutics* 288 (1): 81–87.

Harvey, N.D., Craigon, P.J., Shaw, S.C. et al. (2019). Behavioural differences in dogs with atopic dermatitis suggest stress could be a significant problem associated with chronic pruritus. *Animals* 9 (10): 813.

Hrovat, A., De Keuster, T., Kooistra, H., et al. (2018). Behavior in dogs with spontaneous hypothyroidism during treatment with levothyroxine. *Journal of Veterinary Internal Medicine* 33 (1): 64–71. Wiley, https://doi.org/10.1111/jvim.15342.

Klink, M.P., Shofer, F.S., and Reisner, I.R. (2008). Association of pruritus with anxiety or aggression in dogs. *Journal of the American Veterinary Medical Association* 233 (7): 1105–1111.

Landsberg, G.M., Shaw, J., Donaldson, J. et al. (2008). Handling behavior problems in the practice setting. *The Veterinary Clinics of North America. Small Animal Practice* 38 (5): 951–969 v.

Lopes Fagundes, A., Hewison, L., McPeake, K. et al. (2018). Noise sensitivities in dogs: an exploration of signs in dogs with and without musculoskeletal pain using qualitative content analysis. *Frontiers in Veterinary Science* 5: https://doi.org/10.3389/fvets.2018.00017.

Lue, T.W., Pantenburg, D.P., and Crawford, P.M. (2008). Impact of the owner-pet and client-veterinarian bond on the care that pets receive. *Journal of the American Veterinary Medical Association* 232 (4): 531–540.

Luescher, A.U. and Reisner, I.R. (2008). Canine aggression toward familiar people: a new look at an old problem. *The Veterinary Clinics of North America. Small Animal Practice* 38 (5): 1107–1130 vii.

Luescher, A.U., Flannigan, G., Frank, D. et al. (2007). The role and limitations of trainers in behavior treatment and therapy. *Journal of Veterinary Behavior: Clinical Applications and Research* 2 (1): 26–27.

Patronek, G.J. and Dodman, N.H. (1999). Attitudes, procedures, and delivery of behavior services by veterinarians in small animal practice. *Journal of the American Veterinary Medical Association* 215: 1606–1611.

Radosta-Huntley, L.A., Shofer, F.S., Reisner, I.R. et al. (2006). Comparison of thyroid values in aggressive and non-aggressive dogs. Poster presented at the American College of Veterinary Behaviorists and American Veterinary Society of Animal Behavior Scientific Symposium, Honolulu (July 17, 2006).

Shore, E.R., Burdsal, C., Douglas, D.K. et al. (2008). Pet owners' views of pet behavior problems and willingness to consult experts for assistance. *Journal of Applied Animal Welfare Science* 11 (1): 63–73.

The PowerPoint of figures, appendices, MCQ's are available at www.wiley.com/go/martin/behavior

2 Canine behavior and development

Lisa Radosta
Florida Veterinary Behavior Service, West Palm Beach, FL, USA

CHAPTER MENU

Veterinary technicians and nurses are the educators of the veterinary healthcare team. They educate pet parents, their peers, and veterinarians. As primary care veterinary appointments get shorter, the technician's role becomes even more essential. A technician's time observing the patient navigating the hospital and exam room may be lengthier than the veterinarian's. An understanding of normal

Canine and Feline Behavior for Veterinary Technicians and Nurses, Second Edition. Edited by Debbie Martin and Julie K. Shaw.

Companion website: www.wiley.com/go/martin/behavior

development and capabilities of our patients is the foundation for understanding abnormalities and providing high-quality patient care.

- An understanding of normal development and capabilities of our patients is the foundation for understanding abnormalities and providing high-quality patient care.

Canine sensory capacities

Dogs are observers of the world around them. Those observations help them cope with stressors and gain resources. They link what they see, hear, touch, taste and smell with antecedents (stimuli preceding an event) with consequences (stimuli following an event). Deficits in any of the aforementioned senses can contribute to changes in behavior and reduction in quality of life. There is debate regarding whether dogs rely more on vision or smell to navigate their environment. Some argue that as dogs were domesticated, they were selected for the ability to visually take cues from humans. This is supported by studies that show that dogs are less successful in finding their handler via scent alone (Polgar et al. 2015). Still other studies show that dogs rely more on scent than vision when performing certain tasks (Gazit and Terkel 2003). At this time, we can't say for certain that one sense is more important to the dog than another.

Vision

Canis familiaris is the most diverse species on earth. One example of the diversity of the species is the huge differences in skull shape and length. These differences result in differences in the neurons in the area centralis of the retina (involved in visual acuity) contributing to the differences in vision between breeds (McGreevy et al. 2004). Visual acuity, a measure of the sharpness of vision, is eight times worse in dogs when compared to humans meaning that dogs are not as able as humans to distinguish fine details at a distance.

Contrary to popular belief, dogs can see colors in the blue – violet and the yellow – green ranges, (i.e. dichromatic vision) (Neitz et al. 1989) with cones comprising 20% of the central portion of the retina (Parry 1953). Dogs can distinguish colors within their scope of vision well enough to be successful in discrimination tests. Dogs may see colors outside of this range as shades of gray.

Brightness discrimination (ability to distinguish between shades of gray) is somewhat dependent on visual acuity and is about two times worse in dogs than in humans, varying between breeds (Pretterer et al. 2004).

Dogs have good vision in dim light because of the wealth of rods in the central area of the retina when compared to humans who have predominantly cones (Miller and Murphy 1995) and the unique tapetum lucidum in the back of the eye which reflects light back onto the retina a second time. Pet parents often report that their dog doesn't like to be photographed. That may be due to differences between humans and dogs in the function of the photopigment rhodopsin. In dogs, after exposure to bright light (e.g. flash) rhodopsin takes over an hour to completely regenerate (Jacobs et al. 1991; Kemp and Jacobson 1992; Parkes et al. 1982). This apparent loss of some of the elements of vision may be frightening to dogs causing them to avoid being in photographs by moving away or averting their gaze when presented with the antecedents (e.g. phone, camera) to being in a photograph.

A dog's total binocular field of vision is about 250°, which is about 60–70° greater than a human's enabling dogs to visualize the horizon more completely.

Compared to humans, dogs see less of the color spectrum, have a greater degree of binocular vision, cannot distinguish fine details at a distance, see better in low light and are not as able as humans to distinguish between subtle differences in gray scale.

- Compared to humans, dogs see less of the color spectrum, have a greater degree of binocular vision, cannot distinguish fine details at a distance, see better in low light and are not as able as humans to distinguish between subtle differences in gray scale.

Hearing

Dogs can hear higher pitched sounds (up to 65 000 Hz) compared to humans (20 000 Hz). In addition, dogs have more sensitive ears than ours. They can hear sounds between −5 and −15 dB (0 dB is the softest sound that can be heard by a human). These differences may contribute to the prevalence of noise and storm phobia in dogs as well as the frequent report by pet parents that their dogs know that a storm is coming before any visual cues (e.g. gray clouds, rain, thunder). Dogs can localize the source of a noise by moving their pinnae. Like humans, they can also derive the direction from which a sound is coming from the time difference between the left and the right ear perceiving the sound.

Olfaction

Dogs are 10 000–100 000 times better than humans at recognizing a scent in the environment having between 220 million and 2 billion neurons in the olfactory epithelium (humans have 2–5 million) (Moulton 1977; Siniscalchi et al. 2018). This superior ability has led to training dogs for search and rescue, bomb detection, cancer detection, and hypoglycemia alert. Dog sports have also emerged to exploit most dogs' apparent love for sniffing (e.g. nosework, tracking). Although outside the scope of this text, it should be noted that the olfactory system is intimately linked to the limbic system (emotional system in the brain). The processing of the information from this part of the environment is like no other, triggering cascades of neurotransmitters involved in the physiologic actions related to emotions. This partially explains the strong emotional reactions that dogs have to the veterinary clinic.

It is unknown whether dogs use olfaction to a greater degree in their daily life or whether through domestication while the ability to detect scent in small amounts remains, the usefulness to the domestic dog has diminished. However, it is accepted that dogs use their sense of smell in food selection (Houpt et al. 1978).

Vomeronasal organ

The vomeronasal organ is a pair of channels lined with an epithelium containing chemoreceptors that open into the mouth just behind the upper incisors. Unlike other species such as horses, dogs do not show flehmen (lip-curling behavior) when investigating a substance; rather, they lick substances they want to test (such as urine of another dog), and "tongue" them (rub the tongue against the roof of the mouth).

The vomeronasal organ is important for detecting pheromones and therefore for social communication. Because it is connected to the limbic system, perception via the vomeronasal organ affects emotions. This is the basis for the use of pheromone analogues for behavior modification. Processing of olfactory sensory input whether via the vomeronasal organ or the olfactory epithelium is intimately linked to the processing of emotions. This is the basis for the use of pheromone analogues as a way to decrease fear, anxiety and stress.

- Because it is connected to the limbic system, perception via the vomeronasal organ affects emotions.

Taste

Dogs like any other animal can develop a taste preference or taste aversion to almost any substance. Their sense of taste is already functional at birth. Aside from taste, palatability is largely based on smell, temperature, and texture. Dogs have about 1700 taste buds compared to humans who have approximately 9000. Dogs can perceive six types of tastes: sweet, sour, salty, bitter, umami, and water (Kumazawa and Kurihara 1990; Kurihara and Kashiwayanagi 2000; Lindemann 1996). Dogs prefer sweet tasting foods over bitter and salty foods. Preferences develop in puppyhood and may be congenital (Stokke 2014).

Touch

The skin has receptors to sense touch, pressure, pain, body movement and position, temperature, vibration, and chemical stimulation. Touch receptors are located at the base of every hair, and especially the vibrissae. Touch can be calming, arousing, or aversive, depending on type and circumstance. Dogs can be conditioned to appreciate and enjoy touch. The reverse (touch being regarded by the dog as aversive) is also true and is seen regularly at the veterinary clinic. It shouldn't be assumed that touch of any particular type is reinforcing (pleasurable) to any individual dog. In addition, while it may seem counterintuitive, some dogs appear in puppyhood to develop preferences and aversions to touch without any overt trauma noted. Any time that a patient presents with an intolerance of touch, pain or discomfort should always be considered a factor until proven otherwise.

Canine communication

Dogs communicate with visual, auditory, and olfactory cues. Humans are a mostly visual species, therefore knowledge of the body language of dogs is particularly important for us to be able to understand their intentions or emotions. For dogs, the language is simple and easy to understand if both the sender and the recipient have normal behavior patterns because many signals are highly ritualized and preserved genetically. That is to say that they have become part of the normal behavior repertoire of dogs and have taken on a specific meaning in dog–dog communication. Body language signals when understood by the recipient (e.g. other dogs) will then influence the recipient's behavior. They are used as a means of communication primarily to avoid conflict and resolve challenges over resources without injury to either party and first and foremost are an expression of fear, anxiety, stress, and conflict (FASC) and frustration.

Different postures may indicate fear, anxiety, conflict, aggression, play, happiness or appeasement among other things. One body language signal may be made up of many signals originating from several body parts including the ears, musculature, tail, and mouth. Some body language displays can be interpreted differently depending on the accompanying individual body language signals and the context. To further complicate matters, the conformation, coat color and coat length of the dog may limit or enhance that individual's ability to display a certain body language signal and for the intended recipient to receive an accurate message. This can contribute to FASC and aggression in the sender and recipient dog.

Like any other behavior, body language signals while seemingly innate, can be learned, punished (decreased) or reinforced (increased). For example, if a dog who leans away from a person (indicating FASC) while on a walk, is then petted by that person, the behavior of leaning away will be punished reducing the likelihood that it will be displayed in the future. With enough repetition, leaning away in this circumstance may very well be abandoned as a tool for communication. In this example, however, the dog's motivation (FASC) has not been addressed. For this reason, the dog is likely to find another body language signal that is louder such as growling or barking to repel the stimulus of which it is afraid (Figure 2.1).

- Think of canine body language signals as requests. Your job is to figure out the dog's "ask."

Think of canine body language signals as requests. Your job is to figure out the dog's "ask." Does the dog want you to approach? Move away? Play? Learning another species' language is complicated, but with study and practice, it is possible to better understand the intentions and emotions of our canine patients.

Body language classifications

Body language postures can be classified in many ways depending on the discipline. Ethologists may characterize them as offensive or defensive, distance

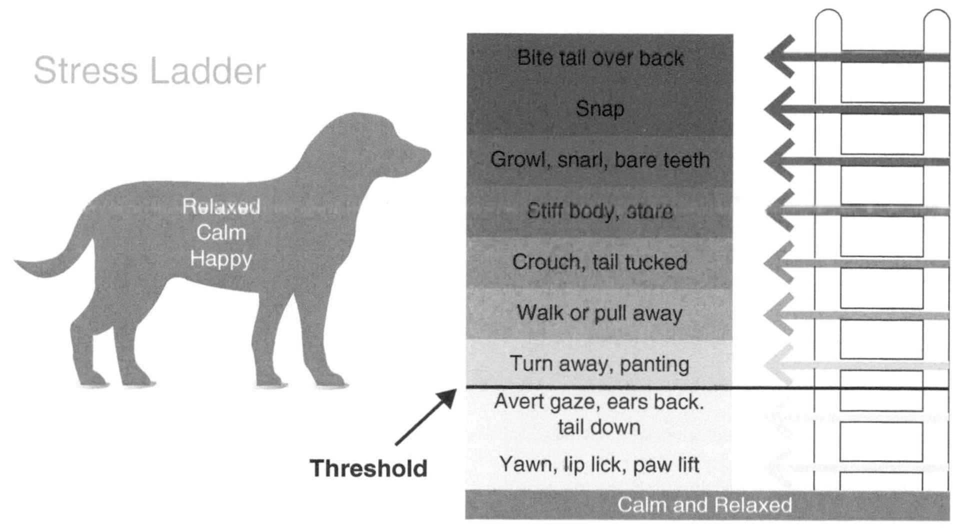

Figure 2.1 Canine stress ladder. *Source:* Courtesy of Lisa Radosta, DVM, DACVB.

increasing or distance decreasing. Most often in veterinary medicine they will be classified as relaxed, fearful, anxious, stressed, conflicted, and aggressive. Familiarity with the different terms while not essential is interesting and allows for a deeper understanding of the dog's intention. In this text, we will most often characterize body language as relaxed or FASC; however, distance increasing or decreasing may be used. What you will notice is absent from this text is the use of dominance or submission. These terms have been overused and incorrectly used in the lay literature to such an extent that they have lost their association with the scientific meaning. Below, you will find an explanation of these terms.

Body postures

Body posture may be the easiest body language signal to assess. A tense or stiff body posture (e.g. muscles tense, body still) indicates neurochemical arousal. Neurochemical arousal describes the activation of the fight or flight system (sympathetic nervous system). Despite the name (fight or flight), this system can become activated when the dog is excited as well. Arousal can occur with almost any emotional state. The resultant behavior may be one of interaction with the environment in a positive way (play) or a negative one (aggression). A tense body posture should cause the observer to stop and assess the situation considering context, additional body language and conformation.

The dog's weight might be shifted forward, down, or back whether the dog is standing, sitting, or lying down. Weight shifted away from the stimulus or toward the ground, generally indicates a decreased interest in interacting with the stimulus (e.g. fear, anxiety, conflict, stress) while weight shifted forward indicates an interest in interaction (e.g. play, excitement, predation, aggression) (Figure 2.2). It should be noted that interest in interaction can be friendly or unfriendly. Dogs with weight shifted away or down should cause the observer to decrease stress by backing away or removing the stimulus. Dogs with body weight shifted forward should cause the observer to assess the situation based on context, conformation and additional body language.

- Piloerection (raised hackles) indicates neurochemical arousal, which can be associated with conflict, fear, anxiety, or excitement and could result in friendly or unfriendly interactions.

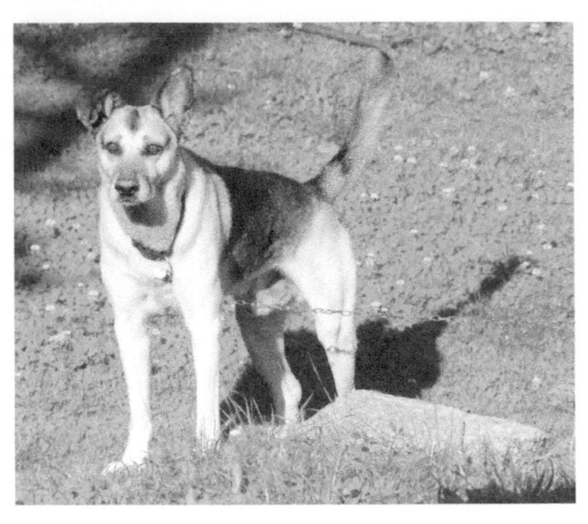

Figure 2.2 The tail is held high, the dog is leaning forward with a direct stare, and the ears are pricked forward indicating arousal which may be associated with attention to a stimulus, predation, fear, anxiety, stress, conflict or frustration.

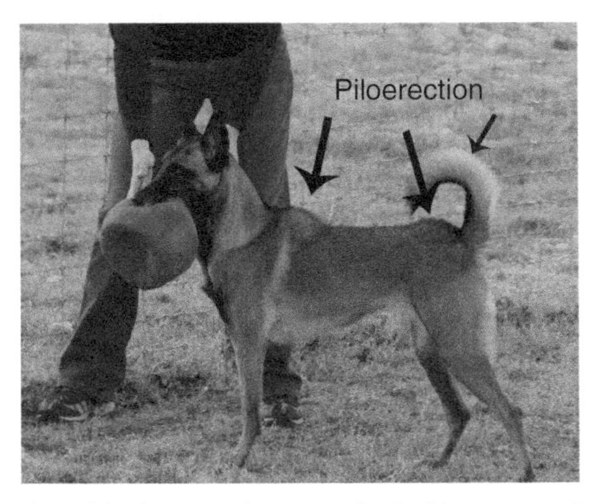

Figure 2.3 Piloerection shown over the shoulders, rump, and tail, indicating arousal and uncertainty.

Piloerection (raised hackles) indicates neurochemical arousal, which can be associated with conflict, fear, anxiety or excitement and could result in friendly or unfriendly interactions. As with other body language signals, piloerection should cause the observer to assess the situation (Figure 2.3).

Mounting can be sexual; however, in gonadectomized dogs it is most often a displacement or conflict behavior indicating a level of excitement and uncertainty, not a desire to dominate the mountee. The observer should try to redirect the dog calmly to another behavior that is inconsistent with mounting.

Lifting of one of the front paws is an indication of anticipation of either an action on the dog's part or an action on the part of something in the environment. It may indicate excitement that a treat will be tossed or an intention to lunge and bite. As with many other signals, a paw lift should cause the observer to stop and assess the situation considering context, additional body language and conformation.

The play bow (rump in the air, front legs lowered to ground) is a play solicitation (Figure 2.4). The play bow can also be seen in other situations such as aggression in which the dog's movement is restricted. It is a combination of moving forward and an intention to jump backward. While the play bow is almost always associated with play, it can be associated with other emotional states such as conflict. Action on the observer's part should be based on other body language signals and context.

A step back or step away is an indication that the dog is requesting more space from the stimulus. It may be preceded by an avert gaze (see below). As with any body posture in which weight shifted back or down with the exception of the play bow, the dog should be given space.

The shake off where the dog rotates the body side to side (similar to what is displayed after a bath) indicates that the preceding incident was exciting, stressful, or arousing. This is often displayed during play when a particular dog needs a break or after a physical examination has been completed. The observer should wait for the dog to recover and approach when he is ready.

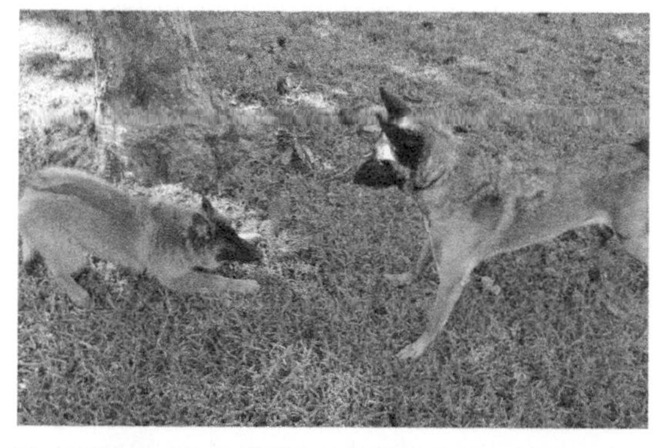

Figure 2.4 A puppy offering a play bow to an adult dog. The puppy is signaling nonthreat and an invitation to play but is also ready to retreat pending the adult dog's response.

Tail

The tail may be the most misunderstood part of the dog's body. A wagging tail is inaccurately interpreted by most pet parents and many veterinary healthcare team members as a sign of friendly interaction. In fact, a wagging tail is consistent with neurochemical arousal and a willingness to interact. As above, neurochemical arousal can be associated with FASC, joy, or aggression.

- A wagging tail is inaccurately interpreted by most pet parents and many veterinary healthcare team members as a sign of friendly interaction. In fact, a wagging tail is consistent with neurochemical arousal and a willingness to interact. As above, neurochemical arousal can be associated with FASC, joy, or aggression.

The carriage, laterality, intensity of movement, engagement of entire or parts of the tail as well as other body language signals will elucidate in most situations, the meaning of the tail wag.

When analyzing the position of the tail, the breed's normal carriage should be considered. For example, a Labrador Retriever will carry the tail level with the back when it is relaxed whereas a German Shepherd will often hold their tail below the back when relaxed. When the tail is held below the natural carriage for an individual dog, it indicates FASC. When it is held very far under the body, the FASC is severe. When it is positioned above the normal carriage for that individual, it indicates neurochemical arousal, which most often indicates aggression or overarousal, not friendly intent. Another consideration aside from carriage is the level of stiffness, amplitude and intensity of tail movement. A stiff tail indicates FASC (Bradshaw and Rooney 2016; Hecht and Horowitz 2015). A slow wagging tail generally indicates uncertainty while a very fast wagging tail or a stiff tail with just the tip wagging indicates high arousal. A large amplitude wag where the caudal part of the body moves with the tail indicates excited and friendly interaction. A study published in 2017 suggests that the laterality (the direction of largest amplitude) can indicate emotional state in dogs (Quaranta et al. 2007). Dogs who have a positive emotional state wag their tails more to the right and dogs with a negative emotional state wag their tail more to the left.

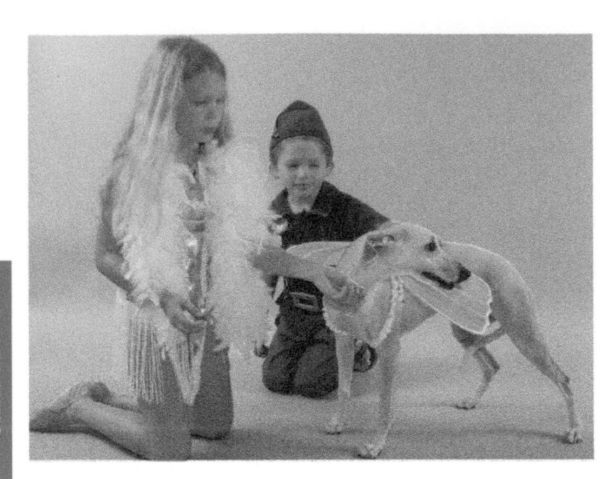

Figure 2.5 The dog turns away, licks her lips, while refusing a treat from the child. These are signs the dog is stressed about the situation or interaction.

In addition, there is evidence that in fact dogs can interpret tail wags, effectively assessing the emotional state of other dogs (Siniscalchi et al. 2013).

Head

Dogs who move their head away (e.g. avert gaze, look away) are indicating that they want distance from the stimulus (Figure 2.5). They do not want to interact. An avert gaze is characterized by a movement of the head away from the stimulus, but the body stays still. Often the eyes will continue to engage the stimulus. In this case, the observer should move away.

Ears

Ear carriage is dependent on the conformation of the dog. With that said, there are some generalizations that can be made. Ears that are pricked up (or raised at their base in lop-eared dogs) indicate attentiveness. Ears that are folded back and flattened indicate FASC (Table 2.1) or play. The farther back the ears fold, the more intense the motivation whether that be fear or play. Because the same ear carriages can be associated with different emotional states, the observer should analyze them in context considering other body language signals displayed concurrently (Figure 2.6).

Eyes

A direct eye stare indicates an alert and potentially highly aroused dog and may precede aggression. Most dogs will not maintain direct eye contact for long if they are not neurochemically aroused, have not been taught to do so (e.g. watch me), or were not reinforced for this behavior (e.g. ball toss, treat). Completely avoiding eye contact usually indicates some degree of FASC although if a dog has been punished for looking at a person, that can cause him to avoid eye contact. Dilated pupils in a well-lit environment, in a normal-sighted dog are a sign of neurochemical arousal. When a dog orients his nose toward a stimulus and moves his eyes laterally exposing more of the sclera (i.e. whale eye), he is indicating FASC and neurochemical arousal. The dog does not want to look away from the stimulus as it is too dangerous (in his mind) to do so, but he intends to indicate that he needs space or distance (averting the gaze). This is often accompanied by a tense body posture and is displayed just before an aggressive display. Dilated pupils, direct stare, and whale eye all indicate arousal except in the situations mentioned above. The observer should analyze them in context with the situation and concurrent body language signals (Figure 2.7).

Mouth

A lip curl that exposes the teeth indicates aggression or play (see Figure 2.8). It does not indicate a motivation of FASC or confidence. It indicates that the dog is asking for distance from the stimulus and is threatening to do harm if the interactions are not terminated (aggressive lip curl) or that he is soliciting play. Licking or nuzzling the mouth of a dog or a person is an appeasement behavior, or a way to initiate social contact in a friendly, nonthreatening way. It has also been reinforced by many pet parents as "kisses." Yawning can be displayed when the dog first wakes up from sleep or because of FASC. Lip licking when not eating or anticipating food is a distance increasing signal indicating a level of FASC. Yawning, lip licking are displays of FASC. Lip curls and snarls generally indicated aggression. These behaviors should cause the observer to increase distance.

Clinical interpretation

Play

Play is muted predatory behavior. Not all dogs know how to play appropriately. Matter of fact if puppies aren't socialized with other dogs before 20 weeks of age, they avoid social play (Fox and Stelzner 1966). The game of dog play is neurochemically arousing

Table 2.1 Body language signals, possible meanings, and observer action.

Signal	Meaning	Observer action
Tense	Neurochemical arousal	Assess with context, conformation and other body language signals
Weight shifted down or back	Decreased interaction with environment or stimulus, FASC	Increase distance from stimulus, move away
Weight shifted forward	Increased interaction with environment or stimulus,	Assess with context, conformation and other body language signals
Piloerection	Neurochemical arousal	Assess with context, conformation and other body language signals
Mounting	Conflict, excitement, displacement	Redirect to another action
Paw lift	Anticipation	Assess with context, conformation and other body language signals
Tail over 45° above normal carriage	Neurochemical arousal	Assess with context, conformation and other body language signals
Tail below normal carriage	Fear, anxiety, stress, conflict	Increase distance from stimulus, move away
Tail wagging	Willingness to interact, neurochemical arousal	Assess with context, conformation and other body language signals
Tail tucked	Severe FASC	Increase distance from stimulus, move away
Step back/step away	FASC	Increase distance from stimulus, move away
Ears forward	Alert, attentive	Assess with context, conformation and other body language signals
Ears back	FASC, play	Increase distance from stimulus, move away, assess for play body postures
Avert gaze/head turn	FASC	Increase distance from stimulus, move away
Dilated pupils	Neurochemical arousal, play	Assess with context, conformation and other body language signals
Whale eye	FASC, neurochemical arousal, often precedes aggression.	Increase distance
Yawn	Sleep, FASC	Assess with context, conformation and other body language signals
Shake off	Previous interaction was arousing or exciting	Give the dog a break to recover
Lip lick	Distance increasing, FASC	Assess with context, conformation and other body language signals

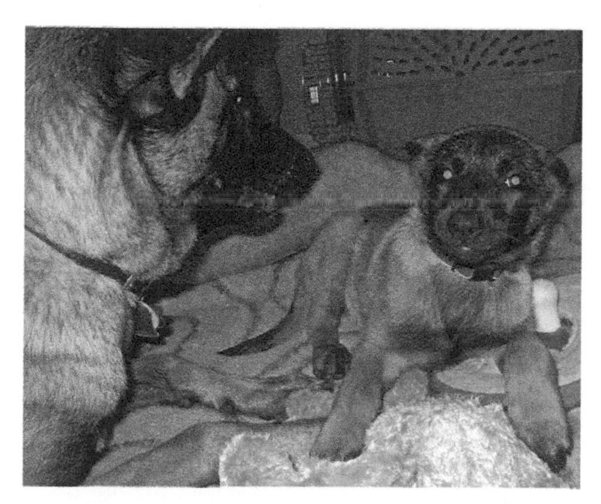

Figure 2.6 The puppy is pulling her ears back, most likely due to fear, in response to the adult dog.

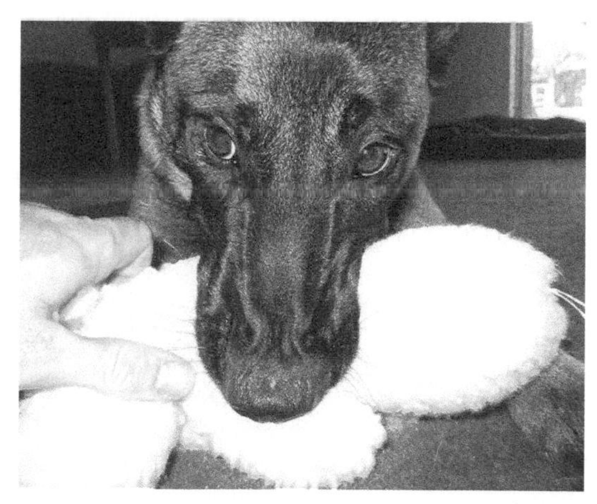

Figure 2.7 A dog displaying a stiff posture, normal pupil dilation, ears back, and whale eye.

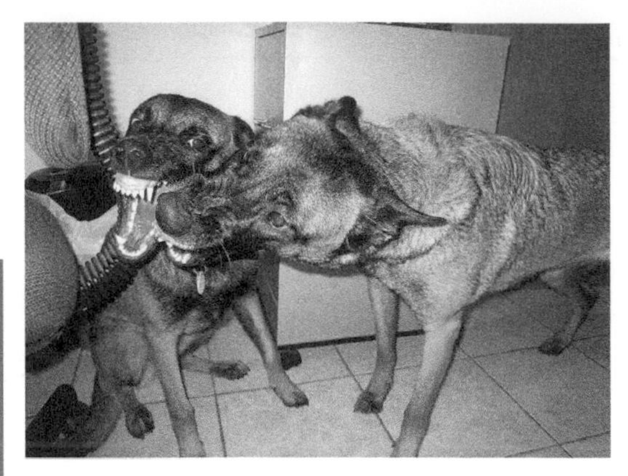

Figure 2.8 Teeth exposed can indicate aggression or play.

and can include pawing with a front foot, twisting jumps, open-mouth panting, tail wagging, tail over, lower or at the back, chase, inguinal presentation, wrestling, biting, and growling. As you can see, play can look like almost anything! Because during play dogs are neurochemically aroused they can move into more aggressive and injurious interactions fairly quickly. Observers should look for self-handicapping (one dog assuming inguinal presentation), role reversals (chaser vs. being chased), loose tail carriage, relaxed body postures, quick changes from lying to standing to chasing and inhibited bites and growls.

Conflict

Conflict is a state of stress and is defined as a psychological struggle, often unconscious, resulting from the opposition or simultaneous functioning of mutually exclusive impulses, desires, or tendencies. Conflict behaviors are often shown in situations of frustration, uncertainty and/or motivational conflict and may or may not have an effect on the receiver. It often has components of fear and anxiety. It can arise from an unpredictable environment where the dog lacks control over pleasant or unpleasant outcomes including social interactions, schedule and time of feeding. The dog may display motivational conflict where he experiences two opposing motivations, such as the motivation to approach and the motivation to withdraw. For example, a dog that wants to socialize with a person but at the same time is afraid of how the person might react may approach with a tail below the normal body carriage, wagging slowly, ears slightly back as he licks his lips. Then, when reached for he may retreat. Conflict behaviors can be recognized because the dog will display opposing body language signals (Table 2.2).

Table 2.2 Signs of fear, anxiety, stress, and conflict.

Ears back or to the side
Tail down or tucked
Weight shifted back
Lowered head/neck (common when guarding)
Leaning or backing away
Hiding
Trembling/shaking
Pacing, running, or escape behavior
Seeking close human contact
"Grabbing" treats or not taking treats at all
Hackles raised-piloerection
Scanning
Furrowed brow
"Whale" eye
Dry, squeaky pant
Barking
Growling
Snapping
Freezing
Glassy eyed stare
Turning away
Turning the head
Averting eyes
Shifting eyes/brows
Licking
Squinting
Scratching
Sneezing
Sitting down
Lying down
Yawning
Mounting
Wet dog shake
Many others. . .

- Conflict is a state of stress and is defined as a psychological struggle, often unconscious, resulting from the opposition or simultaneous functioning of mutually exclusive impulses, desires, or tendencies.
- The dog may display motivational conflict where he experiences two opposing motivations, such as the motivation to approach and the motivation to withdraw.

Aggression

Dogs generally avoid conflict and use aggression as a last resort. As in people, aggression can be a conflict behavior in dogs. An aggressive outburst is a common mammalian reaction to the stress of having lost control and the ability to predict what is going to happen. Similarly, dogs that lose control, are frustrated or displaying FASC may become aggressive. Aggression at its core is a distance increasing signal with an intent to do harm if the social pressure is not reduced.

Pet parents often report that their dog became aggressive "without warning." Fortunately for us and for dogs, this is rarely the case. Aggression is almost always directly or historically preceded by body language signals that indicate FASC and frustration. Consider the following example. You are on an elevator with several other people. One person steps close enough that they are touching you. You turn to them and ask politely if they can take a step back. The person does not take a step back as you requested. You may raise your voice and place a hand in front of yourself which may be considered threatening (aggressive) to the other person. If the person remains too close, you may become more aggressive and threatening with the hope they will retreat. As previously discussed, body language signals can be punished or reinforced, decreasing or increasing their likelihood of being exhibited in any given circumstance. Once a body language signal has been successful in achieving a return to homeostasis or a more relaxed state free of FACS and frustration, that body language signal or group of signals has been reinforced and will be exhibited more frequently. This is one of the ways that dogs whose motivation is FACS come to display aggression and body language that is more consistent with tension and arousal than fear. They have learned that aggressive displays are effective and fearful body language is not. Once this has been "learned" it cannot be completely "unlearned." Consider your own life. You have learned your multiplication tables. Now, if I ask you to unlearn them, can you do so? You can decrease your practice of those tables, but the original learning has been laid down as a memory in your brain. That cannot be undone. As in Figure 2.1, if the lower rungs of the ladder have been punished, consider them to have disappeared. Rebuilding those rungs in the dog's mind is very difficult.

- Once a body language signal has been successful in achieving a return to homeostasis or a more relaxed state free of FACS and frustration, that body language signal or group of signals has been reinforced and will be exhibited more frequently.

Fear, anxiety, and stress and/or conflict

Over the past decade, it has become clear that FASC are the cause of almost all behavior disorders in dogs. A relaxed dog who is in homeostasis physically, physiologically, and emotionally generally does not get involved in or cause conflict. The individual behaviors associated with fear, anxiety, and stress have been described above. Generally, a dog displaying signs of fear or anxiety has a low body posture, weight shifted back, ears back, tail down or tucked and may attempt to escape. A stressed dog has an increased heart rate, respiratory rate, body temperature, dilated pupils, and may display any or all of the body language signals listed in this text associated with fear, anxiety, and stress. Fear, anxiety, and stress are closely related and cannot generally be separated by gross observation. If you observe body language associated with fear or anxiety, assume that stress is also present and vice versa (Table 2.2).

- Over the past decade, it has become clear that fear, anxiety, stress, and conflict are the cause of almost all behavior disorders in dogs.

Auditory communication

Dogs bark, growl, whimper, whine, grunt, and cry to communicate; indicating distress, need for attention, territorial threat, solicitation of play, greeting, pain, or excitement among other things (Bradshaw and Nott 1995). The production of vocal signals depends on the size and anatomy specific to that individual dog and is influenced by breed. In addition, domestication by humans as in every other aspect of the life of dogs has influenced the tone and purpose of certain dog vocalizations. The structure of growls in dogs and wolves is identical and both use growls during conflict and displays of aggression although that is where the similarities end. Adult wolves do not growl in play as dogs do demonstrating the effect of domestication and neoteny on dogs (Cohen and Fox 1976). Whimpers and whines are high pitched and often indicate a need for attention, greeting or distress (Fox 1984). Vocalization of any kind can also be used in situations of conflict or frustration.

Olfactory communication

Olfactory communication can take place through direct contact (e.g. sniffing an individual) and investigation of scent left behind (e.g. urine marking). Dogs deposit scent via feces, urine, and glandular secretions. Dogs can recognize individuals and distinguish that scent from their own (Bekoff 2001; Bradshaw and Rooney 2016). It is unclear what information the dog can glean from this type of communication, but the interest of dogs in the scents in their environment implies that the information at minimum is enriching if not essential. Raised-leg urination (posture of urine marking) serves to leave a scent communication, and is a social display and a sign of anxiety. Many dogs with separation anxiety, for example, exhibit this behavior. Ground scratching is a form of scent (sweat glands on feet) and visual marking (Handelman 2012). Dogs also roll in odiferous items such as feces of other species or carrion (Figure 2.9). The function of this behavior is not understood.

- It is unclear what information the dog can glean from this type of communication, but the interest of dogs in the scents in their environment implies that the information at minimum is enriching if not essential.

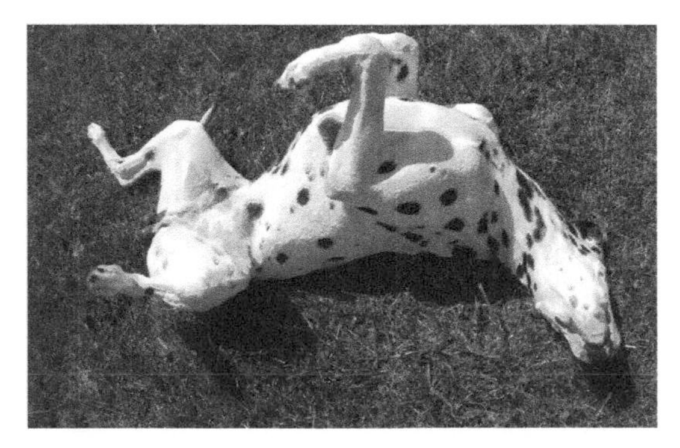

Figure 2.9 The Dalmatian has found an interesting scent to roll in.

Canine social structure

Domestication and canine behavior

Domestic dogs as we know them are a product of human domestication of wild gray wolves (*Canis lupus*) 15 000 years ago (Sablin and Khlopachev 2002). Wolves who were most likely to possess the characteristics necessary to live and work with humans were selected for domestication. Those characteristics might include being good scavengers (cleaning up the area where humans lived to keep away pests), good protectors and sociability (warm companions). Domestication appears to have affected the likelihood of dogs to seek out other dogs for social interaction. Dogs can prefer petting from humans to food and may prefer the company of humans to other dogs (even those that they know well). Conversely, some dogs prefer to play with another dog over a human and to most dogs food is more important than touch.

Through domestication, traits present in wolf pups, but not present in adult wolves such as engagement in play, seeking physical contact, desire to be social and interact, barking, pawing, and nuzzling have been retained in adult dogs. This is called neoteny, and the resulting retention of juvenile characteristics by adult animals is called pedomorphosis. Some breeds are more highly neotenized than others.

While the DNA sequence in dogs and wolves is similar, it is not identical. The forces of domestication have affected the expression of the domestic dog's genes (i.e. epigenetics) to cause changes including: the size and shape of the head, frequency of heat cycles, social structure, visual and auditory communication, response of the hypothalamic–pituitary axis to stressors, levels of oxytocin and oxytocin signaling (Nagasawa et al. 2015; Wirobski et al. 2021), digestive enzymes (e.g. carbohydrate digestion) (Axelsson et al. 2013), frequency and context of vocalizations and behavior patterns (i.e. domestication syndrome). Dogs are not friendly wolves. Regarding them as such leads to assumptions and misinterpretations that are inaccurate and dangerous.

- Dogs are not friendly wolves. Regarding them as such leads to assumptions and misinterpretations that are inaccurate and dangerous.

Social organization of feral and/or free-ranging dogs

In contrast to wild wolves, free-ranging unowned dogs do not live in well-structured family groups or packs (van Kerkhove 2004). Instead, they live in small, loosely coherent groups of two to five unrelated dogs. Upon the loss of members of the group, the number regenerates through the addition of abandoned or escaped pets. The range occupied by a group of dogs is less than 0.1 sq. mile in urban areas where there are many food sources, but no high concentration of food anywhere. In these urban areas, dogs tend to be territorial, that is, they defend their territory against other dogs that might try to intrude. Dogs, unlike wolves, attempt to raise the puppies alone. As a result, pups born to stray dogs seldom survive to adulthood (one study showed 1 in 20 puppies born survived) and rarely account for growth or regeneration of a pack.

Predatory behavior is poorly developed in dogs compared to wolves and depends on the degree of neotenization of a breed. Dogs are predominantly scavengers, and when they hunt, they do not hunt in a cooperative way.

Scientific findings overwhelmingly show that the extrapolation of wolf social behavior to dogs, and especially to dogs and their relation to their human family, is inappropriate. What sense does it make, really, to claim that an infantile form (puppy) of a highly neotenized species (a species that "never grows up") tries to dominate all their social partners to rise to the top and lead the group? That is akin to saying that a toddler is inherently interested in leading the family. Like many dogs, toddlers are interested in acquiring the skills and resources necessary to be happy and safe (Table 2.3).

Table 2.3 Comparison of domestic dog and wolf behaviors.

Domestic dog	Wolf
Loosely structured packs generally contain between 2 and 5 unrelated members	Tightly structured packs generally contain between 2 and 20 related members
Females come into estrus twice a year. All intact females are bred	Females come into estrus once a year. Generally only high-ranking female is bred
Bitch rears puppies alone and experiences low survival rate	Pack cooperatively rears pups to ensure high survival rate
Exhibit pedomorphic behaviors throughout adult life	Pedomorphic behaviors absent in adult wolves
Generally scavengers	Highly developed predatory behavior
No real cooperative hunting	Hunt as a cohesive unit

The role of dominance in the social structure of the dog

Dominant describes the comparison of two individuals, not a character trait that is always displayed in every situation. Think of your own life. Maybe at work, you are the leader, your make decisions and advise the owners of the hospital where you work. How does your behavior, relationship or relative dominance change when you visit your parents as an adult child? Do you feel dominant? Do they follow all of your recommendations? If you are like most of us, you have a different relationship with your parents than you do with your partner and your boss. Your behavior changes depending on your comfort level, your willingness to engage in conflict due to a risk assessment and your relationship with the individual with whom you are interacting. This is also true of dogs. This is not to say that dogs are dominant in some situations and not in others. It is to say that dogs modify their behavior to avoid conflict and retain resources no matter where they are and with whom they are interacting. For example, when a dog is working with a dog training professional, he sits quietly when asked and calmly takes the food reward. When he is with his pet parent, he barks incessantly until the food reward is given. Why the difference? Is he dominant over the pet parent? The explanation is simpler than that. The dog training professional has reinforced calm behavior and has not reinforced barking. The pet parent has reinforced barking and as a result the dog barks. Simple learning theory. The dog doesn't have great plans to take over the household, he has learned how to gain the resources that he needs to be happy and healthy from each individual. These interactions can lead to a structure within the household as the dog learns the patterns of which behaviors to exhibit with which individuals in which situations.

Dominance hierarchies are evident throughout our society and animal societies. Depending on the species being studied, the most dominant animal may be the most aggressive or they may be the least likely to engage in aggressive encounters (Furuichi 1997; Premnath et al. 1996). Therefore, it is a misconception to always assume that the most dominant individual is the most aggressive individual in the group. In dogs, the most aggressive individual is most likely to be the most uncertain dog in the interaction (Silk et al. 2019). In addition, the concept that a dog is constantly driven to strive for a higher rank is unsubstantiated in the literature. The strongest evidence for aggression between dogs in the same household comes from two areas: FASC (discussed above) and resource holding potential (RHP). RHP can be understood as the traits possessed by an individual which affect ability to win a competitive contest over a limited resource (Allen and Krofel 2017). RHP may be a factor in aggression between dogs in the same household as some resources such as the attention from the pet parent are considered by the dogs as scarce or limited.

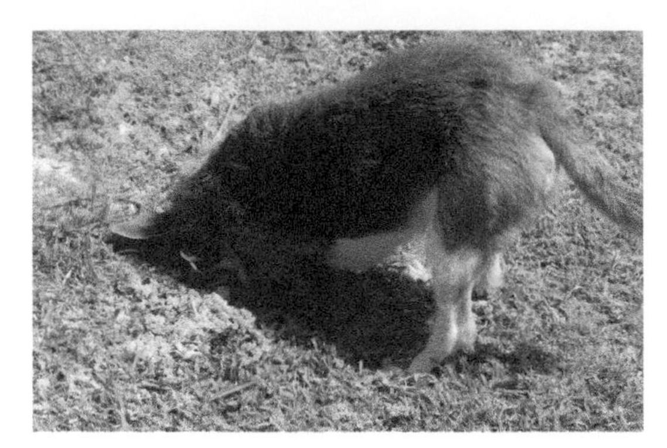

Figure 2.10 Digging is a common exploratory behavior of dogs.

- It is a misconception to always assume that the most dominant individual is the most aggressive individual in the group. In dogs, the most aggressive individual is most likely to be the most uncertain dog in the interaction (Silk et al. 2019).

Social organization of dogs living in a human household

The behavior of animals with others of their species is generally more straightforward than their interspecies behavior patterns as a result of shared communication strategies. Tensions between dogs in the household tend to coincide with lack of structure, presence of FASC, and miscommunication leading to a sense of threat and consequently aggression. It is beyond the scope of this chapter to fully explore inter-dog aggression, however it is clear that the factors for aggression between household dogs have little to do with dominance and more to do with fear, lack of structure and control over resources viewed as necessary for homeostasis and survival.

- Tensions between dogs in the household tend to coincide with lack of structure, presence of FASC, and miscommunication leading to a sense of threat and consequently aggression.

Exploratory behavior

Exploratory behavior is evident in the puppy with the beginning of locomotion. Through exploratory behavior, the dog learns details of its environment (e.g. what is food, escape pathways, location of nest, water). Exploration consumes a significant part of dogs' time and is of great importance to them. Dogs will work for the opportunity to investigate a novel stimulus: dogs have been trained to press a lever in a skinner box and as reinforcement a door would open with a different object behind it each time. This leads to the conclusion that dogs have an inherited motivation to satisfy curiosity or maintain a certain level of sensory input. Roaming may in part be rewarding for the same reason, in addition to providing the opportunity to scavenge, socialize, and maybe even reproduce (Figure 2.10).

Ingestive behavior

Since dogs have associated with human settlements, they have been selected to be good scavengers while they have become much less proficient at hunting. They still have the potential for predatory behavior and show many of the motor patterns associated with it, especially during play even when they are not hungry implying that this behavior serves a greater function than acquisition of food.

Free-roaming dogs normally eat one large meal every few days, although they may eat small animals, carrion, fecal material, and plants in-between if available. Dogs who are free fed will often eat many small meals throughout the day (Mugford 1977). Whether restricted or free feeding is recommended is dependent on the individual animal and environment. Free feeding can contribute to obesity as competition over food increases consumption. In addition, inter-dog aggression can evolve over resources. Conversely, free feeding may reduce possessive aggression by decreasing the value of the resource by making it plentiful. Alternatively, reducing access to food or use of a restrictive diet can cause aggression, decreased working ability and irritability. Care should be taken before changing the diet or feeding schedule of a dog so as not to induce behavior problems.

Dogs are not stress eaters. The refusal of food can be the first indication of FASC, which is why dogs don't eat as well in the veterinary hospital or boarding kennel. Competition over food often increases consumption. Palatability is largely based on smell. Dogs also generally prefer novel food.

- Care should be taken before changing the diet or feeding schedule of a dog so as not to induce behavior problems.

Eliminative behavior

Eliminative behavior includes defecation, urination, and pre- and post-eliminative behaviors (smelling, exploring for a location, circling before elimination, and scratching the ground after elimination). Bitches stimulate puppies to urinate and defecate by licking the perineal area and ingesting the excrement. Puppies begin to eliminate on their own at two to three weeks of age at which time bitches discontinue digesting the excrement. By three weeks of age, the pups begin to leave the nest and gradually start to defecate outside the nest. By approximately three months of age, males lean forward, at six months they occasionally lift their leg. Leg lifting progressively increases in males until two years of age. Castration before puberty may delay the onset of leg lifting, but most castrated males still develop leg lifting due to the priming of their brain with testosterone while *in utero*. The typical female urination posture is squatting. However, females can adopt a wide breadth of body postures when urinating including leg lifting. This should be considered normal behavior.

Stimuli that affect elimination

It is important to know what stimuli affect elimination in order to house train a dog. Elimination is most common after waking up from sleep, after eating and drinking, and after exercise. The smell of previous elimination also stimulates further urination or defecation. The amount of time since a dog eliminated last also affects the likelihood of elimination. While most dogs are able to refrain from eliminating all day, puppies, older dogs, and sick dogs often need to eliminate more frequently. A rule of thumb for puppies is that they can refrain from eliminating for as many hours as they are months old, plus one. Puppies confined for long periods and thus forced to urinate and defecate in their cage, and lie in it, may completely lose their ability to be house-trained. There may be a sensitive period when the puppy needs to be able to avoid its excrements in order to be trainable, but this has not been scientifically established; however, by eight to nine weeks of age, puppies are attracted by the odors of urine and feces to specific areas for elimination and begin to avoid soiling their den (sleeping quarters) (Ross 1950; Scott and Fuller 1965).

- Puppies confined for long periods and thus forced to urinate and defecate in their cage, and lie in it, may completely lose their ability to be house-trained.

Sexual behavior

Most males sexually mature from 9 to 12 months of age. While smaller breeds may mature sooner (6–9 months old), giant breeds generally mature later (12 months or older). Females are sexually mature (first estrus) at six to nine months, although larger breeds frequently experience first estrus at a later age. Precopulatory behavior is ritualized with great individual variation. It may include joint play-running, chasing, vocalizing, head-to-head nosing and sniffing of the female's body, particularly genitalia. The female may present to the male and solicit play. At first, the female avoids the male; then becomes more tolerant. She urinates frequently and examines the male. The bitch may mount the male, particularly if the male is inexperienced. The female becomes increasingly docile, "flagging" or moving her tail to the side. A female is ready to be bred when she adopts a mating stance and allows the male to mount her. At this point, she shows less soliciting behavior. Coital lock occurs after penetration. The male turns during the "tie" and the coital lock persists for 10–30 minutes. Separation occurs after muscular relaxation of the vagina and contraction of the bulbus glandis. Nonestrous bitches may mount estrous bitches or vice versa. Estrous bitches may mount males. Estrus may increase general activity, nervousness, and vocalization. Pregnancy lasts about 63 days.

Maternal behavior

Increased time licking nipples and genital area may be seen as parturition approaches. The bitch lactates (milk can be expressed) one to seven days prepartum. Her appetite may be noticeably decreased 24–48 hours before parturition. Restlessness of the bitch increases 12–24 hours before parturition and body temperature drops by 2–3 °F approximately 24 hours before birth (most reliable indicator of imminent parturition). Nest building is seen along with a potential for aggression toward strangers. Labor signs include respiration varying from panting to slow and deep respiration, decreased activity, and agitation, particularly when not given adequate privacy. During parturition the bitch licks her vulva and expels the puppy in the amnion. She then licks/chews through the amnion, and bites through the umbilical cord (brachiocephalic breeds are unable to do so). The puppies are licked to stimulate urination and defecation. Average time between births is 30 minutes but this is very variable. Long intervals may be associated with stillbirths. Disturbances, such as strange people, can cause delays from one to six hours. The delay can come during rest, active labor, or actual delivery with a pup in the vagina. Excitement produces adrenaline, which inhibits uterine activity.

Parent–offspring behavior

Care-giving behavior

Licking the puppy serves three functions: stimulates eating, urination, and defecation; guides the puppy to the nest by licking its head, rather than by carrying, which is seldom done by dogs; and it may also "label" the puppy with maternal pheromones.

Care-soliciting behavior

Postpartum grooming includes the bitch licking, tearing, and ingesting the placenta and severing the umbilical cord. The length of time for placental removal varies. The bitch removes fluid from the head and mouth of the puppy and cleans herself and the bedding. Dead pups are treated the same as live pups until they are cold, then pushed aside or eaten. Nursing is initiated by the mother from 0 to 14 days and initiated by puppies after that until weaned (around 5–6 weeks).

Puppy activity and vocalization

Newborn puppies move only a few inches at a time and are not usually moved by the dam. Head movements are from side to side and they are attracted by heat and repelled by cold (their nose is used as a temperature probe). The puppies move against the grain of the hair and against pressure when the mother licks them. Vocalization occurs one to four minutes after birth. Whines decrease when the pups are warm or nursing; grunts can signify pleasure. The dam is insensitive to whines during whelping; if out of sight, she will not retrieve the puppy. If the dam sits on a pup, she will ignore cries unless she feels or sees it.

Play behavior

Play is for learning, muscular development and coordination, as well as being inherently pleasurable. Play-fighting begins around five to six weeks of age. Play is a major mechanism by which social relationships are established and maintained. Play signals include the play bow, exaggerated approach, repeated barking, approach and withdrawal, pouncing, and leaping. Social play is more common than solitary play in dogs with the exception of those not socialized with other dogs before 20 weeks. Behavior sequences are mixed up (predatory, mating, etc.). Role reversal occurs in play, with an adult often participating in play with a younger, weaker conspecific.

- Social play is more common than solitary play in dogs with the exception of those not socialized with other dogs before 20 weeks.

Canine behavioral development

Experiences during development have long-lasting effects on temperament and adult behavior. It is therefore important to appreciate normal and

Table 2.4 Developmental periods and life stages of dogs.

Period	Duration
Prenatal	Up to birth
Neonatal	0–10 to 14 days
Transitional	11–21 days
Socialization	3–4 wk to 12–14 wk
Juvenile	~3–4 mo to sexual maturity (~5–14 mo)
Adolescence	Sexual maturity to social maturity (~2–3 yr)
Adult	Social maturity to 7–10 yr
Senior	7–10 yr to geriatric
Geriatric	Life expectancy for breed to death

abnormal development in order to prevent, understand, and resolve behavior issues. There are eight postnatal developmental and life stages in dogs: neonatal (birth to 10–14 days); transitional (11–21 days); socialization (3–4 weeks until approximately 12–14 weeks); juvenile (3–4 months to sexual maturity); adolescence (sexual maturity to 2–3 years); adult (from social maturity to 7–10 years); senior (7–10 years to geriatric); geriatric (life expectancy to death) (Table 2.4). Much has been said about the importance of the sensitive period for socialization; however, the juvenile period, sexual maturity, and social maturity are times of development and sweeping changes in the dog's psyche. Training and positive exposure to environments and stimuli should continue throughout the dog's life especially during the first 36 months.

- Much has been said about the importance of the sensitive period for socialization; however, the juvenile period, sexual maturity, and social maturity are times of development and sweeping changes in the dog's psyche. Training and positive exposure to environments and stimuli should continue throughout the dog's life especially during the first 36 months.

Complexity of early environment

An animal's central nervous system develops its genetically predetermined functions only if exposed to appropriate environmental stimulation, especially early in life. A restricted environment early in life will result in an animal with abnormal sensory perception. The animal may not be able to perceive stimuli to which it was not exposed during development. An animal reared in a restrictive environment will also be emotionally unstable. In addition to emotionality, the complexity of the early environment also greatly influences learning ability. A restricted early environment may result in reduced learning ability and trainability. It is therefore important to provide an interesting and stimulating early environment. In addition, it is also important that the early environment be predictable and consistent. If not, the animal will not only be frustrated and under stress, but it will also learn that its behavior has no impact on what is happening around it. Such animals are exceedingly difficult to train later.

- A restricted environment early in life will result in an animal with abnormal sensory perception.

Effect of neonatal stress

Some degree of stress (e.g. handling, cold temperature, very brief separation) in the neonatal period may accelerate hair growth, weight gain, and maturation of the nervous system; reduce emotionality later in life, increase problem-solving ability and social confidence; decrease reactivity and emotionality and promote resistance to some diseases (Serpell and Jagoe 2016). Handling sessions from the first days of a puppy's life are therefore recommended. They will not only expose the puppy to a mild stress, but also facilitate socialization when the puppy gets older. In addition to handling sessions, puppies may be removed from the nest (best while someone else walks the mother) and placed singly on a cool vinyl floor for a brief time (30 seconds) before being put back into the warm nest. Flashing light, noises, and motion have also been used as mild stress.

When is the best time to adopt a puppy?

For those who adopt from shelters or rescues, the option to adopt earlier or later is a moot point. Shelters are inherently stressful places so movement of puppies out of the shelter via adoption or foster immediately is imperative. However, for those who adopt from a breeder, there may be an option to take the puppy home earlier or later than the traditional age of eight weeks. In one study, puppies taken from the litter earlier (at six weeks) had more health and developmental problems and showed increased stress at separation from the dam. They did not socialize any better to humans than puppies taken away from the mother at a later date and provided human contact on a daily basis while with the dam. Conversely, if the environment is very stressful, the puppy will fare better if removed. If the breeder is able to adequately socialize the puppy, it may be better to adopt the puppy around 10–14 weeks so that he can have more time to interact with his peers. This would also avoid adoption during a fear period (see below). As is the case for much of life, there is no blanket right or wrong answer, only the right or wrong answer for that individual puppy.

Sensitive periods of development and life stages

It is well documented that there are "sensitive periods" in the behavioral development of a dog. These are periods of development during which certain experiences need to be made to achieve normal development. Lack of these experiences during the sensitive periods has lifelong irreversible effects. For instance, between 4 and 12 weeks of age, a puppy learns how a social partner looks. During this time, the brain develops a sort of filter system in the visual cortex, which becomes sensitized to the shapes of the social partners of the puppy. In the dog, they include humans and other pets. This filter system ensures that certain neurons in the visual brain are only activated when the puppy sees a social partner. After 12 weeks, this system can hardly be further modified so that the puppy will not learn (or learn only with difficulty) to accept previously unknown species as social partners.

- Lack of these experiences during the sensitive periods has lifelong irreversible effects.

The recognition of sensitive periods in canine behavioral development may be one of the most important discoveries about dogs. By controlling the puppy's environment during its early life, we can influence the emotionality, temperament, sociability, confidence, and learning ability of the dog. Early and appropriate intervention can result in the dog being more adaptable, easier to train, and physically and emotionally healthier. The exact time course of development varies between authors (and probably between dogs to some degree!) as the sensitive periods do not start abruptly but rather phase in and out gradually. Although there are some variations in the literature, for this book the development of dogs has been divided into the periods and life stages shown in Table 2.4.

- By controlling the puppy's environment during its early life, we can influence the emotionality, temperament, sociability, confidence, and learning ability of the dog.

Prenatal

The prenatal period includes development of the fetus up to parturition. Human parents-to-be are often told that the pregnant mother should keep her stress level low. This recommendation is not only true for humans but for all mammals. If the dam is under psychologic or physiologic stress, the puppies are more reactive (emotional), abnormal socially, fearful and unable to cope with stress (Braastad 1998; Clarke and Schneider 1993; Lehmann et al. 2000; Tuber et al. 1999). These changes are most likely due to changes in the development of the hypothalamic–pituitary-axis (HPA). Many puppies adopted from shelters and rescues as well as puppies that are purchased from pet stores were born to dams under physiologic or psychologic stress (McMillian et al. 2013). While it makes common sense that a stressed dam grows a stressed puppy, pet parents may not know this information. In puppy appointments, education of pet parents as to the potential etiologies of their puppy's behavior and any predisposing factors to the development of behavior problems in the future is essential.

- If the dam is under psychologic or physiologic stress, the puppies are more reactive (emotional), abnormal socially, fearful and unable to cope with stress (Braastad 1998; Clarke and Schneider 1993; Lehmann et al. 2000; Tuber et al. 1999).

During the prenatal period, the male brain undergoes a process that determines gender differences in behavior. Shortly before parturition, the male fetus produces a burst of testosterone which masculinizes and defeminizes the brain.

This results in the organization of typical male behavior such as roaming, urine marking, intermale aggression, and male sexual behavior. The priming of the fetal male brain is irreversible and affects all behavior that is gender-dimorphic even in a gonadectomized dog.

Neonatal

The neonatal period extends approximately during the first 10–14 days of the puppy's life (Figure 2.11). During the neonatal period, puppies spend the majority of the day nursing, sleeping, and interacting with the dam; however, that should not lead to the assumption that during this stage the puppy doesn't have the capacity to learn or that interactions during this stage are not important. A puppy is born both blind and deaf but is capable of whining to attract attention from its mother. It is born with the senses of balance, taste, smell, touch, and temperature. Until three weeks of age, the puppy is not able to urinate and defecate spontaneously and is dependent on stimulation (licking) by the mother to fulfill these functions. Its nervous system is poorly developed; for the first three days it has "flexor dominance," that is, it curls up when picked up by the neck, and from day 4 to day 21, it has "extensor dominance," that is, it stretches when picked up. Although puppies are dependent on the mother for thermoregulation, they are born with sensitivity to temperature and will root against a warm object. Newborn puppies will also move against the grain of the hair of their mother so they will get closer to the teat, and also turn or move toward the side they are touched.

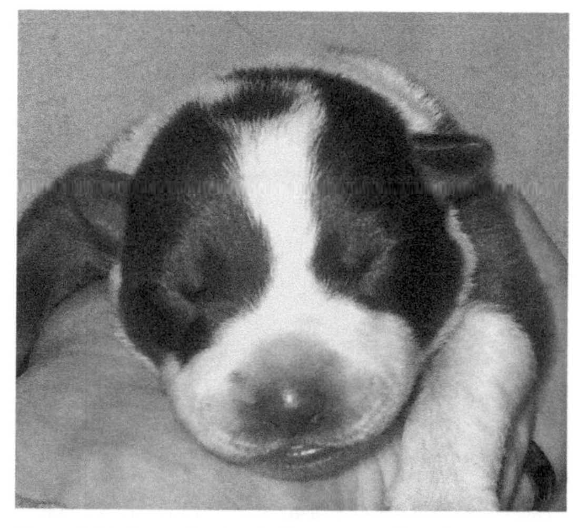

Figure 2.11 Rye, a Border Collie puppy, at four days of age.

From about two to three days of age, a puppy is able to crawl moving its head from side to side, using its nose as a touch and temperature probe. Again, all of the puppy's behaviors are designed to get it back into the heap of littermates and to the teat. Already during this early stage, human contact and handling are important as environmental enrichment and for inducing a mild stress, as mentioned above. Puppies may vocalize when hurt, when cold, or uncomfortable, or when they lose contact with their littermates or the mother. However, most bitches will not react to these vocalizations. Learning with positive reinforcement is already possible, although the puppies' responses are very limited. Conditioned aversion has also been achieved in very young puppies.

Transitional

The transitional period follows the neonatal period and reaches to about three weeks of age. It is characterized by fast maturation. Puppies are born in a very early stage of development. Such animals are called altricial. In the transitional period, a puppy catches up with those animals that are born in a much more developed state, such as foals or calves that are examples of "precocial" animals. The puppy begins to develop its senses, gains control over thermoregulation, and at the end of the transitional period, becomes able to eliminate spontaneously (and the mother stops eating its stool). From this point on, the puppies should have the possibility to leave the nest site to eliminate. Puppies that are thwarted from doing so may become almost impossible to house train. The puppy's nervous system is developing at a rapid pace. However, it does so only in reaction to a stimulating environment. During the transitional period, the puppy begins to develop its senses of vision and of hearing (Figure 2.12). The eyes begin to open around 12–14 days, but vision is poor. Later during this period, around 20–21 days, the ears open. The development of vision and hearing makes the puppy more responsive to environmental stimuli. Since the puppy is also able to habituate to stimuli, and still profits from environmental complexity for normal neurological development, the provision of sensory, visual, and auditory stimuli is very important. This can be done through handling, placing the puppy for short periods in a play pen with toys, platforms, tunnels, and so on (under supervision!),

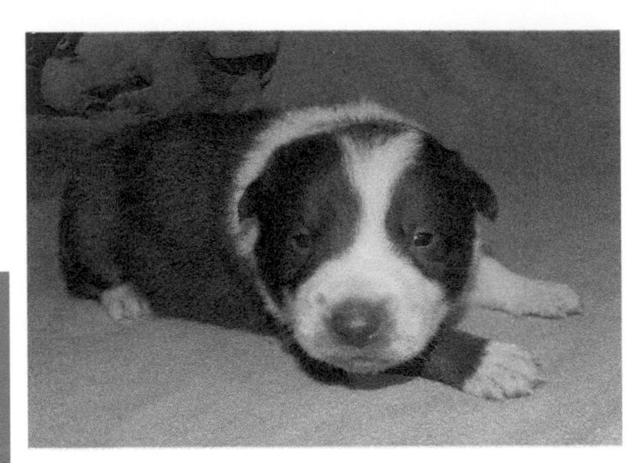

Figure 2.12 Rye, a Border Collie puppy, at two weeks of age.

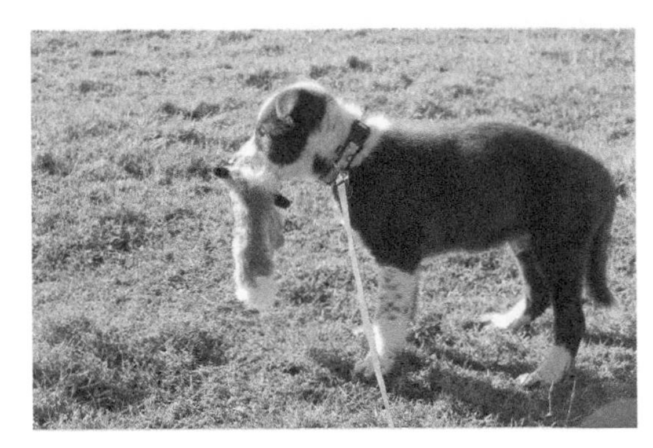

Figure 2.13 Rye, a Border Collie puppy, at nine weeks of age.

and playing recordings (commercially available) of various noises. Puppies might begin to walk unsteadily as early as day 12. Puppies will also begin to play-fight, and are better able to learn, especially with positive reinforcement. At around three weeks of age, the mother and father may start to regurgitate food for the puppies. Probably as an effect of domestication, not all dogs will do that. The puppies will solicit food regurgitation by pushing their noses into the corners of the parents' mouths, a behavior that later develops into an appeasement behavior. At three weeks of age, it is appropriate to begin feeding solid food to puppies.

Socialization

The socialization period extends from about 3 weeks to 12–14 weeks although more study is necessary to determine if this period is shorter or longer in individual dogs and specific breeds (Figure 2.13). This period is one of tremendous physical and psychological change. During this time, dogs gain the ability to stand, sit (day 28), eat solid food, eliminate outside of the den (eight to nine weeks) (Houpt 2011), form social attachments (attachments to individuals and species), form site attachments (attachment to a location), learn normal play postures, use body language signals to communicate and avoid conflict, and offer affiliative behaviors. Teeth erupt during this period and puppies are consequently weaned at about four to six weeks.

In addition, the socialization period is marked by a willingness to approach novel objects or people, explore new environments and chase moving objects. Over this time the mother withdraws from social interactions as the puppy interacts more with his peers. Puppies develop their social personality during this period, sleeping in groups at about four weeks and showing more independence by sleeping alone at six weeks. They can learn as well as adults via operant and classical conditioning during this period (four to five weeks) and their brain waves are similar to adult brain wave patterns by eight weeks (Fox 1968). It goes without saying that all training should be positive reinforcement, science-based training.

But all is not positive during this period. By 8 weeks of age, puppies show fear postures, by 12 weeks sociability decreases with fear signals being more prominent in the unsocialized puppy and by 20 weeks socialization isn't possible. The magnitude of this period is matched only with the urgency of the puppy's needs. Puppies that present with behavior problems related to FASC must be treated immediately as time is of the essence.

Much has been written about this period in a puppy's development and with good reason. The development of behavior during this time is turbo-charged with small experiences whether positive or negative causing huge, long-term changes in behavior which last well into adulthood. Socialization is the positive exposure to stimuli that will be a part of the puppy's environment in the future in small increments without causing anything greater than mild stress. When socialization is done correctly, the result is a well-adjusted, behaviorally appropriate puppy. When it is done incorrectly or not at all, the result can be disastrous. Puppies who are not well or properly socialized are more fearful, aggressive and reactive (Vaterlaws-Whiteside and Hartmann 2017). They avoid social play and cannot form social bonds.

- The development of behavior during this time is turbo-charged with small experiences whether positive or negative causing huge, long-term changes in behavior which last well into adulthood.

Puppy classes can be a great way to start the socialization process (Figures 2.14–2.16). They result in increased retention in the home, decreased behavior problems and increased obedience (Duxbury et al. 2003). Puppies should be enrolled in puppy class after their first vaccination and deworming provided that they are healthy. Not all puppy classes are created equal. Ideal puppy classes would be indoors so that the facility can be cleaned properly and have designated elimination areas which are picked up regularly. Puppy class curriculums should include socialization, impulse control, education and play. There may also be training in puppy classes, however a puppy class isn't an obedience class. Puppies are able to obtain new behaviors easily although they may have a short attention span.

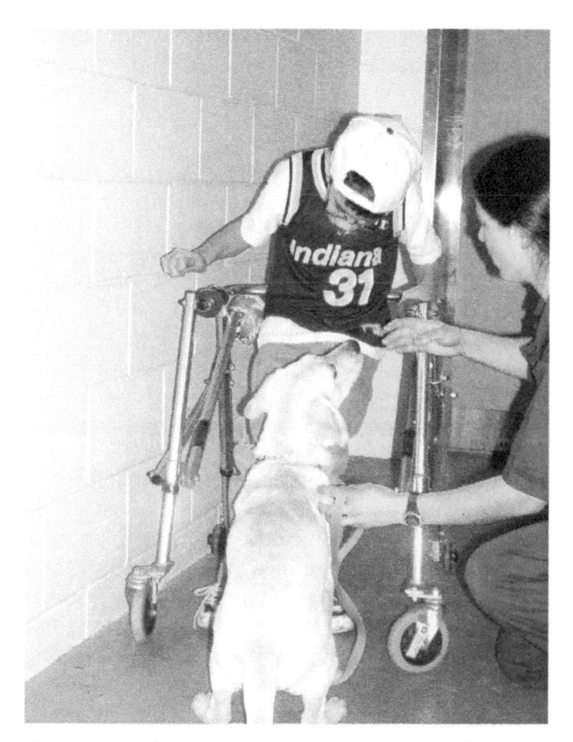

Figure 2.14 Physically challenged child socializing with puppies in a puppy class.

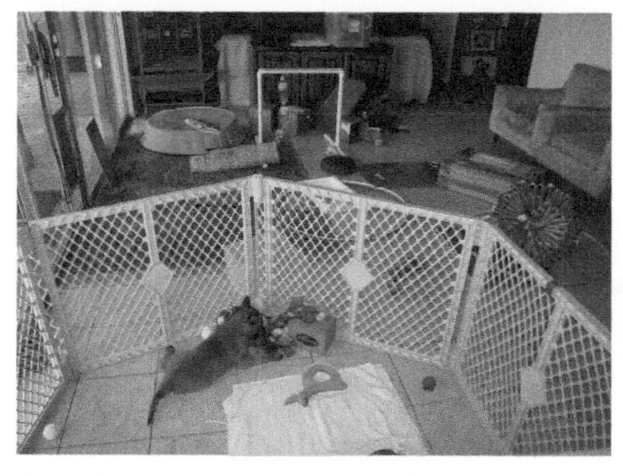

Figure 2.15 The environment is enriched with an entire "puppy park" of novelties for this youngster to explore with human supervision.

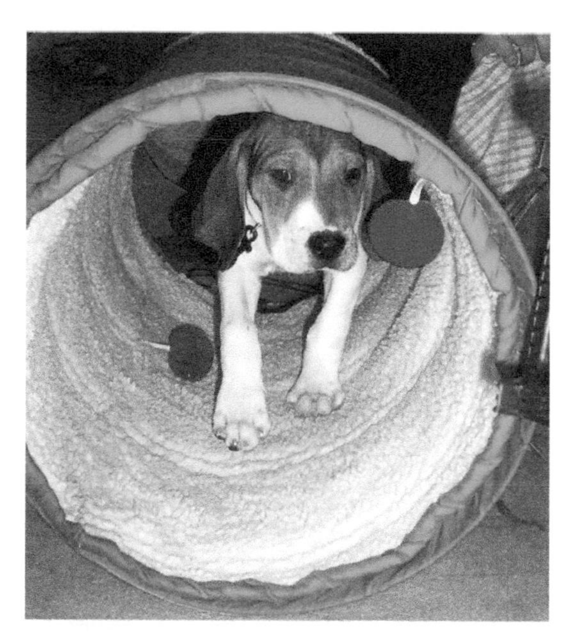

Figure 2.16 A puppy exploring a tunnel at puppy class.

Veterinarians and pet parents alike may be concerned about infectious disease spread in puppies that attend puppy classes. In a study comparing puppies who received one vaccination for Canine Parvovirus (CPV) that attended class and those that did not, there was no difference in the incidence of CPV between the two groups (Stepita et al. 2013). See Chapter 7 for more information on puppy classes.

Socialization can be successful without puppy classes. Matter of fact, puppy classes while helpful and recommended should be regarded as a supplement to socialization, not the only form of socialization. Resources exist (see recommended reading) to assist with socialization. Socialization can be divided up into places, living things and non-living things. Pet parents should make a comprehensive list or utilize one provided online or in a puppy training book of every stimulus in those three categories that their puppy might encounter over the course of their lives. Then, the work of slow, positive exposure can happen. This type of exposure can and should occur in the case of sick puppies that are well enough to be outside of the house but cannot necessarily go to puppy class. For example, a puppy who has intestinal parasites and is being treated but cannot yet go to puppy class can at a minimum walk in the neighborhood, be exposed to the vacuum cleaner, cars in the neighborhood, rides in the car, images of animals on television, sounds of thunderstorms and fireworks, sight of people, dogs and children from a distance and traffic sounds. Even that list isn't exhaustive. Time is of the essence when it comes to socialization to avoid serious behavior problems.

Socialization sounds like a magic pill doesn't it? A cure all for behavior problems. Unfortunately, that isn't the case. Life experience, general wellness, and genetics shape behavior throughout the dog's life. Socialization generally doesn't cure fear in a puppy who is fearful or reactive genetically or due to prenatal stress. It will help. It is a start. For those puppies with behavioral pathology, socialization must be carefully completed so that the puppy is not overwhelmed. For example, puppies that are showing aggression to other dogs who are brought around unfamiliar dogs are more likely to show aggression to unfamiliar dogs as adults. This may be because those interactions are not monitored closely by the pet parent. As a result, negative interactions occurring during that time cause negative changes in behavior later on.

- Life experience, general wellness, and genetics shape behavior throughout the dog's life.

Within the socialization period lies the first fear period. It is generally regarded as occurring between 8 and 10 weeks of age, but the ages of onset and end seem to vary considerably between breeds and individuals. In one study, Cavalier King Charles Spaniels had a later onset of fear when compared to German Shepherd Dogs and Yorkshire Terriers in the same age group (Morrow et al. 2015). In that same study, Cavaliers were more likely to show fear and German Shepherds were least likely.

The fear period is characterized by increased fearfulness, and likely permanent retention of the fear. Any aversive experience during that time, including shipping a puppy, is to be avoided as it may have lifelong effects on emotionality, anxiety, fear, hyperactivity and reactivity, and aggressiveness. If five-week-old puppies are punished, that is, with an electric shock for approaching a person, they will show fear, but approach that person again when retested later. If the puppies are between eight and nine weeks of age, they retain the fear of that person. Puppies older than 12 weeks are less influenced by a mild shock and may approach the person in spite of the shock, or at least can overcome their fear. Because of the increased fearfulness and the enhanced learning from bad experiences during the fear period, extra caution should be used to safeguard puppies from possibly lifelong effects of a negative experience during this time. Some dogs that are genetically predisposed to fearfulness may start to show fear during the fear period and remain fearful even in the absence of any trauma.

- The fear period is characterized by increased fearfulness, and likely permanent retention of the fear. Any aversive experience during that time, including shipping a puppy, is to be avoided as it may have lifelong effects on emotionality, anxiety, fear, hyperactivity and reactivity, and aggressiveness.

Juvenile

The juvenile period starts at approximately three to four months and extends to sexual maturity (~5–14 months). It is characterized by rapid physical growth and increasing activity, excitability, and independence. This is a difficult stage to go through (for the pet parent), in particular if the puppy has yet to receive any training. Pet parents of young puppies often do not see the need to take their dog to puppy class or to start training at all. Their puppy may appear to be well behaved, following them everywhere voluntarily and with no training at all!

Once the puppy reaches about four months of age, they are often greatly disappointed. Their once so voluntarily compliant puppy suddenly does not seem to care much about them anymore, and it becomes a chore to keep it under control. This is a reason why many dogs are relinquished around five to six months of age.

During the juvenile period, dogs may go through one or several more fear periods, lasting around two to three weeks each, during which the dog is much more easily frightened and adverse experiences can be more difficult for the dog to overcome. During these fear periods, dogs may suddenly show fear of familiar objects or situations. For example, a dog that encountered garbage cans twice a week on his daily walk, may suddenly be frightened by their sight, and not dare to go near, become piloerect, and bark. Because we can't easily discern a puppy's genetic makeup and how any given situation will cause expression of those genes, every encounter in which the puppy expresses FASC should be taken seriously. Counterconditioning, response substitution, and in severe cases, systematic desensitization can be used to help the animal to get through this. Aversive training techniques, punishment, and other traumatic experiences could have a long-lasting effect on fearfulness, aggressiveness, and emotionality and should be avoided.

Adolescence

The adolescence period starts with puberty and ends with attainment of social maturity which is somewhere around two to three years of age. Different breeds and individuals within those breeds may come into social maturity at different times. Dogs become increasingly more independent at this stage and cute puppy behaviors might be less tolerated by pet parents of the adolescent dog. Prevention and management of behaviors that are not under the pet parent's control will keep the dog from learning unwanted behaviors. Physical and mental exercise for the dog is essential to making this stage more enjoyable. Training problems and behavior disorders are likely to become more pronounced during this stage of development. For example, dogs might start barking at strangers entering the home or become territorial during adolescence.

Adult

The adult life stage starts at the end of social maturity, which is typically around two to three years of age but may be earlier or later depending on the breed or individual dog. Play behavior and social tolerances to other familiar and unfamiliar dogs can change as a dog reaches adulthood. The adolescent dog that thrived at the dog park or doggy daycare, as an adult might become less accepting of and less interested in playing with unfamiliar dogs. Play with known dogs with which they have an established relationship is often more enjoyable. Changes in the dynamics and relationships within a multidog household might change as a dog reaches adulthood. In the author's experience many of these changes are due to pain, systemic disease or discomfort. As with all behavior disorders, when a dog presents with a behavior change, systemic disease should be considered.

- The adolescent dog that thrived at the dog park or doggy daycare, as an adult might become less accepting of and less interested in playing with unfamiliar dogs.

Senior

Dogs become senior at 7+ years of age. Small-breed dogs live longer and become senior at a later age (10–12 years), than large-breed dogs. Some consider the senior life stage to be the last 25% of the dog's expected lifespan based on the breed. As dogs age, their activity level will decrease. This might be associated with degenerative processes such as arthritis, reduced hearing, normal clouding of the cornea and/or reduced visual acuity, and muscle atrophy. Senior dogs should be screened at least annually by a veterinarian for systemic disease as well as behavioral changes associated with aging. Some senior dogs will develop cognitive dysfunction syndrome, similar to Alzheimer's disease or dementia in humans. Early medical and behavioral treatment can greatly benefit the welfare of these dogs. Mental stimulation is important for physical and behavioral wellness of all senior dogs.

- Senior dogs should be screened at least annually by a veterinarian for systemic disease as well as behavioral changes associated with aging.

Geriatric

The geriatric life stage is considered to last from life expectancy for the breed until death. This stage is not always recognized in the literature and is often included in the senior life stage. The same considerations for physical and behavioral care of senior patients should be applied to geriatric patients. Enrichment and activities appropriate for the individual should be maintained.

Conclusion

By having a clear understanding of normal development and behavior in dogs, the veterinary technician will become astute at recognizing abnormal behavior. Through early prevention training and intervention before the development of serious behavior disorders, often the veterinary nurse can assist in maintaining and enhancing the human – dog bond and prevent relinquishment of the dog.

References

Allen, A.L. and Krofel, M. (2017). Resource holding potential. In: *Encyclopedia of Animal Cognition and Behavior* (ed. J. Vonk and T.K. Shackelford). # Springer International Publishing AG https://doi.org/10.1007/978-3-319-47829-6_444-1.

Axelsson, E. et al. (2013). The genomic signature of dog domestication reveals adaptation to a starch-rich diet. *Nature* 495 (7441): 360–364.

Bekoff, M. (2001). Observations of scent-marking and discriminating self from others by a domestic dog (*Canis familiaris*): tales of displaced yellow snow. *Behavioural Processes* 55: 75–79.

Braastad, B.O. (1998). Effects of prenatal stress on behavior of offspring of laboratory and farmed mammals. *Applied Animal Behaviour Science* 61: 159–180.

Bradshaw, J.W.S. and Nott, H.M.R. (1995). Social and communication behavior of companion dogs. In: *The Domestic Dog: Its Evolution, Behavior and Interactions with People* (ed. J. Serpell), 117. Cambridge: Cambridge University Press.

Bradshaw, J.W. and Rooney, N. (2016). Dog social behavior and communication. In: *The Domestic Dog* (ed. J. Serpell), 133–159. Cambridge, UK: Cambridge University Press. ISBN: 978-0521425377.

Clarke, A.S. and Schneider, M.L. (1993). Prenatal stress has long-term effects on behavioral responses to stress in juvenile rhesus monkeys. *Developmental Psychobiology* 26: 293–304.

Cohen, J.A. and Fox, M.A. (1976). Vocalizations in wild canids and possible effects of domestication. *Behavioural Processes* 1 (1): 77–92.

Duxbury, M.M., Jackson, J.A., Line, S.W. et al. (2003). Evaluation of association between retention in the home and attendance at puppy socialization classes. *Journal of the American Veterinary Medical Association* 223: 61–66.

Fox, M.W. (1968). Socialization, environmental factors, and abnormal behavioral development in animals. In: *Abnormal Behavior in Animals* (ed. M.W. Fox). Philadelphia: WB Saunders.

Fox, M.W. (1984). *Behaviour of Wolves, Dogs, and Related Canids*. Malabar, FL: Krieger Publishing Co.

Fox, M.W. and Stelzner, D. (1966). Behavioural effects of differential early experience in the dog. *Animal Behavior* 14: 273–281.

Furuichi, T. (1997). Agonistic interactions and matrifocal dominance rank of wild bonobos (*Pan paniscus*) at Wamba. *International Journal of Primatology* 18: 855–875. https://doi.org/10.1023/A:1026327627943.

Gazit, I. and Terkel, J. (2003). Domination of olfaction over vision in explosives detection by dogs. *Applied Animal Behaviour Science* 82: 65–73.

Handelman, B. (2012). *Canine Behavior: A Photo Illustrated Handbook*. Wenatchee, WA, USA: Dogwise Publishing. ISBN 0976511827.

Hecht, J. and Horowitz, A. (2015). Introduction to dog behaviour. In: *Animal Behaviour for Shelter Veterinarians and Staff*, 1e (ed. E. Weiss, H. Mohan-Gibbons and S. Zawistowski), 5–30. London, UK: Wiley-Blackwell. ISBN 978-1118711118.

Houpt, K.A. (2011). *Domestic Animal Behavior for Veterinarians and Animal Scientists*. Ames, IA: Iowa State University Press.

Houpt, K.A., Hintz, H.F., and Shepherd, P. (1978). The role of olfaction in canine food preferences. *Chemical Senses* 3: 281–290.

Jacobs, G., Deegan, J., Crognale, M., & Fenwick, J. (1993). Photopigments of dogs and foxes and their implications for canid vision. *Visual Neuroscience*, 10(1), 173–180. doi:10.1017/S0952523800003291.

Kemp, C.M. and Jacobson, S.G. (1992). Rhodopsin levels in the central retinas of normal miniature poodles and those with progressive rod-cone degeneration. *Experimental Eye Research* 54: 947–956.

van Kerkhove, W. (2004). A fresh look at the wolf-pack theory of companion-animal behavior. *Journal of Applied Animal Welfare Science* 7 (4): 279–285.

Kumazawa, T. and Kurihara, K. (1990). Large synergism between monosodium glutamate and 5′-nucleotides in canine taste nerve responses. *American Journal of Physiology. Regulatory, Integrative and Comparative Physiology* 259 (3): R420–R426.

Kurihara, K. and Kashiwayanagi, M. (2000). Physiological studies on umami taste. *The Journal of Nutrition* 130 (4): 931S–934S.

Lehmann, J., Stöhr, T., and Feldon, J. (2000). Long-term effects of prenatal stress experience and postnatal maternal separation on emotionality and attentional processes. *Behavioural Brain Research* 107: 133–144.

Lindemann, B. (1996). Taste reception. *Physiological Reviews* 76 (3): 719–766.

McGreevy, P., Grassi, T.D., and Harman, A.M. (2004). A strong correlation exists between the distribution of retinal ganglion cells and nose length in the dog. *Brain, Behavior and Evolution* 63: 13–22.

McMillan, F.D., Serpell, J.A., Duffy, D.L., Masaoud, E., Dohoo, I.R. Differences in behavioral characteristics between dogs obtained as puppies from pet stores and those obtained from noncommercial breeders. *J Am Vet Med Assoc.* 2013 May 15;242(10):1359–63. doi: 10.2460/javma.242.10.1359. PMID: 23634679.

Miller, P.E. and Murphy, C.J. (1995). Vision in dogs. *Journal of the American Veterinary Medical Association* 207: 1623–1634.

Morrow, M., Ottobre, J., Ottobre, A., Neville, P., St-Pierre, N., Dreschel, N., Pate, J., Breed-Dependent Differences in the Onset of Fear-Related Avoidance Behavior in Puppies, *Journal of Veterinary Behavior* (2015), doi: 10.1016/j.jveb.2015.03.002.

Moulton, D.G. (1977). Minimum odorant concentrations detectable by the dog and their implications for olfactory receptor sensitivity. In: *Chemical Signals in Vertebrates* (ed. D. Muller-Schwarz and M.M. Mozell), 455–464. New York: Plenum Press.

Mugford, R.A. (1977). External influences on the feeding of carnivores. In: *The Chemical Senses and Nutrition* (ed. M.R. Kare and O. Maller), 25–50. New Your, NY: Academic press.

Nagasawa, M. et al. (2015). Social evolution. Oxytocin-gaze positive loop and the coevolution of human–dog bonds. *Science* 348 (6232): 333–336.

Neitz, J., Geist, T., and Jacobs, G. (1989). Color vision in the dog. *Visual Neuroscience* 3: 119–125.

Parkes, J.H., Aguirre, G., Rockey, J.H., Liebman, P.A. Progressive rod-cone degeneration in the dog: characterization of the visual pigment. *Invest Ophthalmol Vis Sci.* 1982 Nov;23(5):674–8. PMID: 7129812.

Parry, H.B. (1953). Degeneration of the dog retina, I: structure and development of the retina of the normal dog. *British Journal of Ophthalmology* 37: 385–404.

Polgar, Z., Miklosi, A., and Gacsi, M. (2015). Strategies used by pet dogs for solving olfaction-based problems at various distances. *PLoS One* 10 (7): e0131610. https://doi.org/10.1371/journal.pone.0131610.

Premnath, S., Sinha, A., and Gadagkar, R. (1996). Dominance relationship in the establishment of reproductive division of labour in a primitively eusocial wasp (Ropalidia marginata). *Behavioral Ecology and Sociobiology* 39: 125–132. https://doi.org/10.1007/s002650050274.

Pretterer, G., Bubna-Littitz, H., Windischbauer, G., Gabler, C., Griebel, U. Brightness discrimination in the dog. *J Vis.* 2004 Apr 6;4(3):241–9. doi: 10.1167/4.3.10. PMID: 15086313.

Quaranta, A., Siniscalchi, M., and Vallortigara, G. (2007). Asymmetric tail-wagging responses by dogs to different emotive stimuli. *Current Biology* 17: R199–R201.

Ross, S. (1950). Some observations on the lair dwelling behavior of dogs. *Behaviour* 2: 144–162.

Sablin, M.V. and Khlopachev, G.A. (2002). *The earliest Ice Age dogs: evidence from Eliseevichi. Current Anthropology* 43: 795–799.

Scott, J.P. and Fuller, J.L. (1965). *Genetics and the Social Behavior of the Dog.* Chicago and London: University of Chicago Press.

Serpell, J. and Jagoe, J.A. (2016). Early experience and the development of behavior. In: *The Domestic Dog* (ed. J. Serpell), 81. Cambridge, UK: Cambridge University Press. ISBN: 978-0521425377.

Silk, M.J., Cant, M.A., Cafazzo, S., Natoli, E., McDonald, R.A. Elevated aggression is associated with uncertainty in a network of dog dominance interactions. *Proc Biol Sci.* 2019 Jul 10;286(1906):20190536. doi: 10.1098/rspb.2019.0536. Epub 2019 Jul 3. PMID: 31266423; PMCID: PMC6650704.

Siniscalchi, M., Lusito, R., Vallortigara, G., and Quaranta, A. (2013). Seeing left-or right-asymmetric tail wagging produces different emotional responses in dogs. *Current Biology* 23: 2279–2282.

Siniscalchi, M., d'Ingeo, S., Minunno, M., and Quaranta, A. (2018). Communication in dogs. *Animals* 8 (131): https://doi.org/10.3390/ani8080131.

Stepita, M.E., Bain, M.J., and Kass, P.H. (2013). Frequency of CPV infection in vaccinated puppies that attended puppy socialization classes. *Journal of the American Animal Hospital Association* 49: 95–100.

Stokke, T. (2014). The effect of reward type and reward preference on the performance of detection dogs Master's thesis, Norwegian University of Life Sciences, Ås.

Tuber, D.S., Miller, D.D., Caris, K.A. et al. (1999). Dogs in animal shelters: problems, suggestions, and needed expertise. *Psychological Science* 10: 379–386.

Vaterlaws-Whiteside, H. and Hartmann, A. (2017). Improving puppy behavior using a new standardized socialization program. *Applied Animal Behavior Science* 197: 55–61.

Wirobski, G., Range, F., Schaebs, F. et al. (2021). Endocrine changes related to dog domestication: comparing urinary cortisol and oxytocin in hand-raised pack-living dogs and wolves. *Hormones and Behavior* 128: 104901.

Further reading

Martin, K. and Martin, D. (2011). *Puppy Start Right: Foundation Training for the Companion Dog, Karen Pryor Clicker Training*. Waltham, MA: Sunshine Books, Inc.

Peterson, M.E. and Kutzler, M.A. (ed.) (2011). *Small Animal Pediatrics*. St. Louis: Elsevier.

Rogers, M. and Anderson, E. (2021). *Puppy Socialization. What it Is and how to Do it*. Bright Friends Productions.

The PowerPoint of figures, appendices, MCQ's are available at www.wiley.com/go/martin/behavior

3 Feline behavior and development

Debbie Martin[1,2]
[1]*TEAM Education in Animal Behavior, LLC, Spicewood, TX, USA*
[2]*Veterinary Behavior Consultations, LLC, Spicewood, TX, USA*

CHAPTER MENU

Understanding how cats perceive the world and their social nature helps us to better understand their tendencies for specific behaviors. In order to be able to recognize abnormal behavior, one must first have knowledge of normal behavior for the species. As of 2022 over 45 million United State households have a pet cat (American Pet Products Association's 2021–2022 National Pet Owners Survey). Relinquishment of cats to animal shelters is also common. About a third of cats relinquished are surrendered due to behavior problems, including Inappropriate Elimination (IE), problems between other pets in the household, aggression toward humans, and destructive behavior (Salman et al. 2000).

The veterinary behavior technician needs to be fluent in understanding felines, including their

Canine and Feline Behavior for Veterinary Technicians and Nurses, Second Edition. Edited by Debbie Martin and Julie K. Shaw.

Companion website: www.wiley.com/go/martin/behavior

sensory capacities, communication, social behavior, and development. This knowledge will allow the technician to educate and assist cat owners.

- The veterinary behavior technician needs to be fluent in understanding felines, including their sensory capacities, communication, social behavior, and development.

Feline sensory capacities

Cats are born with tactile, olfactory, gustatory, and vestibular abilities. Hearing, vision, and thermoregulation develop during the first weeks to months after birth (Bradshaw 1992).

Vision

There is a wide range reported for the time period a kitten opens its eyes. It may occur anytime between 2 and 16 days (Villablanca and Olmstead 1979). The average is 7–10 days. Although determined primarily by genetics, female kittens generally open their eyes earlier than males. Vision is not completely developed and adult-like until around four to five weeks of age (Bradshaw 1992).

Cats are adept at noticing motion, which is advantageous when hunting field mice or preying on other small animals. As ambush predators who are active during the day and night, the vertical elongated pupil of the domestic cat gives it an advantage. The pupil can quickly constrict to a thin slit to protect the light sensitive retina. The elongated vertical pupil results in better visual acuity with things in vertical contours; thus, improving success in capturing prey. In contrast, horizontal elongated pupils, think sheep and goats, result in better visual acuity in the horizontal contours, improving predator detection along a wider horizontal plane (Banks et al. 2015) (Figure 3.1).

Compared to humans, cats have poor visual acuity, a slightly wider field of view, and a smaller area of binocular vision (Table 3.1). The visual acuity of the cat is about 20/100 to 20/200 with a field of view of 200° and binocular overlap of only 90° to 100° (Bradshaw 1992). In comparison, a normal

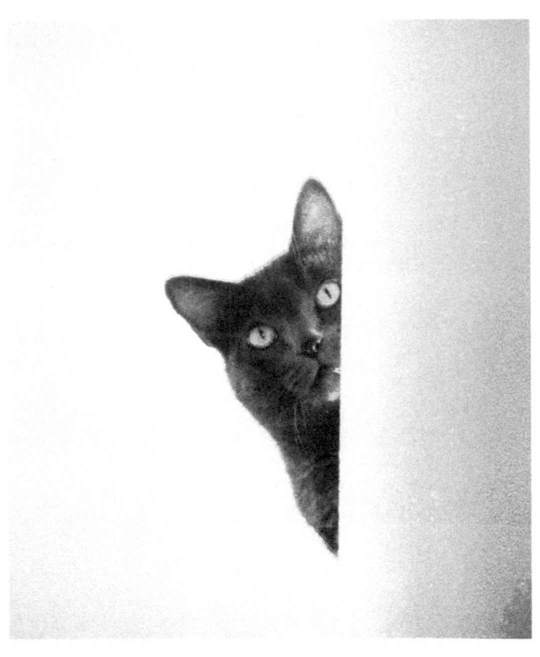

Figure 3.1 The cat is capable of quickly constricting the pupils into narrow slits to protect the retina. *Source*: Danielle G. Theule.

Table 3.1 Comparison of domestic cat and human vision.

Type of vision	Average domestic cat	Average human
Color vision	Dichromatic, red–green colorblind, likely able to see some UV	"Full" spectrum[a]
Field of view	200°	180°
Binocular vision	90° to 100° overlap	140° overlap
Visual acuity	Relatively poor (20/100–200); acuity is best along vertical planes due to vertical pupil	Standard 20/20 vision; round pupil
Dim light	Good vision	Poor vision

[a] Full spectrum refers to the typical colors humans can perceive. This does not include ultraviolet.

human sees 20/20, has a field of view of 180° with a binocular field of vision overlap of 140°. The field of view and binocular field of vision overlap is not as significantly different between cats and humans as it is between dogs (depending on breed morphology) and humans. Cats increased binocular vision results in better depth perception than dogs.

The cat's eyes are adapted for hunting in low light and have superior low-light vision. This is due to a combination of the large lens, pupil, and cornea, the tapetum lucidum, and a large number of rods. The tapetum lucidum, a layer of reflective cells behind the retina, reflects light back through the eye, allowing for a second chance of absorption by the rods and cones. Cats have about three times more rods (important for low-light vision) than humans and only about a sixth of the number of cones (used for color vision) (Berkley 1976). Because of the blurring caused by the tapetum lucidum and decreased resolution due to the increased number of rods, the cat's visual acuity is limited (Beaver 2003).

Cats have limited color vision, even more limited color vision than dogs. Most likely, cats have dichromatic vision with sensitivity to greenish-yellow and blue. The neutral point is nearly identical to humans with red–green color blindness, known as deuteranopia (Clark and Clark 2016). The domestic cat's eye is not specialized for color vision and the importance of color is likely minimal for the species.

- The domestic cat's eye is not specialized for color vision and the importance of color is likely minimal for the species.

Domestic cats are among several mammals thought to be able to process some ultraviolet light (Douglas and Jeffery 2014).

The physiological composition of the eyes of Siamese and Burmese cats shows a difference in the ganglion cells (compared to non-oriental breeds of cats) and also a lack of stereoscopic vision resulting in poor depth perception. However, they do have a normal field of vision and no difference in acuity compared to other breeds (Bradshaw 1992).

Hearing

At birth, kittens have the neurological ability to hear. However, the ear canals are blocked by skin folds. As the kitten develops and the pinnae extend, the ability to hear increases. By three to four weeks of age, the hearing ability is comparable to an adult cat.

Cats can perceive a wider range of frequencies than humans or dogs. The hearing range for cats is estimated to be 48 Hz to up to 85 000 Hz (Heffner and Heffner 1985) while the range for humans is 64 Hz up to 23 000 Hz. The functional or useful upper limit is likely around 60 000 Hz (Beaver 2003; Bradshaw 1992). Because cats have moveable pinnae and the ability to rotate the ears independent of each other up to 180° they are better able to locate the source of sounds. The shape of the pinna also amplifies the sound (Bradshaw 1992). This increased hearing range and mobility of the ears, allows cats to detect prey such as mice with outstanding accuracy.

Congenital deafness is often found in non-purebred white cats. Reviewing two studies from the 1970s, 64.9% to 85% of white cats with two blue eyes were found to be unilaterally or bilaterally deaf. Whereas approximately 40% of white cats with one blue eye and 16.7% to 22% of white cats with no blue eyes were found to have either unilateral or bilateral deafness (Mair 1973; Bergsma and Brown 1971).

- This increased hearing range and mobility of the ears, allows cats to detect prey such as mice with outstanding accuracy.

Olfaction

The sense of smell is present at birth. Compared to people, a cat's sensitivity to smells is much higher. A person's olfactory epithelium is approximately 2–4 cm² whereas a cat's is approximately 20 cm² (dog's range 20–200 cm²) (Bradshaw 1992).

Cats mainly rely on visual, auditory, and tactile senses for hunting. Unlike the dog, cats do not track prey utilizing olfaction. However, olfactory cues are an important means of social communication between cats.

- Olfactory cues are an important means of social communication between cats.

Vomeronasal organ

The vomeronasal organ (VNO) is located in the roof of the mouth behind the incisors and opens into the nasal cavity. When investigating a smell such as urine from another cat, the cat will open its mouth and show a "flehmen-like" response or gape; the upper lip is retracted, and the mouth is held open about a quarter inch for a few seconds. This allows the scent to travel through the VNO, which is neurologically connected to the limbic system (emotional center) of the brain. The gape response is performed on nonfood-based scents and generally only in response to odors of other cats; thus, it likely is used for social information gathering (Turner and Bateson 2000).

Social chemical messages are processed through the VNO to the accessory olfactory bulb, which is part of the limbic system. Pheromones are chemical compounds secreted or excreted by individuals of the same species (conspecifics). Pheromone detection can result in innate behaviors associated with safety, reproduction, aggression, and fear. There is evidence that some receptors can detect chemical compounds from other species.

Cats are more adept at distinguishing pheromones than humans or dogs. G protein-coupled receptors (GPCR) act as chemosensory receptors in olfactory sensory neurons. Mammalian noses have three different types of GPCR in the VNO. Vomeronasal receptors type 1, which will be referred to as V1R, are found in the apical VNO. They are distantly related to bitter taste receptors (Dulac and Axel 1995) and have a strong affinity for detecting chemical messages from urine and reproductive pheromones. Dogs have nine variants of the V1R; humans have two and cats have 30! An interesting fact, mice have approximately 180 V1R! It appears some V1R are also able to detect other species pheromones as well. Pheromones and chemical messages play an important role in the cat's environment. Perhaps the relationship of the V1R with bitter taste receptors heightens the cat's sensitivity to bitter tasting substances.

Taste

Cats have a limited sense of taste compared to humans. Humans have nine thousand or more taste buds, whereas cats only have about 480. Dogs have about 3.5 times more taste buds than cats. The taste buds of the cat are located on the outer edges of the tongue. A cat's perception of taste is certainly different than our own. However, a cat's enhanced olfactory abilities likely play a significant role in the cat's sense of taste. Cats will use smell first then taste to select food (Hullar et al. 2001). Cats smell their food before eating it.

Cats appear to lack functioning receptors for sweet stimuli (Li et al. 2006). They are obligate carnivores, so the need for sugary plant-based carbohydrates is not necessary from an evolutionary perspective. Some cats will be interested in sugary foods, but this may be due to the fat content or texture of the food (whipping cream seems to be a favorite for many cats!).

Cats seem to be particularly good at detecting bitter tastes. This may be enhanced through their complex olfactory system. Sensing bitter substances help cats to avoid potentially toxic substances and likely contributes to difficulty with administering oral medications. Regardless of how well we attempt to disguise medications, cats can detect, through smell and taste, the hidden medications. Taste aversion can quickly develop, and a cat will avoid anything that smells similar to the food used to disguise medication. This phenomenon (conditioned taste aversion) will be discussed in further detail in Chapter 6.

Cats may prefer novel foods depending on the cat's level of neophobia and the circumstances in which the food is presented (Bradshaw 1992). Interest in new foods may be associated with what they were exposed to by their mother (Bradshaw 1992). If medically appropriate, it is suggested to feed a variety of foods with different meat bases and texture. Not only can this be enriching but also can facilitate the acceptance of a variety of foods by the cat.

Touch

Tactile sensitivity is the first sense to develop in the cat. In fact, it is functional *in utero* (Turner and Bateson 2000). Although not able to regulate their body temperature at birth, kittens respond to temperature fluctuations and as neonatal kittens (first one to two weeks) will root or bury their head in warm objects (Beaver 2003). At birth, when touched on the side of the face or abdomen, kittens will turn their head in the direction of the touch.

Perhaps adapted to aid in the feline's hunting ability and manipulation of prey, the pads, especially the front pads, have an increased sensitivity to touch and vibrations. Not only are the feet and pads

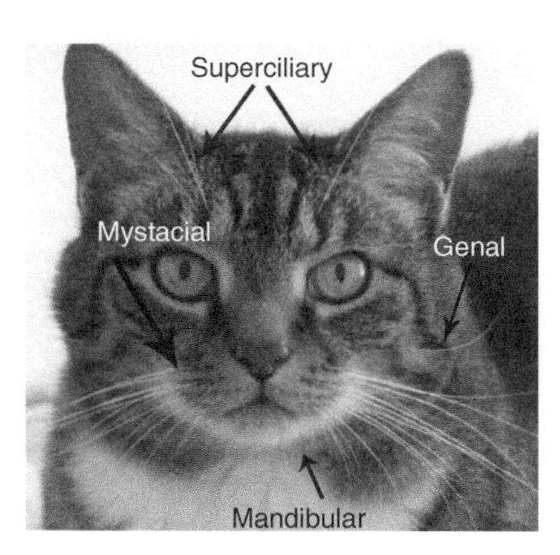

Figure 3.2 Facial vibrissae: superciliary, mandibular, genal, and mystacial marked by arrows.

densely packed with receptors, but the claws also have specialized sensory cells (Bradshaw 1992).

Cats have specialized hairs called vibrissae. The cranial and carpal vibrissae provide sensory information regarding the surroundings and may aid the cat in nocturnal hunting (Beaver 2003). The carpal vibrissae are located on the caudal surface of the wrist. The cranial vibrissae include the mystacial – located on the upper lip and arranged in rows, the superciliary – located above each eye, the genal tufts 1 and 2 – located below each ear near the mandibular angle, and the mandibular – located on the chin (Figure 3.2).

A few studies have looked at the domestic cat's preferences for petting. A 2002 study of nine cats, indicated the temporal region (between the eyes and ears) was preferred. Intermediate preference was the perioral (including the chin and lips) and the least preferred area was the caudal (tail) region (Soennichsen and Chamove 2002). These results were comparable to another study performed in 2000 with 90 cats and owner-described petting preferences. This study found the head area was preferred and only 8% of cats were described as preferring to be petted on the stomach or tail (Bernstein 2000).

Feline communication

With an understanding of how a cat's sensory perception is similar and different to our own, let's turn our focus to how cats communicate. The cat's main forms of communication are through olfactory signals (pheromones), auditory signals (vocalizations), and visual body language signals. The importance of each may vary depending on the context, the individual cat, and previous learning history. Cats also communicate using tactile signals or touch, but this form of communication will not be discussed.

Olfactory communication

Olfactory cues, including pheromones and odors, are an important means for social communication between cats as well as providing information regarding the safety of a given situation.

Each cat has its own signature scent. When it grooms itself, it transfers scent from its saliva and from glands around the head and pads to the fur. It is hypothesized that a feline colony establishes a communal scent, and it is used to recognize and identify members of the colony. Allorubbing refers to a tactile exchange between cats, whereby one cat will rub against the other, usually starting at the neck. This behavior likely is used to mix their scents and appears to be a friendly behavior. In one large farm study, females and younger cats initiated allorubbing more often than males or older cats (Bradshaw 1992). Cats will often rub their cheeks on a person returning home or on novel objects in the environment.

- Olfactory cues, including pheromones and odors, are an important means for social communication between cats as well as providing information regarding the safety of a given situation.

Because scent is so important, in multiple cat households when one cat goes to the veterinarian, he may be initially rejected by the other cats upon returning home. Failure of recognition may in large part be due to a change in scent. Preventive measures should be taken to avoid negative encounters when reintroducing a cat (specific recommendations will be provided in Chapter 7).

Scent glands are located on the chin, corners of the lips, temples, tail base, pads, and the external reproductive organs. Cats will rub scent glands on objects within the core area of their territory to mark it with their scent. When marking with the front claws, not only is a scent from the glands deposited, but a visual mark is also left from the claws.

Cats may use urine to mark the outskirts and high traffic areas of a territory. One motivation for urine marking is territoriality or stress/anxiety associated with the presence of other cats inside or outside the home. Urine marking is also associated with sexual behavior. An intact male will mark more frequently in response to an estrus female. With marking, the urine is usually deposited on vertical surfaces, but it also can be deposited horizontally on novel items or objects with concentrated scent. During marking behavior, the tail is held high and may quiver back and forth. Middening is the term used for marking with feces. It is relatively uncommon but if it occurs, the feces are usually deposited in high traffic locations or pathways.

The use of synthetic calming pheromones and odors for behavioral calming and marking behaviors may be beneficial.

Auditory communication

Cats are more likely to communicate using vocalizations with people than conspecifics. Cats appear to have their own distinct "voices" and their owners are better able to interpret the meaning of their cat's vocalizations than a stranger (Saito and Shinozuka 2013). Cats also recognize their owner's voice (Saito and Shinozuka 2013).

Domestic cats have a wide range of vocalizations; up to 21 different vocalizations have been described. Box 3.1 lists some of them.

BOX 3.1: COMMON TYPES OF VOCALIZATIONS OF ADULT DOMESTIC CATS

- Calls are a broad category of different vocalizations used in a variety of interactions between the sender and receiver. They may vary by the context and include meows and other sounds.
- Chatters refer to sounds that are emitted in association with prey and includes chattering of the teeth. These sounds are often considered voiceless because they are made without the use of the vocal cords.
- Chirps, tweedles, and tweets appear to be similar in sound and function with variations in duration or intensity. These sounds are likely to occur when the cat wants or desires something.
- The gurgle is considered to reflect friendly intentions and non-threat (Peters and Tonkin-Leyhausen 1999).
- The mew, meow, or miaow appears to be used most often in play or associated with feeding but they also may occur in various contexts. A 2019 study indicates a mew with a higher pitch, shorter duration, and rising melody occurs in a positive context (Schötz et al. 2019) rather than a negative context.
- The murmur and murmur-mew vocalizations occur in friendly contexts and is the most used vocalization.
- The purr can be heard in a variety of contexts and will have slight tonal variations pending the context. Queen and neonatal kittens will purr. Purring might reflect contentment (cat relaxed and lying in the sun), anticipation or excitement (mealtime), or self-soothing and healing (a cat in discomfort or pain). The purr is a low-pitch vocalization. While a low-pitch vocalization is more likely to be a distance increasing signal (go away), that is not usually the case with purring.
- The growl is a low-pitched, guttural sound meant to increase distance. It is given in agonist interactions and might be combined with other distance increasing sounds such as the moan, spit, hiss, yowl, or howl (Schötz et al. 2019).
- The spit and hiss are similar. The spit is a shorter duration than the hiss. Both are exhibited in startling and agonistic interactions. They are considered voiceless and may be involuntary (Tavernier et al. 2020).
- The yowl and howl are also similar. The howl is of shorter duration than the yowl. These sounds are heard in threatening situation or in the case of the yowl, also during reproductive situations (Stanton et al. 2015).
- The pain shriek is a short, loud, and high-pitched sound emitted during fights between cats. Although high-pitched, this sound is not meant to decrease distance or signal come closer.

Source: Adapted from Tavernier et al., 2020.

Vocalizations need to be evaluated in context. In general, high-pitched vocalizations are distance decreasing sounds meaning come closer. Examples include the mew or meow, chirp, tweedle, and tweet. An exception to the rule is the pain-shriek, which is high-pitched and seen during agonistic interactions. Conversely, in general, low-pitched vocalizations are distance increasing sounds meaning go away. Examples may include the spit, hiss, and growl. In contrast the purr is a low-pitched sound and, in most contexts, indicates a come closer signal (Table 3.2).

Table 3.2 Common auditory communication.

Meaning	Vocalization
Distance increasing (go away)	Hiss, growl, shriek, spit, yowl, or howl
Distance decreasing (come closer)	Sexual mating calls (can include a yowl), meow, purr, chirp, tweedle, tweet, murmur, mew, gurgle

Cats will also produce a variety of chirps and trills and unique vocalizations specific to each individual cat.

Visual communication

Cats are known for using subtle body language to express their intentions and mood and communicate with others. A glance or look may communicate to an approaching cat to find an alternate route. Many owners recognize outward signs of tension between cats such as hissing, growling, or swatting. The more subtle visual communication, such as a prolonged stare or twitching tail, leading up to more intense communication may be completely overlooked. Once people are aware of the signals, they no longer seem subtle. Cats will use body language to avoid or end confrontation and invite or avoid interactions. The veterinary behavior technician can help educate owners on typical feline communication and likely interpretations.

Although the individual components of body postures will be discussed, it is necessary to look at the entire picture including the context, to attempt to hypothesize the intended message. Cats may display a combination of body cues that seem to contradict each other, thus making it difficult to interpret the message. It is important to look at the entire cat and the context. The same body expression could have two entirely different messages depending on the circumstances. Evaluating feline communication involves interpreting all forms of observable communication as well as the behavioral history of the individual animal and the current context.

In general, cats have fewer morphological changes than breeds of dogs. However, some cat breeds with changes in skull shape due to brachycephaly, changes in tail length, such as the bobbed tails, or changes in ear conformation, such as folded ears, will have varying signaling abilities, which may result in miscommunication.

- Cats will use body language to avoid or end confrontation and invite or avoid interactions.

Facial expressions

The head and facial expression of the cat are complex. We will look at each individual aspect of facial expression, the eyes, brow, ears, mouth, and the whiskers before putting it all together.

Eyes

The eyes are very expressive and can tell us a lot about the possible emotional status of the cat. Table 3.3 summarizes eye positions of a cat and possible meanings. When the eyes are relaxed, they may be half open indicating the cat is calm and not worried. A right gaze and head turn bias is associated with relaxation (Bennett et al. 2017). Prolonged staring, also known as a "hard stare" could mean threat and challenge or interest and fixation on something depending on the context.

- The eyes are very expressive and can tell us a lot about the possible emotional status of the cat.

Dilated pupils could be a fear response, displayed in fear aggression but also could be associated with excitement, interest in something, or just adjusting to dim light. Constricted pupils can indicate high arousal, threat or challenge, or just an adjustment

Table 3.3 Feline eye positions and possible meanings.

Display description	Possible meanings
Half open	Relaxed; calm and not worried
Prolonged staring	Threatening or challenging; interested and staring at something
Dilated pupils	Fear; defensive aggression; excitement; play; high arousal; dim light
Constricted pupils	Aroused; threat/challenge; bright light
Avoiding eye contact	Polite greeting signaling no threat; avoidance; "leave me alone"; lack of interest
Blinking slowly, looking away	Conflict; signaling non-threat; fear; calming

to bright light. Avoiding eye contact can be a polite greeting, signaling non-threat. A lateralization bias of shifting the gaze to the left is seen in domestic cats, and many other species including dogs, when presented with more negative stimuli. This bias appears to be used to signal from a distance because the loss of the bias occurs with close encounters. It could be avoidance or meant to signal "leave me alone", or just a lack of interest. Blinking slowly and looking away is thought to be a conflict behavior meant to defuse tension and signal non-threat.

Blinking and half-blinking along with left head and gaze bias are likely associated with fear (Bennett et al. 2017). These behaviors may also help to calm the cat.

Brow

Table 3.4 summarizes brow positions of a cat, and possible meanings. When the brow is relaxed the muscles in the forehead will appear relaxed and smooth. This usually occurs when a cat is calm and relaxed.

A furrowed brow refers to tension in the muscles between the eyes. This expression can be seen in a variety of contexts including when a cat might be afraid, worried, focused on something, or thinking. Consider when you furrow your own brow. It can be in concentration or in concerning situations.

When a cat is in an active fight or attempting to avoid a confrontation, they will often pull their ears to the side or back resulting in flattening of the brow.

Ears

Each cat ear has 32 muscles associated with movement of the pinnae. The cat can move its ears independently of each other, rotate 180°, and move them up and down. Not only are the ears utilized in locating small prey while hunting, but they are also used to communicate.

Table 3.5 summarizes ear positions of a cat, and possible meanings. Unlike dogs, there is less variation in the morphology of the cat's ears. The exceptions would be specific breeds such as the Scottish Fold and American Curl, which are named based on their distinct ear morphology.

The normal calm or relaxed ear carriage for most cats is with the ears oriented forward but relaxed or slightly to the side. Cats will perk their ears forward in an alert response, when curious about something, but also when displaying offensive aggression and intending to create distance. The context and other body language indicators will help determine the possible meaning.

If the ears are to the side and slightly down and this is not the normal carriage for the cat, it could indicate some worry or concern. To the side and perked could indicate alertness and listening to something in the direction the ear is pointing. Flattening of the ears to the side may also be a sign of frustration (Bennett et al. 2017).

Cats might pin their ears back against the side of the head when afraid or worried. You might also see a cat hold one ear up and one ear down. This can happen when the cat is ambivalent about the situation or interested in two different things and the ears are pointing in the directions of their interests.

Table 3.4 Feline brow positions and possible meanings.

Display description	Possible meanings
Relaxed brow (muscles in forehead are relaxed)	Calm and relaxed
Furrowed brow (muscles in forehead area are tense)	Tense or worried; focused on something; thinking
Flattened brow (with ears pulled back or to side)	Attempting to avoid confrontation; in a fight

Table 3.5 Feline ear positions and possible meanings.

Display description	Possible meanings
Forward or slightly to the side	Calm or relaxed
Perked forward	Alert; interested; curious; possibly threatening
To the side; flattened	Worried; concern; alert and listening; frustrated
Pinned back	Worried and fearful
One ear up, one ear down	Ambivalent; interested in two different things (ears may point in direction of interest)

- Each cat ear has 32 muscles associated with movement of the pinnae. The cat can move its ears independently of each other, rotate 180°, and move them up and down.

Mouth

The mouth and lips of the cat can also convey information regarding the cat's potential emotional state. The mouth position often correlates with vocalizations (open or closed mouth vocalizations). Table 3.6 summarizes mouth positions of a cat, and possible meanings. A relaxed or soft mouth occurs when the muscles around the lips are relaxed. The mouth is closed, and the rest of the facial expression indicates relaxation. Unlike dogs who will open mouth pant when stressed, rarely do cats pant unless they are in respiratory distress. Increased respiratory rate due to stress would be observed through thoracic movements.

Cats will open their mouth slightly to take in pheromones, known as the flehmen or gape response. This display is not necessarily indicating signals of the emotional state of the cat.

When a cat yawns the mouth is opened wide, the lips are pulled back, the tip of the tongue curls up and may extend out of the mouth briefly (Figure 3.3). Depending on the context it could indicate uneasiness with the situation, be a polite gesture to signal non-threat, a way of coping with stress or frustration, or when not associated with social interactions, could be because the cat is content or tired.

When hissing a cat will pull the lower lip back, lower the mandible, the upper lip raises slightly making the nose wrinkle, the mouth opens wide, and the sides of the tongue curl up, but the tongue remains in the mouth. The hiss is considered a fear or frustration response meant to increase distance or signal "go away."

Table 3.6 Feline mouth positions and possible meanings.

Display description	Possible meanings
Relaxed "soft" closed mouth	Calm and not worried
Held slightly open	Flehmen or gape response when taking in pheromones
Yawning – mouth wide, lips pulled back, tongue curls up	Could be a sign of uneasiness; polite gesture to signal non-threat; cat's way of handling stress or frustration; content; tired
Hissing – lower lips back, mandible dropped, raised upper lip, wrinkled nose, mouth wide, sides of tongue curled	Fear; frustration; distance increasing signal
Nose or lip licking	Could be a sign of uneasiness; polite gesture to signal non-threat; cat's way of handling stress or frustration

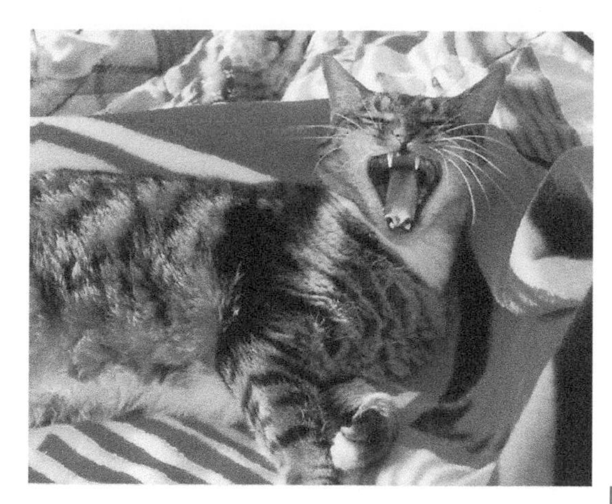

Figure 3.3 A cat yawning in contentment or to defuse tension. More information about the situation is necessary to determine motivation.

Nose or lip licking, like yawning, might be a sign of uneasiness, used as a polite gesture to signal non-threat, or the cat's way of handling stress or frustration. Nose or lip licking often proceeds and follows yawning and hissing. Licking associated with yawning involves more of the tongue and is a slower movement sweeping across the lips, whereas the lip or nose lick with the hiss just the tip of the tongue will quickly appear straight in front rather than sweeping across the mouth.

According to Bennett et al. (2017), nose licking, dropping of the jaw, raising of the upper lip, nose wrinkling, lower lip depression, parting of the lips, yawning and showing the tongue may be expressions of frustration.

Whiskers

The whiskers of the cat can also communicate information about the emotional state of the cat (Table 3.7). In a relaxed state, the cat will hold the

Table 3.7 Feline whiskers positions and possible meanings.

Display description	Possible meanings
To the side, neutral	Relaxed; calm
Perk forward and fan out	Interested; aroused; hunting
Perked forward and stiff	Offensive threat
Held back against the cheeks	Fear; non-threat; defensive aggression

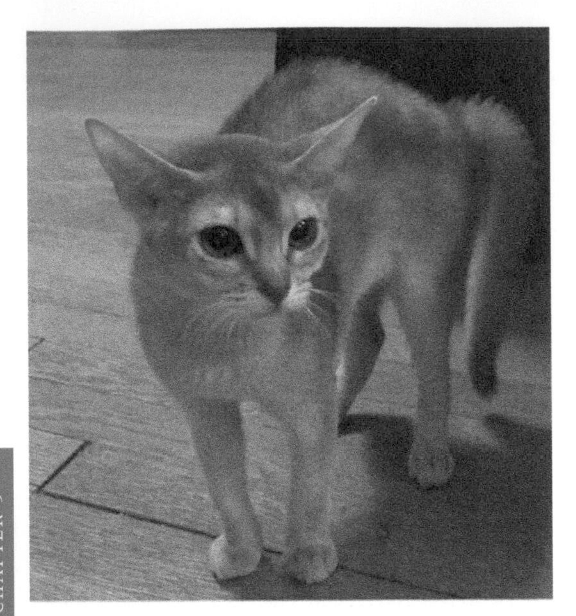

Figure 3.4 This cat displays a variety of body language. Notice the inverted L tail position, slightly raised hindlegs, piloerection along the spine and tail, direct stare, ears slightly to the side, and the whiskers forward, all indicating a more offensive threat (fear related). However, the body is turned slightly sideways and the pupils are dilated, signs indicative of defensive aggression and fear.

whiskers just to the side in a neutral position. The whiskers perk forward and fan out and might appear to curve forward when the cat is interested in or aroused by something. In a display of offensive threat, the whiskers are likely to come forward and be stiff (see Figure 3.4). In contrast, when the whiskers are pulled back tight against the cheeks, this can indicate fear, attempting to communicate non-threat, or defensive aggression. For a link to an article on feline whiskers and mood, check out the additional resources at the end of this chapter.

Feline Grimace Scale

A validated feline grimace scale to assess pain has been developed (Evangelista et al. 2019). Fear, anxiety, stress, and pain are integrally connected. Pain automatically increases fear, anxiety, and stress. This study examined changes in feline facial expressions of mesocephalic and dolichocephalic cats. Brachycephalic cats were excluded from this study. Five areas of facial changes were assessed. These five areas included ear position, orbital tightening, muzzle tension, whiskers position, and head position. For more information on the feline grimace scale please refer to the additional resources at the end of this chapter.

Tail positions

The tail not only has a functional purpose as an organ of balance in hunting and stalking prey but is also used to signal and communicate information regarding a cat's mood or intentions (Table 3.8).

- The tail not only has a functional purpose as an organ of balance in hunting and stalking prey but is also used to signal and communicate information regarding a cat's mood or intentions.

When in a neutral position the base of the tail is relaxed, and the tail will hang toward the ground often with the end in a slight U shape. This tail carriage with the tail raising slightly higher could indicate interest in something.

A tail held vertically without piloerection and with the last third of the tail slowly curving back and forth, known as a flagpole or winding tail, is seen in friendly greetings. This signal can be seen at a great distance. The tail is often involved in signaling from

Table 3.8 Feline tail positions and possible meanings.

Display description	Possible meanings
Neutral position-base is relaxed, tail down with the end curling up slightly in a U shape	Relaxed or slightly alert
Held vertically without piloerection, last 3rd of tail may slowly curve back and forth; flagpole or winding	Friendly greeting
Vertical with piloerection, upright bottle brush	Fear and defensive aggression; kitten play
Tucked to side close to the body or between legs	Fear and defensive aggression
Inverted L – first inch is horizontal, and remainder points down with or without piloerection. Rump is usually raised.	Fear and offensive aggression
Twitching or flicking	High arousal; agitation; distance-increasing signal

a distance and plays an important role in communication. Cats with bobbed or missing tails will be limited or lack this communication tool.

If the tail is vertical with piloerection, also known as upright bottle brush appearance, the cat may be afraid and displaying defensive aggression. When kittens play and mock fight, the tail may be bristled, held up, and curved in an inverted U. If the tail is tucked to the side, held close to the body or between the legs, with or without piloerection, this can be an indication of fear and defensive aggression.

When the first inch of the tail is horizontal with the remainder pointing straight down, also known as an inverted L, with or without piloerection, this can be an indication of fear and offensive aggression (see Figure 3.4). The hind end is often raised and higher than the forelegs. Although a distance-increasing signal, the inverted L tail may also be a sign of conflict. The cat may not appear to be as overtly afraid as the cat with a tucked tail but is still feeling threatened and likely attempting to defuse aggression.

A twitching tail or flicking tip of the tail can indicate agitation or high arousal and is usually meant to increase distance. A cat who appears to be resting calmly but with the tail thrashing or tip flicking, should be approached with caution or not at all.

- A cat who appears to be resting calmly but with the tail thrashing or tip flicking, should be approached with caution or not at all.

Body postures and hair coat

The overall posture of the cat can be indicative of the general demeanor of the cat (Table 3.9). Body posture refers to the overall position of the entire body. This can include the head, torso, legs, and hair coat.

A cat in a relaxed state will often rest on their side, with their limbs extended, tail still and relaxed, ears forward but relaxed, pupil dilation appropriate for the environment, and brow, eyes, mouth, and whiskers relaxed.

Piloerection refers to the hair being raised. Sometimes it might just be the tail or spine but other times it can be the entire body. This is a chemical response fueled by adrenaline that signals high arousal, excitement, fear, or uncertainty.

If the hindlegs and rump are being carried slightly higher than the forelegs and the cat is moving directly forward or even slightly to the side, this could signal threat, challenge, offensive aggression, or interest (Figure 3.4). Looking at the tail, facial expression, as well as the context will help you interpret this body posture.

Table 3.9 Feline body postures and hair coat and possible meanings.

Display description	Possible meanings
Resting on side, ears up but relaxed, eyes half open, pupils normal for environment, tail still, mouth, whiskers, and brow relaxed	Relaxed state
Piloerection (hair is raised between shoulder blades, down the spine, over the rump and/or tail)	A chemical response that signals high arousal, excitement, fear, or uncertainty
Hindlegs carried slightly higher than the forelegs; moving directly forward or slightly to the side	Threat or challenge; offensive aggression; interest (look at the tail to gain more information)
Lowering entire body, leaning backwards(weight on hindlegs), or turning sideways, the back might be hunched or arched	Fear; defensive aggression; desire to avoid confrontation; "leave me alone"

Another possible body posture a cat might display is lowering the entire body, leaning weight on the hindlegs, or turning sideways with the back either hunched or arched. This posture likely signals fear, defensive aggression, a desire to avoid confrontation or a "leave me alone" signal.

Rolling refers to a cat that rolls on its side and back exposing the abdomen (Figure 3.5). This posture

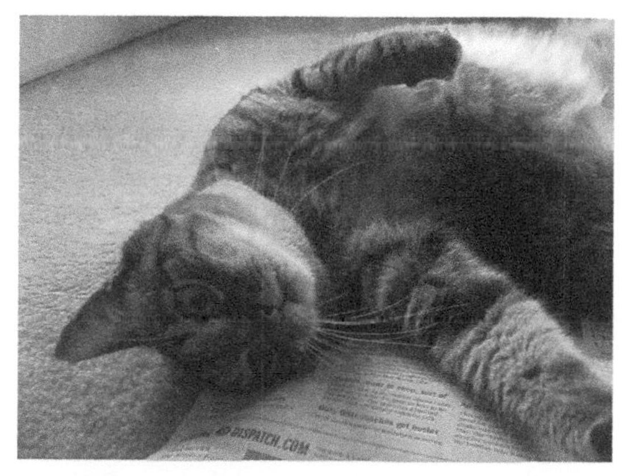

Figure 3.5 A cat rolling on its back as a possible invitation for an amicable interaction.

can be seen in kittens as an invitation for play, during proestrus in females (Bradshaw 1992), and also at times in response to a social encounter. It is generally seen in times of nonaggressive encounters (Bradshaw 1992). However, it does not necessarily communicate a cat wants to be petted on the abdomen. Many cats will become agitated or overstimulated if rubbed on the belly and may turn and nip or scratch the person.

Play postures

Social play is most prevalent between 4 and 16 weeks of age (Beaver 2003). Through play, kittens often display body language associated with predatory and aggressive behavior. For example, a kitten may crouch and then spring at the other kitten (predatory) or piloerect the hair along the spine and tail and side step around the other cat (defensive aggressive displays) in mock play fighting. Perhaps other subtle signals such as facial expression and tail movement and rate, modify the meaning of the signals and signify play rather than true aggression.

Veterinary behaviorist Bonnie Beaver describes eight different play behaviors seen in kittens in her book, *Feline Behavior: A Guide for Veterinarians*. These postures include belly-up, stand-up, side-step, pounce, vertical stance or rearing, chase, horizontal leap, and face-off. Some of these same behaviors are displayed in play with objects as well.

Conflict behaviors

Conflict behaviors refer to body language used to signal uneasiness in a given context and are used in an attempt to neutralize the situation or avoid further conflict. They might include behaviors that could be termed displacement behaviors or calming signals. The animal maybe experiences competing emotions and motivations. For example, they are curious and social but afraid at the same time. The following are examples of potential conflict behaviors in cats. Many of these behaviors were described in the previous section when looking at specific body part signals and their potential meanings and some are considered polite communication between cats; a kind of social "nicety" used to avoid conflict. Box 3.2 identifies some possible feline conflict behaviors.

Cats certainly will display some of these behaviors when they are relaxed, but when they are displayed in response to a specific stimulus or interaction, it could mean the cat is uneasy with the situation. These subtle cues might be inadvertently overlooked or misinterpreted, and that can lead to miscommunication.

BOX 3.2: POSSIBLE FELINE CONFLICT BEHAVIORS

- Yawning
- Lip licking
- Grooming
- Averting gaze
- Dilated pupils
- Blinking eyes or squinting
- Ears back
- One ear up and one down
- Turning sideways
- Rolling to the side
- Freezing
- Shake off as if wet

Look for these behaviors in cats. Conflict behaviors are used to decrease social tension and decrease aggression. In some cats, they are a precursor to aggression, especially when the message is not effectively understood or responded to appropriately by the receiver. They are a way for the cat to tell us or another animal, "Please back off or calm down; you are making me uneasy. I am a little afraid and unsure."

- Look for these behaviors in cats. Conflict behaviors are used to decrease social tension and decrease aggression. In some cats, they are a precursor to aggression, especially when the message is not effectively understood or responded to appropriately by the receiver.

Reading the entire cat

The neutral and content cat will display half-open eyes, pupils appropriate for the environment, tail relaxed and still, brow relaxed, and ears forward or mostly forward (Figure 3.6). He may purr or meow as well.

The playful cat displays partially dilated pupils, whiskers and ears forward, and tail up.

Fear and anxiety may be displayed with the pupils dilated, head tucked, ears back or to the side, body

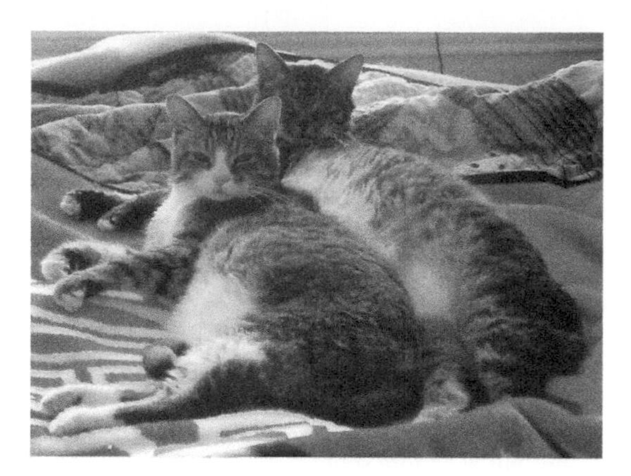

Figure 3.6 Relaxed state: resting on side, ears up but neutral, eyes half opened, tail still.

tucked or turned sideways, tail tucked or between the legs, complete piloerection, furrowed brow, and whiskers held back. A defensive cat may growl, hiss, or spit.

Offensive aggression, which is also modulated by fear or a perceived threat, may be displayed with constricted pupils, direct eye contact, ears back, inverted L tail, piloerection along the spine, and head up or moving from side to side. The offensive cat may growl or yowl.

Just a reminder, when we are attempting to infer the emotional state of another, it is just that, inference. We cannot know the internal states of an individual. We are attempting to identify behavioral indicators associated with potential emotional states based on observable expressions and contexts.

For video examples of feline body language, please review the companion website Videos 3.1, 3.2, and 3.3.

- Just a reminder, when we are attempting to infer the emotional state of another, it is just that, inference. We cannot know the internal states of an individual. We are attempting to identify behavioral indicators associated with potential emotional states based on observable expressions and contexts.

Feline domestication, social structure, and behavior

Domestication

The domestic cat is thought to be descendent from the wild cat *Felis silverstris* and specifically the African or Arabian wild cat, *Felis silverstris lybica* (Clutton-Brock 1987). The oriental breeds may have descended from the Indian Desert Cat, *Felis silverstris ornata* (Bradshaw 1992). *F.s. ornata* was a leaner cat compared to the stockier *F.s. lybica*. The formal classification of the domestic cat is *Felis silverstris catus*.

Domestication was a gradual process but likely started around 4000 BCE in Egypt. Around 1600 BCE, cats appear to have become involved in everyday human activities as depicted in artwork during that time. Domestication of the cat resulted in less behavioral changes compared to other domesticated animals. The notable changes included a reduced brain size, a change in hormone balance (decreased adrenals), and retention of juvenile behavior characteristics into adulthood (neoteny) (Bradshaw 1992). What is unique to the domestication of the cat is that domestication may have occurred as a result of religious beliefs rather than just utilitarian purposes. Although cats certainly were instrumental in controlling rodent populations, they were also considered sacred by the ancient Egyptians. Recognition of a cat goddess was even part of the ancient Egyptian religion (Bradshaw 1992).

- Domestication of the cat resulted in less behavioral changes compared to other domesticated animals.

Domestication results from an ongoing relationship between humans and animals that has proved to be mutually beneficial to both parties. Sociability is an important determinant of domestication. For animals to be domesticated, they must breed and reproduce in the proximity of man. In Egypt, cats were primarily used in granaries to control rodents, but they were also used to hunt, fish, and retrieve birds.

It is possible that cats are "self-domesticated" because selective breeding by humans has done little to produce physiologic, morphologic, or behavioral changes and domestic cats readily revert to being self-sufficient without human intervention and care. Agricultural stores of feed attract wild rodents, and with prey plentiful, wildcats were attracted to early human settlements. Early mankind likely tolerated the wildcats' proximity near human settlements for their beneficial mousing ability and cats became tolerant of human company. Throughout history, human views toward cats have varied from intolerance and the extermination of the "devilish" little creatures to being revered and considered God-like religious symbols.

Social organization of domestic cats

How social are domestic cats and how does it affect cat–cat and cat–human relationships? Many issues arise in the human domestic environment when the innate behavior of the cat is not understood or taken into consideration. By studying the natural tendencies of the domestic cat in a less restricted environment than a human household, we can identify trends in behavior when given a choice. Information regarding the dynamics of intraspecies relationships of cats has mainly been obtained through studies of groups of cats living together outdoors.

Although *Felis silvestris lybica* was solitary, the domestic cat appears to vary widely in regard to sociability. The domestic cat has the ability to be either solitary or social, known as social flexibility, depending on early experiences and genetics. In cats, friendliness may be genetically related to the behavior of the tom. Even though the tom is often absent during the raising of the kittens, his boldness of behavior and his friendliness toward unfamiliar people may be more influential than the behavior of the queen and the early rearing environment (Reisner et al. 1994). Studies from the 1980s on the socialization of cats found that approximately 15% of cats have a temperament that is resistant to socialization; some cats have unfriendly tendencies (Karsh 1984).

- The domestic cat has the ability to be either solitary or social, known as social flexibility, depending on early experiences and genetics.

Free-ranging domestic cats are solitary hunters meaning they rarely cooperate to catch prey and they don't share meals. This is because meals primarily consist of small mammals such as a mouse. Because meals are small, they must eat frequently, and a large portion of their time is spent hunting.

Free-ranging feline groups or colonies will form dependent on the availability of resources, primarily food. A colony may consist of 30 to 50 cats, but a majority of colonies consist of 10 or fewer. The colonies mainly consist of females and their young. Within a colony, cats will have preferred associations (Macdonald et al. 2000; Crowell-Davis et al. 2004).

This matrilineal group will cooperatively rear litters together and may defend their core territory from unknown cats (male or female). Females tend to stay their entire life with the colony in which they were born. Males will usually leave the colony by two to three years of age. Mature males may form loose associations with a group or multiple groups but are more solitary than females.

A study by Barry and Crowell-Davis from 1999 investigated factors which might influence affiliative and aggressive behaviors between indoor-only neutered domestic cats. Sixty households comprised of dyads of either two males, two females, or a male and female ranging from six months to eight years of age were observed for 10 hours. The study found, "... no significant differences in affiliative or aggressive behavior based on cat gender. However, females were never observed to allorub other females. The male/male households did spend more time in close proximity. The amount of time the cats had lived together was negatively correlated with the amount of aggression observed during the study." Meaning the shorter the duration that the cats had lived together the more aggression was observed. The study also found, "Factors such as size of the house and weight difference between the cats did not correlate with the aggression rate. Large standard deviations and the correlations of social behavior between housemates indicated the importance of individual differences in behavior" (Barry and Crowell-Davis 1999).

A study by Knowles et al. conducted during 2001 and 2002 sought to determine whether the direction of dominance as determined by agonistic interactions away from food was different from the direction of dominance as determined by access to food in cats. A colony of 28 neutered cats living in a residential home with outdoor access to a confined yard were observed. "Dyadic relationships and hierarchy formed from observation of agonistic interactions away from food were compared with those formed from interactions at the food bowl. A cat was scored as subordinate to another cat if it lost three of three interactions or lost greater or equal to 75% of the interactions when greater than three interactions occurred." This study found a positive correlation between hierarchy rank between dyads based on agonistic interactions away from food and rank at the food bowl.

The study also found, "In post hoc analyses, when considering the relationship between two cats, the heavier cat most likely ranked higher in each hierarchy; however, age was not significantly correlated with either hierarchy. On the basis of dyadic information, the older cat in a dyad was more often dominant in agonistic interactions. Males had a higher mean dominance rank than females; however, sex had no effect on rank determined by interactions at the food bowl" (Knowles et al. 2004).

Although research of animals, including dogs and cats, may seek to identify dominance hierarchies among groups or pairs of animals, in the clinical treatment of behavior conditions, this information is often of little use. A definitive linear dominance hierarchy is not displayed among free-ranging groups of cats (Bernstein 2006).

- Although research of animals, including dogs and cats, may seek to identify dominance hierarchies among groups or pairs of animals, in the clinical treatment of behavior conditions, this information is often of little use.

Strong bonds can form between cats if they are together as kittens whether related or not. They are more likely to maintain close relationships, sharing space, and allogroom each other (Bernstein 2006). Littermates will have a closer relationship with each other than two unrelated individuals (Bradshaw and Hall 1999).

Another study sought to determine the effects of relatedness and familiarity on proximity and grooming in cats in a multicat household (Curtis et al. 2003). The study found that familiarity and relatedness were significantly associated with time spent within 1 m of each other and time spent allogrooming. When comparing familiar cats, familiar relatives were significantly more likely to be within 1 m and to be groomed compared to familiar non-relatives. The study concluded, "This may be important when considering adoption of one or more kittens and when adding a new cat to a household in which other cats are present. Adopting small family groups may result in higher rates of affiliative behavior, stronger bonding, and lower incidence of conflict than periodically adopting single unrelated adult cats."

Territorial behavior

There is some debate as to whether cats are truly "territorial." What we do know is that domestic free-ranging cats and housecats tend to be unaccepting of unfamiliar cats in or near their core territory. This tendency can certainly be a challenge when cat owners desire to have a multiple cat household.

When discussing home range and core territory, the home range will be larger than the core territory of the cat (Figure 3.7). The exception is the house cat for which the home range and core territory will often be the same. The home range of several free-ranging males may overlap but it is the core territory that will be defended against other cats (Beaver 2003). Both male and female cats may be unaccepting of intruders in their core territory.

With free-ranging domestic cats, home ranges vary greatly in size depending on the availability of resources. On average, a male cat will have a home range 3.5 times larger than females in the same area (Liberg and Sandell 1988).

A study by Bernstein and Strack observed 14 unrelated neutered cats living in a 10-room house. Although the cats had access to the entire house, not all rooms were used. The home range of the individual cats was defined as the number of specific rooms used regularly by the cat. The cats in this house had overlapping but distinct home ranges. Males tended to have slightly larger home ranges; they utilized more rooms of the house on a regular basis. The ranges seemed to correlate with

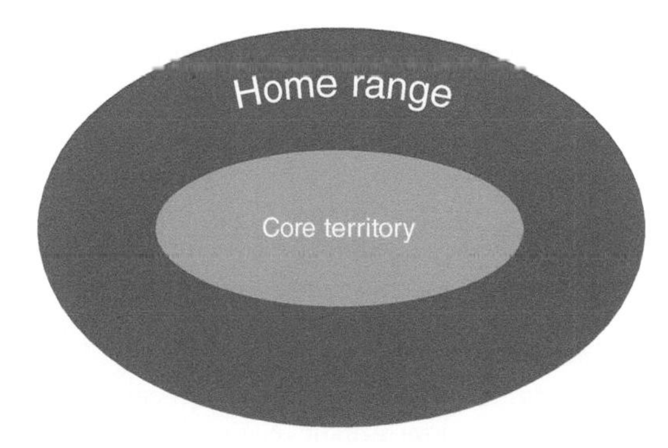

Figure 3.7 Home range versus core territory.

individual preferences for particular rooms and approach or avoidance of particular cats. Cats shared favored resting spots on a rotational basis. Rather than sharing a space simultaneously, they would often time-share spots (Bernstein and Strack 1996).

Let's apply some basic guidelines for attempting to successfully house multiple cats in a household (https://purrfectlove.net/how-many-cats-is-too-many). One method is to not exceed the number of bedrooms in the residence. A two-bedroom residence would accommodate up to two cats. However, additional levels in the house can extend this number by an additional cat. For example, a two-story home with two bedrooms could accommodate three cats.

Another option is to base it on square footage. Anything under 1000 square feet should not have more than two cats. For every 500 square feet over 1000, you can add one cat. So, a home that is 1500 square feet, could potentially house three cats comfortably. A home that is 2000 square feet could house up to four cats.

However, it is important to recognize harmonious cohabitation will also be dependent on many additional factors including age and temperament.

Because of possible territorial behavior, it is important in multiple-cat households to provide ample resources, such as multiple feeding, water, and litter box locations, scratching posts, and vertical living space. In essence this creates multiple core territories, thus decreasing social tension. Cat trees and perches add additional square footage to the territory (Figures 3.8 and 3.9).

- Because of possible territorial behavior, it is important in multiple-cat households to provide ample resources, such as multiple feeding, water, and litter box locations, scratching posts, and vertical living space.

When introducing a new cat to a household with existing cats, a systematic approach should be taken to provide for the best chance of successful integration. A detailed process of how to properly introduce cats will be provided in Chapter 7.

The cat–human relationship

The cat–human relationship has not been studied as much as the dog–human relationship. Research as of 2022 has been geared toward the types of interactions between familiar and unfamiliar people (tolerance to handling and time spent interacting), variations in cat personalities, and the role the cat plays in a person's life. However, very little has been studied regarding the effects of human interactions on the well-being of the cat, except to indicate that we provide cats with food, security, and companionship.

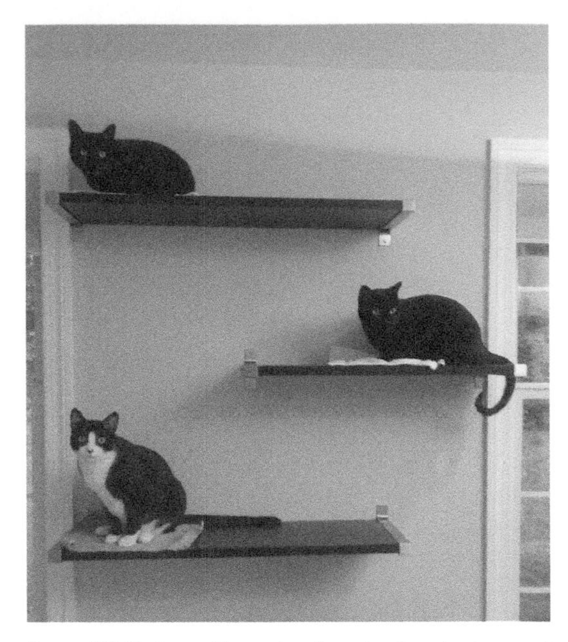

Figure 3.8 Shelves with perches for cats allow for increased vertical living space.

Pet cats provide both social and emotional support to humans. People can develop very strong bonds with cats and cats can decrease a human's negative mood (Rieger and Turner 1999; Turner and Rieger 2001; Turner et al. 2003). Cats often fill the role of a significant partner for older people who live alone (Turner 2000).

Interestingly, the risk for cardiovascular disease for current and past cat owners was significantly lower than for people who had not owned cats (even in comparison to owning other pets) (Qureshi et al. 2009).

Cat owners are better able to interpret their cat's vocalizations than a person not familiar with the cat. Cats tend to use more vocalizations in communications with people than with conspecifics. This is likely due to learning. Cats learn that people respond to vocalizations more

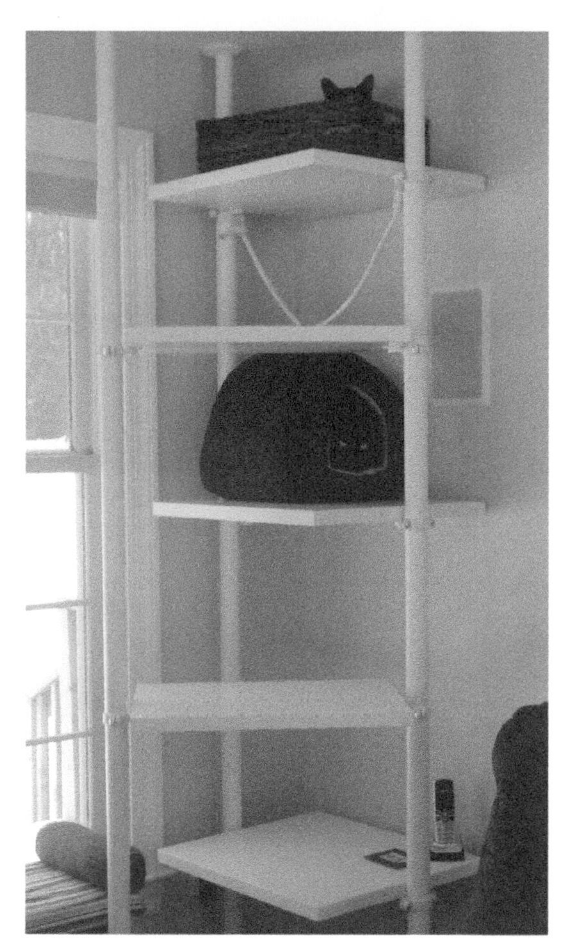

Figure 3.9 Floor-to-ceiling cat perches.

often than to their more subtle and silent communication.

When comparing cat-initiated versus human initiated interactions, there is some seemingly contradictory information in the literature. Turner (1991) recorded that cat initiated interactions with the owner resulted in longer interaction times versus owner-initiated interactions. Based on this information, it has often been suggested to "play hard-to-get" with cats and allow them to choose to interact with us.

However, a study comparing shelter and pet cats, indicated cats in both groups interacted more with attentive humans than inattentive ones (Vitale and Udell 2019). In this study the attentive humans could encourage the cat to approach them, but they could not approach the cat. Most likely it is about finding the right balance between the two extremes; showing interest through visual and vocal interactions but also allowing the cat to choose to approach or not. When encouragement, such as looking at the cat and providing vocal enticements is not having the desired effect, then acting as if the cat doesn't exist (playing hard to get) might be a better strategy. Either way, in the clinical setting it is best to allow the cat to choose to approach and interact with us rather than us approaching and initiating physical contact with the cat. The best strategy, attentiveness or ignoring, will depend on the individual cat's response.

Sexual behavior

The female cat will reach sexual maturity on average between 3.5 and 12 months of age. Cats are seasonally polyestrous, meaning they will have several estrous cycles per season. Although some individual cats will cycle year-round, most cats in the United States cycle from February to April and June to August (Beaver 2003). Most cats are anestrous in the Fall from September through December.

Proestrus is accompanied by an increase in activity, object rubbing, and less aggression toward an approaching male. Within a 24-hour period, the female will increase rolling, rubbing, and kneading. At this point, she will allow close contact from a male but not tolerate any attempts at being mounted (Bradshaw 1992).

In estrus, rolling is discontinued and instead the female assumes a lordosis position whereby her head is close to the ground, the back is arched ventrally, the hind limbs are up and the tail is raised and to the side. She is receptive to being mounted by a male. During copulation, the male will grasp the female by the nape of the neck with his jaws. Multiple copulations are necessary to induce ovulation (Bradshaw 1992). Cats are considered induced ovulators because of the need for copulation to trigger ovulation. The reproductive cycle of the cat is an efficient one. It is estimated that in seven years, one female cat and her offspring could be responsible for 781 250 kittens (Mahlow and Slater 1996; Olson and Johnston 1993).

Cats are polygamous and the estrus female may be bred by multiple males. In fact, several males will congregate around a receptive female. According to one source, when this occurs, there is less aggression between the males (Bradshaw 1992). One would think that competition for an estrous female would elicit increased aggressive encounters in the toms. Along those lines of thinking, another source indicated males may be aggressive to one another when in proximity to a female in estrus, but that is not always the case (Crowell-Davis et al. 2004).

Males become sexually mature around 9–12 months of age. A surge in testosterone at around 3.5 months of age can be evidenced by testosterone-induced behaviors such as mounting in play as early as four months of age. Although there has been at least one report of infanticide (tom cat killing kittens sired by other males in a colony), it does not appear to be common practice in domestic feral cats (Bradshaw 1992).

Regarding sexual selection and mating success, a female will choose a familiar male over an unfamiliar male. If choosing between unfamiliar males, she is more likely to choose the larger male. However, a smaller familiar male is more likely to be successful than an unfamiliar male whether larger or smaller (Crowell-Davis et al. 2004; Clutton-Brock 1989).

Maternal behavior

Gestation lasts about 63 days. About one week prior to parturition, the queen will select a den site. As mentioned earlier, cat colonies consist primarily of a matrilineal group. A communal den near the food source is a successful strategy that results in a lower mortality rate when compared to individual dens further from the food source (Bradshaw 1992). Adult female cats in the group will assist with the care of the young. Even during parturition, another female cat may assist with cleaning and drying the young immediately postpartum.

Epimeletic, care-giving, behaviors exhibited by the queen include

- licking the kittens to clean them and stimulate urination and defecation during the first weeks of life,
- initiating nursing,
- retrieving kittens that have wandered from the litter, and
- responding to kitten vocalizations.

Kittens will exhibit care-seeking, et-epimeletic, behaviors such as distress vocalization when cold or hungry.

The cat–human relationship is probably similar to a kitten–mother relationship whereby the people act as the care giver and the cat will display care-seeking behavior.

- The cat–human relationship is probably similar to a kitten–mother relationship whereby the people act as the care giver and the cat will display care-seeking behavior.

Ingestive and predatory behavior

The suckling reflex is present at birth. During the first three weeks of life, the queen initiates nursing. Teat preference is established during the first few days of life and lasts approximately one month (Beaver 2003). Kittens will continue to nurse on average until 8–10 weeks of age. Weaning is a gradual process. Kittens can start to eat solid food at around one month.

Cats are carnivores and if raised in a feral or semi-feral setting, the queen must teach the kittens how to hunt. When the kittens are around a month old, the mother will bring dead prey back to the litter and later (around two months) injured but live prey. Chasing and catching prey is an innate behavior that needs to be practiced to be perfected. However, manipulating, killing, and ingesting prey is learned (Beaver 2003). Kittens will hunt what their mother hunted. If a cat was not taught to hunt as a young kitten, only about half will be able to learn to hunt as an adult and it is a much lengthier process (Beaver 2003).

Cats prefer to eat small meals frequently. Consequently, free-choice feeding is less stressful for the cat (Finco et al. 1986). However, feeding needs to be managed with portion control to prevent obesity.

- Cats prefer to eat small meals frequently. Consequently, free-choice feeding is less stressful for the cat. However, feeding needs to be managed with portion control to prevent obesity.

Eliminative behavior

During the first three weeks of life, urination and defecation must be stimulated by the urogenital reflex. This is generally accomplished by the queen licking the perineal region. The queen also ingests the excrement, thus keeping the nest clean and odor free. Kittens begin to be able to eliminate on their own by three weeks of age. By one month of age, kittens will start to explore dirt and litter and dig or rake the substrate with their forepaws. Because ingestion of substrate may also occur during this early exploration, caution should be used with clumping and expanding litters with young kittens (Marder 1997).

Cats generally prefer large, open, liner-less litter boxes with an unscented fine-grained substrate. (More information on litter box training and preference can be found in Chapter 7.) A typical urination includes digging a small hole in the substrate, squatting to urinate, and then covering the urine by pulling the substrate over the spot with the forepaws. Not all cats perform the digging or covering behavior. The adult cat urinates on average two to three times a day.

Cats may not dig as much prior to defecation (Pannaman 1981). Within the core area, it is common for the feces to be covered following defecation. Although it has been noted that uncovered feces may be left along hunting paths and elevated surfaces and is more common in territorial males (Cooper 1997), it is generally thought that marking with feces, middening, does not occur (Beaver 2003) or is rare in the domestic cat. The number of defecations in a 24-hour period is variable and dependent on diet and the individual. Commercially available condensed diet may limit defecation to less than once a day.

Feline inappropriate elimination (FIE) problems, including periuria (urinating outside of the litter box), account for a vast number of behavioral complaints by owners. Inappropriate elimination damages the human–animal bond and often results in relinquishment. A thorough medical workup is warranted for any cat exhibiting inappropriate elimination. Medical factors may cause or exacerbate an FIE issue. At the very least, they will undermine the success of treatment if not identified and addressed. Generally, FIE when attributed to behavioral causes will fall into one of two categories:

1. House soiling: The cat has either a preference for a different substrate than what is being provided or an aversion to the existing options. An aversion or avoidance of the box can be facilitated by social or environmental stress in the household.
2. Marking: It is a sexual or an anxiety-driven inappropriate elimination issue.

Often a case will present that is a combination of house soiling, marking, and medical factors rather than one or the other.

- Feline inappropriate elimination (FIE) problems, including periuria (urinating outside of the litter box), account for a vast number of behavioral complaints by owners.
- FIE damages the human–animal bond and often results in relinquishment.
- A thorough medical workup is warranted for any cat exhibiting inappropriate elimination.

Urine marking

Although urine marking often occurs on vertical surfaces on the outskirts of the territory, it can also be performed on horizontal surfaces within the territory. Anxiety associated with a novel item brought into the house may stimulate a cat to urinate on the object. The concentrated scent of an absent owner could produce frustration or anxiety resulting in urine marking of the person's side of the bed. Stress associated with changes in routine, other cats in or around the home, social tension between existing cats or other pets, novel items or smells could all be triggers that result in urine marking.

Urine marking occurs in males and females, as well as intact and neutered cats. However, prevalence is higher in intact males due to urine spraying associated with sexual behavior. Urine marking has a genetic component to it (Halip et al. 1992). Neutering of the male and female cat can considerably decrease marking: 90% in males and 95% in females (Hart and Cooper 1984).

Urine marking serves a different function than normal micturition and defection. Consequently, many cats who urine mark will also use the litter box for normal toileting behavior (Dantas 2018).

Exploratory behavior and activity levels

Domestic cats are likely partially diurnal (Bradshaw 1992). They generally disperse their activity throughout a 24-hour period with a majority of activity occurring during the day, rather than being crepuscular (active at dusk and dawn) or nocturnal (active at night). Depending on the environment of the cat (house cat vs. free-ranging cat), an individual cat's circadian rhythm may be affected by the activity level of a household or availability of food or prey. A free-ranging cat will be forced to hunt at a time that its preferred prey is active. However, many free-ranging cats hunt a variety of small animals that have various peak activity levels

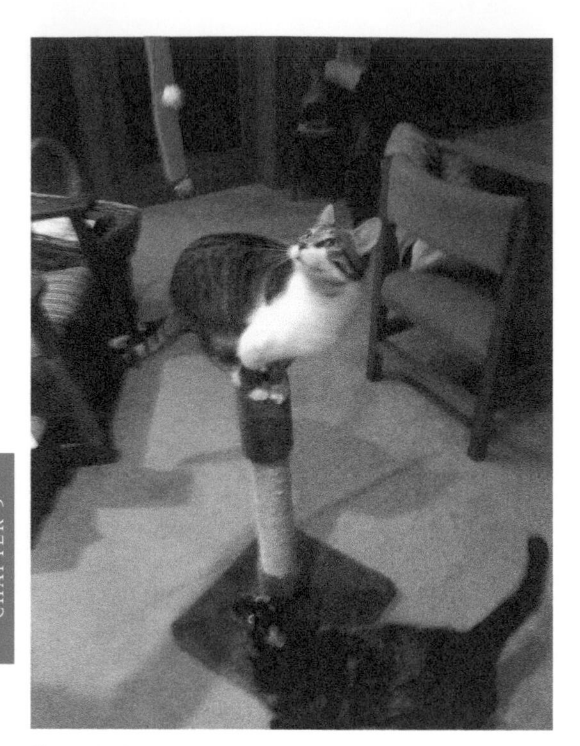

Figure 3.10 Providing exploration and enrichment: two cats exploring ways to dislodge the balls from the hanging fabric.

within a 24-hour period. Domestic house cats have basically adapted to our lifestyle; when there is activity in the house, they are more active.

- Domestic cats generally spread their activity throughout a 24-hour period with a majority of activity occurring during the day. Rather than being crepuscular (active at dusk and dawn) or nocturnal, they are likely partially diurnal.

To provide the indoor cat with appropriate exploration and activity, cat owners will need to provide enrichment to meet the cat's needs (Figure 3.10). Specific strategies will be covered in Chapter 7, including providing a variety of interactive toys and food storage devices, scheduling set play and training times, and providing vertical living space for exploration and hiding.

Grooming behavior

Cats spend a large amount of their awake-time grooming. In fact, about 50% of awake-time or about 3.6 hours of a 24-hour period is spent grooming (Eckstein and Hart 2000; Pannaman 1981).

During the first few weeks of life, the queen grooms the kittens until they learn to perform it on their own. Self-grooming starts at around two weeks of age. Beaver reports that kittens that were not well groomed early in life, are more likely to be less fastidious groomers as adults (Beaver 2003). Cleanliness is likely learned and strongly influenced by experience during the first few weeks of life.

Grooming appears to have four main functions (Beaver 2003). The most obvious is maintenance of healthy skin and coat. Grooming will remove extra hair to prevent matting and also remove ectoparasites. Another function of grooming is to dissipate heat as it provides for evaporative cooling (Hart 1976). The third purpose may be an affiliative behavior between cats when one cat grooms another. The final purpose of grooming may be as a calming behavior for the cat or a communicative one. A cat when placed in a stressful situation may start to groom. Perhaps self-grooming is used to help soothe the cat, or decrease tension. Rather than reacting to the stimuli, the cat stops what it is doing and begins to groom. This is an example of a displacement behavior or a possible conflict behavior.

- The four main functions of grooming:
  1. Maintain healthy skin and coat
  2. Dissipate heat
  3. Affiliative behavior between cats
  4. Calming or communicative

With normal self-grooming, a majority of it is performed with the tongue and teeth: oral grooming. It is usually performed from the fore body to the tail. The forepaws and hindpaws are used to reach areas that the cat is unable to reach with its mouth. The cat will lick its forepaws and then wipe its neck, ears, head, and face. Utilizing the hindpaws to scratch the neck and behind the ears is the least frequent grooming behavior performed.

The front nails will be maintained by scratching them along a surface. This behavior has a dual purpose of maintaining nail health as well as use in olfactory and visual communication.

A decrease or increase in self-grooming behavior may be a sign of medical and/or behavioral conditions and warrants investigation by a veterinarian.

- A decrease or increase in self-grooming behavior may be a sign of medical and/or behavioral conditions and warrants investigation by a veterinarian.

Mutual grooming or allogrooming is performed by one cat to another cat. The head and neck areas are the most frequent locations groomed. Allogrooming occurs while the cats are at rest. Some cats will rest next to each other but not groom one another (Bradshaw 1992). It appears to be a friendly behavior by the initiator; however, some recipients may not be accepting of being groomed.

Breed differences

As of 2022 few studies on cat breed differences exist. There appear to be some discernable personality predilections among breeds with variability within breeds. Oriental cats seem to be genetically more susceptible to developing stereotypies than other pedigree and non-pedigree cats (Bradshaw et al. 1997).

Some behaviors of cats are moderately heritable depending on the breed (Salonen et al. 2019). This is similar to hereditability findings with canine behavior. About half of the differences in cats' behaviors might be attributed to genetic variations among populations of cats. Nature and nurture play a significant role in cat personality. For more information about cat breed differences, see the article link under additional resources at the end of this chapter.

Feline behavioral development

Feline behavioral development is affected by numerous factors. Genetics play a role. However, early experience and learning also has a profound effect. Behavior is a combination of genetics and experience or learning. The research exploring the role of epigenetics in development and the expression of genes is ongoing. Epigenetics is defined as: the study of how behaviors and environment can cause changes that affect the way genes work (modified from https://www.cdc.gov/genomics/disease/epigenetics.htm). Unlike genetic changes, epigenetic changes are reversible and do not change the DNA sequence, but they can change how the body reads a DNA sequence. Gene expression refers to how often or when proteins are created from the instructions within genes. While genetic changes can alter which protein is made, epigenetic changes affect gene expression to turn genes "on" and "off."

The genetic platform may prime the individual for specific behaviors or diseases, but without environmental factors and experiences those characteristics or diseases might not reach fruition.

- The genetic platform may prime the individual for specific behaviors or diseases, but without environmental factors and experiences those characteristics or diseases might not reach fruition.

For example, at birth, the nervous system is still developing. Without appropriate stimuli, sensory perception may not develop normally. To optimize development, an enriched environment is necessary.

Developmental periods and life stages

The developmental periods of cats have not been as clearly defined as with dogs. The Humane Society of the United States and Denver Dumb Friends League identify a neonatal period (0–2 weeks), socialization period (2–7 weeks), most active play period (7–14 weeks), ranking period (3–6 months), and adolescence (6–18 months). AAFP-AAHA: Feline Life Stage Guidelines (Vogt et al. 2010) suggest a broader age classification system to help focus attention on specific physical and behavioral characteristics. They are: Kitten (birth to 6 months), Junior (7 months to 2 years), Prime (3 to 6 years), Mature (7–10 years), Senior (11–14 years), and Geriatric (15+ years).

Classification of age ranges can help guide the veterinary professional in regard to typical life changes that may occur during a specific time. Sensitive periods of development are different from classification by life stages. Cats have some sensitive periods early in development when, if particular stimuli are not provided, normal development cannot occur. A sensitive period represents a time that is conducive to specific learning or experiences. The most sensitive period of development in cats is from birth to three to four months of age.

In an attempt to simplify terminology, this author will use the same terms that were used to define the

Table 3.10 Developmental periods and life stages of cats.

Period	Duration
Prenatal	Up to birth
Neonatal	Birth to 9–14 days
Transitional	~10 to 21 days
Socialization	2 to 7–10 wk
Juvenile	~2 mo to sexual maturity (~4–10 mo)
Adolescent	Sexual maturity to social maturity (~2–4 yr)
Adult	Social maturity to 11 yr
Senior	11–14 yr
Geriatric	Life expectancy (~15 yr) to death

canine developmental periods of life and apply these periods and life stages to cats. Obvious differences will be the demarcation of age for specific stages and developmental milestones specific to the species.

Although ages will be used to define a period, these are only guidelines. Each individual will develop at slightly different rates (Table 3.10).

Prenatal

The prenatal period occurs *in utero* and ends at birth. The nutritional, emotional, and physical status of the queen will have a profound impact on the development of the fetuses. Stress in the queen during pregnancy, whether nutritional, physical, or emotional, can have a profound impact on the developing fetuses. The environment can negatively affect the developing fetuses when the pregnant mother experiences prolonged fear, anxiety, or stress. Stress hormones secreted by the mother will cross the placenta and affect the offspring. Chronic stress and poor nutrition of the queen can affect not only the physical development but also the psychological development of the kittens.

A malnourished queen (both prenatally and during lactation) is more likely to have kittens with poor learning abilities, poor social skills with other cats, and increased emotionality, including abnormal levels of fear and aggression (Turner and Bateson 2000).

- A malnourished queen (both prenatally and during lactation) is more likely to have kittens with poor learning abilities, poor social skills with other cats, and increased emotionality, including abnormal levels of fear and aggression.

Neonatal

The neonatal period is from birth to about 9–14 days of age. The kittens are completely dependent on the queen for survival: nursing, thermoregulation, and elimination. Time is spent sleeping and nursing. Although cats are born with tactile, olfactory, gustatory, and vestibular abilities (ability to right themselves), they are blind and mostly deaf. Consequently, they are fairly insulated from the world during this period. The most developed senses are associated with smell and taste for suckling. Kittens are able to smell *in utero*, and food preferences of the mother may influence the preferences of offspring.

Maternal nutrition and quality of milk influence the developmental rate of the kittens and deficits can produce lifelong deficiencies.

In contrast, mild stressors including gentle handling of the kittens or placing them on a cool surface for a few seconds, may have beneficial effects. A study with Siamese kittens revealed kittens that were held and stroked gently for a brief time every day during the first few weeks of life, opened their eyes earlier, left the nest sooner, and developed color points faster (Meier 1961). Mild neonatal stress can produce beneficial effects including decreased emotionality and increased resistance to some diseases. Sensory stimulation involving tactile, thermal, and olfactory senses should begin at birth.

- Mild stressors including gentle handling of the kittens or placing them on a cool surface for a few seconds, may have beneficial effects. Sensory stimulation involving tactile, thermal, and olfactory senses should begin at birth.

Transitional

The transition or transitional period overlaps with the neonatal and socialization periods. This period of development in cats is somewhat variable and it overlaps the neonatal and socialization period. In cats the period begins at 10 to 14 days and ends at 2 to 3 weeks of age. The transitional stage is a transition from complete reliance on the mother to the beginning of independence. The transitional period readies kittens for the socialization period and continued sensory development. The transitional period is important because it is a time of rapid neurological changes influencing mobility and sensory perception. The eyes open around 7–10 days (range 2 to 16 days). The ears begin to open by five days with a response to loud sounds noted at that time. By two weeks of age, kittens will orient toward natural sounds (Olmstead and Villablanca 1980). The teeth begin to erupt just before two weeks of age. At around two weeks they begin to walk unsteadily and by three weeks, can walk. Also, at around three weeks of age, the kitten is better able to regulate its body temperature and can eliminate voluntarily. Thermoregulation is fully developed by seven weeks of age (Turner and Bateson 2000).

Because of the developing senses and increased mobility, kittens become more aware of their surroundings and begin to interact more with stimuli (Figure 3.11).

Socialization

The socialization period lasts from 2 to 7 weeks of age and perhaps up to 10 weeks. This period is marked by decreasing reliance on the queen for survival and increased interaction with social and environmental stimuli. The socialization period is the most important sensitive period in the cat in regard to living in the human domestic household. It is a time when social learning is enhanced, and social experiences have a strong influence on future behavior. The cat is primed to be able to bond with a variety of species through this time. Positive social experiences with other species allow the cat to become socialized and more accepting of those species throughout its lifetime. Although not impossible after this sensitive period, socialization is more difficult and less effective. Handling prior to two weeks of age does not have an effect on acceptance of humans. However, handling by humans after two weeks and before seven weeks of age produces cats that are more responsive to people than those that were not handled (Beaver 2003). If during the socialization period, kittens are gently handled by multiple people rather than just one person, they will be less fearful of people.

According to *Domestic Animal Behavior for Veterinarians and Animal Scientists* (Houpt 2018, p. 172), "A litter of kittens isolated for the first month will be reluctant to approach people even if they are genetically friendly. Handling for 15 minutes per day from two to six weeks will result in friendly kittens." Interestingly, a study also found that if kittens were handled for less than 30 minutes twice a week between five and eight weeks, it did not increase their friendliness (Reisner et al. 1994). Based on numerous studies, it is suggested kittens should be handled in a gentle way by as many people as possible for a minimum of five minutes a day from two to seven weeks of age and there is a benefit to continuing up to 14 weeks of age (Peterson and Kutzler 2011). It has been suggested that kittens' responses to being handled by an unfamiliar person are stable from eight weeks of age up to three years of age (Lowe and Bradshaw 2002).

- The socialization period is the most important sensitive period in the cat in regard to living in the human domestic household.

- If during the socialization period, kittens are gently handled by multiple people rather than just one person, they will be less fearful of people.

Three to six weeks of age is the most influential time in regard to intraspecies (cat–cat) social development (Overall 1992). Early weaning (before five weeks of age) and removal from the litter will cause inadequate socialization with other cats. Possible behavioral consequences to early weaning include over-attachment to humans, self-mutilation, lack of bite or claw inhibition, abnormal mating or maternal behavior, timidity, and fearfulness with or without aggression (Beaver 2003). Social play with littermates is prevalent at four weeks of age and continues throughout the socialization period.

- Possible behavioral consequences to early weaning include over-attachment to humans, self-mutilation, lack of bite or claw inhibition, abnormal mating or maternal behavior, timidity, and fearfulness with or without aggression.

During the socialization period, kittens begin to eat solid food by 4 weeks of age and are completely weaned by 7–10 weeks. Starting around three weeks and cumulating at five to six weeks, kittens are able to voluntarily eliminate, thus no longer being dependent on the queen for stimulation. By six to eight weeks of age, kittens will display an adult-like response to threatening social stimuli

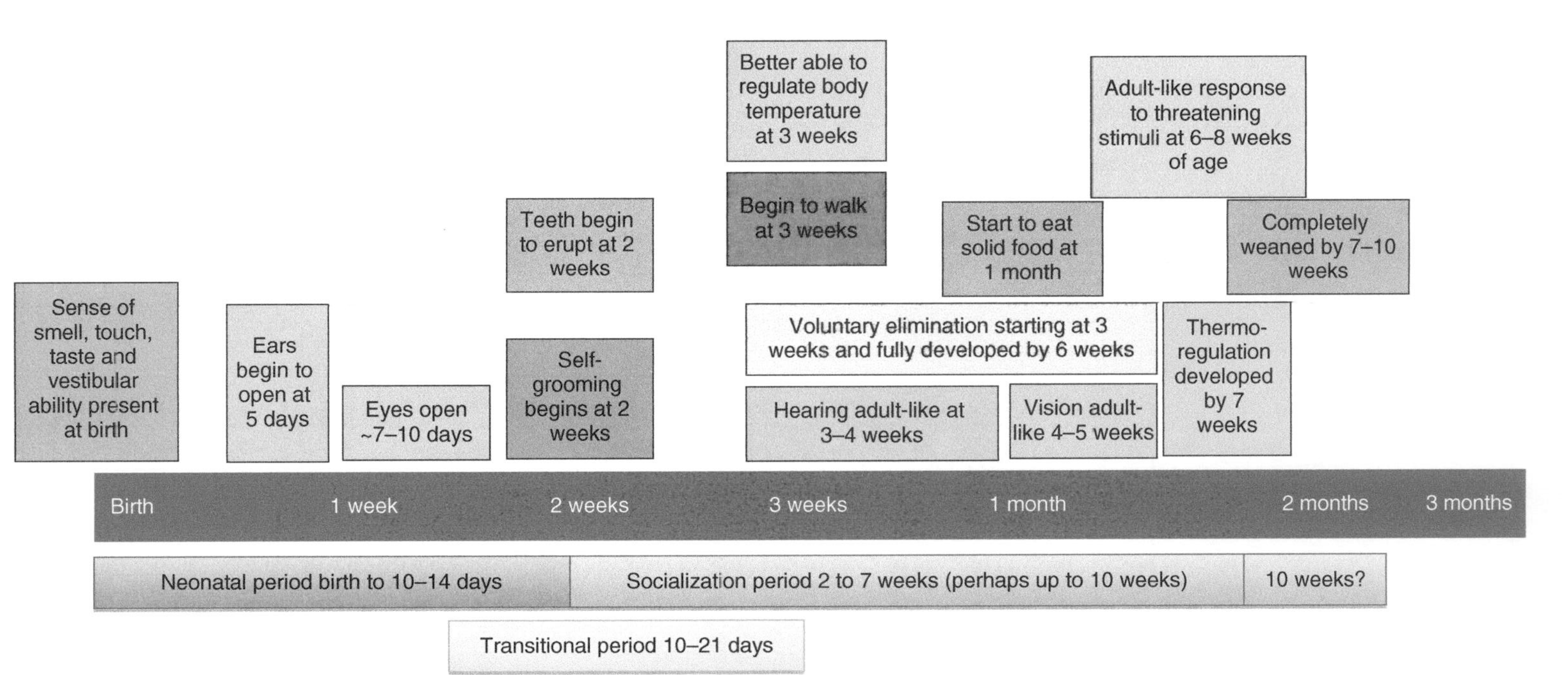

Figure 3.11 Developmental changes in the first three months of life.

(Kolb and Nonneman 1975). The end of this period is marked by the development of a fear response. See Figure 3.11 for a summary of developmental milestones during the first three months of life.

Juvenile

The juvenile stage is approximately from 2 months to sexual maturity (average 4–10 months of age). During this stage, object play becomes more prevalent and social play begins to slowly decrease by 12–14 weeks of age (West 1974). Perhaps this is in part due to the need to develop fluent hunting skills in a free-range setting. Thus, the cat is perhaps genetically programmed to evolve in this manner for survival. Dexterity and motor skills are perfected during this stage. Proper and appropriate play with objects and wand toys can minimize the likelihood of human-directed aggression associated with play.

Dr. Bonnie Beaver notes a normal period of human avoidance occurring around seven weeks of age. Even kittens that have been socialized well with humans will show avoidance. However, the well-socialized kitten will rebound around 10 weeks of age and no longer display avoidance (Beaver 2003).

Positive social and environmental experiences are important during the juvenile period and beyond. Stopping positive socialization experiences after 14 weeks of age will result in cats regressing in regard to their social skills and comfort level in novel situations.

Through the juvenile and into the adolescence stage, cats become less accepting of unfamiliar cats. Integration of a new cat into a household after a cat has reached sexual maturity can be more challenging. The bond between the cats may not be as strong if they were not introduced as young kittens. The end of this period is recognized by reaching sexual maturity.

Adolescence

The adolescence stage occurs from sexual maturity to social maturity. Social maturity is probably reached around two to four years of age (Overall 2013). During adolescence, the cat continues to develop independence and males will often disperse from the colony.

Adolescence and sexual maturity are a common time for relinquishment of cats because of associated behavior problems. Adolescent felines living in the human household will require sufficient mental and physical activity through environmental enrichment. Positive-based training not only provides enrichment and is fun but also enhances the human–animal bond (Figure 3.12a, b).

Adult

The adult stage is defined as commencing around social maturity and concluding around 11 years of age or at about 25% of the cat's life expectancy. The adult period coincides with social maturity and possible changes in cat-to-cat relationships. Cats may become less playful and therefore less accepting of unfamiliar members of their species.

Moderate physical exercise, social play with humans, and mental stimulation in the form of exploration and positive-reinforcement training are important for maintaining optimal behavioral and physical health.

Senior and geriatric

The senior stage for cats begins at the last 25% of life expectancy for the species and ends with death or the geriatric stage, which is life expectancy and beyond. For cats, the senior stage begins around 11 years of age and ends at 14 years of age, which is life expectancy. The geriatric stage begins at life expectancy and continues beyond life expectancy until the death of the individual.

Special care should be taken to ensure that a harmonious relationship continues between the aging cat and the owners. Identifying and addressing medical issues that may have an impact on behavior help to maintain a strong human–animal bond. It might be necessary to educate clients that cats with mobility issues due to osteoarthritis may find a tall litter box located down a flight of stairs too difficult to navigate. Identifying and treating pain conditions is imperative for the emotional and physical welfare of aging cats. Screening should occur at each visit and the owners should be educated on the signs of pain in cats. It is estimated that 90% of cats over the age of 12 years are affected by osteoarthritis (Hardie et al. 2002). Cats might display difficulty with jumping up or down, climbing up or down stairs, chasing moving objects, or running.

Cognition issues in aging cats can lead to changes in sleep–wake cycles, excessive vocalization, pacing or restlessness, anxiety, and elimination outside of the litter box. Detecting early signs of cognitive dysfunction and providing early treatment may help to alleviate signs and slow the progression. The risk of clinical signs increases with age, so cats should be

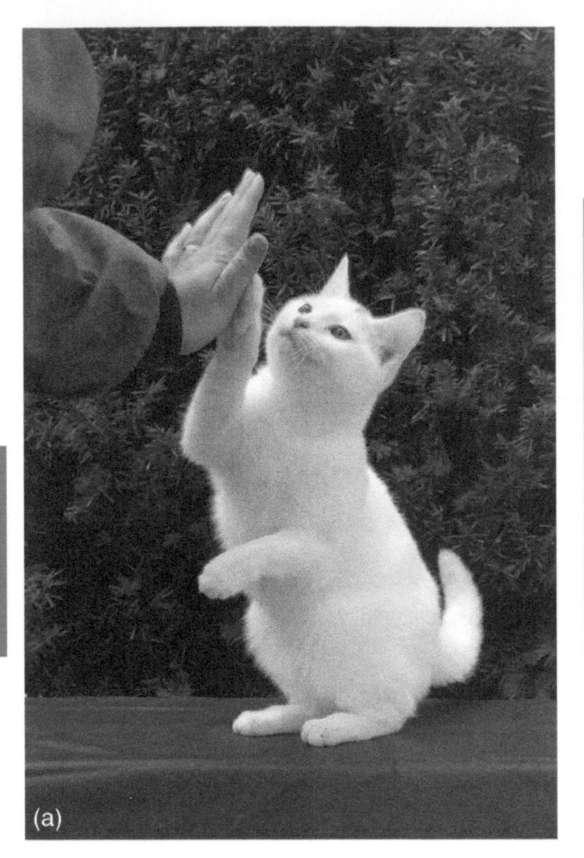

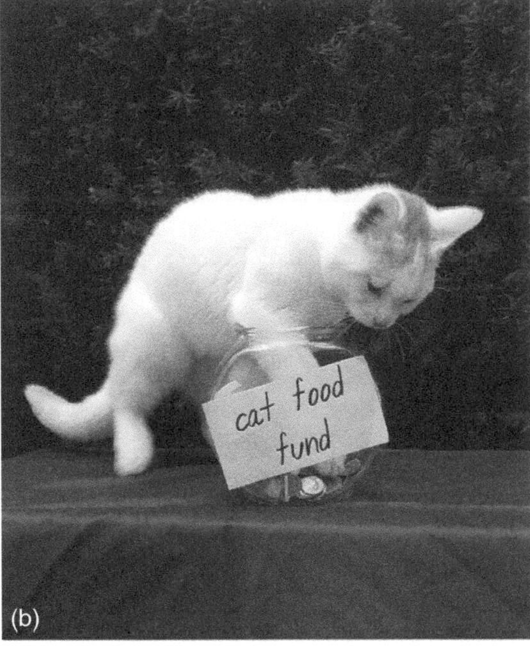

Figure 3.12 (a) and (b) Examples of behaviors a young cat has been trained to perform using positive reinforcement. *Source*: Courtesy of M. Heigl.

screened for the condition at least annually. Early identification and treatment are recommended.

Senior and geriatric cats may benefit from daily mental and physical stimulation in the form of moderate exercise and training. Mental and physical stimulation may delay signs of dementia and improve behavioral and physiological wellness. Positive-reinforcement training can help to keep older pets socially engaged with their humans. Schedule interactive play sessions tailored to the activity level of the cat.

Conclusion

The domestic feline is an adaptive animal that can live in groups or solitarily, depending on early experience. Cats have a complex communication system involving visual, auditory, and olfactory communication. Colonies of cats are generally comprised of females and their young. Cats are not accepting of unfamiliar cats and will protect their core territory.

As you will learn in Chapter 7, the veterinary technician can play a pivotal role in the prevention of behavior problems and disorders. Through a thorough understanding of normal development, sensory perception, social behavior, and innate behavior for a species, the veterinary behavior technician can empower others with this knowledge. Knowledge provides understanding and empathy and creates a client who is more likely to implement changes to help the cat be successful, improve the cat's welfare, and maintain the human–animal bond.

- Knowledge provides understanding and empathy and creates a client who is more likely to implement changes to help the cat be successful, improve the cat's welfare, and maintain the human–animal bond.

Additional resources

Differences in cat breeds: https://www.psychologytoday.com/us/blog/the-modern-heart/202006/cat-breeds-and-their-personalities-according-research

Epigenetics: https://www.cdc.gov/genomics/disease/epigenetics.htm

Feline Grimace Scale: https://www.felinegrimacescale.com

Fear Free Happy Homes Cat Body Language 101 video: https://www.fearfreehappyhomes.com/video/cat-body-language-101

Guidelines for housing cats in a household: https://purrfectlove.net/how-many-cats-is-too-many

Pheromone and V1R information: https://www.ncbi.nlm.nih.gov/books/NBK200993; https://www.ncbi.nlm.nih.gov/pmc/articles/PMC4310675

Whiskers: https://fearfreehappyhomes.com/face-talk-what-your-cats-whiskers-tell-you-about-his-mood

The Humane Society of the United States (2010). Cat chat: understanding feline language, February 5, 2010. https://napahumane.org/wp-content/uploads/2017/07/Cat-Chat.pdf (accessed November 3, 2022).

Video 3.1 This video is muted so you focus on the cat's body language. Note the following body language: tail swinging and flicking back and forth, licking lips, turning head, ears neutral or slightly forward, the pupils are normal dilation, whiskers neutral, twitching of the skin over the lower spine and rump.

Based on the body language indicators what might the cat be attempting to communicate? The tail certainly was saying "I am highly aroused" but the rest of the body seemed relatively neutral. However, the cat did not initiate interaction with the person filming and actually turned his back to her. More information is needed to ascertain the cat's interest.

Video 3.2 Here is another short-muted video of the same cat just a few seconds later. Notice the tip of tail moves, then the entire tail wags, ears go to the side and back, and the cat turns his head away from the camera.

The cat started to wag his tail, ears went to the side and back, and he turned away from the camera in response to the videographer talking to the cat and passively encouraging interaction.

Based on the body language this cat was indicating please leave him alone as he was not interested in interacting at the time.

Video 3.3 This video was taken in front of the author's house. The grey cat was owned by neighbors about a block away. The cat was a frequent visitor to the house and sought out attention from people. However, she was seen giving chase to many small dogs and cats throughout years of observing her. Watch this short interaction between the grey cat and the unfamiliar orange tabby. Prior to filming this interaction, an attempt to interrupt the interactions with food distractions was unsuccessful. The orange cat eventually left the area without a physical altercation with the grey cat. Watch this video as many times as you like while noting the differences in body language.

The grey cat displays more offensive behavior. Note the following: rump raised (0:15), direct approach but then would slow and turn to the side to avoid confrontation. Ears forward (0:15), tip of tail wags, tail held out then dropped down. Vocalization-Growling/Yowling.

The orange cat displays more defensive and fear related behaviors. At 0:06 in the video his ears are to the side and back. The tail is curled close to the body and the body is turned sideways. The pupils are partially dilated. At 0:15 in the video he is moving slowly and hunched in the rear. He avoids eye contact, stops, turns sideways, sits with the tail close to his body and ears back while yowling (0:46).

References

Banks, M. S., Sprague, W.W., Jürgen, S., et al. (2015). Why do animal eyes have pupils of different shapes? *Science Advances* 1 (7): https://doi.org/10.1126/sciadv.1500391.

Barry, K.J. and Crowell-Davis, S.L. (1999). Gender differences in the social behavior of the neutered indoor-only domestic cat. *Applied Animal Behaviour Science* 64 (3): 193–211.

Beaver, B.V. (2003). *Feline Behavior: A Guide for Veterinarians*, 2e. Philadelphia: W. B. Saunders Company.

Bennett, V., Gourkow, N., and Mills, D.S. (2017). Facial correlates of emotional behaviour in the domestic cat (*Felis catus*). *Behavioural Processes* 141 (Pt 3): 342–350.

Bergsma, D.R. and Brown, K.S. (1971). White fur, blue eyes, and deafness in the domestic cat. *Journal of Heredity* 62: 171–185.

Berkley, M.A. (1976). Cat visual psychophysics: neural correlates and comparisons with man. *Progress in Psychobiology and Physiological Psychology* 6: 63–119.

Bernstein, P.L. (2000). People petting cats: a complex interaction. Abstracts of the Animal Behaviour Society, Annual Conference, Atlanta, GA, USA, 9.

Bernstein, P.L. (2006). Behavior of single cats and groups in the home. *Consultations in Feline Internal Medicine* 2006: 675–685.

Bernstein, P.L. and Strack, M. (1996). A game of cat and house: spatial patterns and behavior of 14 cats (*Felis catus*) in the home. *Anthrozoös* 9: 25–39.

Bradshaw, J.W.S. (1992). *The Behaviour of the Domestic Cat*. Wallingford: CABI Publishing.

Bradshaw, J.W.S. and Hall, S.L. (1999). Affiliative behaviour of related and unrelated pairs of cats in catteries: a preliminary report. *Applied Animal Behaviour Science* 63 (3): 251–255.

Bradshaw, J.W.S., Neville, P.F., and Sawyer, D. (1997). Factors affecting pica in the domestic cat. *Applied Animal Behaviour Science* 52: 373–379.

Clark, D.L. and Clark, R.A. (2016). Neutral point testing of color vision in the domestic cat. *Experimental Eye Research* 153: 23–26. https://doi.org/10.1016/j.exer.2016.10.002.

Clutton-Brock, J. (1987). *A Natural History of Domesticated Mammals*. Cambridge, and the British Museum (Natural History), London: Cambridge University Press.

Clutton-Brock, T.H. (1989). Review Lecture: Mammalian mating systems. *Proceedings of the Royal Society of London. Series B, Biological Sciences* 236 (1285): 339–372.

Cooper, L.L. (1997). Feline inappropriate elimination. *The Veterinary Clinics of North America Small Animal Practice* 27 (3): 569–600.

Crowell-Davis, S.L., Curtis, T.M., and Knowles, R.J. (2004). Social organization in the cat: a modern understanding. *Journal of Feline Medicine and Surgery* 6: 19–28.

Curtis, T.M., Knowles, R.J., and Crowell-Davis, S.L. (2003). Influence of familiarity and relatedness on proximity/allogrooming in domestic cats (*Felis catus*). *American Journal of Veterinary Research* 64 (9): 1151–1154.

Dantas, L. (2018). Vertical or horizontal? Diagnosing and treating cats who urinate outside the box. *Veterinary Clinics of North America: Small Animal Practice* 48 (3): 403–417.

Douglas, R.H. and Jeffery, G. (2014). The spectral transmission of ocular media suggests ultraviolet sensitivity is widespread among mammals. *Proceedings of the Royal Society B: Biological Sciences. Royal Society Publishing: Proceedings B* 281 (1780): 20132995.

Dulac, C. and Axel, R. (1995). A novel family of genes encoding putative pheromone receptors in mammals. *Cell* 83: 195–206.

Eckstein, R.A. and Hart, B.L. (2000). The organization and control of grooming in cats. *Applied Animal Behaviour Science* 68 (2): 131–140.

Evangelista, M.C., Watanabe, R., Leung, V.S.Y. et al. (2019). Facial expressions of pain in cats: the development and validation of a feline grimace scale. *Scientific Reports* 9: 19128.

Finco, D.R., Adams, D.D., Crowell, W.A. et al. (1986). Food and water intake and urine composition in cats: influence of continuous versus periodic feeding. *American Journal of Veterinary Research* 47 (7): 1638–1642.

Halip, J.W., Luescher, U.A., and McKeown, D.B. (1992). Inappropriate elimination in cats, part 1. *Feline Practice* 20 (3): 17–21.

Hardie, E.M., Roe, S.C., and Martin, F.R. (2002). Radiographic evidence of degenerative joint disease in geriatric cats: 100 cases (1994–1997). *Journal of the American Veterinary Medical Association* 220: 628–632.

Hart, B.L. (1976). The role of grooming activity. *Feline Practice* 6 (4): 14, 16.

Hart, B.L. and Cooper, L. (1984). Factors relating to urine spraying and fighting in prepubertally gonadectomized cats. *Journal of the American Veterinary Medical Association* 184 (10): 1255–1258.

Heffner, R.S. and Heffner, H.E. (1985). Hearing range of the domestic cat. *Hearing Research* 19 (1): 85–88. https://doi.org/10.1016/0378-5955(85)90100-5.

Houpt, K.A. (2018). *Domestic Animal Behavior for Veterinarians and Animal Scientists*. Hoboken: John Wiley & Sons, Incorporated.

Hullar, I., Fekete, S., Andrasofszky, E. et al. (2001). Factors influencing the food preference of cats. *Journal of Animal Physiology and Animal Nutrition* 85 (7–8): 205–211.

Karsh, E. (1984). Factors influencing the socialization of cats to people. In: *The Pet Connection: Its Influence on Our Health and Quality of Life* (ed. R.K. Anderson, B.L. Hart and L.A. Hart), 207–215. Minneapolis: University of Minnesota Press.

Knowles, R.J., Curtis, T.M., and Crowell-Davis, S.L. (2004). Correlation of dominance as determined by agonistic interactions with feeding order in cats. *American Journal of Veterinary Research* 65 (11): 1548–1556.

Kolb, B. and Nonneman, A.J. (1975). The development of social responsiveness in kittens. *Animal Behaviour* 23: 368–374.

Li, X., Li, W., Wang, H. et al. (2006). Cats lack a sweet taste receptor. *The Journal of Nutrition* 136 (7): 1932S–1934S. https://doi.org/10.1093/jn/136.7.1932S.

Liberg, O. and Sandell, M. (1988). Spatial organisation and reproductive tactics in the domestic cat and other felids. In: *The Domestic Cat: The Biology of its Behaviour* (ed. D.C. Turner and P. Bateson), 83–98. Cambridge: Cambridge University Press.

Lowe, S.E. and Bradshaw, J.W.S. (2002). Responses of pet cats to being held by an unfamiliar person, from weaning to three years of age. *Anthrozoös* 15 (1): 69–79.

Macdonald, D.W. and Yamaguchi, N. (2000). Group-living in the domestic cat: its sociobiology and epidemiology. In: *The Domestic Cat: The Biology of its Behaviour*, 2e (ed. D. Turner and P. Bateson), 96–118. Cambridge: Cambridge University Press.

Mahlow, J.C. and Slater, M.R. (1996). Current issues in the control of stray and feral cats. *Journal of the American Veterinary Medical Association* 209 (12): 2016–2020.

Mair, I.W.S. (1973). Hereditary deafness in the white cat. *Acta Oto-Laryngologica* (Suppl. 314): 1–48.

Marder, A. (1997). Managing behavioural problems in puppies and kittens. *Friskies Pet Care Symposium Small Animal Behavior Proceedings* 15–24.

Meier, G.W. (1961). Infantile handling and development in Siamese kittens. *Journal of Comparative Physiology and Psychology* 54: 284–286.

Olmstead, C.E. and Villablanca, J.R. (1980). Development of behavioral audition in the kitten. *Physiology and Behavior* 24: 705–712.

Olson, P.N. and Johnston, S.D. (1993). New developments in small animal population control. *Journal of the American Veterinary Medical Association* 202 (6): 904–909.

Overall, K.L. (1992). Preventing behavior problems: early prevention and recognition in puppies and kittens. *Purina Specialty Review* 13–29.

Overall, K.L. (2013). *Manual of Clinical Behavioral Medicine for Dogs and Cats*, 3e. St. Louis, MO: Elsevier.

Pannaman, R. (1981). Behavior and ecology of free-ranging female farm cats (*Felis catus* L.). *Zeitschrift für Tierpsychologie* 56: 59–73.

Peters, G. and Tonkin-Leyhausen, B.A. (1999). Evolution of acoustic communication signals of mammals: friendly close-range vocalizations in Felidae (Carnivora). *Journal of Mammalian Evolution* 6: 129–159.

Peterson, M.E. and Kutzler, M.A. (2011). *Small Animal Pediatrics: The First 12 Months of Life*. Saunders/Elsevier.

Qureshi, A., Zeeshan Memon, M., Vazquez, G., and Suri, M.F. (2009). Cat ownership and the risk of fatal cardiovascular diseases. Results from the second national health and nutrition examination study. Mortality follow-up study. *Journal of Vascular and Interventional Neurology* 2 (1): 132–135.

Reisner, I.R., Houpt, K.A., Hollis, N.E., and Quimby, F.W. (1994). Friendliness to humans and defensive aggression in cats: the influence of handling and paternity. *Physiology and Behavior* 55 (6): 1119–1124.

Rieger, G. and Turner, D.C. (1999). How depressive moods affect the behaviour of singly living persons toward their cats. *Anthrozoös* 12 (4): 224–233.

Saito, A. and Shinozuka, K. (2013). Vocal recognition of owners by domestic cats (*Felis catus*). *Animal Cognition* 16: 685–690.

Salman, M.D., Hutchison, J., Buch-Gallie, R. et al. (2000). Behavioral reasons for relinquishment of dogs and cats to 12 shelters. *Journal of Applied Animal Welfare Science* 3 (2): 93–106.

Salonen, M., Vapalahti, K., Tiira, K. et al. (2019). Breed differences of heritable behaviour traits in cats. *Scientific Reports* 9: 1–10.

Schötz, S., van de Weijer, J., and Eklund, R. (2019). Melody matters: an acoustic study of domestic cat meows in six contexts and four mental states. In: *Proceedings of VIHAR 2019; August 29–30, 2019, London, UK*.

Soennichsen, S. and Chamove, A.S. (2002). Responses of cats to petting by humans. *Anthrozoös* 15: 258–265.

Stanton, L.A., Sullivan, M.S., and Fazio, J.M. (2015). A standardized ethogram for the Felidae: a tool for behavioral researchers. *Applied Animal Behaviour Science* 173: 3–16.

Tavernier, C., Ahmed, S., Houpt, K.A., and Yeon, S.C. (2020). Feline vocal communication. *Journal of Veterinary Science* 21 (1): e18.

Turner, D.C. (1991). The ethology of the human–cat relationship. *Swiss Archive for Veterinary Medicine* 133: 63–70.

Turner, D.C. (2000). Human–cat interactions: relationships with, and breed differences between, non-pedigree, Persian and Siamese cats. In: *Companion Animals and Us: Exploring the Relationships Between People & Pets* (ed. A.L. Podberscek, E.S. Paul and J.A. Serpell), 257–271. Cambridge: Cambridge University Press.

Turner, D.C. and Bateson, P. (2000). *The Domestic Cat: The Biology of its Behaviour*, 2e. Cambridge: Cambridge University Press.

Turner, D.C. and Rieger, G. (2001). Singly living people and their cats: a study of human mood and subsequent behavior. *Anthrozoös* 14 (1): 38–46.

Turner, D.C., Rieger, G., and Gygax, L. (2003). Spouses and cats and their effects on human mood. *Anthrozoös* 16 (3): 213–228.

Villablanca, J.R. and Olmstead, C.E. (1979). Neurological development in kittens. *Developmental Psychobiology* 12: 101–127.

Vitale, K.R. and Udell, M.A. (2019). The quality of being sociable: the influence of human attentional state, population, and human familiarity on domestic cat sociability. *Behavioural Processes* 158: 11–17.

Vogt, A.H., Rodan, I., Brown, M. et al. (2010). AAFP-AAHA: feline life stage guidelines. *Journal of Feline Medicine and Surgery* 12: 43. https://doi.org/10.1016/j.jfms.2009.12.006.

West, M. (1974). Social play in the domestic cat. *American Zoologist* 14: 427–436.

The PowerPoint of figures, appendices, MCQ's, cited videos are available at www.wiley.com/go/martin/behavior

4 The human–animal bond – a brief look at its richness and complexities

Julie K. Shaw[1] and Sarah Lahrman[2]
[1]Julie Shaw Consulting, Lafayette, IN, USA
[2]Purdue Comparative Oncology Program, Purdue University, West Lafayette, IN, USA

The celebration, protection and nurturing of the human–animal bond is veterinary medicine's North Star. It is the reason our profession exists and thrives and is trusted and admired. Veterinary practice must be a blend of science and soul. Successful veterinarians [veterinary technicians] know that the human–animal bond is the fuel that powers the emotional side of our profession. The bond allows us to thrive and not just survive in the greatest profession on earth.

Marty Becker, DVM and author, as quoted from the mission and vision statement of the Association of Human–Animal Bond Veterinarians.

CHAPTER MENU

The human–animal bond (HAB) was defined in a statement from the American Veterinary Medical Association in 1998 as

> A mutually beneficial and dynamic relationship between people and other animals that is influenced by behaviors that are essential to the health and well-being of both. This includes but is not limited to, emotional, psychological, and physical interactions of people, other animals, and the environment.
>
> The veterinarian's [veterinary technician's] role in the human–animal bond is to maximize the potentials of this relationship between people and other animals.
>
> (Statement from the Committee on the Human–Animal Bond in JAVMA vol. 212, No. 11, p. 1675, June 1, 1998)

The primary aim of veterinary behavioral medicine is to strengthen and protect the HAB while allowing both the human and the animal to live a high-quality life. The strength of the HAB is directly related to the animal's behavior (Sherman and Serpell 2008). A well-behaved animal improves people's lives by improving their general health and sense of well-being (Serpell 1995). Animal behavioral problems place enormous stress on the HAB and are often the reason for the pet's relinquishment (Patronek et al. 1996).

Veterinary technicians are in the ideal position to support pet owners in building a strong HAB by assisting them to choose the best pet for their lifestyle during pet-selection counseling (see Chapter 7)

Canine and Feline Behavior for Veterinary Technicians and Nurses, Second Edition. Edited by Debbie Martin and Julie K. Shaw.

Companion website: www.wiley.com/go/martin/behavior

and continuing to strengthen the bond through problem-prevention strategies, including puppy and kitten classes (Chapter 7). The primary goal of developing and strengthening the HAB must stay in the forefront of our minds, especially when very difficult situations arise, including removal of a pet from a home or euthanasia for a behavioral disorder. The veterinary technician can support the client during such times by assisting the grief process, continuing to promote, support, and protect the HAB (see section titled **Grief counseling** in Chapter 5). The ultimate goal of companion animal behavior is to promote, support, and protect the human–animal bond. That must never be forgotten.

- The ultimate goal of companion animal behavior is to promote, support, and protect the human–animal bond. That must never be forgotten.

Julie Shaw, RVT, VTS (Behavior)

The HAB past, present, and future

An animal was first distinguished as a pet when it was begun to be seen as "humanized." Three characteristics occurred to elevate an animal to the "pet" category: it was allowed in the house, given a name, and not eaten (Levi-Strauss 1966).

The concept of a special connection between animals and people (the HAB) was met with significant resistance when it was presented by Dr. Leo K. Bustad in the 1980s. His first attempts to bring the HAB to the forefront were met with scorn, disbelief (Hines 2003), and skepticism. Initially, the veterinary field was also disbelieving of his ideas.

The pioneers of the HAB movement campaigned and with the assistance of the media, provided research for their theories. Working with veterinary medicine, the media, conferences, and publications, the special bond noted between a pet and its owner became widely accepted by society (Hines 2003). Research on the health benefits of animals began in the 1960s. The majority of research focused on the effects of animals on human health, cardiac benefits, alerts of health emergencies, and the health of the elderly and children (Hering 2008). Further studies came to similar conclusions reporting that people with some type of animal exposure typically had lower blood pressure and decreased stress levels (Pachana et al. 2011; Siegel et al. 2011).

Let's look at a brief history of the human–animal bond and the research regarding health benefits. Humans, throughout history, have always shared a special connection with animals. Only the time from when the relationship may be considered mutually beneficial can be debated. Prior to the domestication of animals, human cultures around the world have shared various spiritual and religious connections with animals, with some animals even revered as sacred. That relationship has evolved from the time of species domestication. Our relationship has grown from more intensive human–animal interaction, from a time when animals were used primarily for food and utilitarian purposes on the farm to the companions living in our homes today.

In the late 1970s and early 1980s in Scotland, the concept of the "human–animal bond" was used by Konrad Lorenz and Boris Levinson. The first study published in a medical journal, which reported benefits to human cardiovascular health, occurred in 1980. In that study, pet owners experienced an increased one-year survival after discharge from a coronary care unit (Friedmann et al. 1980). In 1983, the term "human–animal bond" was popularized by veterinarian, Leo K. Bustad. Dr. Bustad delivered a summary lecture on the human–pet relationship at the International Symposium in Vienna.

In the 1990s, a study reported that pet owners had slightly lower systolic blood pressures, plasma cholesterol, and triglyceride values than non-pet owners (Anderson et al. 1992). A National Institute of Health Clinical Trial found that dog ownership lowers anxiety and provides human social support, which are associated with an increased likelihood of one-year survival after a myocardial infarction (Friedmann and Thomas 1995).

In the 2000s, studies found that oxytocin levels in the brain are increased by human–animal interaction (Miller et al. 2009; Odendaal 2000; Odendaal and Meintjes 2003). Studies also demonstrated that decreases in blood pressure occur in both dogs and humans, in addition to neurophysiological changes, such as increased levels of beta endorphin, oxytocin, prolactin, dopamine, and phenylacetic acid were affected (Odendaal 2000; Odendaal and Lehmann 2000; Odendaal and Meintjes 2003).

In the 2010s, research indicated the presence of a therapy dog reduces pain and improves mood or levels of satisfaction in medical facilities (Harper et al. 2014; Marcus et al. 2013). The reduction of subjective psychological stress (fear, anxiety) due to animal contact, as well as the dampening of physiological stress parameters in connection with activation of the oxytocinergic system represent a core mechanism in explaining many of the positive effects of human–animal interaction (Beetz et al. 2012). An economic study on the human health-care cost savings associated with pet ownership found $11.7 billion in savings as a result of pet ownership (Clower and Neaves 2015).

Now we will take a look at the science behind the human–animal bond. The benefits of human–animal interaction are neurochemical. Oxytocin levels in the brain are increased by human–animal interaction (Miller et al. 2009; Odendaal 2000; Odendaal and Meintjes 2003). Oxytocin promotes maternal care in mammals and plays a role in emotional bonding, social behavior, and stress relief. Human–animal interaction is related to positive changes in physiological variables both in humans and animals, in particular dogs. Benefits include decreases in heart rate and blood pressure, decreases in cortisol, and increases in hormones correlated with well-being such as oxytocin, beta endorphin, prolactin, phenylacetic acid, and dopamine (Pop et al. 2014; Odendaal and Meintjes 2003). Scientific evidence suggests that positive social interactions with pets are good for our health (Box 4.1).

BOX 4.1: HUMAN–ANIMAL INTERACTION HAS THE FOLLOWING BENEFITS

- Improves cardiovascular health and reduces obesity (lowers blood pressure, increases physical activity, reduces stress, and improves cardiovascular recovery)
- Prevents allergy and strengthens immune responses
- Improves quality of life in cancer patients (reduces stress and anxiety)
- Improves pain perception
- Reduces the number of doctor visits
- Improves children's physical, social, emotional and cognitive development
- Improves social behavior and interaction in sufferers of autism
- Improves quality of life in sufferers of Alzheimer's/dementia (reduces aggression, agitation and depression, improves nutrition and social behavior)
- Improves mental health (reduces stress and anxiety, provides social support, reduces loneliness, improves mood and reduces symptoms of depression)
- Improves quality of life and workplace wellness
- Improves recovery from trauma and alleviates signs of PTSD

(Source: Adapted from Human Animal Bond Research Institute n.d.; https://habri.org/research)

Well-documented animal effects on humans include medical, or mental health benefits for: social attention, social behavior, interpersonal interactions, and mood; stress-related parameters such as cortisol, heart rate, and blood pressure; self-reported fear and anxiety; and mental and physical health, especially cardiovascular diseases (Beetz et al. 2012). Limited evidence exists for: reduction of stress-related parameters such as epinephrine and norepinephrine; improvement of immune system functioning and pain management; increased trustworthiness of and trust toward other persons; reduced aggression; enhanced empathy and improved learning (Beetz et al. 2012).

The HAB is the reason why billions of US dollars are spent on pets annually. See Box 4.2 for examples of evidence of pets' special relationship with humans. Let's look at actual sales spent on pets within the US market. This is a steadily increasing number from $55.7 billion in 2013, $69.5 billion in 2017, and $123.6 billion in 2021.

- Food: $50.0 billion
- Veterinary care and product sales: $34.3 billion
- Supplies, live animals, and over-the-counter medicine: $29.8 billion
- Other services: $9.5 billion (Other services include boarding, grooming, insurance, training, pet sitting and walking and all services outside of veterinary care)

Source: American Pet Products Association. U.S. Pet Industry Market Size and Ownership Statistics. Available online at: https://www.americanpetproducts.org/press_industrytrends.asp (accessed June 10, 2022).

Future US census reports may include questions pertaining to family pets, allowing exploration of subtle positive effects of animals on the family unit (Beck and Katcher 2003). Future data may indicate that the HAB is growing in strength because of an increase in life expectancy (Miniño 2011), people marrying later in life (Census 2010), choosing to not have children, or to have children later in life (Livingston 2010). The role of veterinary medicine will likely change and increase in scope as the HAB continues to advance. The mental and emotional health of pets must become a routine component of the animal's holistic treatment. Pet insurance companies may play a more prominent role in our profession and begin to readily include behavioral health, including prevention such as puppy and kitten classes, into their insurance policies.

It is certain the HAB will continue to gain strength and depth as companion animals continue to fill the

BOX 4.2: THE FOLLOWING ARE EXAMPLES THAT MAY BE TAKEN AS EVIDENCE OF A PET'S SPECIAL RELATIONSHIP WITH A HUMAN

- Pets may have human names and/or special nicknames. We name our pets after special people and many pets have many alternate and cute nicknames.
- Pets may have their own theme song or online presence. We give pets their own online identity on social media or even their own website. Some pet owners have theme songs for their pets that reflect the pet's individual personality.
- People travel with their pets and spend time incorporating them into their daily lives. At the very least, our pets are with us when we rise in the morning, and some accompany us when we go to bed. They often even share our beds.
- We purchase vehicles and homes with our pets in mind. We make sure there is room in the car for the family dog and/or his crate. We look for homes with a sunroom for the cat and a large, fenced backyard for the dog to run, play, and stay safe.
- We dress our pets in clothing, sometimes ours or their very own clothes.
- We celebrate their birthdays with cakes and parties. We purchase gifts for pets on holidays because we want them to feel special. It makes us feel good to do so. (Figure 4.1)
- We share our food with our pets and provide them with special meals. The word *companion* is derived from the Latin word "com", meaning "together," and "panis" – another Latin word, meaning "bread."
- We spend large amounts of money on their routine health and daily care. For some of us, our pets are our "children."

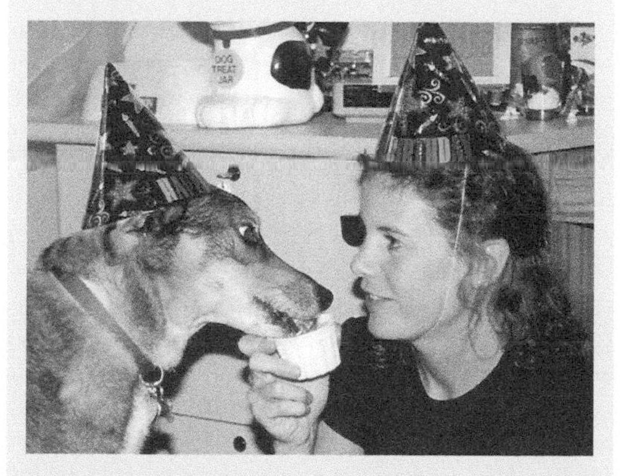

Figure 4.1 Evidence of the human–animal bond; celebrating the dog's birthday.

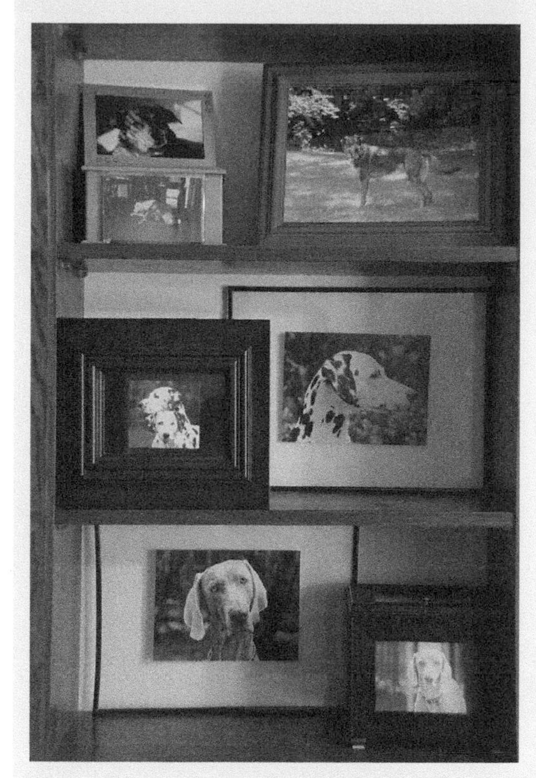

Figure 4.2 Further evidence of the human–animal bond; memorial wall of deceased pets.

- We treat them when they have veterinary emergencies and major illnesses. We do what we can to try to save them.
- We care about their emotional well-being and behavior. We educate and train them and don't want them to experience fear, anxiety, or stress. We want them to have a good quality of life and to enjoy themselves.
- We grieve over their loss similar to and sometimes more than the passing of a close family member or friend.
- We remember and honor our deceased pets with cemeteries, crematories, and memorials. (Figure 4.2)

voids that we sometimes feel as humans. Veterinary medicine must be prepared to meet the expanded needs that are required to support the HAB.

- The mental and emotional health of pets must become a routine component of the animal's holistic treatment.

The veterinary team's role in behavioral medicine is to strengthen and protect the special relationship between people and their animals, thereby improving the quality of life for human and animal alike.

Medical health and mental health are inseparable with each directly affecting the other.

The emotional well-being of companion animals is important; fear, anxiety, and aggression can be symptoms of compromised welfare and they most certainly can negatively affect the human and animal relationship.

- The veterinary team's role in behavioral medicine is to strengthen and protect the special relationship between people and their animals, thereby improving the quality of life for human and animal alike.

The HAB during the COVID-19 pandemic

Pets often provide their humans profound emotional support and distraction (requiring the pet guardian to focus on the pet's care and routine) in the face of disasters (hurricanes, fires, floods, earthquakes, etc.) and events that result in a drastic change in life circumstances (divorce, death of a spouse or family member, loss of job, war, etc.). Usually, these events are either a personal experience or a local phenomenon. However, in 2020 when the SARS-CoV-2 virus resulted in the COVID-19 pandemic, we saw the effects of a disaster/drastic change in life circumstances on a global scale.

The resulting lockdowns and work from home orders, creating an extended period of social isolation for many people. Survey results from several studies indicate that people with pets had significantly higher levels of mental well-being during the pandemic and that pets provided a social connection decreasing the sense of isolation and loneliness (Ng et al. 2021; Grajfoner et al. 2021; Bussolari et al. 2021).

Social isolation can lead to loneliness and boredom and can be a risk factor for physical and mental health issues. Our connection with pets can be strong, even stronger than human connection, and has been shown to positively affect human physical and mental health problems as well as decrease isolation and loneliness (Bussolari et al. 2021).

With pet guardians being home and spending more time with their pets during the pandemic, there is concern that as people begin to spend more time away from home, pets might have a difficult time adjusting to less contact with their people.

The changes to our relationships with our pets that have occurred and that will remain post pandemic are yet to be determined. It is clear human beings have realized to an even greater degree the importance of the HAB.

Special bonds – Animal-assisted interventions

Animal-assisted interventions (AAI) are broadly defined as any intervention that included an animal in the process (Kruger and Serpell 2010). AAI include animal-assisted therapy (AAT), animal-assisted activities (AAA), and assistance (service) animals (O'Haire et al. 2015a).

Animal-assisted therapy

The earliest animal-assisted therapy (AAT) programs dated back to 1790 in England, where companion animals were used to treat mental health patients. During World War II, soldiers with mental and emotional trauma worked on farms at the hospital as therapy (Hering 2008). Today, animals are being integrated into hospitals, nursing homes, and schools. When animals are brought into these settings, those involved feel more at home, and some normalcy is brought into their lives (Butler 2004).

AAT describes therapy involving an animal, with specific therapeutic goals for the patient and measured progress reports. For instance, during the AAT, asking a patient to throw a ball to an animal to retrieve to improve the patient's range of motion. Animal-assisted activities (AAA) are more spontaneous activities without specific patient treatment goals (Walsh 2009; Kruger and Serpell 2010; O'Haire et al. 2015a).Children with autism spectrum disorder have demonstrated increased social behaviors toward their peers and received more social approaches from their peers when an animal was present versus when a toy was present (O'Haire et al. 2013). Animals may act as a social buffer conferring unique anxiolytic effects on children with autism (O'Haire et al. 2015b).

Animals to be used in an AAA/AAT program should be qualified through programs such as Therapy Dogs International, Inc. (TDI) or Pet Partners. Qualifying organizations evaluate both the handler and the animal for suitability for therapy work. AAA/AAT benefits the

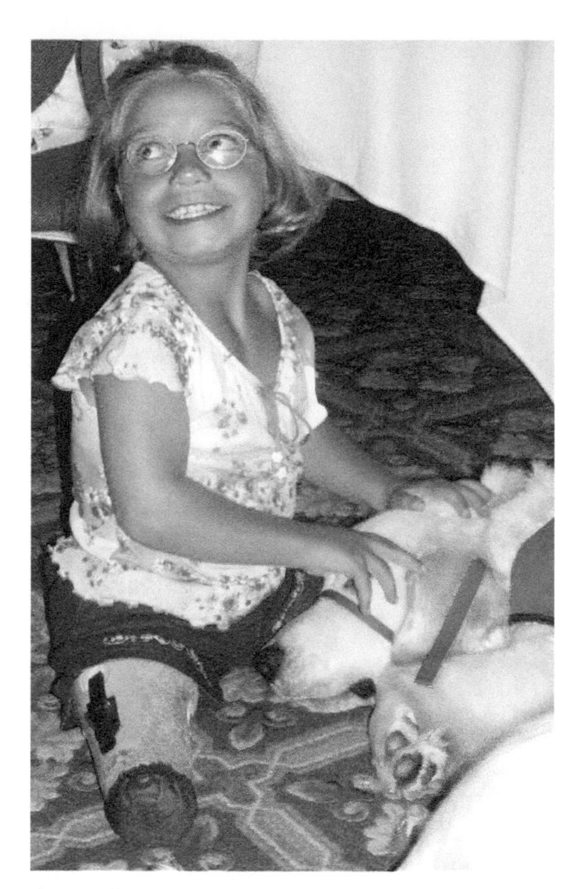

Figure 4.3 AAA/AAT benefits the handler, the animal, the facility staff, and the patient.

handler, the animal, the facility staff, and, most importantly, the patient (Figure 4.3) (Ensminger 2010).

The use of AAA/AAT will continue to proliferate in our most innovative schools, prisons, and community programs (Walsh 2009), and research data from such programs will continue to define the benefits of AAT.

Assistance (service) dogs

An assistance animal is any animal that performs tasks for the benefit of a person with a disability. On March 15, 2011, the Department of Justice published revised final regulations to the Americans with Disabilities Act (ADA.gov 2011), clarifying and refining issues that arose over the last 20 years pertaining to the use of assistance (service) animals. The term "assistance animal" is a broad term, whereas the ADA defines "service animals" as dogs that are individually trained to perform work or perform tasks for people with a disability. Examples of such work include guiding people who are blind, alerting people who are deaf, pulling a wheelchair, alerting and protecting a person who is having a seizure, reminding a person with mental illness to take prescribed medications, calming a person with post-traumatic stress disorder during an anxiety attack, or performing other duties (ADA.gov 2011). "Other duties" may include alerting to a diabetic crisis or assisting a child with autism. Dogs whose sole function is to provide comfort or emotional support do not qualify as service animals under the current revised ADA.

The ADA includes only dogs as service animals, although a new, separate provision pertaining to miniature horses has been included. Miniature horses are most often used in guide work because of their long life expectancy. Entities covered by the ADA must modify their policies to permit miniature horses where reasonable.

When it is not obvious what service the animal provides, only two questions may be asked by the staff: is this dog a service animal required because of a disability? What work or task has the dog been trained to perform? Questions pertaining to the person's disability, requirement of medical or training documentation, or a request for demonstration of the ability of the animal to perform work are not allowed and are prohibited by law.

The clarification and change to the ADA pertaining to service animals are a testament to the growing value of the HAB. There is no doubt these highly trained animals benefit their challenged partners in a multitude of ways. To quote one child on the death of his service dog, "It is like losing a Mom, a best-friend and an arm all at the same time." (Quote from Dylan Shaw, who used a service dog from the age of 3–18 years) (Figures 4.4 and 4.5).

Difficult to understand relationships

It would be easy and more palatable to focus only on the most common and acceptable human–animal relationships as described previously. As veterinary technicians, we should also be able to detect potential situations in which animals and/or people might be at risk. By educating ourselves in these areas we may be able to take steps toward preventing such relationships from occurring.

Motives for animal abuse

Possibly, the most difficult to understand and the largest distortion of the human–animal relationship is animal abuse or cruelty. Animal cruelty can be

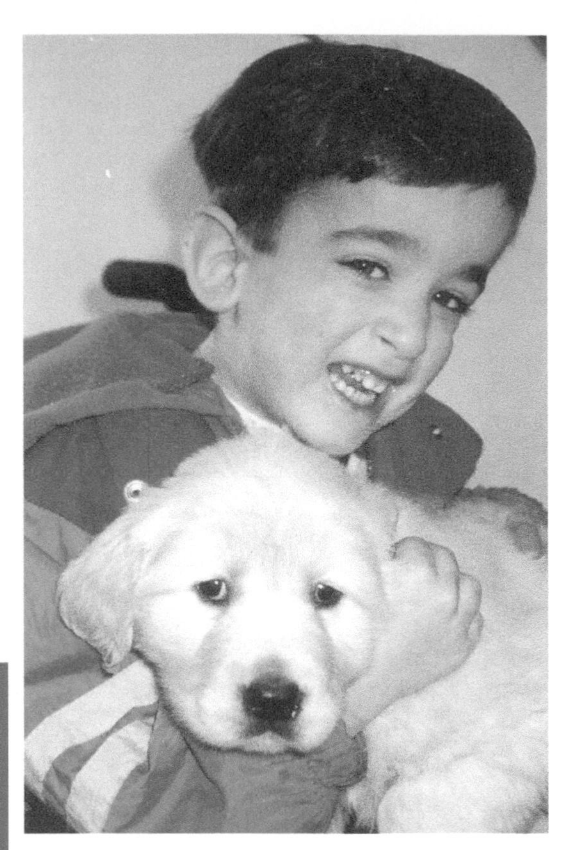

Figure 4.4 Dylan Shaw (aged three years) with his first service dog "Faith" (aged eight weeks).

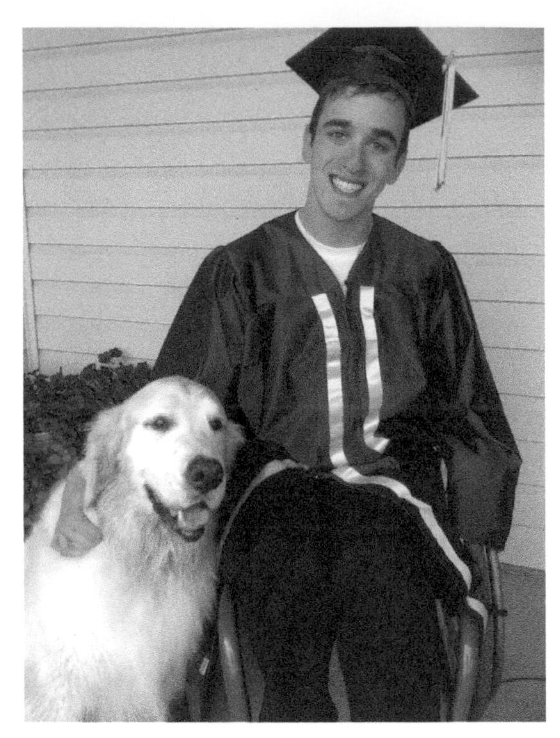

Figure 4.5 Dylan Shaw (aged 19 years) with his second service dog "Hero" (aged 10 years).

somewhat a subjective judgment, but in this chapter, it is defined as willful infliction of pain, injury, or harm on a nonhuman animal (Kellert and Felthous 1985).

Kellert and Felthous determined motivations for animal cruelty among criminals and noncriminals during their childhoods. It should be noted that motives are usually multidimensional, with multiple motives occurring. The following nine motivation categories were identified in their research:

1. To control or gain compliance from the animal. Excessive use of violence or punishment to shape an animal's behavior.
2. To retaliate against the animal for a previous infraction. Taking obvious delight in excessively punishing a "wrong" behavior, such as digging in the garden.
3. To satisfy a prejudice against the animal or species. Designating groups of animals as "good" or "bad," such as all cats are evil. This type of prejudice is often culturally related.
4. To express aggression through the animal. Using cruelty or violence in an attempt to "make the animal mean" or to "toughen it up." This motivation is often seen in the dogfighting culture.
5. To enhance one's own aggression. Some subjects in the study described "practicing" their techniques on animals before attempting aggression on humans or to impress others (e.g. friends or gang members).
6. To shock for amusement, usually in an attempt to "be funny" to gain attention.
7. To retaliate against another person. This is a technique often used in spousal abuse cases to control the spouse. The abuser threatens to hurt the animal if their demands are not followed (Faver and Strand 2003). National and state surveys of domestic violence victims consistently find that as many as 71% of battered women report that their male partners had threatened to or had, in fact, harmed or killed their pets (Randour and Hardiman 2007). An early study found that there was animal abuse in 88% of families who were under state supervision for the physical abuse of their children (DeViney 1983). Animals may be used by

perpetrators to coerce children into silence by threatening to harm the animal (Davidson 1998).

8. Displacement of hostility from a person to an animal. An example of this is a person, driven by frustration or aggression toward a "feared" authority figure, hurts an animal "to get even" with the authority figure. One study stated two out of five children who were bullied and victimized at school performed some type of cruelty toward an animal to let out their frustration and anger. A study by Baldry indicated that children who lived in a home in which violence against a parent, themselves, or an animal occurred were three times more likely to abuse animals. Whether the cruelty to animals occurred because of displacement or because violence was normalized is not known (Baldry 2005).

   One of the earliest reported symptoms of childhood conduct disorder is cruelty to animals (Frick and Paul 1993). Conduct disorder in children refers to a group of behavioral and emotional problems, including great difficulty following rules and behaving in a socially acceptable way. Other children, adults, and social agencies unfortunately, view them as "bad" or delinquent, rather than mentally ill (AACAP 2004). Children who are cruel to animals are also more likely to exhibit more severe conduct disorder problems than other children (Luk et al. 1999).

9. Nonspecific sadism. A desire to inflict injury, suffering, and death without provocation, with the primary goal of gaining pleasure from the act. Sadism is often used to compensate a person's feeling of weakness (Kellert and Felthous 1985; Perez-Merz et al. 2001).

On January 1, 2016, the Federal Bureau of Investigation (FBI) began tracking crimes against animals via the National Incident-Based Reporting System (NIBRS), listing animal cruelty crimes as Group A offenses – the same category as arson, rape, and murder. The NIBRS database will now include all animal cruelty cases investigated by participating law enforcement agencies, which will fall under four categories: gross neglect, torture, organized abuse (such as dogfighting and cockfighting), and sexual abuse (bestiality).

Dogfighting

The Humane Society of the United States estimates that there are at least 40 000 dogfighters in America, although that number seems to underestimate the street-fighting epidemic in urban areas (Gibson 2005). Dogfighters are violent criminals who engage in a multitude of peripheral criminal activities, including organized crime, racketeering, drug distribution, and gang activity (Gibson 2005; Randour and Hardiman 2007). Dogfighting is a cunning and insidious type of underground, organized crime and is an incredible source of income for gangs and drug trafficking (Gibson 2005).

Children – The other victims

The atrocities seen in dogfighting environments appall seasoned law enforcement officials, yet children who grow up in a dogfighting lifestyle believe violence is normal. Over time, their exposure causes them to be calloused to suffering and desensitized to criminalization.

The routine exposure of the children to animal abuse and neglect is a major contributing factor for those children to later develop social deviance. Children between the ages of 8 and 10 years living in neighborhoods with strong gang activity can be found holding their own fights or as spectators at fights that are being held. Dogfighting is a desensitization tool for young gang members. Gene Mueller, DVM and past President of the Anti-Cruelty Society in Chicago, Illinois said, "You want to find the perfect way to desensitize a kid so he'll kill that anonymous gangbanger from three blocks over? Give him a puppy and let him raise it. Then let him kill it. I guarantee that will desensitize that kid" (Gibson 2005). Young gang members are often required to kill their own losing dog to regain lost respect (Blazina et al. 2011).

As children become desensitized to violence, the cycle is perpetuated and passed on to another generation.

The "dogmen"

Dogmen are individuals who fight their pit bulls against others in "matches" (Evans and Forsynth 1998).

A study by the Society of Animals determined five major characteristics dogmen use to justify dogfighting.

1. Denial that the dogs are victims. Dogmen believe their dogs "like" to fight and denying them the opportunity would be cruel. They rationalize the dog does not have to fight, it chooses to, therefore it cannot be a victim.
2. Denial of responsibility. Dogmen interviewed believed they were not hurting anyone and there

was no harm in the "sport." They compared themselves to being a "coach" to an athlete.

3. Denial of injury. Many dogmen contest their dogs are well taken care of before and after the fight and what happens in the ring is pleasurable to the dog.
4. Appeal to higher loyalties. Dogfighters contend their "sport" dates back to the eighteenth century and was attended by European aristocracy. They argue they are not criminals but "good people." They compare dogfighting laws to being "penalized for jaywalking."
5. Condemnation of the condemners. Dogmen believe dogfighting is a cultural tradition and they are being prevented from practicing their tradition, in turn causing "cultural genocide." They believe they are "normal folks" who are different in some ways and try to rationalize their behavior as reasonable if not conventional. They believe the animal humane organizations are extremist and are causing their dogs to suffer by not allowing them to fight (Evans and Forsynth 1998; Evans et al. 1998; Gibson 2005).

It is rare that fighting dogs will be seen in a veterinary hospital for fear of arrest, but characteristics to be aware of are pattern of bite wounds on head, neck, and legs (Patronek 1997).

Animal hoarders

By definition, an animal hoarder is a person who continues to obtain animals (usually one species) without providing the proper care for the animals already present, ignoring the deteriorating environment and denying there is a problem present (Patronek and Nathanson 2009).

Animal hoarders frequently believe themselves to be rescues or "no kill" shelters and often live isolated or secretive lives. When questions or concerns are raised, they may become defensive. It is estimated that there are approximately 600–2000 cases reported each year, with 60% being repeat offenders. Hoarders are most commonly female, middle aged to older, and live alone. Male hoarders often live in homes with their families (frequently multigenerational) (Arluke and Killeen 2009; Patronek and Nathanson 2009).

Although hoarders are represented as criminals in the media, research of those affected by the disorder has found many hoarders develop symptoms of personality disorders, delusions, dementia, addiction, attachment disorder, control issues, and obsessive–compulsive disorder. Animal hoarders perceive themselves as animal caregivers, suggesting animal hoarding is largely an egosyntonic disorder (Patronek and Nathanson 2009).

Animal hoarding can be brought on by difficult childhood experiences (i.e. absent parents, several relocations, divorce, etc.). Other traumas have included loss of a stabilizing adult relationship, a serious health crisis, or loss of a major bodily function. It has also been noted that persons with personality traits suggesting self-regulatory defects may be at a greater risk for complicated grief (pathological grief), with symptoms resembling post-traumatic stress disorder and often associated with extreme fear of abandonment. Hoarders appear to become enmeshed in a grief that incorporates animals as a method of healing (Patronek and Nathanson 2009). Those affected with this condition see animals as the one stable factor in their lives (Vaca-Guzman and Arluke 2005; Arluke and Killeen 2009).

State laws require pet owners to provide sufficient food and water, a sanitary environment, and the minimal necessary veterinary care. Animal hoarding cases often end in the euthanasia of multiple animals because of the lack of these requirements and the condition of the animals when the hoarders are discovered. Hoarders often do not recognize they are living in an unhealthy environment that includes excrement in the living space. Indifference to the squalor and animal suffering appears to indicate a severe lack of insight indicative of disassociation (Patronek and Nathanson 2009).

Most counseling for animal hoarding is not patient initiated but rather court ordered and therefore has low compliance. Treatment is difficult with many complicating factors, including impairments of cognition, lack of insight, poor abstract thinking, difficulty understanding cause and effect, poor problem-solving skills, and difficulty organizing and completing a task. Exaggerated perception of threat, hypervigilance, and distrust of authoritative figures makes developing a therapeutic relationship difficult. It is challenging for them to relate to another person when animals have been their primary relationship (Patronek and Nathanson 2009).

Client characteristics to be aware of include clients who bring in multiple pets at different times and seem to have a large number of animals. Clients may request a medication for a pet the veterinarian has no record of seeing (i.e. ear medications or antibiotics), and animals may smell of urine and feces (Arluke and Killeen 2009). Watch for a lack of continuity of care for individual animals, office visits for trauma, and preventable contagious and parasitic diseases may be common. The client may request heroic efforts for a newly acquired pet with a poor prognosis and may visit many different veterinary hospitals.

In such cases of neglect, it is often productive to educate rather than condemn. When possible, framing discussions on whether the needs of the animal are being met rather than on the "bad" behavior of the owner helps to depersonalize the discussion, allowing the veterinary professional to become an educator and animal advocate rather than passing judgment on a person (Patronek 1997).

Defining healthy versus unhealthy bonds

The relationship we share with our pet is unlike any other relationship in our lives. It has the complexities, challenges, and rewards of a parent–child relationship, teacher–student relationship, and deep friendship.

Defining and developing a healthy HAB

Healthy relationships add to the well-being of everyone in the relationship and should be pervasively positive in their nature. Mutually healthy relationships meet both the human and the pet's psychological, emotional, and physical needs.

The foundation of a healthy human–animal relationship includes respect and trust. Respect develops through consistent clear communication and predictability. Respect of the animal's unique and specific species differences are valued. Appreciating those differences encourages pet owners to be fair in their expectations of the pet. For example, teaching an animal not to drink from the toilet is an easy task to train, but owners need to realize drinking from the toilet is "normal" or innate behavior for the animal.

Trust develops when the relationship is consistent and based on looking for the "good" in the relationship. There is no place for fear, intimidation, or coercion. Anxiety and fear develop when animals, human, or nonhuman cannot predict "what will happen next." There should be a "balance of power" in which mutual goals are met. The ability to exercise some control over the environment is empowering and a primary survival behavior. People and animals should have the ability to remove themselves from a frightening or stressful situation when possible.

BOX 4.3: SIGNS OF AN EMOTIONALLY HEALTHY PET

- ☐ Affectionate without being needy
- ☐ Not overly attention seeking
- ☐ Can be separated from people without undue stress
- ☐ Friendly or at least tolerant to conspecifics, children, family members, and strangers
- ☐ Plays well with others and exhibits impulse control in play
- ☐ Confidence to be inquisitive
- ☐ Not overly fearful of new objects, places, people, or events
- ☐ Rebounds from "scary" events or stimulus
- ☐ Change does not cause undue anxiety or stress

Source: With permission from Suzanne Hetts, PhD and Daniel Q. Estep, PhD and modified from Animal Behavior Associates, Inc., Copyright 2022 All Rights Reserved. For the complete Behavior Wellness Evaluations, see: http://animalbehaviorassociates.com/dog-behavior-wellness-quiz/; https://animalbehaviorassociates.com/cat-behavior-wellness-quiz

Emotionally healthy animals are affectionate without being needy or overly attention seeking (Box 4.3). They can be separated from people without undue stress. They are friendly or at least tolerant of their own species, children, family members, and strangers. They should be able to play well with others and exhibit impulse control during play. They have the confidence to be inquisitive and are not overly fearful of new objects, places, people, or events. An emotionally stable animal will "rebound" quickly from a "scary" event or stimulus. Change does not cause extreme or long-lasting anxiety and stress (McCurnin 2010).

Ironically, emotionally healthy humans share many of the same qualities of emotionally healthy pets, including the ability to deal with stress and bounce back from adversity. They show flexibility to learn new things and adapt to changes in the environment. Emotionally healthy humans are also self-confident, independent, and not overly fearful (http://Helpguide.org 2010).

Potential unhealthy pet relationships

If we accept that animals benefit humans, we must also examine potentials for adverse responses in some populations (Beck and Katcher 2003).

Unhealthy relationships commonly bring out stress and leave a feeling of being "used up" with an overall negative outlook. Signs of an unhealthy relationship include neglecting self-care, routinely giving up activities or relationships that make you happy for the pet's emotional and psychological needs. Feelings of pressure and persistent anxiety when away from the pet may occur. Other signs may include feelings of anxiety "walking on eggshells" and uncertainty of what may happen next. Fear for yourself or others (including other pets) or having a feeling of being unsafe when around your pet is a constant stress. Fear in any relationship is a strong indicator that the relationship is not healthy and a significant sign the HAB has been seriously damaged or broken (see Table 4.1).

Identifying at-risk populations for unhealthy HAB

More research needs to be performed to fully define at-risk populations, but it has been suggested that an over-attachment to animals could decrease bonds to people. Research by Brown and Katcher found people with high levels of pet attachment had a three times greater chance of showing clinical levels of dissociation compared to those with low levels of pet attachment. Dissociation is defined as the inability to integrate various parts of an experience, such as thoughts, feelings, or images into their stream of consciousness (Carlson et al. 1993). People with an already impaired ability to connect with other humans may substitute the connection with animals and therefore lose the human social support system (Brown and Katcher 1997, 2001). High levels of dissociation have been strongly correlated with traumatic experience, including childhood abuse or exposure to combat. It is therefore plausible that a subset of people highly attached to animals may have histories of abuse or trauma. It is speculated that some people with both high pet attachment and high dissociation may be attempting to create a reparative relationship from trauma and find animals a safe, stable, and trusting relationship substitute for a human relationship (Brown and Katcher 1997).

Participants from animal-related professions, including veterinary technicians, had dissociation scores much higher than people from non-animal-related fields. The 113 veterinary technicians in the study had clinical dissociative experiences scale (DES) (Bernstein and Putnam 1986) scores of 22%, which are five times higher than that in the normal population.

Previous research has found no significant personality type or trait to predict attachment to pets. It is possible that until the research by Brown and Katcher, no one had looked at the relationship to trauma and dissociation correlating the HAB. These findings are important as we interact with our

Table 4.1 Pet owner strain related to a pet's behavioral disorder and possible indications of an unhealthy HAB.

Life area	Manifestation of strain
Mental and emotional	□ Stress and a feeling of being "used up" □ Worry or anxiety □ Anger toward your pet □ Fear your pet may hurt you or a loved one □ "Aloneness" and alienation □ Feelings of "hopelessness" when it comes to your pet □ Feelings of "not being able to go on" if your pet were to die
Health	□ Health issues because of stress (weight loss or gain, headaches, etc.) □ Declined self-care □ Decreased energy □ Injury from your pet
Social	□ Embarrassment □ Shame or guilt □ Fear of stigma/social disapproval □ Alienation □ Limit or cease having house guests □ Guilt when socializing outside the home □ Neglected relationships or giving up relationships that make you happy to tend to your pet's psychological and emotional needs □ Fear of being away from your pet □ Giving up hobbies □ Fear of injury to strangers
Financial	□ Distraction during work day □ Financial liability/lawsuits □ Property damage and destruction □ Cost for treatment, medication, training, and so on
Family environment	□ Fear for safety of family members □ Discord with significant other □ Strained relationship with extended family members □ Alienation by extended family

Available as a fillable form in Appendix 7.

Source: Adapted from Mendenhall and Mount 2011; Anon. 2011 *Client Essays*.

clients. Although most attachments may not have an underlying dissociative connection, it is an association that should be at least passively acknowledged. Our clients may be using their attachment to their pet as a bridge to attachments with humans or to avoid human relationships.

- High levels of dissociation have been strongly correlated with traumatic experience, including childhood abuse or exposure to combat. It is therefore plausible that a subset of people highly attached to animals may have histories of abuse or trauma.

Strengthening the HAB and preventing pet relinquishment

Pets with behavioral problems are more likely to be euthanized, abandoned, rehomed, or relinquished to animal shelters (Sherman and Serpell 2008). Nearly 90% of owners report behavioral concerns with their pet, and "behavior problem" is the primary reason cited for relinquishment. In this case, "behavior problem" was not differentiated from a true affective behavioral disorder. Another important reason for relinquishment includes false expectations in regard to the time, effort, and cost of care for a pet.

Characteristics that increase the potential for relinquishment include mixed breeds, unneutered dogs younger than six months, dogs not obtained as puppies, and dogs obtained from shelters at low or no cost.

The National Council on Pet Overpopulation discovered 96% of dogs relinquished to shelters had no proper training (Miller 2001). First-time owners were less likely to give up their pet, whereas men younger than 35 years were more likely to relinquish their pet. Dogs kept for extensive amounts of time in a crate, basement, or garage were at higher risk likely because of a weak owner attachment.

Veterinary care and advice are the most important protective factors. Dogs that were taken to a veterinarian at least once a year were 23 times less likely to be relinquished than those that were not. Dogs were less likely to be surrendered if advice came from a veterinary versus a nonveterinary professional. Surprisingly, dogs given as gifts were at less risk. Those obtained at a high price also had a lower risk factor. Dogs that were allowed in the living area of the home and that received training were also more protected from relinquishment (Salman et al. 1998; Scarlett et al. 1999; Salman et al. 2000; Luescher and Martin 2010).

The risk factors for cat relinquishment differ somewhat from those of dogs. First-time cat owners, intact cats, mixed-breed cats, and cats younger than six months were at a higher risk. Inappropriate expectations and lack of information on cat behavior contributed to relinquishment. Behavioral problems and disorders that increased risk included inappropriate elimination, scratching in unwanted areas, and aggression toward people. Cats that did not visit the veterinarian, were kept in a basement or garage, or had access to the outdoors were at a higher risk to lose their homes. Cats found as strays or acquired with little planning were at less risk, and cats that were declawed and visit their veterinarian were more protected from relinquishment (Salman et al. 1998; Scarlett et al. 1999; Salman et al. 2000; Luescher and Martin 2010). Veterinary technicians play a key role in preventing pet relinquishment by educating clients and building a relationship of trust that will be maintained throughout the pet's life. Pet-selection counseling (detailed in Chapter 7) assists the client in choosing a pet that is appropriate for their lifestyle and desires, although relinquishment has not been associated with lack of planning. Pet-selection counseling is also an educational tool to prevent behavioral problems and disorders from developing by assessing areas of concern or possible inappropriate expectations. New pet-owner counseling can occur immediately after a client obtains a pet and should include a systematic approach that includes the important points for behavior management and problem prevention. Every veterinary visit should include specific questions pertaining to behavioral health (Box 4.4).

- Veterinary technicians play a key role in preventing pet relinquishment by educating clients and building a relationship of trust that will be maintained throughout the pet's life.

The key is prevention when possible and early detection of pet behavior concerns before they have had a detrimental effect on the HAB. Inform pet owners of preventive behavioral services the hospital offers, including training classes and preferred educational sources as soon as possible. Puppy and kitten classes (described in detail in

BOX 4.4: BEHAVIOR-RELATED QUESTIONS A TECHNICIAN SHOULD ASK AT *EVERY* APPOINTMENT

	General behavior health assessment
	Is your pet having accidents in the house?
Is there anything your pet does not "like you to do," for example,	
	Hugging or restraining?
	Touching his/her collar or other body part?
	Brushing, bathing, nail trimming?
	Picking him/her up?
	Removing his/her food bowl or toy?
	Moving him when he/she is sleeping?
	Has your pet growled or hissed at anyone or anything lately?
	Does your pet readily interact with family members?
	Does your pet readily interact with strangers?
	Is there anything your pet seems afraid of?
	Has there been any destruction by your pet?
	How do you stop unwanted behavior?*
What type of training are you using to teach your pet? ◻ Food treats ◻ Clicker training ◻ Choke or pinch collar ◻ Shock	
If there was any behavior you would like to change in your pet, what would it be?	

*Note: This question could be smoothly incorporated into another question, for example: What did you do when you found the destruction? The goal is to determine whether the owner is using punishment and to then educate them on the side effects and give them alternate methods for changing behavior.

Chapter 7) are instrumental in strengthening the HAB. Classes also bond the client to the hospital and the staff. Early education can prevent problems from developing. High-risk puppies or kittens can be identified quickly, and treatment prescribed.

- The key is prevention when possible and early detection of pet behavior concerns before they have had a detrimental effect on the HAB.

All veterinary hospitals should either have a qualified trainer on staff (could also be the veterinary technician) or be associated with a qualified trainer. A qualified trainer is defined as an animal trainer who is certified from a standardized positive-based curriculum and is policed by an organization in which certification can be revoked if the trainer acts unprofessionally or outside the organization's code of ethics (Shaw 2011).

- A qualified trainer is defined as an animal trainer who is certified from a standardized positive-based curriculum and is policed by an organization in which certification can be revoked if the trainer acts unprofessionally or outside the organization's code of ethics.

Training classes (detailed in Chapter 7) should be based on positive training techniques and should not use or encourage punishment. Punishment almost always damages the HAB, has serious side effects (see Chapters 6 and 7), and usually does not work. Classes should be based on clear, concise, and consistent interactions. Classes should teach the client to look for what they want their pet to do, rather than focus on "wrong behavior" or "pack leadership" theories.

With the number of families sharing their homes and lives with pets, veterinary colleges must strive to incorporate and educate students on the importance of animal behavior (Salman et al. 1998). As of 2008, only one-third of veterinary colleges include animal behavior training in their curriculum (Sherman and Serpell 2008).

One survey indicated only 26.8% of graduating veterinary students felt prepared to handle behavior-related cases on "Day 1" of practice. A lack of behavior courses and clinical offerings exists in veterinary colleges and schools (Calder et al. 2017).

An online survey of over 1000 practicing veterinarians found that only 42.8% felt they received a significant amount of training in the field of animal behavior during veterinary school. The majority of survey participants reported participating in post-graduation continuing education sessions about behavior (Kogan et al. 2020). A total of 57.2% indicated they received none or only a few hours of student lectures focused on animal behavior in veterinary school. The vast majority of survey participants reported feeling they did not receive enough behavior or behavior medicine training for canines (90.8%) or felines (92.7%). Despite these results, which validate other studies that veterinary students want more exposure to behavioral medicine, the number of veterinary behavioral medicine programs in the United States veterinary schools is decreasing.

As of 2022, nearly 60% of veterinary teaching hospitals in the United States require or highly encourage Fear Free® education in their curriculums (Fear Free LLC 2022).

The goal for any veterinary professional should be more than just practicing medicine. Focusing on maintaining a healthy relationship and preserving the bond between clients and pets is the key. Clients make a commitment to their pets the day they bring them home. It is of upmost importance that they are educated on normal and abnormal behavior, counseled on appropriate training techniques/modifications, given proper resources, and in some cases, referral to an animal behaviorist. Offering behavioral services shows you value the relationship between pet and client and the importance of preserving the bond (Sherman and Serpell 2008).

Behavioral problems and disorders chip away at the HAB if undetected, inappropriately addressed, or unaddressed. The research clearly shows that pets are less likely to suffer the consequences of relinquishment if up-to-date information from veterinary professionals is provided to pet owners. There may be no other area in veterinary medicine that technicians have such a significant role in keeping pets in their homes than by helping owners develop a strong HAB.

Animals with behavioral disorders and the people who love them

The relationship between a client and a pet with a serious affective behavioral disorder is one that is multidimensional and affects all members of the family unit. In this chapter, "behavioral disorder" is defined as psychological or behavioral patterns outside behavioral "norms" that usually have an affective aspect (Shaw 2011). A "behavior problem" in veterinary medicine is defined as the animal's behavior that causes a problem for the owner. The issues could be lack of training, conditioned unwanted behavior, a behavioral disorder, or a combination of issues. A veterinarian's diagnosis may be required.

- A "behavior problem" in veterinary medicine is defined as the animal's behavior that causes a problem for the owner.
- The issues could be lack of training, conditioned unwanted behavior, a behavioral disorder, or a combination of issues. A veterinarian's diagnosis may be required.
- A "behavioral disorder" is defined as psychological or behavioral patterns outside behavioral "norms" that usually have an affective aspect and require a diagnosis by a veterinarian.

There has been almost nothing written on the intricacies of such a relationship (Buller and Ballantyne 2020). Clients have compared it to living with a child with an emotional disorder, a parent with Alzheimer's disease, or even living in an abusive relationship as a victim. One person wrote, ". . . I expected understanding but was blamed instead of supported. I was accused of being a weak [pet owner] and I endured lots of unwanted and inappropriate advice. These messages came from close friends, family members, [trainers, and veterinary professionals]. The blame and judgment came from so many directions that it was hard to believe they weren't true. On top of this, I felt guilty that I somehow caused my [pet's] condition and I searched for explanations. Did I discipline too hard? Was this genetics? Had there been abuse by someone and I didn't know about it?"

The aforementioned selection was only slightly modified from the book *Raising Troubled Kids* by Margaret Puckette. Ms. Puckette was writing about her child with an emotional disorder. By changing only a few words, the excerpt could easily be the words of a person living with a pet with a behavioral disorder. The references for this section have come from the experts – pet owners who have coexisted and loved an animal with significant and serious behavioral disorders (Anon. 2011).

The stigma

Stigma or stigmatizing occurs when shame and ridicule are placed on someone for breaking a societal "taboo." Stigma is manifested by bias, distrust, prejudgments, fear, embarrassment, and anger, and lead to the stigmatized person having low self-esteem, isolation, and hopelessness. It is a barrier in the treatment of human mental health issues both from the patient and the family's standpoints and similarly felt among pet owners who live with a pet that has a serious behavioral disorder. One pet owner described the stigma she suffered when keeping her aggressive dog, "Family members and neighbors called him 'mean' or 'Cujo'." She reported feeling shameful and embarrassed but also felt guilty if she considered euthanizing him. A prevalent and common thread described by pet owners was a desperation that if "others could only see what he is like with us they would understand." Many felt as though they had caused their pet's disorder by being "bad pet owners" or that they "let their pet down" in some way.

The impact on the pet owner

Caregiver burden has been described as an individual's distress response to the difficulties encountered while providing care for an ill individual (Zarit et al. 1980). The strain of caring for a child with mental illness contributes to caregiver burden (Mendenhall and Mount 2011). Pet owners living with a pet with a significant behavioral disorder have described similar stresses and difficulties (Table 4.1).

Pet guardians caring for animals with behavioral disorders may be affected comparably to people caring for family members with mental illness and chronic illness (Buller and Ballantyne 2020). Research published in 2020 indicated stresses that contributed to caregiver burden specific to animals with behavior disorders included extra time required for management and training, difficulty managing the pet in public or when left alone, increased planning and vigilance required to keep their pet and others safe, cost for behavioral support for the pet and the pet parent being limited on the time they could be away from home (Buller and Ballantyne 2020).

Clients have described feelings of hopelessness in finding help for their pet after being given advice to "not let him get away with that" and to be a stronger "pack leader" only to have such advice cause the pet's issues to worsen. Others were left feeling completely alone when they were told by a family member, friend, neighbor, trainer or veterinarian to "put the animal down" without giving them a diagnosis or explanation for the animal's behavior. They express shock, fear, and anger if they were injured by their pet both because of the injury and because of the emotional strife it caused in their family. Some describe a loss of trust and deep confusion. A common description is that "he is so loving and wonderful 90% of the time. Yet, there were times we were afraid of him. We never knew when his aggression would strike again. We were 'on guard' all of the time and we loved him at the same time." These exceptional pet owners are often willing to dramatically modify their own lives for the well-being of their pet, sometimes to the point it may not be entirely beneficial to their own well-being. One pet owner admits, "The unexpected is our enemy. I do not have my grandchildren spend the night. I rarely have visitors. I have specially built primary and secondary gates to manage any interactions that may occur. While I know of no one who lives in this manner, I have grown accustomed to it so there are no regrets on my choice for him to live out his life as it is today. I only regret the harsh treatment I administered early on without understanding his disorder."

Conclusion

Unfortunately, the mental health field has undervalued the importance of the HAB (Walsh 2009), therefore general mental health professionals may not be prepared to assist pet parents in addressing caregiver burden and other related issues.

As of 2022 a few HAB training programs, such as the Veterinary Social Work program at the University of Tennessee, are becoming available to help increase understanding within the mental health profession about pet guardians' experiences.

Recent research indicates a team-based collaborative approach in caring for pets and their people is needed. This collaborative effort may include mental health professionals with certification in veterinary social work, veterinarians, veterinary behaviorists or certified applied animal behaviorist, veterinary nurses, and trainers to create a collaborative relationship that meets the needs of both pets and the pet parents (Buller and Ballantyne 2020).

The veterinary behavior technician can be a vital part of the support system for clients who live with a pet with a serious behavioral disorder. Pet owners may struggle with conflicting advice from the media, trainers, neighbors, and family members. It is imperative they feel connected and confident with the veterinary behavior technician. It is one of the most personal, intense, and rewarding relationships a veterinary technician will have with a pet owner.

References

AACAP (2004). Conduct disorder, "Facts for families," No. 33.

ADA.gov (2011). 2010 Revised requirements: Service animals. U.S. Department of Justice, Civil Rights Division, Disability Rights Section.

American Pet Products Association (n.d.). U.S. pet industry market size and ownership statistics. https://www.americanpetproducts.org/press_industrytrends.asp (accessed June 10, 2022).

Anderson, W.P., Reid, C.M., and Jennings, G.L. (1992). Pet ownership and risk factors for cardiovascular disease. *Medical Journal of Australia* 157: 298–301.

Anonymous (2011). *Client Essays*. West Lafayette, IN: J. Shaw.

Arluke, A. and Killeen, C. (2009). *Inside Animal Hoarding: The Case of Barbara Erickson*, 167–220. West Lafayette, IN USA: Purdue University Press.

Baldry, A.C. (2005). Animal abuse among preadolescents directly and indirectly victimized at school and at home. *Criminal Behaviour and Mental Health* 15 (2): 97–110.

Beck, A.M. and Katcher, A.H. (2003). Future directions in human–animal bond research. *American Behavioral Scientist* 47 (1): 79–93.

Beetz, A., Uvnäs-Moberg, K., Julius, H., and Kotrschal, K. (2012). Psychosocial and psychophysiological effects of human–animal interactions: the possible role of oxytocin. *Frontiers in Psychology* 3: 234.

Bernstein, E.M. and Putnam, F.W. (1986). Development, reliability, and validity of a dissociation scale. *Journal of Nervous and Mental Disease* 174 (12): 727–735.

Blazina, C., Boyra, G., and Shen-Miller, D. and Springer Link (Online Service) (2011). *The Psychology of the Human–Animal Bond A Resource for Clinicians and Researchers*. New York, NY: Springer Science+Business Media, LLC.

Brown, S.E. and Katcher, A.H. (1997). The contribution of attachment to pets and attachment to nature to dissociation and absorption. *Dissociation* 10 (2): 125–129.

Brown, S. and Katcher, A. (2001). Pet attachment and dissociation. *Society and Animals* 9: 25–42.

Buller, K. and Ballantyne, K. (2020). Living with and loving a pet with behavioral problems: pet owners' experiences. *Journal of Veterinary Behavior.* 37: https://doi.org/10.1016/j.jveb.2020.04.003.

Bussolari, C., Currin-McCulloch, J., Packman, W. et al. (2021). "I couldn't have asked for a better quarantine partner!": experiences with companion dogs during Covid-19. *Animals* 11 (2): 330.

Butler, K. (2004). *Therapy Dogs Today: Their Gifts, Our Obligation*. Norman, Oklahoma, USA: Funpuddle Publishing Associates.

Calder, C.D., Albright, J.D., and Koch, C. (2017). Evaluating graduating veterinary students' perception of preparedness in clinical veterinary behavior for "Day-1" of practice and the factors which influence that perception: a questionnaire-based survey. *Journal of Veterinary Behavior* 20: 116–120.

Carlson, E.B., Putnam, F.W., Ross, C.A. et al. (1993). Validity of the dissociative experience scale in screening for multiple personality disorder: a multicenter study. *American Journal of Psychiatry* 150: 1030–1036.

Clower, T.L. and Neaves, T.T. (2015). The health care cost savings of pet ownership. The Human–Animal Bond Research Initiative (HABRI) Foundation, December 2015.

Davidson, H. (1998). What lawyers and judges should know about the link between child abuse and animal cruelty. *ABA Child Law Practice* 17: 60–63.

DeViney, D.L. (1983). The care of pets within child abusing families. *International Journal for the Study of Animal Problems* 4: 321–329.

Ensminger, J.J. (2010). *Service and Therapy Dogs in American Society*. IL, USA: Charles C. Thomas Publishing.

Evans, R.D. and Forsynth, C.J. (1998). Dogmen: the rationalization of deviance. *Society and Animals: Journal of Human Animal Studies* 6 (3): 203–218.

Evans, R., Gauthler, D.K., and Forsyth, C.J. (1998). Dog fighting: symbolic expression and validation of masculinity. *Sex Roles* 39 (11/12): 825–838.

Faver, C.A. and Strand, E.B. (2003). To leave or to stay?: battered women's concern for vulnerable pets. *Journal of Interpersonal Violence* 18 (12): 1367–1377.

Fear Free LLC (2022). Statistics on Fear free in universities, veterinary practices and professionals. https://fearfreepets.com (accessed June 1, 2022).

Frick Benjamin, B. and Paul, J. (1993). Oppositional defiant disorder and conduct disorder: a meta-analytic review of factor analyses and cross-validation in a clinic sample. *Clinical Psychology Review* 13 (4): 319–340.

Friedmann, E. and Thomas, S.A. (1995). Pet ownership, social support, and one-year survival after acute myocardial infarction in the cardiac arrhythmia suppression trial (CAST). *American Journal of Cardiology* 76: 1213–1217.

Friedmann, E., Katcher, A.H., Lynch, J.J., and Thomas, S.A. (1980). Animal companions and one year survival of patients after discharge from a coronary care unit. *Public Health Reports* 95: 307–312.

Gibson, H. (2005). *Dog Fighting Detailed Discussion*. Animal Legal and Historical Center.

Grajfoner, D., Ke, G.N., and Wong, R. (2021). The effect of pets on human mental health and wellbeing during COVID-19 lockdown in Malaysia. *Animals: An*

Open Access Journal from MDPI 11 (9): 2689. https://doi.org/10.3390/ani11092689.

Harper, C.M., Dong, Y., Thornhill, T.S. et al. (2014). Can therapy dogs improve pain and satisfaction after total joint arthroplasty? A randomized controlled trial. *Clinical Orthopaedics and Related Research* 473 (1): 372–379.

HelpGuide.org (2010). Improving emotional health: strategies and tips for good mental health. https://www.helpguide.org/articles/mental-health/building-better-mental-health.htm (accessed November 4, 2022).

Hering, C. (2008). *Health benefits of companion animals. Health Insights Today: A Service of the Cleveland College Foundation* 1 (2): 1–4.

Hines, L.M. (2003). Historical perspectives on the human animal bond. *American Behavioral Scientist* 47 (1): 7–15.

Kellert, S.R. and Felthous, A.R. (1985). Childhood cruelty toward animals among criminals and non-criminals. *Human Relations* 38 (12): 1113–1129.

Kogan, L.R., Hellyer, P.W., Rishniw, M., and Schoenfeld-Tacher, R. (2020). Veterinary behavior: assessment of veterinarians' training, experience, and comfort level with cases. *Journal of Veterinary Medical Education* 47 (2): 158–169.

Kruger, K.A. and Serpell, J.A. (2010). *Handbook on Animal-Assisted Therapy (Third Edition): Animal-Assisted Interventions in Mental Health: Definitions and Theoretical Foundations*, 33–48. Cambridge, Massachusetts: Academic Press.

Levi-Strauss, C. (1966). Anthropology: its achievements and future. *Nature* 209 (5018): 10–13.

Livingston, G. (2010). *The New Demography of American Motherhood*. Pew Research Center: A Social and Demographic Trends Report.

Luescher, A. and Martin, K.M. (2010). *Dogs! & Cats: Diagnosis and Treatment of Behavior Problems*. West Lafayette: Purdue University.

Luk, E.S.L., Staiger, P.K., Wong, L., and Mathai, J. (1999). Children who are cruel to animals: a revisit. *Australian and New Zealand Journal of Psychiatry* 33 (1): 29–36.

Marcus, D.A., Bernstein, C.D., Constantin, J.M. et al. (2013). Impact of animal-assisted therapy for outpatients with fibromyalgia. *Pain Medicine* 14 (1): 43–51.

McCurnin, D.M. (2010). *Clinical Textbook for Veterinary Technicians*. Philadelphia: Saunders.

Mendenhall, A.N. and Mount, K. (2011). Parents of children with mental illness: exploring the caregiver experience and caregiver-focused interventions. *Families in Society* 92 (2): 183–190.

Miller, P. (2001). *The Power of Positive Dog Training*. New York, NY: Wiley.

Miller, S.C., Kennedy, C.C., DeVoe, D.C., et al. (2009). An examination of changes in oxytocin levels in men and women before and after interaction with a bonded dog. *Anthrozoös* 22 (1): 31–42.

Minino, A.M. (2011). *Death in the United States, 2009. NCHS Data Brief, No. 64*, 2011. Hyattsville, MD: National Center for Health Statistics.

Ng, Z., Griffin, T.C., and Braun, L. (2021). The new status quo: enhancing access to human–animal interactions to alleviate social isolation & loneliness in the time of COVID-19. *Animals* 11 (10): 2769.

Odendaal, J.S.J. (2000). Animal-assisted therapy—magic or medicine? *Journal of Psychosomatic Research* 49 (4): 275–280.

Odendaal, J.S.J. and Lehmann, S.M.C. (2000). The role of phenylethylamine during positive human–dog interaction. *Acta Veterinaria* 69: 183–188.

Odendaal, J.S.J. and Meintjes, R.A. (2003). Neurophysiological correlates of affiliative behaviour between humans and dogs. *The Veterinary Journal* 165 (3): 296–301.

O'Haire, M.E., McKenzie, S.J., Beck, A.M., and Slaughter, V. (2013). Social behaviors increase in children with autism in the presence of animals compared to toys. *PLoS One* 8 (2): e57010.

O'Haire, M.E., Noémie, G., and Kirkham, A. (2015a). Animal-assisted intervention for trauma: a systematic literature review. *Frontiers in Psychology* 6 (1121).

O'Haire, M.E., McKenzie, S.J., Beck, A.M., and Slaughter, V. (2015b). Animals may act as social buffers: skin conductance arousal in children with autism spectrum disorder in a social context. *Developmental Psychobiology* 57 (5): 584–595.

Pachana, N.A., Massavelli, B.M., and Robleda-Gomez, S. (2011). A developmental psychological perspective on the human–animal bond. In: *The Psychology of the Human–Animal Bond* (ed. C. Blazina, G. Boyra and D. Shen-Miller), 151–165. New York: Springer.

Patronek, G.J. (1997). Issues for veterinarians in recognizing and reporting animal neglect and abuse. *Society and Animals* 5 (3): 267–280.

Patronek, G.J. and Nathanson, J.N. (2009). A theoretical perspective to inform assessment and treatment strategies for animal hoarders. *Clinical Psychology Review* 29 (3): 274–281.

Patronek, G.J., Glickman, L.T., Beck, A.M. et al. (1996). Risk factors for relinquishment of dogs to an animal shelter. *Journal of the American Veterinary Medical Association* 209 (3): 572–581.

Perez-Merz, L., Heide, K.M., and Silverman, I.J. (2001). Childhood cruelty to animals and subsequent violence against humans. *International Journal of Offender Therapy and Comparative Criminology* 45 (5): 556.

Pop, D., Rusu, A.S., Pop-Vancia, V. et al. (2014). Physiological effects of human–animal positive interaction in dogs – review of the literature. *Bulletin UASVM Animal Science and Biotechnologies* 71 (2).

Randour, M.L. and Hardiman, T. (2007). Creating synergy for gang prevention: taking a look at animal fighting and gangs. In: *Proceedings of Persistently Safe Schools,* 199. Washington, DC: Hamilton Fish Institute, The George Washington University.

Salman, M.D., New, J.G. Jr., Scarlett, J.M. et al. (1998). Human and animal factors related to relinquishment of dogs and cats in 12 selected animal shelters in the United States. *Journal of Applied Animal Welfare Science* 1 (3): 207–226.

Salman, M.D., Hutchinson, J.M., Ruch-Gallie, R. et al. (2000). Behavioral reasons for relinquishment of dogs and cats to 12 shelters. *Journal of Applied Animal Welfare Science* 3 (2): 93–106.

Scarlett, J.M., Slaman, M., New, J., and Kass, P. (1999). Reasons for relinquishment of companion animals in U.S. animal shelters; selected health and personal issues. *Journal of Applied Animal Welfare Science* 1 (1): 41–57.

Serpell, J. (1995). *The Domestic Dog: Its Evolution, Behaviour, and Interactions with People*. Cambridge, NY: Cambridge University Press.

Shaw, J. (2011). Should you or shouldn't you: when is a veterinarian's diagnosis required. In: *Purdue University Veterinary Fall Conference*. W. Lafayette, IN: Purdue University.

Sherman, B.L. and Serpell, J.A. (2008). Training veterinary students in animal behavior to preserve the human–animal bond. *Journal of Veterinary Medical Education* 35 (4): 496–502.

Siegel, J.M., Blazina, C., Boyra, G., and Shen-Miller, D. (2011). Pet ownership and health. In: *The Psychology of the Human–Animal Bond,* 167–177. New York: Springer.

U.S. Census (2010). United States Census Bureau. https://www.census.gov/ (accessed 28 December 2022).

Vaca-Guzman, M. and Arluke, A. (2005). Normalizing passive cruelty: the excuses and justifications of animal hoarders. *Anthrozoos: A Multidisciplinary Journal of The Interactions of People & Animals* 18 (4): 338–357.

Walsh, F. (2009). Human–animal bonds II: the role of pets in family systems and family therapy. *Family Process* 48 (3): 481–499.

Zarit, S.H., Reever, K.E., and Bach-Peterson, J. (1980). Relatives of the impaired elderly: correlates of feelings of burden. *The Gerontologist* 20 (6): 649–655.

The PowerPoint of figures, appendices, MCQ's are available at www.wiley.com/go/martin/behavior

5 Communication and connecting the animal behavior team

Julie K. Shaw[1] and Lindsey M. Fourez[2]
[1]*Julie Shaw Consulting, Lafayette, IN, USA*
[2]*Purdue Comparative Oncology Program, Purdue University, West Lafayette, IN, USA*

CHAPTER MENU

Characteristics of a strong and empowered animal behavior technician–client–patient relationship begins with a technician who has the ability to communicate knowledge, demonstrate technical skill, and is able to teach in multiple different styles dependent on the style the patient and the client need at any particular moment. The communication relationship is comparable to that of a

Canine and Feline Behavior for Veterinary Technicians and Nurses, Second Edition. Edited by Debbie Martin and Julie K. Shaw.

Companion website: www.wiley.com/go/martin/behavior

nurse–parent–child relationship. The relationship is often laden with high emotion but also reaps deep and long-lasting rewards.

The animal behavior technician must also be able to connect and coordinate the behavior team to work together for the benefit of the pet owner and the pet.

A comparison between marriage and family therapist and the role of the animal behavior technician

Strong commonalities between the counseling aspects of animal behavior therapy and the field of marriage and family therapy (MFT) have been found (Canino et al. 2007).

Four major parallels were found between marriage and family counseling and the role of an animal behavior technician.

(1) One of the most striking similarities between the work of the animal behavior team and emotionally focused marriage and family therapists involves how change occurs in the context of treatment. Both professions seek to change the emotional experience of the clients, although in veterinary behavioral medicine the goal is often to also change the emotional experience of the pet along with that of the pet owners. Couples, for instance, often find themselves in a destructive interaction cycle that repeats itself in times of stress. In comparison, pet owners may have developed a general negativity toward their pet. The content of the problem is irrelevant until a more positive interaction can be developed. For instance, restructuring the emotional process of the owner toward understanding their pet is not directly attempting to get back at them when destruction occurs when left alone, but rather that their pet is having a panic attack that they will not return home. This type of restructuring can dramatically change the emotional experience for the pet owner.

    Assisting the client in developing clear and predictable communication skills and stopping punishment-type techniques can be the foundation for changing the emotional state of the animal.

(2) There are also similarities in the methods for obtaining information from the client. A detailed history, including input from all pertinent family members, is obtained in both disciplines. The idea is predicated on the belief that all people in the family system are affected by the problem, regardless of how individual in nature the problem may appear. It is important to determine if a specific event triggered the call for an appointment and if the current stress is underlying the presenting problem or is only a symptom of it. The simple question of "what triggered you to seek help now?" will often obtain the required information. The answer may be that the pet owners only recently found there were services to assist with their pet's disorder or they may have been a sudden change in their lifestyle, a change in the family dynamics (birth of a child, divorce, etc.), or a more serious incident of the behavior.

(3) Similar difficulties and barriers encountered with clients are found between MFT and veterinary animal behavior. In general, clients enter a therapy room with some level of anxiety about the process they are about to undertake. Frequently, pet owners believe they have "caused" the problem to their pet and feel deep shame or guilt, causing a reluctance to impart information. This fear may come from the concern that they will be blamed or that they may be told to euthanize their pet. In order to build a rapport with clients, the technician must gain their trust. Trust is gained by effectively and genuinely opening up to the client, and in turn, the client begins to feel safe and becomes open. It is helpful if the technician perceives that these concerns may be an issue to directly communicate to the pet owner that you are not going to tell them to euthanize their pet but that you are there to assist them and that withholding information will make it more difficult for you to assist them. Gaining the trust of the pet owner is imperative. At no point is it useful to place blame on the pet owner. They are seeking your help now, and regardless of the information they were given in the past, that should be the focus.

    Asking the client to change how they currently interact with their pet involves significant effort on the part of the client and includes asking them to take a risk into unfamiliar territory. It is critical that the veterinary technician creates a safe, non-judgmental, and positive environment with the owner. The veterinary technician's assistance can be critical for the positive outcome of the case by instructing the owners not only on how they can successfully implement the veterinarian's prescribed treatment plan in their daily lives but also to ensure that the owners understand specifically how the prescribed techniques will modify the pet's behavior. The veterinary technician may feel resistance from the client if the client feels coerced into bringing their pet for treatment. Such situations may occur if the client was given an ultimatum by the legal system, other family member, or another authoritative figure.

Resistance may be exhibited when clients who continually disagree and protest make excuses or show no effort to implement the therapeutic recommendations or terminate treatment prematurely (Egan 2002). This result can occur if the veterinary behavior team places guilt or blame on the client or implies that the owner is the sole cause of the problem (Hetts 1999). Clients who are resistant appear to be those who believe they are not entering into the therapeutic process voluntarily, but resistance can be counteracted by identifying and pointing out areas where their pet is showing fear and anxiety, often without the owner's knowledge. Fear and anxiety on the owner's part can be decreased by giving them choices and input into the creation of the treatment plan, therefore empowering the owner and creating a team effort. In addition, it is helpful to let the clients know that their fears and concerns are normal and to be expected. Letting clients know that you have seen the problem before and that there is treatment is often enough to initiate the process of change.

(4) Presenting problems seen in marriage and family counseling and animal behavior consultations are similar. Anxiety-related behavioral disorders and problems (lack of training or conditioned unwanted behaviors in pets) are the two common problems that seem to cut across the field of animal behavior and MFT. Marriage and family therapists, in particular, report that anxiety and child behavior problems are among the five most commonly seen problems in the therapy room (Northey 2002).

Communication

Communication skills have to be taught, learned, applied, and then adapted to fit one's personal style. When information is inadequately presented to the client, trust is lost, and the client becomes stressed and anxious (Chun et al. 2009).

Nonverbal communication

Just as a veterinary behavior technician must accurately read the body language of their patient, they must also be adept at interpreting that of the pet owner. Eighty percent of communication with another individual is given through nonverbal cues, whereas only 7–20% of the message is actually sent through words (Durrance and Lagoni 1998; Carson 2007).

Often, body language can give direct insight into the status of the human–animal bond (HAB). Observe whether the pet owner leans away from their pet or is constantly reaching to touch the pet.

The technician must then combine what they see in nonverbal with verbal communication to determine if both verbal and nonverbal cues match up. If the pet owner appears open to your suggestions and is sending the correct words and vocal cues, but is standing with arms crossed against the body, a mixed message is sent (Durrance and Lagoni 1998). Attending to both verbal and nonverbal cues is critical to interpreting the full scope of the pet owner's thoughts.

Nonverbal communication includes essentially all forms of communication other than words, such as facial expressions, body postures, tone of voice, eye contact, gestures, and hand movements.

When working with a pet owner, it is important to pick up on closed body language. For example, if the pet owner's arms are crossed against their chest and they are diverting their eyes, most likely they are having feelings of conflict toward what you are saying. Likewise, it is important to be aware of your own body language and the messages you are conveying back to the owner (Durrance and Lagoni 1998).

There will be times when speaking with a client that their nonverbal and verbal communication differs from each other. Research has shown that when words are not compatible with nonverbal cues, the receiver should give more focus to the nonverbal cues. Mixed communication can often be seen when we say things we believe others want to hear. For instance, Ms. Smith might tell you Fluffy has been acting fine, but her body language (tone of voice, lack of eye contact, and slumped posture) speaks quite differently. In this case, dismissing such nonverbal cues may bring about feelings of carelessness and lack of empathy. By noticing a pet owner's mismatched communication, you convey good listening skills and can evoke feelings of trust.

Nonverbal cues can be placed into four categories: kinesics, proxemics, paralanguage, and autonomic shifts. *Kinesics* focuses on body gestures, movement, and position. Facial expressions and touch can also be placed in this group. *Proxemics* pertains to personal space and to how the environment is set up. If the clinic or even the examination room is not welcoming, the client will automatically put up a barrier. *Paralanguage* focuses on how the voice is controlled. This is the category in which the focus is put on the tone, pace, volume, and emphasis. Research shows that when information is given in a soft and slower pace than normal, it will be taken as soothing to the receiver. The last category is *autonomic shifts*. These are items that are out of our control, such as blushing, sweating, or increased breathing. If autonomic shifts occur, the client may be upset, and recovery mode should start immediately. The four categories of nonverbal communication should be used to help determine whether the pet owner feels safe. If a client becomes extremely uncomfortable, they may go into a "fight or flight" agenda (Carson 2007).

If a client starts to go into "fight or flight" mode, damage control should take place quickly. A client in fight mode may have a tense stance, clenched teeth, and fists, and narrow eyes. If a client is entering the flight mode, they will have increased body tension, push, or step back, change in voice volume, increase in breathing rate, and change in facial color. These are the clients who will start to create barriers and hold onto the animal tighter (Carson 2007). If a client starts to go into "fight or flight," the goal is to get them back to a safe place quickly.

Clients can be brought back to the safety zone by perceiving and addressing any mismatched information. Pet owners have often researched their presenting problem on the internet, and there is a chance the information you are presenting is not the same as that previously discovered by the client, therefore causing confusion.

It is important to understand that when a client is upset, it is not a reflection of how they feel about you personally. In this situation, the STOP format can be beneficial (Ryan 2005) (Figure 5.1).

Verbal communication

The effectiveness of verbal communication depends on the words chosen, emphasis, grammar, tone, and pace (Durrance and Lagoni 1998). There are eight communication techniques required for proper verbal communication. The first is *acknowledging*. This is the act of noticing someone and making a person feel they exist. Examples include saying, "I understand," "Is that right?," and so on. The second technique is *normalizing*. This allows one to acknowledge and let them know that there is an understanding of

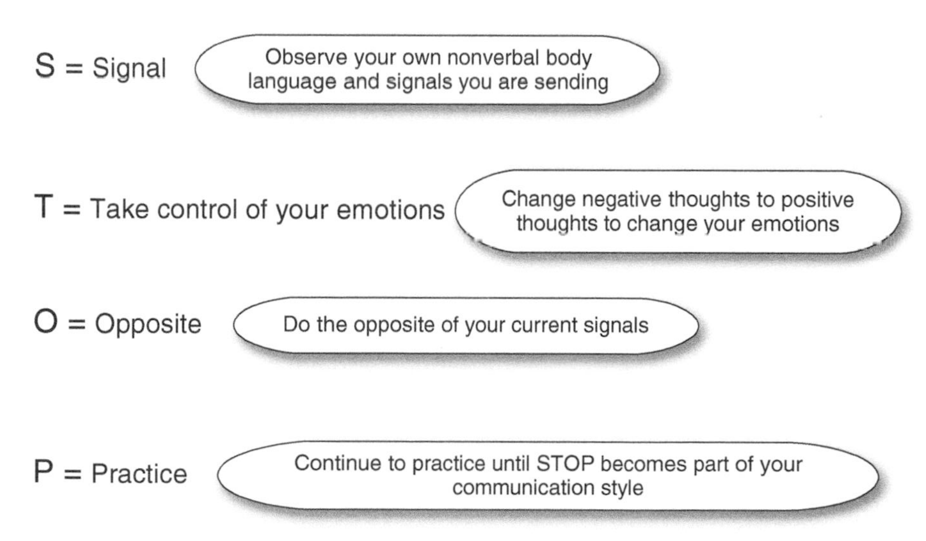

Figure 5.1 STOP when responding to an upset client.

previous experiences and gives them credibility. The third technique is giving *permission*. This helps people perform what they feel needs to be done. Fourth is asking *appropriate questions* of a person. This technique allows one to get the information needed. Technique number five is *paraphrasing* what has been discussed. In a conversation, this helps let the person talking know that the listener understands what has been said. The sixth technique is *self-disclosing* to a client. Sharing a personal story or analogy with a client helps make a connection. With this technique, the client knows that you have been through a similar experience and that you know what they are feeling. The seventh technique is *gentle confrontation*. This technique is used to point out a problem or inconsistencies in a statement. Sometimes, when a client is upset or angry, this technique can be used to let them recognize their limits. The final technique is *immediacy*. Immediacy is a combination of gentle confrontation and self-disclosure. It is often used in an emergency situation when large amounts of information are being given quickly (Durrance and Lagoni 1998).

Road blocks to verbal communication

Do not take an adversarial role when communicating with the pet owner. When people feel that their beliefs or attitudes are being attacked, they become uncomfortable and defensive, closing down communication. Avoid direct threats such as "If you do not stop Fluffy's aggression, she will likely have to be euthanized." Do not be judgmental or blaming such as "Fluffy's aggression is because of the way you have trained her"; this will not create a team-building atmosphere. "Commanding" a person or dog creates a "do-it-or-else" atmosphere, which is not optimum for the learning process. A good teacher understands that although the pet owner's current attitude may differ from what you are attempting to teach, it is likely only transient. Simply accept the pet owner's current perceptions as information and continue to build a rapport with them (Ryan 2005).

Active listening

Much of our life is spent listening; yet to be a skilled listener takes practice. Listeners usually interpret what they hear through a protective filter formed through life experiences; therefore, no two people hear things exactly the same (Ryan 2005). Active listening focuses on the emotional content of the conversation. By asking questions, paraphrasing, and using open body language, you encourage clients to further discuss those feelings. Necessary silences and minimal encouragers are techniques used in active listening. Necessary silence allows clients to vent their feelings or gather their thoughts. Minimal encouragers are used to keep the conversation going. Minimal encouragers can be head nods, eye blinks, or a simple "yes," "uh-huh," or "I see" to let the client know you are listening and an active part of the conversation (Durrance and Lagoni 1998).

Establishing an alliance with the family (pet owner and significant family members) in a noncritical manner is frequently a key to the success of the case. A partnership relationship style provides an equal separation of the power between the client and the veterinary behavior team (Gray and Moffett 2010). This technique gives control to the client by allowing them to openly discuss and choose aspects of the treatment plan.

In the past, owners may have been blamed for the issues their pet was having rather than being reinforced for seeking help to alleviate the issue. Listen to the family's experiences and specific areas of stress. Often the patient's owners have been put in a position of being damned if they do too much or too little. They may have restricted taking the pet outside to avoid conflicts but were then told that they needed to socialize their pet more (Abosh and Collins 1996). They may have attended many training classes and read many books only to find that the training they were taught and the books they read were outdated and may have worsened the problem.

Areas of stress should be acknowledged during the creation of the treatment plan. For instance, if one family member indicates they are frightened of the pet, that person may be asked to ignore the patient completely until the follow-up appointment. Or, they may be asked to toss treats from a distance when another person is clicker training the patient. Finding a safe indirect interaction can be the first step in repairing the HAB. In some cases, it may be recommended that the patient be boarded for a time to give the family respite. In some cases, in which the HAB has been seriously damaged, this respite gives the family time to adjust to not having the pet in the home and can be the first step in the grief process, although some owners may feel "relieved" with the pet out of the home and then feel remorse for the feelings of relief.

Connective communication techniques

The four-habits communication model

Pet owners are less concerned with how much their pet's medical caregivers know than with how much they care (Stein et al. 1998). The four-habits model is a tool that can be applied and used to perfect communication skills and focuses on relationship-centered care. The goal of the four-habits model is to establish rapport and build trust rapidly to expedite the effective exchange of information, demonstrate concern and care, and increase compliance.

The model has four main goals that are established when applied correctly. The first is Invest in the Beginning by building rapport with the client, thus ensuring a higher level of trust with the behavior team that helps move the proper exchange of information. It makes it easier to discuss issues with clients, giving more accurate information in the end. The second goal is to Elicit the Patient's [Client's] Perspective. The third goal is to Demonstrate Empathy by showing care and concern for the client and the patient. The last goal is to Invest in the End to increase compliance, therefore increasing the chances for a positive outcome (Frankel and Stein 1999; Adams and Frankel 2007). See Table 5.1 for a modified guide of the four-habits model for client communication between the veterinary behavior team during a behavior consultation.

Table 5.1 Modified four-habits model for client communication between the entire behavior team in a behavior consultation.

Skill	Task	Example
Invest in the beginning		
Create rapport quickly	Introduce the behavior team to everyone in the room Acknowledge any wait	Explain roles in the appointment
	Convey knowledge of patient's history by commenting on previous visit or problem	
	Attend to client and pet's comfort	Include a water bowl and blanket for the patient
	Make a social comment or ask a nonmedical question to put the client at ease	Let the client know "there is nothing Fluffy can do 'wrong' here."
	Adjust your language, pace, and posture to that of the client's	
Elicit client's concerns	Start with open-ended questions	
	Repeat concerns back to check understanding and prioritize the client's concerns	"I understand you are most concerned about Fluffy's aggression to children but also her urinating in the house, is that correct?"
Plan the visit with the client	Let the client know what to expect	"The doctor will get more information from you while I work with Fluffy. Once we have the full history, our behavior team will create your treatment plan, and I will show you some training techniques."
Elicit the client's perspectives		
Ask for the client's thoughts	Determine the status of the HAB, including all family members' input	"How do you feel about Fluffy?"
Ask for a specific goal	Determine if the client's expectations are appropriate	"If we could improve the aggression by 50%, would that be enough?"
Explore the impact on the client's life		"How are YOU doing?"
Demonstrate empathy		
Be open to the client's emotions	Assess the client's changes in body language and voice tone	"How do you feel about what we have talked about so far?"

(Continued)

Table 5.1 (*Continued*)

Skill	Task	Example
	Look for opportunities to use brief empathic comments or gestures	"Living with an animal with a serious behavior disorder is very difficult and can be very emotionally draining."
Make at least one empathic statement	Name a likely emotion the client may be feeling Compliment the client on efforts to address problem	"It is understandable if you are afraid of Fluffy." "It is obvious how much you love Fluffy."
Convey empathy nonverbally	Use a pause, touch, or facial expression to convey your understanding and empathy	
Be aware of your own reactions	Be genuine in your own emotional response Take a brief break if necessary	
Invest in the end		
Deliver diagnostic information	Frame diagnosis in terms of the client's original concerns Test client's comprehension	"We will address Fluffy's general anxiety issues first, which will also help with her aggression and accidents in the house, does this make sense to you?"
Provide education	Explain rationale for tests and treatments Review possible side effects and expected course of recovery Recommend management techniques Provide written materials and refer to other resources	"To prevent Fluffy from continuing to practice her unwanted behaviors while we work on the issue, we would like you to avoid triggers. . ."
Involve client in making decisions	Discuss treatment goals and realistic expectations for progress	"I understand ignoring Fluffy's attention seeking will be difficult but this is only temporary while we work on her issues."
Complete the visit	Explore options, listening for the patient's preferences Assess patient's ability and motivation to carry out plan Ask for additional questions and concerns Assess satisfaction Reassure patient of ongoing care	"What do you feel will be the most difficult aspect of Fluffy's treatment plan for you to follow?" "How do you feel about what we have talked about?" "We will see you back in 4 weeks, in the meantime, we will be following up with you and your trainer."

Source: Adapted from Frankel and Stein 1999.

Validation

Validation occurs when the veterinary behavior team truly understands what the clients are experiencing and gives them permission to feel upset, angry, and so on. The pet owner should be told there is nothing wrong, shameful, or irrational about their emotional responses to this situation. A veterinarian or veterinary technician might say, "This must be very difficult for you. It has to be exhausting to be on guard and worried. Those feelings are quite understandable." During the interview process, the client may admit to hitting their animal when it injured them or a family member. This statement is frequently presented with intense feelings of guilt. The veterinarian or veterinary technician can alleviate this guilt by normalizing with a statement such as, "That is quite a normal and understandable response." Validation helps build trust between the client and the behavior team.

Normalizing

As stated earlier in Chapter 4, clients often feel alone and alienated. Many times they have not found others who have dealt with the specific problem their pet is facing before, and they desperately want to hear, "We have seen this problem before and there is hope." Simply knowing that they are not alone can change the course of the consultation and is likely to give the client relief and open them to potential treatment strategies.

Guiding the conversation

Sometimes it becomes necessary to interrupt a client's story. This should not be thought of as interrupting as much as guiding the conversation to the pertinent information and is a critical therapeutic skill (Canino et al. 2007). Guiding the conversation can be done is such a way that it does not feel like an interruption. Saying something such as, "Hold on to that thought, we will come back to it. Please tell me more about. . ." or "Back up a second, tell me more about the first time he growled at you." Usually, such statements are not perceived as impolite but a way to obtain the specific information needed.

Reframing

Two common communication issues that can significantly contribute to relationship issues between pet owners and their pet are inaccurate owner interpretations of behavior and unrealistic expectations (McCurnin 2010).

Anthropomorphic interpretations distract from the needed objective observations required to accurately assess a situation, and unrealistic expectations create a scenario for failure and a weak HAB by setting up both the animal and client for the failure, although it may be necessary to reframe some comments in order to obtain a better understanding of the problem. However, many pet owner interpretations may simply be ignored but noted and addressed later in the education process (Table 5.2).

Table 5.2 Reframing anthropomorphic interpretations.

Client statement	Technician's response	Client's rephrasing	Technician's reframing[a]
He hates men	What does he do that tells you he does not like men?	He backs up and growls	So he is worried about men and feels he has to defend himself
He knows he should not get into the trash	What does he do that tells you he "knows" he should not get into the trash?	He runs away when I come into the room, and the trash is on the floor	So, he has learned when trash is on the floor you may be upset
He gets mad if I try to move him	What does he do when you try to move him?	He growls at us	First let us make sure he is not in pain, then we can teach him to move to the place you want him to without creating conflict
He tries to dominate me when I brush him	What does that look like?	He tries to get away from me when I brush him	So, he is uncomfortable with brushing
He knows I do not like it when he gets on the couch	What does he do that tells you he knows the couch is off limits?	He puts his ears back and growls when I approach him	So, he expects a conflict when he is on the couch and he does not know what to do
He knows what I want him to do, he is just being stubborn	What makes you believe he is stubborn?	He would not do what I want him to do	It is likely he does not understand what you want because something has gone wrong in the training process
He is a very dominant dog	What does that look like?	He walks in front of me when we go on walks	Has he been taught loose leash walking?
He pees on the floor when he is mad at me for leaving him	What makes you believe he is angry at you?	He does not like it when I leave and paces and pants when I am getting dressed for work, and he only does it when I leave	He is likely so upset and anxious when you leave that he cannot control himself. Can you imagine how afraid he must be to lose control of his bladder?

(Continued)

CHAPTER 5

Table 5.2 (*Continued*)

Client statement	Technician's response	Client's rephrasing	Technician's reframing[a]
He knows what he did wrong because he looks guilty	What does "guilty" look like?	He puts his ears back, tucks his tail, and hides from me	So he suspects you are upset and he does not know what you will do next so he is afraid
He tries to dominate us when we punish him	When do you need to punish him?	When he has something we do not want him to have	It sounds like he is afraid and unsure what is expected of him. Let us teach him he does not have to be afraid when he has something and then we will teach him to not pick up certain objects
We have spoiled her and that is why she would not listen to us	Can you give me an example of when she acts "spoiled"?	She climbs on the dinner table no matter how many times we tell her not to	Let us control the times she is near the table unsupervised and teach her to go to a mat
She is bossy	What does she do when she is "bossy"?	She barks at me when I tell her to sit	Barking can be a sign of frustration. Let us reteach the sit and see if we can decrease her frustration
He is protecting me that is why he is aggressive	What does that look like?	When a stranger approaches, he growls and stands behind me	It sounds as though he may be unsure of strangers and feels safer when you are nearby or he may be more confident that you will protect him and be his "back up" support system

[a] Responses may be phrased in a question format in the attempt to gain agreement from the pet owner. In addition, many pet owner interpretations may simply be ignored but noted in the education process.

The dominance theory

The dominance theory may be the greatest interpretative miscommunication in companion animal behavior. The dominance theory was originally based on studies performed on wolf packs in the 1940s. It was extrapolated that dogs had social hierarchies comparable to wolves. The adapted theory went as far as to assume that a human family replaces a dog pack. It was theorized that a dog tries to gain the top position over family members and may become aggressive to lower ranking "members of the pack."

There were three significant flaws in the early research.

(1) The initial wolf studies were short term and only focused on about 1% of a wolf's life, namely hunting (Murie and Etats-Unis. National Park Service 1944). Wildlife biologist, Dr. David Mech, an internationally recognized expert on wolves, points out that the notion of "alpha wolf" and the struggle to be "top dog" were based on observations of captive groups of unrelated wolves. These artificial social groups bear little resemblance to a pack of free-living wolves that (except for the breeding pair) are all related to one another. The idea that individuals in a family of wolves are engaged in constant daily struggles to best one another, and that our dogs do the same with us, is simply not true (Mech 2008).

(2) Sweeping conclusions were made from this misinformation and then generalized to dogs, ignoring 15 000 years of domestication, and then generalized again to the human–dog relationship. Veterinarian Ian Dunbar made the comparison that trying to understand dogs better by looking at wolf behavior is comparable to humans attempting to improve their parenting skills by observing primates.

(3) The researchers observed what are now known to be ritualistic displays and misinterpreted them into forcible dominance displays. For example, researchers determined that a higher ranking wolf forcibly pins a "subordinate" wolf to the ground. We now know that the "subordinate" wolf is not forced to the ground but voluntarily assumes the position as part of ritualized appeasement behavior – a method of avoiding conflict.

This dominance theory has been overused, complicates the relationship we have with dogs, and puts pet owners in an adversarial role. Pet owners are led to believe that their dog is trying to "take over" and therefore "must not be allowed to get away with things."

In the past, puppies were considered "dominant" when they demanded petting, pushed through doorways, jumped up to greet people, or guarded objects. It is now understood that when a puppy "demands petting" or paws at the owner, it is simply performing a conditioned behavior. The puppy is rewarded for pawing when the owner gives it attention. Pushing through a doorway is simply an indication that sitting at the door has not been taught – it is an issue of lack of training. Jumping on people is a greeting behavior and is conditioned by people responding to the behavior with touch and attention. Guarding of a resource is almost always initially fear or anxiety related but becomes conditioned through avoidance conditioning. The puppy then becomes more offensive after experiencing the success of getting out of the stressful situation and eventually no longer shows anxiousness. Guarding of a resource can be an early indication that a puppy is at risk of developing conflict-induced aggression (Guy et al. 2001c) (Box 5.1).

An alternate explanation is that whenever the dog is uncertain or uncomfortable in a situation (i.e. conflict situation), it has learned to use aggression to avoid the situation (i.e. avoidance conditioning). The dog becomes less fearful because it learns how to avoid the fear-provoking situation. The aggression has nothing to do with the debunked "dominance theory."

The "dominance theory" often damages the HAB because owners believe that their puppy views them as a lower ranking "pack member." Owners often feel they need to practice techniques such as "scruff shaking," "alpha roll overs," and other domination techniques to control their puppy. These techniques increase anxiety and fear for both the owner and the puppy and are counterproductive in the treatment process. Owners are often relieved and compliant with the treatment plan when they understand that the puppy is not trying to "dominate" them but is anxious and uncertain (Shaw 2005).

BOX 5.1: RISK FACTORS FOR DEVELOPING OWNER-DIRECTED AGGRESSION (CONFLICT-INDUCED AGGRESSION)

Risk factors
Suffered a serious illness under four months of age
Not walked off property regularly
Higher level of excitement, reactivity, and fearfulness
Inappropriate or overly aggressive play
Guarding (objects, food, or space)
Handling issues
Shows conflict behaviors

Empathy

Empathy is the ability to have a deep emotional understanding of another's feelings and experiences. The ability to empathize both with the patient and with the pet owner is the greatest attribute of the veterinary behavior technician and one of the most challenging skills to obtain.

- Seek first to understand then to be understood. Stephen Covey

Ancient Toltec wisdom may give us the most simplified principles for clear empathetic communication. The Toltec tradition is about freedom from a belief system, in other words, not being attached to any particular point of view (Rosenthal 2005). Being able to perceive and understand a client's perspective allows you to "walk in the shoes" of the client. Attempting to empathize with the pet includes understanding the deep fear and confusion that often create or add to a pet's behavior disorder. Empathy for the pet allows the technician to see the pet in a light other than as an aggressive or fearful animal.

Empathy builds trust and creates a platform for effective communication and relationship development. Developing the ability to empathize requires the ability to "step back" from our own emotions and beliefs to let the other's emotions and viewpoint in. Letting go of your own perspective, even temporarily, requires courage on your part but is essential in developing the ability to sincerely empathize with others.

Empathy and understanding for the client carry over to the patient. Philosopher Marcha C. Nussbaum said that as we learn to imagine what another creature might feel in response to various events and we begin to identify with the other creature, we learn something about ourselves. Being able to identify and empathize with the fear and anxiety many of our patients exhibit is the first step in modifying their behavior. When a pet is described as a "mean dog" or a "mean cat," the label ends the process to genuinely empathize. Recognizing that the animal is trying to protect itself from the stimulus (you) and emphasizing with them changes your motivation and enhances your ability to teach both the animal and the client.

- When we understand the needs that motivate our own and other's behavior, we have no enemies. Marshall B. Rosenberg

The following four Toltec principles are the foundation for genuine empathetic and unambiguous communication (Figure 5.2).

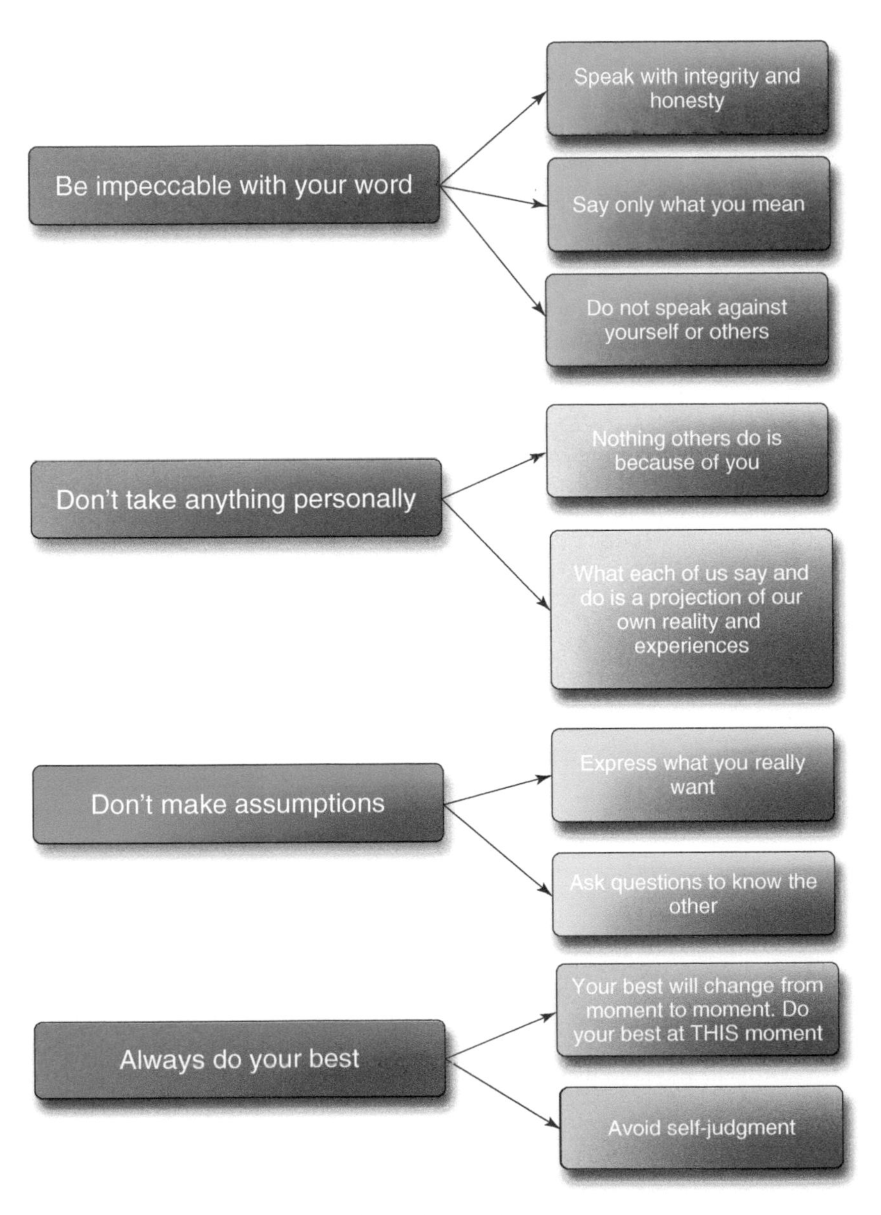

Figure 5.2 Toltec principles for empathetic communication and interactions.

Teaching

A veterinary animal behavior technician is a teacher, a leader, and a mentor to the pet owners. The following are attributes of an excellent teacher.

Enthusiasm and passion are contagious to whomever you teach. If you love what you do, it will show. *Kindness and humility* will guide your teaching away from condescending actions or remarks. Understanding that there is no "one way" to perform things creates an open learning environment for both the student and the teacher. *Be patient and flexible.* If your student is not "getting it," it means you need to be comfortable enough with the material to modify your teaching technique for that specific learner. Being able to modify "on the run" also keeps the material fresh and interesting for you. A sense of humor will keep what you are teaching light and fun. Remember to laugh at yourself and at your own mistakes. This often helps the student to relax and understand that making a mistake is learning. *Make each student feel special and important.* Shaping human behavior is no different from shaping a pet's behavior. Find something to reinforce that is heading toward the goal behavior (Ryan 2005).

TAGteach®

TAGteach (McKeon 2012) is a package of tools that emphasizes the use of positive reinforcement and incorporates several well-established behavioral principles and practices. Although the purpose of TAGteach is to improve skill acquisition for the student, its first benefit goes to the teacher. Teachers quickly learn to identify, highlight, and reinforce vital skills for the student and deliver information in a learner-accessible manner. When teaching the pet owner specific goals, it is important to keep the learning goals specific, measurable, attainable, realistic, and timely (Meyer2003; Cornell 2012) (Figure 5.3).

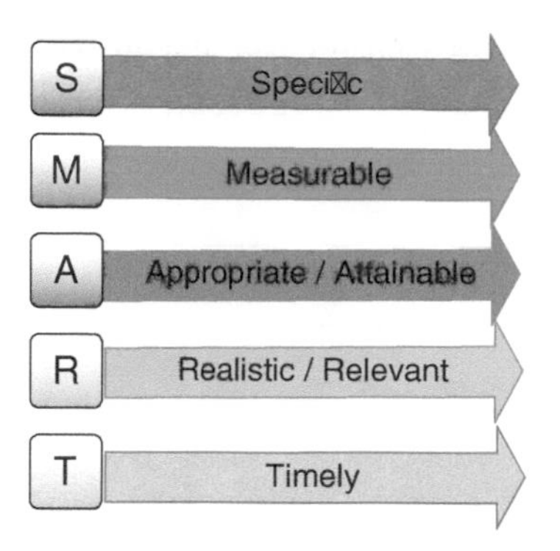

Figure 5.3 Smart learning goals.

The Focus Funnel

Analogous to a common household funnel, the job of the Focus Funnel is to channel and reduce. The Focus Funnel encourages teachers to distill potentially confusing information into critical sound bites that can be easily absorbed by students. It starts with "the lesson." The teacher gives a lesson containing the largest amount of material, including all information pertinent to learning a skill. Next, the teacher delivers "the directions." The directions contain only information vital to the performance of the skill. Finally, immediately before the student performs the new skill, the teacher gives the student a single goal or "Tag Point" that when performed, will be marked with an audible marker (Figure 5.4).

The Reverse Focus Funnel

Turn the focus funnel upside down and then you have the Reverse Focus Funnel. The TAGteach website defines the reverse focus funnel as, "Deliver the least amount of information necessary for success first (tag point). Once the behavior has been accomplished, and the learner is more confident, additional information can be delivered. This is useful in situations where too much information may overwhelm the learner and cause a loss of concentration" (accessed August 1, 2022 at https://tagteach.com/widget/TAGteach_lexicon).

The tag point

The Tag Point is uniquely constructed to be the pivotal point of focus for the student and the teacher. Tag Points support a positive student–teacher relationship by clearly stating a single criterion for success (Box 5.2).

BOX 5.2:

Tag Points – WOOF

What you want
One thing at a time
Observable and measurable
Five words or less

Source: Adapted from http://www.tagteach.com.

CHAPTER 5

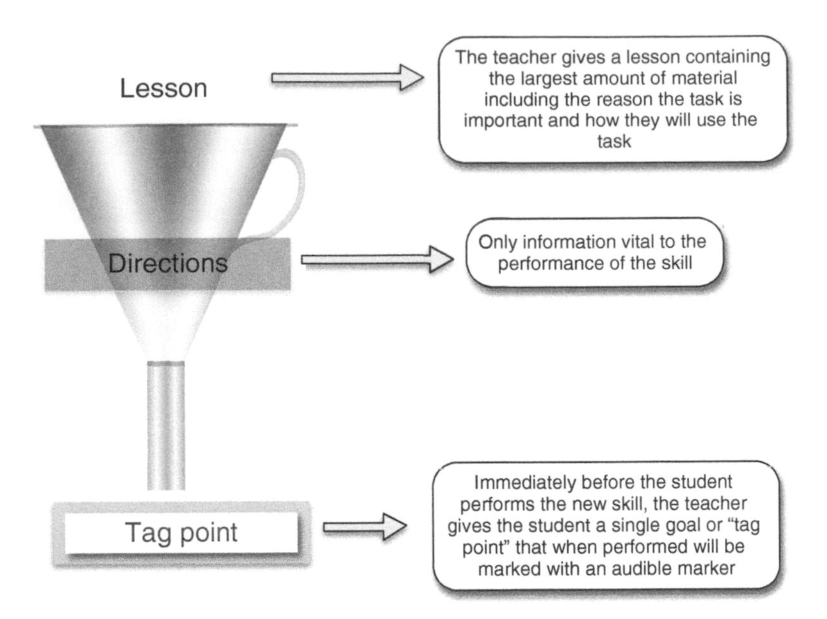

Figure 5.4 The Focus Funnel is used to channel and reduce information.

The focus point is analogous to a Tag Point. It is phrased in the same manner but is referred to as a *focus point* rather than a Tag Point. This can be used when the learner will not be audibly tagged by an observer, but instead the learner focuses on the task and determines on their own if they have met the criteria.

The tag

After the teacher delivers the Tag Point, the student performs the skill. The teacher marks the moment the Tag Point is achieved with an audible sound. The audible mark always means success. Most students are reinforced by success. Therefore, the audible mark becomes reinforcing. Using a short sharp sound such as a clicker or a tone from a cell phone as a marker is preferred over verbal marks such as "yes" or "good." The pure sound is easily processed by the student and reduces the emotions associated with the human voice. The more distractions eliminated during the actual moments before, during, and after learning, the more focus we get from our students. If the teacher notices something else within the skill that needs to be improved, it can be made into a different Tag Point or discussed at a later time. Success is solely contingent on the performance of the designated Tag Point.

An example of using the Focus Funnel in veterinary medicine might be the following:

The lesson is that dogs often communicate with body language. Some of the natural friendly behaviors humans express toward dogs can actually be perceived as a threat. For example, people often greet dogs by looking directly at them, walking toward, and leaning over them. All of these behaviors would be interpreted as a threat if between two dogs.

The directions are that when meeting a dog instead of looking directly at the dog, glance at it then look away.

The Tag Point or focus point is to look at your feet.

Success makes us feel confident. Success makes us want to do it again. Use the Focus Funnel, Tag Points, and an audible marker as tools to quantify and highlight success for you and your students.

The communication cycle

Treating and preventing behavior disorders requires a team approach that includes the veterinary technician as the "case manager," the veterinarian who diagnoses, prescribes, and gives a prognosis, and a qualified trainer who works in the field with the pet owner. A list of included forms for expediting the communication cycle is included in Table 5.3 and the Appendix Section 1.

The veterinary technician is the key to the communication cycle by being in contact with the entire team to keep everyone in the loop. When a client calls in with a "behavior problem," it is the veterinary technician who should perform a phone assessment and triage the case. The technician will

Table 5.3 Form utilization.

Form	Who uses	How to use
Behavior problem list (Table 5.4) + refer to Triage Table 1.2	Completed during first contact with pet owner (veterinary technician/trainer)	Used at first contact to triage and determine if the next contact should be with hospital's qualified trainer (could also be the veterinary technician) or be seen by the veterinarian
Field assessment	Completed by veterinary technician/ qualified trainer working with the pet owner "in the field"	Completed and submitted to the veterinary hospital when the qualified trainer sees the pet owner in the field and suspects the issue may be a behavioral disorder rather than a training issue
Field follow-up form	Completed by the veterinary technician/ trainer	Completed by the qualified trainer after seeing a patient referred to them by the veterinary hospital
History Part 1 – behavior consultation	Completed by the pet owner with/ without assistance from the veterinarian technician	Completed before the behavior consultation
History Part 2 – behavior consultation	Completed by the veterinarian	Completed during the behavior consultation
Observation chart	Completed by the veterinary technician during the initial consultation	Create a second observation chart to be used to determine progress at the follow-up appointment
Plan of care	Completed by the veterinarian	Plan for the veterinary technician/trainer to assist the pet owner with application of the prescribed treatment plan
Follow-up behavior consultation form	Completed by the veterinarian	Completed by the veterinarian after a follow-up behavior consultation

determine from the communication whether the next contact should be a consultation with the veterinarian or a qualified trainer. If it is initially determined that the "behavior problem" is likely a lack of training or a conditioned unwanted behavior it is referred to the hospital's qualified trainer. It is imperative that the veterinary technician and the qualified trainer have an open and clear communication. If the trainer determines that the initial phone assessment was correct and the issue is training or lack of it, the pet owner will remain with the trainer, but the trainer will send a follow-up report to the veterinary technician on the patient's training progress. If the trainer determines that the issue is more complex than first anticipated, then the patient is referred back to the veterinarian for a diagnosis and treatment plan. At that point, the veterinarian may diagnose a behavioral disorder and along with the input from the technician and trainer create a treatment plan or choose to refer the case to a veterinary behaviorist.

If a treatment plan is prescribed, a Plan of Care (see Plan of Care in Appendix 8) should be submitted to the technician or trainer who will be working with the pet owner. The trainer or veterinary technician working with the patient and pet owner then sends follow-up reports back to the veterinary technician (case manager) who then reports follow-up progress to the veterinarian, and the treatment plan is adjusted as discussed by the team (Figure 5.5).

Assessments

Getting an informal impression or evaluation of the situation is the first step in triaging and differentiating a behavioral problem from a behavioral disorder (see Table 1.2).

Preventive care: preventive care refers to the measures taken to prevent a behavioral disorder from occurring rather than curing or treating the symptoms of an existing disorder. It is the primary role for veterinary technicians.

- Preventive care: preventive care refers to the measures taken to prevent a behavioral disorder from occurring rather than curing or treating the symptoms of an existing disorder.
- It is the primary role for veterinary technicians.

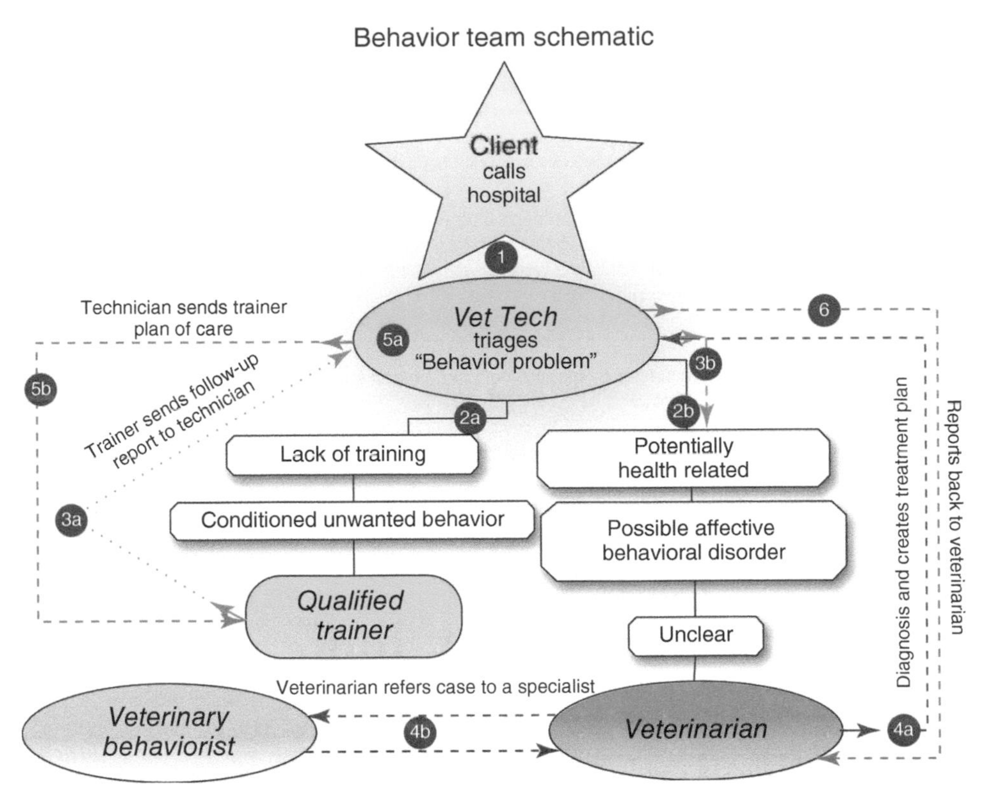

Figure 5.5 1. Client makes the first contact with the veterinary technician. 2a. The veterinary technician assesses the situation and suspects a training issue and sends to the veterinary hospital's qualified trainer. 2b. The veterinary technician assesses the situation and determines case needs to be seen by the veterinarian. 3a. The trainer sends follow-up report to the veterinary technician on patient's training progress. 3b. The trainer determines the issue is more complex than first anticipated, and patient is referred to the veterinarian for a diagnosis and treatment plan. 4a. The veterinarian provides diagnosis and creates treatment plan, or 4b. The veterinarian refers the case to veterinary behaviorist. 5a. The veterinary technician assists the client in applying the prescribed treatment plan. 5b. Plan of care is sent to the trainer to continue to assist the client with the treatment plan. 6. The veterinary technician reports follow-up progress to veterinarian, and the treatment plan is adjusted as needed.

Intervention care: intervention care refers to measures taken to improve or alter an existing behavioral disorder. Intervention requires a veterinarian's diagnosis and treatment plan.

- Intervention care: intervention care refers to measures taken to improve or alter an existing behavioral disorder. Intervention requires a veterinarian's diagnosis and treatment plan.

Initial correspondence

Often, the first contact from the pet owner pertaining to their pet's behavior will be a phone call or email to the veterinary hospital. The initial correspondence is the time to begin building the team approach and bonding the pet owner to the team. During the initial phone or email correspondence, the veterinary technician should obtain brief but specific information to determine the further steps to be taken. The goal is to obtain information regarding the following areas.

Signalment and family orientation

Age of the pet – The age of the pet may help determine the duration of learning history that has occurred. If the issue is aggression, the duration the animal has been "practicing" the aggression may help determine the animal's confidence level. Young animals usually show conflict behaviors before a bite, whereas older ones have developed their own coping skills (i.e. aggression or flight) and practiced them for many years and may no longer demonstrate conflict behaviors because they are no longer in conflict.

Another consideration regarding the age of the pet is the need to rule out medical contributing factors. In general, an adult or senior pet that has an acute change in behavior is indicative of a medical issue.

Breed – The breed of the animal is important for detecting breed predispositions, such as chasing and herding behaviors. The size of the animal may also have an impact on the level of triage needed. For example, giant breeds of dogs can inflict more significant damage than toy breeds; therefore, the situation can have a more immediate need.

Family orientation and other pets in the household – The family orientation, age of children, number of children, and other pets in the household will impact the pet's learning history. Children can increase the opportunities for learning unwanted behaviors and will also impact the risk associated with aggression issues.

Identify high-risk factors

Research from the Ontario Veterinary College (Guy et al. 2001a–c) identified risk factors for puppies developing aggression toward family members, which should be considered "red flags" during initial correspondence (see Box 5.1).

Description and prioritized problem list

The veterinary technician should complete a "problem list" (form in Appendix 9) (Table 5.4). The "problems" are a list of pet owner complaints, not diagnosis.

Ask the pet owner to describe their primary behavior concern and then describe the last incident, including what happened before, during, and after the event. The description the pet owner gives should be comparable to playing a movie. Asking questions such as, "What did that look like?" and

Table 5.4 Behavior problem list.

Eliminative	Social	Ingestive
□ Incontinence	□ Barking/howling/whining	□ Anorexia
□ Diarrhea/vomiting	□ Rolling in unsavory items	□ Chewing objects
□ House soiling	□ Jumps up on people	□ Coprophagia
□ Urine marking	□ Demands attention	□ Compulsive eating
□ Urination on pheromones	□ Demands touch	□ Compulsive drinking
□ Other________	□ Aggressive to owners	□ Eating grass/plants
Grooming	□ Aggressive to strangers	□ Eating garbage
	□ Aggressive to dogs/same household	□ Pica
□ Licking self	□ Aggressive to strange dogs	□ Prey catching
□ Sucking on self	□ Aggressive to other animals	□ Car chasing
□ Chewing on self	□ Other________	□ Light/shadow chasing
□ Scratching self		□ Stealing food
□ Checking hind end		□ Fly snapping
□ Other________		□ Air/mouth licking
		□ Other________
Temperament related	*Reproduction*	*Locomotory*
□ Depressed inappetent	□ Cannibalism	□ Circling/whirling
□ Hyperexcitable/active	□ False pregnancy	□ Tail biting
□ Hyperreactive	□ Masturbation	□ Pacing, figure 8s
□ Nervous/anxious	□ Mounting people	□ Digging
□ Fear of thunder	□ Mounting animals	□ Lameness/cond.
□ Fear of loud noises, e.g. thunder	□ Self nursing	□ Roaming
□ Fear of people	□ Other________	□ Scratching objects
□ Fear of situations		□ Freezing
□ Fear of objects/animals		□ Other________
□ Other________		

Comments:

"What did you do after the behavior occurred?" will give insight into the behavior and steer the conversation away from interpretational descriptions. For example, "He hates it when it storms" is not as helpful as, "When it begins to storm Fluffy hides under the bed and shakes. I pull her out from under the bed and cuddle her," which provides the technician with much more pertinent information (see Table 5.2).

It is helpful to know what initiated the call, especially when the behavior has been ongoing. Inquiring about event changes is one way of assessing the extent to which the pet owner and the pet may be in crisis. A specific recent event may have prompted the call for an appointment. A pet's behavior may have been managed until a recent life change (pregnancy, divorce, extended family addition, etc.) or a significant episode may have caused an escalation in concern. Regardless, it is important to find out if the current issue is acute or a chronic problem. Specific information can help pinpoint whether the stress is underlying the presenting problem or is only a symptom of it (Canino et al. 2007).

Asking the question, "What have you done to treat the problem?" gives the technician insight into the possible frustration level of the pet owner and can determine whether the pet owner is using techniques, including punishment, which could cause the issue to worsen or put the pet owner in a dangerous situation. The pet owner may say, "We've tried everything!" or "I know I'm making it worse. . . ." In these cases, the technician should be supportive and instruct them how to safely interact until the issue can be addressed.

Specific questions to ask pertaining to aggression

During the phone assessment, it is imperative to determine whether the pet owner is in danger of being injured. Asking specifically about past bite history including number of bites, and whether the bites were inhibited is critical. Information as to whether the pet bites once and leaves or continues to aggress during an episode should be obtained. The technician should assist the owner in identifying potential warning signs before the aggression occurs. Pet owners should be asked if they are aware of known triggers for fearful or aggressive behavior, and when those triggers can be identified, they should be avoided until the pet can be seen for a full behavior consultation. If targets cannot be identified or if there are many triggering factors, the pet owner should be asked to interact with the pet as little as possible and in a cue–response–reward format when interaction must occur (see Chapter 9). The goal is to keep the pet owner safe until the consultation and to prevent further deterioration of the HAB.

Status of the HAB

Possibly, the most critical area to obtain information is the status of the HAB. A seriously damaged HAB should be treated as in an emergency situation. Regardless of whether the problem is suspected to be a training issue or behavioral disorder, once the HAB is damaged, it can be difficult to treat the problem. Asking the pet owner how they "feel about their pet" and whether they are afraid of their pet can give critical insight into the current relationship. The technician should also inquire about the relationship with other family members involved with the pet and how their attitudes may affect the current situation.

Assessment in the field

The qualified trainer associated with your veterinary hospital (the qualified trainer could also be the veterinary technician) may be the first contact for the pet owner. When this occurs and the trainer suspects the pet's issues may be based on an affective behavioral disorder, the trainer may either refer the client immediately to the veterinarian or provide a field assessment and then submit their assessment to the veterinary behavior team (see Appendix 30 for a sample field assessment) (Table 5.5).

Parts of a behavior history

A thorough history must be taken to give appropriate and proper recommendations. Without a proper history, wrong advice may be given, and compliance will be low.

It is diagnostically helpful to break the history down into three parts: *signalment and general management history*, including husbandry, *general temperament evaluation*, and *detailed information pertaining to the specific issues*. When discussing specific issues, information concerning when and where the behavior occurs, what triggers the behavior, what behavior is shown, including body language and facial expressions, who or what is the target of the behavior, how people react to the behavior, and how the animal acts and looks after the behavior is obtained. Specific information should also be obtained as to the

Table 5.5 A field assessment should include the following.

Content	Details
Owner's prioritized behavioral concerns	This list should include both training issues and behavioral disorder concerns
General signalment and family orientation	Include changes in family orientation and status changes (divorce etc.)
Problem history	Include pertinent information the veterinary behavior team should know when making their diagnosis and treatment plan, including previously attempted treatment and training techniques
Medical conditions or concerns	Known medications or gross health concerns as reported by the owner (lameness, pain, etc.)
Assessment meeting observations	Include pertinent family interactions, observations, and environmental concerns
Plan training and management suggestions	Include goals, training techniques, training tools, and exercises recommended
Status of the HAB	Note any damage or breaks in the HAB. Comments made by the family such as, "we cannot take much more" or "we are ready to give up" are critical when the behavior team considers a treatment plan
Specific concerns	This section should include the trainer's concerns pertaining to potential compliance issues, lack of progress, or anxiety/aggression issues, which may have an affective basis, including lack of impulse control or difficulty learning

severity, frequency, and what the pet owners have done in attempts to change the behavior.

After obtaining specific details relating to the presenting complaint, clients should be asked to describe the very first time the problem occurred to assess the development of the problem. The clients are also asked to describe in detail the three most recent incidences of the behavior (see Appendices 1–5 for sample history forms and links to sample online history forms).

During the appointment, the veterinary technician should complete an observation form. A second observation form can be completed at follow-up appointments to assess progress (see Technician observation form in Appendix 10) (Table 5.6).

Table 5.6 Veterinary technician's observations during a behavior consultation.

	Start of appointment	15 min	30 min	60 min	End of appointment
Treats	0	Chicken	Anything	Anything	Anything
Treat proximity	0	From owner	From floor 3 ft from owner	Technician's hand	Technician's hand
Interactions	Next to owner	Attention seeking to owner	Walking around room	Greeting people in room	Greeting new people who enter
Trainability (1–10)	0	2	6	8	10
General behavior	Growling	Occasionally growling	Interested in technician	Wagging tail	Sleeping
Restrictions	Muzzle and tie down	Muzzle removed	Allowed off tie down, dragging leash	Off leash	Off leash

Significant events during appointment

Charged door when a noise occurred outside the examination room

Treats – type of treat taken.
Proximity – where took treats (owner's hand, floor, technician's hand, etc.).
Interactions – does the pet interact with others? Interactions with owner?
General behavior – general comments about behavior during appointment.
Restrictions – note any restrictions used during the appointment.
Significant events – note any reactions to stimuli or general comments.
This form can be used to access progress when the patient returns for a follow-up appointment.

Follow-up reports

Follow-up training and behavior modification reports should be sent to the behavior team on a monthly basis or as needed. If major changes in the treatment plan are considered, changes should be discussed before implementation. In a poll conducted on the Veterinary Information Network, veterinarians indicated that it was imperative their treatment plans are not changed by trainers in the field without first discussing those changes (Shaw 2011).

In the same regard, the trainer should be alerted to follow-up appointments at the veterinary hospital and any changes in the treatment plan on a consistent and regular basis (see Follow-up communication form in Appendix 11).

During follow-up appointments, it is helpful to ask the pet owner to rate the problem on a scale of 1–10 (10 being the best the problem has ever been and 1 the worst). The goal is to see a minimum of a 50% improvement at the follow-up appointment. A scale system is helpful for the behavior team and the pet owner to objectively analyze behavior improvements.

Acquiring a behavior history and improving pet owner compliance

Question styles

Clients will commonly not give objective interpretations of their pet's behavior but instead their rationalized interpretations. Therefore, it is important to ask open- and closed-ended questions to distill the information you need. Repeat the information back to the client in a simplified form to verify through reflective listening, the information they have presented. Sometimes, leading questions may be needed. Later, the question can be asked in reverse, giving the clients an opportunity to contradict themselves or provide additional insight.

Closed-ended questions are those that can be answered with a yes or no or a single word or a short phrase. Closed-ended questions are comparable to multiple-choice questions. For example, "Is Fluffy aggressive to strangers?" is a closed-ended question. Closed-ended questions place the control of the conversation with the questioner. They give facts and are easy and quick to answer.

Open-ended questions require the pet owner to answer with more information and are comparable to essay questions. Open-ended questions require the pet owner to think, reflect, and offer opinions and feelings and put the respondent in control of the conversation. When asking open-ended questions, you will not only need to guide the conversation, but also leave openings for the client to digress somewhat so you "can read between the lines." For example, "Toward whom is Fluffy's aggression directed?" pet owner's answer, "He is mostly aggressive to my husband." By reading between the lines, this statement could be interpreted to mean, he is aggressive to the husband most of time but also other people at other times (Table 5.7).

Reflecting is communicating back what you have heard. Reflection is used at a point in the conversation in which a large amount of information has been presented and is intended to help summarize the information to make sure that all information

Table 5.7 Examples of open- and closed-ended questions.

Closed-ended questions	Usage	Example
	Opening question to begin a conversation	"Did you have a nice drive?" "Isn't the weather nice?"
	Testing understanding	"So, you would like to focus on Fluffy's urination in the house today?"
	Setting up a desired frame of mind	"Do you feel better about the current issue you are having with Fluffy?"
	Getting closure of a final agreement	"You can walk Fluffy twice daily, correct?"
Open-ended questions	**Usage**	**Example**
	Follow-up from a closed question	"Are there any other issues you would like to discuss today?"
	To find out more about the client's needs	"How is Fluffy's behavior affecting your family?"
	Assisting clients in understanding the extent of the problem	"How do you feel Fluffy's fear affects your daily activities?"
	Getting the client to trust you	"How are you feeling about Fluffy these days?"

has been provided. Reflection can also be used to get back on track, if a client starts to stray from the specific information being sought.

Improving compliance

In veterinary medicine, the definition of compliance is how consistently and accurately a pet owner completes their pet's prescribed regimen. When there is a lack of compliance, there is an increase in frustration both from the client and from the behavior team.

A study looking at owner compliance found that spending too little time with clients caused a decrease in compliance (Shaw 2007).

The American Animal Hospital Association (AAHA) also performed a study looking at owner compliance with six basic health-care recommendations and found that noncompliance occurred when veterinarians failed to communicate clearly or provide clear recommendations. Both studies indicate that compliance is enhanced when trust and rapport are established with clients. It has also been found that clients are more willing to follow directions when playing an active role in the decision-making process (Shaw 2007).

Compliance enhancers

Empathy – Allow the pet owner to be frustrated or angry at their pet's behavior. Acknowledge and reinforce what they have done so far to improve the issue. Let them know you have seen similar cases and give examples of your past experiences.

Appropriate and clear goals – Ask the owners for their specific goals, what degree of improvement would they be happy with, and what degree of improvement could they live with. Consider the pet owner's limitations, and do not blame them for those limitations. Determine the pet owner's level of commitment to work on the issue. If there are multiple problems to be addressed, set priorities for treatment with the pet owner's input. If certain issues must be addressed ahead of the pet owner's priorities (for example, decreasing anxiety before addressing barking), explain to the pet owner why it is necessary to proceed in the prescribed order (i.e. decreasing the anxiety may also decrease reactivity and barking).

Seeing progress quickly – Owners are more likely to comply with a treatment plan if they see subtle improvement quickly. Simply teaching their pet to target or learn a cue can improve the pet owner's enthusiasm in applying the treatment plan.

Keep explanations and the treatment plan simple and in point form – Small steps are important when providing large amounts of information to clients. Giving small amounts of information intermittently decreases the chance of overwhelming the pet owner. Overwhelmed pet owners do not feel safe (Abood 2007). Be logical and only provide what is completely necessary. Ask the clients if they understand why points of the treatment plan are important (i.e. you are ignoring attention-seeking behaviors so we can decrease hyperexcitability) and have them repeat the key points back. Ask the owners what aspect of the treatment plan they feel will be the most difficult to apply and problem-solve or modify as needed.

Implement the treatment in steps – Start with simple management modifications and training before going into time-consuming and complex behavior modification techniques. Let the pet owners know that this is only the first step in the treatment plan, and more steps will be added in follow-up appointments.

Provide a written discharge and instructions – Include handouts and recommended reading for pet owners to review at their leisure once they have had time to digest the information they have received during the consultation.

Establish realistic expectations for progress – A working rule of thumb is that it takes equally as long to treat a problem as it took to become established. Emphasize the quick improvements that are being seen (i.e. response during the appointment to training). Remind owners that conditioned behaviors may worsen as they go through extinction bursts, and that means the behavior is on its way to improving.

Have the pet owners keep a diary so that progress can be clearly seen – Dealing with an animal with a behavioral disorder on a daily basis can make it difficult for the pet owner to see progress. A behavior diary can be helpful by noting significant stimuli, medications added, and other relevant daily activities. Using a graph format, the pet owner can observe progress that might not be obvious on a daily basis (see Behavior Diary in Appendix 12).

Stay in touch with the pet owner – Follow-up care by the veterinary technician is critical. Checking in with the pet owner about 10–14 days after the appointment to clarify the treatment plan allows the pet owner plenty of time to review the information provided and will reinforce to them that they are not alone. The veterinary technician is the case manager and should also stay in contact with the qualified trainer who is assisting the client "in the field."

Charge enough – Free or under-priced advice is not valued (Luescher and Martin 2010).

The technician is the key to improving pet owner compliance with behavior treatment plans. Spending appropriate time with clients, providing explanations and understanding, answering questions, and allowing collaboration enhance owner compliance and build healthy relationships.

Grief counseling

The relationship we have with our pet overlaps many comparable human relationships such as friend, significant other, family member, and child. "This is not to say that even the most bonded person believes his or her pet is human. Pets seem to occupy an overlapping but different space from humans in a family. Even people who think of their pets as children know this is not literally true. In part, they are identifying their pets as family members by the way in which pets function within the household" (Cohen 2002).

The ultimate goal of grief counseling is to assist the pet owner in the grieving process so the grief can become a positive experience, with the end result being hope for the future.

The "normal" grief process

This section discusses what is considered "normal" or noncomplex grief, which is defined as grief that begins to fade and subside into adequate coping mechanisms within six months.

Grief: an individual's inner emotional feelings occurring because of a loss.

- *Grief*: an individual's inner emotional feelings occurring because of a loss.

Mourning: outward, social expression of the loss. Often the mourning process is dictated by societal norms and impacts. The process of mourning allows a person to move through the grief process and when inhibited can delay the grief process. Ceremony helps you to know what to do when you do not know what to do.

- *Mourning*: outward, social expression of the loss. Often the mourning process is dictated by societal norms and impacts.
- The process of mourning allows a person to move through the grief process and when inhibited can delay the grief process.
- Ceremony helps you to know what to do when you do not know what to do.

Bereavement: the state of events or loss that causes grief.

- ***Bereavement***: the state of events or loss that causes grief.

Grief is a very private and individual process; no two people travel through grief following exactly the same path. Grief is often discussed as occurring in stages, whereas in reality, it occurs more in waves or cycles that come and go depending on triggers in the environment. There are numerous grief paradigms (Table 5.8). In this section, the five stages of coping with dying by Elizabeth Kubler-Ross: denial, anger, bargaining, depression, and acceptance are historically the most commonly used paradigm, although they are being used erroneously in this application as they were developed using information from dying cancer patients rather than survivors of a lost one. Newer clinical approaches include both a more postmodern individualizing of loss and a rejection of predictable stages. "Different individuals grieve in different ways, and counselors should be aware of the diversity of such ways if they are to assist clients to follow their path of grief" (Walter 1996).

The grief model whether you choose to use it will depend on the pet owner and your comfort.

Types of grievers

Intuitive grievers experience grief at an affective level. They work through grief by expressing their deep emotional pain by crying, shouting, and so on. *Instrumental grievers* are more likely to demonstrate their grief in cognitive and physical terms (exercising, talking about their thoughts, etc.) rather than demonstrating intense emotion. They process their thoughts, ruminating and revisiting memories.

CHAPTER 5

Table 5.8 Common grief models.

	Kubler-Ross stages of grief
Denial	"This cannot be happening"
Anger	"Why is this happening? This must be the trainer's fault"
Bargaining	"Maybe if we try a new medication or a different dosage things will get better"
Depression	"This hurts too much, I am overwhelmed with sadness"
Acceptance	"I have done everything I can, and I know that I am giving her a gift of love by letting her go"
	The five stages of grief
Numbness and denial	Numbness or shock can help cushion the blow as you adjust to the loss. This stage can last a few hours, days, or even a few weeks
Yearning and anger	The numbness wears off, and the painful realization of the loss hits full-force; you will ache missing your pet. You may be angry and have regrets
Emotional despair, sadness, and withdrawal	The storm of intense emotions of the second stage gives way to a period of heavy sadness, silence, and withdrawal from family and friends
Reorganization	Reorganization and the beginning of positive emotions. Over time, sadness will lessen, and you will start to perceive your life in a more positive light, although bouts of grief and sadness will persist
Letting go and moving on	The final phase of this model is to let go of your need for the lost pet and begin to move on with your life. Sadness will lessen greatly and you will begin to think of the future
	The seven stages of grief
Shock and denial	You may deny the reality of the loss at some level. Shock provides emotional protection from being overwhelmed
Pain and guilt	As the shock wears off, it is replaced with the suffering of unbelievable pain. You may have feelings of guilt or remorse, life feels chaotic and frightening
Anger and bargaining	Frustration leads to anger, you may lash out and blame others. You may bargain, "I would give up anything to have him back"
Depression, reflection, loneliness	A sad period of reflection, the true magnitude of the loss sets in You may isolate yourself to focus on memories
Upward turn	As you start to adjust to life without your pet and begin to move on
Reconstruction and working through	As you become more functional, your mind starts working again
Acceptance and hope	You learn to accept and deal with the reality of your situation. You will be "different" but able to begin to think about the future
	The new grief stages
Shock	Shock and numbness set in to protect your mind from being overwhelmed. It may feel as though you are sleepwalking, not fully in reality and unable to make the simplest of decisions
	Allow family and friends to give support. Begin mourning rituals
Suffering	As the shock wears off, the pain begins. This is a time of emotional upheaval and extreme pain emotionally and physically
	The hallmarks of this phase are rapid mood swings, intense emotions, and loss of control over your psyche. You may even feel like you are losing your sanity
	This is not only the time the most emotional support is needed, but also the time friends and family begin to get on with their lives
	Late in this stage you will begin to exist again but feel lonely and depressed, alternating between intense grief; the "roller coaster" of grief. Expect fluid and unpredictable changes in emotion. Do not fight the emotions, allow them to be
	This is the active grieving stage. Yield to the grief; experience it fully and openly in your own way
Recovery	Acceptance and full recovery do not happen overnight. Your depression and despair will just slowly begin to dissipate
	Although not the end of the pain, you begin to learn to function with the pain in your life. You begin to reconnect to life and remember what "happy" felt like
	The ability to function and more immediate life demands start to take precedence
	The benefit of grief may be seen – you have a new appreciation for life and a new-found ability to live life in the moment

Because instrumental grievers do not outwardly show intense emotion, it is important their grief is not overlooked. *Intuitive-instrumental grievers* experience a combination of both styles, although one style may be more pronounced, depending on their own personality type and attachment to the pet (Cordaro 2012).

Complex grief

The grief felt when a pet is diagnosed with a behavioral disorder or is eventually euthanized because of it is multifaceted and complex. There has been no research in any mental health or veterinary science journals specifically pertaining to grief directly associated with pet owners living with pets with behavioral disorders (Luiz Adrian et al. 2009). Owing to the complexities and the stigma associated, it can be ascertained that the grief associated in such a situation is complex and convoluted.

Disenfranchised grief

Disenfranchised grief occurs when a loss is not acknowledged or supported by societal norms. In the case of disenfranchised grief, the bereaved feel unsupported and are unable to openly mourn; therefore, the grief process may be delayed. Common disenfranchised losses include pet loss, death of a loved one by suicide, or a death of a loved one because of AIDS (Worden 1991). Most pet owners will likely struggle with some degree of disenfranchised grief as an empathetic failure, making them less likely to share the authenticity of emotional pain (Cordaro 2012).

Society has not acknowledged the relationship we have with pets as a true relationship and has proscribed pet-related bereavement as unacceptable. Instead, society prescribes that pet owners "swiftly overcome grief reactions and replace the deceased pet." Consequently, the implicit norm that is endorsed is that the bonds forged between people and companion pets do not have the same depth and meaning as bonds between people; therefore, the grief felt when a pet dies would not be as intense as when another person dies. It is not recognized as a true loss (Cordaro 2012).

An extension of disenfranchised grief occurs when the person mourning finds it difficult to discuss the loss because of stigmatization (Worden 1991). Stigmatization was mentioned in Chapter 4 in regard to treating an animal with a behavioral disorder but also occurs when an animal is euthanized because of a behavioral disorder. Pet owners are often caught in a complex paradox. Many are criticized for treating the animal "when they could just get another pet," but also if they choose not to treat the disorder or end treatment, they may be ostracized because they "could have done more, he was a healthy dog." When they do euthanize for the disorder, they are left without support. It is often a no-win situation for pet owners, leaving them alone to grieve without the benefit of being allowed to mourn the loss.

Pet owners may not reach out to friends or family members because they fear the stigma placed on them and the pet. It is therefore critical for the pet owner to know that the veterinary technician will support them in whatever decisions they make, with no judgments. By building a strong, safe relationship with the pet owner, the technician can give them the needed solace and comfort that they may not be able to find elsewhere. If this is not the case, the pet owner may choose euthanasia and do so in a secret manner, never making contact with the veterinary hospital or staff again because they feel they will be judged or that they are bad pet owners. If they feel safe and not judged, the choice of euthanasia can be seen as a gift, continuing and deepening the bond with the veterinary hospital and veterinary professionals.

Grieving the pet they thought they had

Families living with a pet with a serious behavioral disorder will grieve; some have compared the grief experience as being analogous to death of the pet they thought they had and accepting the pet they do have. Grief associated with accepting that their pet has a serious behavioral disorder can be difficult because it lacks finality comparable to any chronic health disorder.

Unlike grief owing to death, this type of grief is complex and ongoing. The diagnosis of a serious behavioral disorder may bring initial relief and hope to the pet owner, relief that the problem has been seen before and they are not to blame and hope the issue can be treated. Such feelings may only be temporary as they realize their pet's behavioral disorder is likely lifelong and will therefore have a direct impact on their family. As clinical signs of the behavioral disorder may lessen, pet owners may cling to the hope that the disorder will spontaneously remit (Abosh and Collins 1996). When an animal is diagnosed with an affective behavioral disorder (with a likely brain chemical imbalance), the pet owner must vacillate between attempting to resolve the loss while also adapting to the impact of their pet's issues on their lives. Such grief may not resolve over time but may intensify as the pet owner is confronted with the reality that their pet may always need some degree of management and may be limited in which activities they can participate. The cyclic and ongoing nature of the grief is a result of periodic durations in which the animal is reported to be "wonderful 90% of the time" followed by episodes of the behavioral disorder (aggression, panic, compulsions, etc.). This same type of grief has been reported by parents when their child or family member is diagnosed with a mental illness and it is still highly unrecognized in human medicine by grief counselors (MacGregor 1994). The grief is described as complicated and nonfinite. During this stage of grief, the pet owner has not only lost their pet, but also lost the emotionally healthy pet they thought they had.

Families are affected in ways that include coping with symptoms of the disorder, increased responsibilities, disruption of family life, inability to get help, and the social stigma associated with behavioral disorder (Richardson et al. 2011). This type of grief can resurface at the same intensity as it did at diagnosis when a perceived "set back" occurs and is therefore surface-similar to the "chronic sorrow" of parents of emotionally or mentally challenged children.

Choosing to euthanize because of a behavioral disorder

The specific type of grief discussed in this section is when a physically healthy pet is euthanized when a pet owner is unable to continue to treat or manage a pet with a behavioral disorder.

In these situations, one or more of the following behavioral disorders is likely involved:

1. Aggression
2. Unresolved inappropriate elimination
3. Severe separation anxiety
4. Severe thunderstorm phobia
5. Compulsive disorders – especially self-mutilation (Hetts 1999).

Denial/shock

Denial occurs when the current situation is too unbearable to emotionally accept. Shock follows, which is a numbness and detachment. Denial and shock are protection mechanisms as the griever prepares to move further into the grief process. An appropriate analogy is that shock is comparable to ice covering a raging river (the river being pending grief). Shock allows our psyches to prepare for dealing with the raging river below.

When a pet owner is suddenly presented with information they were not expecting, they may be unable to immediately digest the information presented. Be patient and repeat yourself during the process. The pet owner will likely need to contemplate what they have heard. It is helpful for other family members or friends to be present to also hear the information being presented so that it can be reiterated to the pet owner later. Giving an option for a second opinion may also aid in the client's absorption of the information.

Anger

A pet owner's anger is often directed toward persons or situations that they believe caused or exasperated their pet's issues. They may blame veterinarians, trainers, breeders, pet stores, or others they believe they obtained outdated or incorrect information from.

It is important to focus on what can be done rather than what has happened in the past that cannot be changed. Emphasizing past experiences is information for the future, and simply listening to the pet owner without exasperating their anger is helpful. Anger directed toward you is not personal; it is simply part of the pet owner's grief experience (see Figure 5.1).

Bargaining

As pet owners begin to accept their pet's behavioral disorder and deal with the future, they may begin to bargain, looking for "other options" or ways out of their current circumstance.

Rehoming versus euthanasia

When aggression is directed toward family members, it is generally not a situation in which the pet is rehomeable or adoptable. It is not fair to rehome the pet and have a new family become attached to the pet. Likely, the new family will become the recipient of aggression in similar situations and have to struggle with the decision to rehome or euthanize. This does not benefit the HAB or the welfare of the pet. It places another family at risk of injury and heartbreak. Often, attempts to correct the problem are inappropriate (positive punishment), and this negatively affects the welfare of the pet. Euthanasia would be a responsible decision in this situation. It would be the best decision from a public health standpoint and for the welfare of the pet. Not all companion animals make good pets and enjoy human companionship.

Exceptions may include the following: aggression directed only toward children living in the home or another pet in the home. In this situation, the pet could be rehomed to a child-free or pet-free home, with the new pet owner fully aware of the issue and agreeable to keeping the pet away from children and other animals.

Guilt

While anger is directed toward someone or something, guilt is anger directed at oneself. Holding onto guilty feelings can keep an owner from moving on or having quality relationships with future pets.

Guilt is present in any grief experience but may be exaggerated for pet owners by their heightened sense of responsibility for their pet comparable to that for the well-being of a child. Pet owners often believe they contributed to their pet's disorder by not noticing the extreme symptoms of anxiety, choosing the wrong trainer, or by not being a strong "pack leader" (see section titled **The dominance theory** earlier in this chapter). Often, after explaining to the pet owner that they are not the direct cause of the disorder, they continue to believe that somehow they should have been able to prevent it. The feeling of powerlessness to deal with the problem exacerbates this type of unrealistic guilt. Allowing the pet owner to have an active involvement as a member of the treatment team can give them a bit of empowerment and relief from this type of guilt. Pet owners who feel listened to and supported and receive accurate and up-to-date information feel empowered and may move to take action with a treatment plan or consider other options.

The notion of pet owners being "bad pet owners" if their animal must be euthanized because of a behavioral disorder creates a scenario of grief and guilt that can be overwhelming. Pet owners may have feelings of guilt because of perceived inadequacy as pet owners and feelings of complicity in the development of their pet's disorder. The loss of an animal because of a behavioral disorder can shake a pet owner's belief in themselves as "good" pet owners. Family members may blame each other, causing family tension. "There are no bad dogs, only bad pet owners" is a very hurtful and blaming statement, and in fact, likely to be untrue.

- "There are no bad dogs, only bad pet owners" is a very hurtful and blaming statement, and in fact, likely to be untrue.

Receiving a diagnosis can alleviate the pet owner's feelings of guilt that they directly caused their pet's behavioral disorder. When a pet owner feels guilty, ask them to state exactly what they specifically feel guilty about. Remind them what they have done in an attempt to treat the problem. Acknowledge that the difficult decisions they are making take deep love and courage only a very brave, selfless, and compassionate pet owner can make (Table 5.9).

- Guilt and pet owner self-forgiveness
  1. Identify the reasons you must consider choosing euthanasia.
  2. Accept the fact it is your responsibility to make this decision.
  3. Acknowledge the pain and guilt you may be feeling.
  4. Identify precisely what you feel guilty about.
  5. Compassionately listen to your desire to avoid this decision.
  6. Love yourself and know that you are innocent of any wrong-doing.
  7. Know that it takes tremendous love to consider taking an action that will release your pet from his suffering, while it leaves you with so much pain.

(Peterson 1997)

It can be hypothesized that pet owners who have euthanized a pet due to a behavioral disorder may experience prolonged guilt, although there has to date been no research produced on the subject.

Anticipatory grief and acceptance

Anticipatory grief occurs before the death of the pet and is the beginning stage of coming to terms and accepting euthanasia as the appropriate option (Cordaro 2012). The pet owner may begin to ask

Table 5.9 Common guilt-ridden statements made by pet owners with responses.

Statement	Response
"I did not do enough to help her"	"You have done everything you can to help her. You have done more than most people could have ever achieved. You have given her the happiest moments of her life and for that I know she is deeply grateful"
"People think I am crazy for keeping him"	"They do not see the wonderful moments, the times where he is happy and relaxed with you. They simply do not know him as you do and therefore cannot understand"
"I created the problem; it is my fault"	"Your pet was most likely born with a physical brain chemistry disorder. There are training techniques and communication styles that can increase anxiety, but you did not create your pet's behavior disorder"
"I made the problem worse"	"You cannot do what you do not know. I have done many things to my past pets that I now wish I could go back and change because I have better and newer knowledge. But all we can do is move forward with the up-to-date information we know. Fluffy taught us lessons that we will take with us into the future"

specific questions such as, "How would we 'do it'?," "Would you be there with us?" This is a critical point for the veterinary technician to gain the confidence of the pet owner. Letting them know the details of the process and the steps that would be taken to make sure their pet is comfortable and unafraid, working with the pet owner to make decisions as to who they would like to be in the room, and so on help the pet owner feel in control.

The resolution and acceptance of the loss can be characterized not by forgetting the loss but by being able to remember the pet with a source of warmth and pleasure rather than pain (Wright 2007–2011). Something that can only happen after the anticipation of death can be accepted (Walter 1996).

Breaking the bond

When the "bad times" begin to dramatically subtract from the "good times" and the stress of dealing with potentially dangerous or unpredictable circumstances outweighs the comfort the pet gives to the pet owner are signs that the bond has become unhealthy, and gentle breaking of the bond may need to occur. In general, it is not our role to tell a pet owner when they should choose euthanasia for their pet (Hetts 1999). Choosing euthanasia, specifically in regard to a behavioral disorder, is a very complex and personal decision. It is the role of the technician to support and guide the pet owner in whatever decision they make, whether that is treatment or ending the pet's life. The decision to end the pet's life needs to be that of the pet owner and not made solely on your recommendation.

Coming to terms with such a decision is a process. It is your job to guide the pet owner through the process side by side rather than as an authoritative figure. When a pet owner asks, "What would you do?" they are asking for your guidance, validation, and knowledge that you will not judge them but will support them. I frequently reiterate, "That is a very personal decision and I will support you in whatever decision you make."

Determining the current level of attachment

Understanding the depth of the emotional bond, the role of the pet in the pet owner's life, and the quality of the pet owner's social support system will help understand and predict the depth of the pet owner's grief (Cordaro 2012).

Exceptionally strong and complex attachments may occur in the following situations.

- The pet was rescued from near-death or a traumatic life experience.
- The pet owner believes the pet got them through an intensely difficult experience or time in their life.
- The pet owner had the pet through childhood.
- When the pet owner has had little outside support in their life and believes their pet to be their main support system.
- Service animals that have assisted a physically, mentally, or emotionally challenged individual.
- The pet owner is deeply anthropomorphic toward their pet.
- The pet owner views their pet as a symbolic link to a person they have lost.

- When the pet owner has invested a great deal of time, financial resources, and effort into the treatment of their pet. This can be especially the case when dealing with long-term behavioral disorders or other health-related disorders (Lagoni et al. 1994).

Once the HAB has been damaged, it is very difficult, if not impossible, to repair. Some pet owners have made the comparison of living in an abusive relationship. "I cannot trust him." "He's good most of the time but if I do the 'wrong' thing everything can change. It is like walking on eggshells." "I cannot completely relax even when things are going well." These comments are likely an indication the pet owner is feeling significant caregiver strain (see Table 4.1 and Appendix 7).

In cases in which the pet owner is not ready to consider euthanasia as an option, it will be the task of the behavior team to guide the pet owner slowly and at their pace. Many pet owners need time and the knowledge that they have done everything they can before considering euthanasia as an option. Setting a time frame to revisit and reassess is often the key to the pet owner accepting the thought of euthanasia. Knowing they have tried all treatment possible helps alleviate guilt. Creating goals agreed on and setting a time frame (two to four weeks) to evaluate progress and whether goals have been reached give the pet owner time to step back and have a method for determining progress or lack of it.

A person's reluctance to choose euthanasia for their pet may stem from their own personal past experiences, which do not have a direct correlation with the current circumstance. For instance, a family member may have developed a mental illness or been taken off life support. In these cases, additional professional help may be needed.

Pet owners may desperately feel the need to be validated, asking questions such as, "What would you do?" My response in these situations is honest and direct, "This problem would be very difficult for me to live with in my own home." Often, hearing that a professional who deals with such issues on a daily basis would also find the situation difficult is a clear validation to the pet owner that they have done enough.

The veterinarian should give the medical, diagnostic, and prognostic reports; the technician can then translate that information into "real-life information." Showing concern for the pet owner's emotional, physical, and mental health well-being by saying, "I'm worried about you" "How are you doing? This must be incredibly stressful for you" gives permission for the pet owner to release emotions that are not being expressed.

The technician can emphasize that the behavior team's goal is to promote and protect the HAB and to help create healthy relationships between pets and people. Acknowledge the importance of the pet and its positive qualities. "This is very difficult because Fluffy is such a wonderful companion much of the time." The technician may find it appropriate to say, "Fluffy loves you and does not want to injure you, but her brain chemistry disorder makes it difficult for her to control her behaviors. We've tried everything medically and behaviorally possible to decrease her fear, and we are running out of options. I'm concerned for her quality of life and your quality of life. How do you feel about what I've said?" The pet owner may not be able to respond or be too emotional to respond. The technician should reiterate, "We are here for you and Fluffy, and we will continue to support you regardless of any decision you make. You will not be judged in any way but fully supported."

If the pet owner introduces thoughts of euthanasia before the treatment team is anticipating it, they should not be discouraged. It is an indication, regardless of the pet's issue, that the HAB is tenuous or severed. At this point, the veterinarian must make the decision whether to encourage treatment or support the pet owner. This may be a point in which either the treatment plan is accelerated using every tool available or the treatment may be simplified, while the pet owner makes a decision whether to continue. It is tragic when a pet owner who is already in the grieving process and loosening their attachment to the pet, is encouraged to continue trying, only to be later heading down the same path in the future. Much has to be determined by listening to the pet owner, and in some cases, specifically asking them how they "feel" about the pet. The depth of the damage to the HAB will likely correlate with lack of compliance with the treatment plan.

When considering euthanasia, the following points should be considered:

- Rarely does a decision have to be made at this moment; allow the pet owner time. Sometimes, recommending respite by boarding the pet will give the pet owner time to continue to consider their life without the pet.
- No decision is perfect. If in the least bit unsure of their decision, the pet owner should be encouraged to postpone the decision.
- The decision should not be made in anger or desperation.

- The pet owner should not act or refrain from acting because of what they believe others will think.
- The pet owner should be able to acknowledge and recognize all they have done for their pet, and let it be enough.

It is an indication the pet owner may be moving toward accepting euthanasia as an option when they are able to

- accept the pet is mentally and emotionally suffering, and see evidence that treatment has failed;
- reach the point at which holding on becomes more painful than letting go and the pet owner has come to accept that euthanasia is a loving way to end the pet's suffering; and
- accept their responsibility in the decision without excessive guilt.

"Choosing euthanasia would be a responsible and humane decision." Dr. Andrew Luescher, DVM, DACVB, PhD in response to an owner considering euthanasia.

- "Choosing euthanasia would be a responsible and humane decision."

Dr. Andrew Luescher, DVM, DACVB, PhD in response to an owner considering euthanasia.

All three areas must be dealt with before a pet owner can accept euthanasia with peace (Peterson 1997). "Letting go is not giving up, it is a deliberate decision to end suffering" Peterson (1997).

- "Letting go is not giving up, it is a deliberate decision to end suffering."

Peterson (1997)

The decision

Once the decision for euthanasia has been made, it means the process of creating a special event can begin. The last weeks or days with the pet can be turned into a gift and become filled with positive memories. The pet owner should be encouraged early in the process to begin creating a tribute to their pet. Possibilities could include writing a letter to their pet, constructing a memory book with photos, and keeping a journal about their grief. Some pet owners find it helpful to save tufts of hair and clay paw prints. The technician should follow the pet owner's lead and monitor their needs.

After euthanasia, some form of sentiment and condolence to the pet owner should be arranged. Often, a card is passed among staff members and doctors, allowing for them to share fond memories of the pet, words of testament, and empathy to the client for their loss. Clients are deeply touched by the heartfelt words and appreciate the care and support provided by the practice.

After the loss

As with suicide and other disenfranchised grief situations, often the first question is, "What should we tell people about how 'Fido' died?" Euthanizing a pet because of a mental or behavioral disorder is complex and difficult to grasp for many people. Acceptance, a final stage in grieving, can be difficult to obtain because of the bewilderment and sometimes lack of definite answers to "Why did this happen." Among others blaming the pet owners, the most cutting blame can come from the pet owner themselves. It is common for the pet owner to remember every mistake they made with their pet, every harsh word, and wonder if "that" is what caused the behavioral disorder. Most will have done the best they could with what they had at the time, which is all we can expect of others or ourselves.

The pet owner will need to make a decision as to with whom and how much they share about their pet's death. In reality, if the pet was euthanized because of a serious behavioral disorder, then the animal suffered from the physical problem of having a neurochemical brain disorder.

There is a stigma when euthanasia occurs because of a behavioral disorder comparable to the stigma people feel when a family member has committed suicide; therefore, it is not uncommon for people to be uncomfortable when they find the pet has been euthanized, specifically for a behavioral reason. People may say nothing in fear of saying the wrong thing. Some may blame the pet owner for their animal "parenting" skills. When asked, "How did your pet die?" the answer could simply be, "He had a brain chemistry imbalance that could not be medically corrected." Most behavioral disorders are likely a combination of life experience (or lack of it) and a physical organic brain chemistry disorder.

Pet owners need to be encouraged that they are good people and good pet owners who have suffered a tragedy.

- Most behavior disorders are likely a combination of life experience (or lack of it) and a physical organic brain chemistry disorder.

Pet owners may be told by family or friends to "get over it." If what they mean is that the pet owner will eventually begin moving forward, that will occur in time. If they mean the pet owner should forget the loss, they will not. A pet wiggles its way into a place in our hearts that needed filling. When that pet is no longer present, the space is filled with memories. The pain will recede, eventually to an ache and finally to soft memories (Wolfelt 2004).

Successful grief counseling will have an impact on future HABs. Assisting the client through their own private grief path with no judgments, only honest empathy, will bond the pet owner to the technician and the veterinary hospital. When performed properly, grief counseling means growth for all involved (Table 5.10).

Relief

Feeling guilty for feeling happy is called *recovery guilt*. A sense of relief may occur after the euthanasia, followed by guilt or shame for feeling that relief. Living with an animal with a behavioral disorder can be extremely stressful. The constant worry and anxiety are gone, and the pet owner may now be filled with both relief and guilt for feeling that relief. The relief comes because not only is the pet owner's stress gone but also because the suffering of their pet is also now relieved.

After care – additional support

Signs of abnormal complicated grief (traumatic or prolonged grief) include a powerful pining for the deceased, great difficulty moving on, a sense that life is meaningless, bitterness, and anger pertaining to the loss lasting longer than six months. Other characteristics of complicated grief may include avoiding all reminders of the death, inability to trust others since the death, bitterness, and anger related to the loss, difficulty moving on with life, numbness since the loss, and feelings that life is meaningless since the loss (Ozgul 2004).

Pet owners may focus on wanting to change the past, mulling over what "should have" been done differently When looking at the past becomes exaggerated or excessive, the process of grief may be delayed. Some may hold onto the grief as "punishment" for "letting the animal down." There may come a time when the veterinary practice is ineffective or ill-equipped in providing support to a grieving client. Similarly, clients faced with extreme depression and feelings of hopelessness would better benefit from additional counseling services or support groups.

Table 5.10 Managing grief after the decision to euthanize.

Strategy	Definition	Example
Catharsis	Coaxing client to express emotions	"I will be just outside the door if you would like to talk."
Empathizing	Identifying with the client's experience	"What you are going through is incredibly difficult and courageous. You are not letting Fluffy go because it is what you want, you are doing it because it will end Fluffy's suffering. She never has to be afraid again. What a brave and loving thing you are doing"
Sympathizing	Expressing an emotion for the owner. May include using "body language" or gestures to convey emotional support	Sitting quietly with the client, holding their hand, not being rushed
Reassurance	Talking to instill confidence	"It is very clear how much you love Fluffy and she knows that. This is your last and greatest act of love to her"
Redirecting	Encouraging owners to focus on the positive aspects of their relationship with their pet	"What was Fluffy like as a kitten/puppy? What is your favorite memory?"
Comforting touch	Touching the owner's shoulder and the pet	Pet Fluffy and show your own compassion and comforting touch to both the pet owner and the pet

Source: Adapted from Morris 2012.

Clients may confide in you their feelings of not being able to go on without their pet. In these instances, it is absolutely imperative that the pet owner is referred to appropriate and more aggressive help. Clients should not feel ashamed for the feelings they are having. However, concern for their well-being must be expressed so that additional resources can be recommended.

It is important to have a list of resources readily available. Provide clients with a phone list of counselors and support group hotlines as well as recommended grieving books and valid online resources. Many veterinary universities offer pet-loss support and counseling services.

When equipped with the right resources, you can find comfort in knowing that you are providing your clients with the proper services and support they need to help them through their loss.

Conclusion

- The capacity to love, requires the necessity to mourn.

Wolfelt 2004

Strengthening, protecting, and promoting the HAB should be the primary goal of veterinary medicine. Relieving the sufferings of animals and their owners also includes alleviating emotional and mental sufferings. There will be times when removing a pet from its home either by rehoming or through euthanasia will be the appropriate and most prudent decision to protect future HABs. If we allow pet owners to continue a destructive relationship with their pet, possibly allowing a family member or child to be seriously injured, thus teaching that family member or child to fear animals and they then teach their own children to fear animals, we have done a great disservice to the pet owner and to the HAB and have failed.

Guiding a pet owner through the grief process associated with living with a pet with a serious behavioral disorder is not only a complex, but also a deeply bonding process. "Considering pet loss as a normative grief process is not only an indication to bereaved pet owners that their loss is valued, but also an initial step toward reinstating within our society a stigmatized grief" (Cohen 2002). When the grief process associated with the treatment of behavioral disorders and euthanasia is skillfully, honestly, and sensitively supported, it can be a profound experience for both the pet owner and the veterinary professional. Assisting a pet owner into and through the grief process should be seen as an absolute and ultimate honor.

- Assisting a pet owner into and through the grief process should be seen as an absolute and ultimate honor.

References

Abood, S.K. (2007). Increasing adherence in practice: making your clients partners in care. *Veterinary Clinics of North America: Small Animal Practice* 37 (1): 151–164.

Abosh, B. and Collins, A. (1996). *Mental Illness in the Family: Issues and Trends*. Toronto: University of Toronto Press.

Adams, C.L. and Frankel, R.M. (2007). It may be a dog's life but the relationship with her owners is also key to her health and well being: communication in veterinary medicine. *Veterinary Clinics of North America: Small Animal Practice* 37 (1): 1–17.

Canino, J., Shaw, J., and Beck, A.M. (2007). A look at the role of marriage and family therapy skills within the context of animal behavior therapy. *Journal of Veterinary Behavior: Clinical Applications and Research* 2 (1): 15–22.

Carson, C.A. (2007). Nonverbal communication in veterinary practice. *Veterinary Clinics of North America: Small Animal Practice* 37 (1): 49–63.

Chun, R., Schafer, S., Lotta, C.C. et al. (2009). Didactic and experimental training to teach communication skills: the university of Wisconsin-Madison school of veterinary medicine collaborative experience. *Journal of Veterinary Medical Education* 36 (2): 196–201.

Cohen, S.P. (2002). Can pets function as family members? *Western Journal of Nursing Research* 24 (6): 621.

Cordaro, M. (2012). Pet loss and disenfranchised grief: implications for mental health counseling practice. *Journal of Mental Health Counseling* 34 (4): 283–294.

Cornell, K. (2012). 5 steps to effective feedback. *Exceptional Veterinary Team* 4 (1): 37–40.

Durrance, D. and Lagoni, L. (1998). *Connecting with Clients: Practical Communication for 10 Common Situations*. Lakewood, CO, USA: American Animal Hospital Association Press.

Egan, G. (2002). *The Skilled Helper: A Problem-Management and Opportunity–Development Approach to Helping*. California, Brooks/Cole: Pacific Grove.

Frankel, R.M. and Stein, T. (1999). Getting the most out of the clinical encounter: the four habits model. *The Permanente Journal* 3 (3): 79–88.

Gray, C. and Moffett, J. (2010). *Handbook of Veterinary Communication Skills*. New Jersey, USA: Wiley–Blackwell.

Guy, N.C., Luescher, U.A., Dohoo, S.E. et al. (2001a). A case series of biting dogs: characteristics of the dogs, their behaviour, and their victims. *Applied Animal Behaviour Science* 74 (1): 43–57.

Guy, N.C., Luescher, U.A., Dohoo, S.E. et al. (2001b). Demographic and aggressive characteristics of dogs in a general veterinary caseload. *Applied Animal Behaviour Science* 74 (1): 15–28.

Guy, N.C., Luescher, U.A., Dohoo, S.E. et al. (2001c). Risk factors for dog bites to owners in a general veterinary caseload. *Applied Animal Behaviour Science* 74 (1): 29–42.

Hetts, S. (1999). *Pet Behavior Protocols: What to Say, What to Do, When to Refer*. Lakewood, CO: AAHA Press.

Lagoni, L., Hetts, S., and Butler, C. (1994). *The Human-Animal Bond and Grief*. Philadelphia, PA: W.B. Saunders.

Luescher, A. and Martin, K.M. (2010). *Dogs! & Cats: Diagnosis and Treatment of Behavior Problems*. Lafayette, IN: Purdue University.

Luiz Adrian, J.A., Deliramich, A.N., and Frueh, B.C. (2009). Complicated grief and posttraumatic stress disorder in humans' response to the death of pets/animals. *Bulletin of the Menninger Clinic* 73 (3): 176–187.

MacGregor, P. (1994). Grief: the unrecognized parental response to mental illness in a child. *Social Work* 39 (2): 160–166.

McCurnin, D.M. (2010). *Clinical Textbook for Veterinary Technicians*. Philadelphia: Saunders.

McKeon, T. (2012). TAGteach International. https://www.tagteach.com (accessed November 7, 2012).

Mech, L.D. (2008). *Whatever Happened to the Term Alpha Wolf*, 4–8. Winter: International Wolf Magazine.

Meyer, P.J. (2003). *Attitude Is Everything: If you Want to Succeed above and beyond*. Scotts Valley, CA: The Meyer Resource Group Incorporated.

Morris, P. (2012). Managing pet owners' guilt and grief in veterinary euthanasia encounters. *Journal of Contemporary Ethnography* 41 (3): 337–365.

Murie, A. and Etats-Unis. National park (1944). *The Wolves of Mount McKinley*. Washington: U.S. Government Printing Office.

Northey, W. (2002). Characteristics and clinical practices of marriage and family therapists: a national survey. *Journal of Marital and Family Therapy* 28 (4): 487–494.

Ozgul, S. (2004). Parental grief and serious mental illness: a narrative. (cover story). *Australian and New Zealand Journal of Family Therapy* 25 (4): 183–187.

Peterson, L.M. (1997). *Surviving the Heartbreak of Choosing Death for your Pet*. Las Vegas, Nev: Greentree Publishing.

Richardson, M., Cobham, V., Murray, J., and McDermott, B. (2011). Parents' grief in the context of adult child mental illness: a qualitative review. *Clinical Child and Family Psychology Review* 14 (1): 28–43.

Rosenthal, S.A. (2005). *The Complete Idiot's Guide to Toltec Wisdom*. New York, NY: Alpha Books.

Ryan, T. (2005). *Coaching People to Train their Dogs*. Legacy Canine Behavior and Training: Sequim, WA.

Shaw, J. and Luescher, L. (2005). Problem Puppies: New Theories on Dominance. *Veterinary Technician* 26 (7): 499–502.

Shaw, J. (2007). Is it acceptable for people to be paid to adhere to medication? *BMJ* 335 (7613): 233.

Shaw, J. (2011). A poll to determine veterinarians' current role expectation of dog trainers. ACVB/AVSAB Veterinary Behavior Symposium, St. Louis, MO.

Stein, T., Nagy, V.T., and Jacobs, L. (1998). Caring for patients one conversation at a time. *The Permanente Journal* 2 (4): 62–68.

Walter, T. (1996). A new model of grief: bereavement and biography. *Mortality* 1 (1): 7–25.

Wolfelt, A.D. (2004). *When your Pet Dies: A Guide to Mourning, Remembering & Healing*. Companion: Gazelle, Fort Collins, Colo.; Lancaster.

Worden, J.W. (1991). *Grief Counseling and Grief Therapy: A Handbook for the Mental Health Practitioner*. New York: Springer Publishing Company.

Wright, J. (2007–2011). The stages of grief: understanding the grief cycle. http://www.recover-from-grief.com/new-grief-stages.html (accessed November 3, 2013).

The PowerPoint of figures, appendices, MCQ's are available at www.wiley.com/go/martin/behavior

6 Learning and behavior modification

Virginia L. Price
Saint Petersburg College, College of Veterinary Technology, St. Petersburg, FL, USA

CHAPTER MENU

Learning can be defined as the permanent change in the behavior of an animal after being exposed to a stimulus (Barker 2001). Although the changes may not be apparent immediately, as seen in latent learning (see Tolman and Honzik 1930 for more details about latent learning in rats), they are nevertheless real changes that affect behavior. Animals learn throughout their lifetime and learning is affected by their environment beginning in the uterus. They learn when a person is teaching them behaviors and when they are interacting with their environment or other animals. They even learn while watching people or other animals. Learning is a full-time pursuit for all animals. The flexibility of the animal brain is just becoming apparent in today's research. From research on animal cognition to animal perception, our knowledge about animals has grown tremendously. Because this is a growing area of science, it is vital to keep current by reading new information.

- Learning is a full-time pursuit for all animals.
- The flexibility of the animal brain is just becoming apparent in today's research.

This chapter discusses some of the innate and environmental effects on learning and different ways that animals learn. Behavior modification techniques using these types of learning are defined and discussed. In Chapter 9, the practical uses of these techniques are discussed in detail. No book chapter can capture completely the complexity of animal learning. Students should read a variety of scientific sources and use critical thinking to create their own ideas on how animals learn.

- Students should read a variety of scientific sources and use critical thinking to create their own ideas on how animals learn.

Genetics and learning

Different species and breeds of animals perform species and breed-specific behaviors because of differences in their genetic codes. The effect of genetics on behavior is due to differences in noncoding genes that function as gene regulators (ENCODE Project Consortium 2012 as cited in Grandin and

Canine and Feline Behavior for Veterinary Technicians and Nurses, Second Edition. Edited by Debbie Martin and Julie K. Shaw.

Companion website: www.wiley.com/go/martin/behavior

Deesing 2014). Genetic effects on behavior are complex. Much more complex than their effects on physical traits. One reason could be folding DNA (as it lays naturally in cells) brings traits in close proximity unlike DNA straightened out in a line for analysis (Grandin and Deesing 2014). Another reason for the complexity of genetic origins of behavior is the number of genes involved in creating behaviors (Ilska et al. 2017). Environmental effects on behavior are well known. The combined effects of genetics and environment on expressed behaviors are another complicating factor. Dogs are especially interesting genetically because their evolutionary path has led to a huge variety of genetic material. According to Lord et al., this variety is due to hybridization and a relaxed natural selection associated with their environmental niche of the human village (2014).

Lorenz (1965) spent many years studying innate behaviors he called fixed action patterns. Animals performed these behaviors or behavioral chains after being exposed to a specific stimulus in their environment called a *sign stimulus*. For example, parent birds feed baby birds displaying the red interior of their mouths. Cats exhibit a pattern of predatory behavior after seeing or hearing a prey animal. Behaviors can be thought of as being on a continuum from innate to learned, with behaviors being either innate, learned, or a combination of the two (Lorenz 1965). Many innate behaviors are simple species behaviors corresponding to conserved genetic material across species (Maher 2012 as cited by Grandin and Deesing 2014). Here are a few examples of behaviors thought to be innate: walking, suckling, flehmen lip curl, kneeling in rat estrus, nest building, sexual behavior, and killing and eating behaviors. Other aspects of behavior have learned influences (burrowing in rats) or are influenced by learning alone (foraging behaviors), which increases flexibility related to environmental influences (Grandin and Deesing 2014).

Behaviors generally believed to be reflexes can be affected by the environment through chemical or contextual input. Environmental influences do not always mean visual stimuli; they can be nutritional or chemical influences. Fixed action patterns with learned modifications related to environmental input are called model action patterns. An example of one is seen in honey bee feeding action patterns where bees adjust their feeding behaviors related to learning a conditioned stimulus (CS) for the presence of sugar water (Smith and Mendel 1989). This is an example of a conditioned odorant (chemical stimulus) causing the feeding action pattern of the honey bee without the presence of the sugar water after the bee learned to associate the conditioned odorant with sugar water.

- Behaviors can be thought of as being on a continuum from innate to learned, with behaviors being either innate, learned, or a combination of the two (Lorenz 1965).

Although it would be orderly for all behaviors to be adaptive, this cannot be the case. The basis for evolution is a large number of diverse offspring from which the environment selects the fittest individuals using natural selection (Darwin 1859). Skinner (1966) discussed how behaviors may appear, even though they are counterproductive for an animal. These behaviors are less likely to be passed on to future generations, but they may be passed on if the animal has enough adaptive behaviors to survive long enough to reproduce. It is this capability, reproduction, which judges whether the animal is fit, as in the survival of the fittest, not aggression and not hierarchical placement.

- It is this capability, reproduction, which judges whether the animal is fit, as in the survival of the fittest, not aggression and not hierarchical placement.

Expressed behaviors may appear the same in different animals, but they can still be formed through different combinations of conditioned and unconditioned learning (Krushinskii 1960). These behaviors although developed in a variety of ways, appear the same when elicited. Fixed behavior patterns or behavioral units are the end result, but the environment and other stimuli affect the exact form this pattern takes. These fixed patterns are governed by natural selection (Krushinskii 1960). The ability of animals to behave in varied ways and yet arrive at the same behavioral outcome is beneficial for them. Flexibility allows animals to take advantage of different situations and arrive at the same ends by different means. By allowing conditioned and unconditioned reflexes (behaviors) to be combined, the nervous system becomes more sensitive to the stimuli it encounters (Krushinskii 1960).

Hormones are substances the body secretes that chemically instruct its systems to perform specific actions. Male sex hormones are associated with the genetic code that instructs the fetus to become male, while female hormones are associated with genes instructing the fetus to become female. The theory used to be that female was the default sex, but there is evidence to support biological sex forms through a complex series of biological events. "Studies in mice suggest that the gonad teeters between being male and female throughout life, its identity requiring constant maintenance" (Ainsworth 2015). To illustrate the power of hormones to affect behavior, Kockaya and Demirbas found 19 Kangal bitches, flock-guarding canines from Turkey, who previously cannibalized their offspring no longer did so after receiving oxytocin every 6 hours for 10 days intramuscular beginning postpartum (2020).

The study on dogs by Krushinskii (1960) showed that male dogs more often exhibited active defense reflexes than female dogs, and the former had a stronger nervous system (not defined), but there were no sex differences found in excitability. In a more recent study, Wallis et al. found male dogs to show more aggression toward humans than females as reported by the owners while excitability differences related to sex did not reach statistical significance (2020). In a study on learning abilities in dogs, sex differences varied by breed (Serpell and Hsu 2005). While female dogs in two dog breeds exhibited better learning abilities, male dogs in other dog breeds performed better in learning tasks. Interestingly, the same study found that conformation show dogs exhibited lower learning ability than field trial dogs in two different breeds. In a study of male and female dog puppies, Bekoff (1974) found no differences in play behavior besides the male Beagles mounting during play, whereas the female dogs did not. In comparison, Hart (1995) found that male dogs showed more dominance (the term dominance was not defined) and aggression toward the owner than female dogs. It is interesting that these two traits were found together in male dogs, as they may be assessing the same trait; the term dominance is no longer used to describe behaviors or traits. Female dogs were found to be more easily trained for obedience and house training. In research, comparing the behavior of Beagle male dogs, female dogs, and female dogs that were treated with testosterone propionate (a fast-acting short ester testosterone product), male dogs were found to maintain a resource (bone) more often than both the types of female dogs (Beach et al. 1982). Female dogs treated with the hormone were more likely to maintain the resource than those untreated. Using shelter dogs, Wells and Hepper (1999) found that female dogs spent less time looking at people than male dogs did, and both sexes of dogs looked and barked at male humans more than they did toward female humans. In cats, Barry and Crowell-Davis (1999) found no differences in behavior associated with sex except female cats did not allorub other cats, and male cats did allorub both sexes. Allorubbing is seen when a cat rubs its head, side, and/or tail on another cat, object, or person. The functions of this behavior include scent exchange as well as a pleasurable tactile sensation (Crowell-Davis et al. 2004).

Sexual differences in behavior can be created by environmental factors. People place a great deal of importance on sexual differences, and change in an animal's behavior can be affected by a person's beliefs about how sex affects behavior. People may reinforce unruly behavior in male animals, believing it is normal behavior in male animals. Conversely, they may reinforce quiet, calm behavior in female animals, believing it to be their nature. These manipulations of an animal's behavior may not be conscious. Confirmation bias may affect the behaviors reported by owners or scientists. There could be a bias inherent in the questions scientists ask about sex differences in behavior, which then affects the knowledge we have to draw from. Because behavior is generally a combination of genetic and environmental effects, sexual differences seen in behavior may also be because of the environmental differences. Wallis et al. remind us in their conclusion, the effects of sex on behavior they found were small, "therefore their biological relevance is questionable" (2020). They also point out, even though associations are found between sex and a behavior does not mean the dog's sex causes the behavior. Research supports the updated conception of biological sex to include intersex individuals by describing biological sex as a spectrum instead of a binary system (Ainsworth 2015). There are varying ways biological sex could be determined, anatomy, hormones, cells, and chromosomes (Ainsworth 2015). These possible determinates are not always demonstrating the same biological sex (Ainsworth 2015).

- When experimental variables are associated or correlated, it does not mean one variable causes the other.

- Because behavior is generally a combination of genetic and environmental effects, sexual differences seen in behavior may be because of environmental differences.

Animals are generally better able to learn certain types of behaviors because of the manner in which their brains and bodies are organized and develop. Lord et al. discussed how certain behaviors are enhanced through hybridization of size, shape, and behavior from the general dog population. Dogs performing wanted behaviors are bred to others who perform the wanted behaviors. Their puppies are more likely to exhibit these behaviors. Thus, breed markers are enhanced in breed population by choosing certain puppies for breeding (2014). An example of how brain organization affects learning and behavior includes how Vervet monkeys communicate the type of predator they observe in their territory. Animals learn to categorize predators by the type of predator including their methods of predation, and Seyfarth et al. knew this because the monkeys exhibited prey-specific alarm calls (1980). Vervet monkeys gave three specific predator alarm calls: one for eagles who attack from the sky, one for pythons who attack from the ground, and yet another for leopards who ambush prey from hiding places (Seyfarth et al. 1980). Once the warning call was given the monkeys responded in predicable ways looking up for eagles then running to get under cover, looking on the ground for pythons, and climbing up a tree for leopards (Seyfarth, et al. 1980). Brains are naturally structured to classify and categorize sensory input like vocalizations. This is a time-saving feature of the nervous system used for species survival.

The organization of brain classifications is based on genetic coding, although classifications are modified throughout an animal's life through its experience. Support for this is seen in working dogs in which their natural behavior through breeding may be to herd sheep and through experience may learn to also herd cattle, geese, or human children.

- The organization of brain classifications is based on genetic coding, although classifications are modified throughout an animal's life through its experience.

Animals selected through natural or artificial selection to perform behaviors will tend to better perform these behaviors over generations through this selection process. Evidence of this is seen in wild animals when they take advantage of an environmental niche and is also seen in domestic animals. Wild animals may take advantage of a rainforest or a desert environment, whereas domestic animals may instead take advantage of a farm yard or household environment. Through selection processes, natural or artificial, the animals become better able to take advantage of their niche. We can witness this evolution in action as our dog and cat populations surpass the numbers seen in their closest wild relations, showing their superior fitness.

Animals may feel intrinsic reinforcement for species- or breed-specific behaviors (Coppinger and Coppinger 2001 reported on this phenomenon in dogs). For example, scent hounds appear to feel good when they are tracking a scent, and because of this reinforcement, they are more likely to spend time tracking scent than are dogs from other breed groups, thus perfecting this behavior through learning. They also have better ability to track scent because of the configuration of their olfactory system (genetics). All domestic animals use their olfactory systems to a greater capacity than humans do, and evidence for this lies in the amount of brain space used to evaluate olfactory sensations and the amount of neural tissue in the nose collecting the sensory input. Research in this area is very exciting and will lead us to a better understanding of animal behavior (see Overall and Arnold 2007 – in dogs).

Alleles (Figure 6.1) are the variations of a gene that produce different characteristics in living beings (National Human Genome Research Institute, n.d.). One way in which alleles are involved in variations in behaviors is through the differences in the physical shapes of the animals they help to build (Coppinger and Coppinger 2001). This idea is simplified immensely as genes create proteins, not animal shapes or behaviors, but these small building blocks are where these differences are seen at the most basic level. Coppinger and Coppinger wrote huskies are known for their sled-pulling ability,

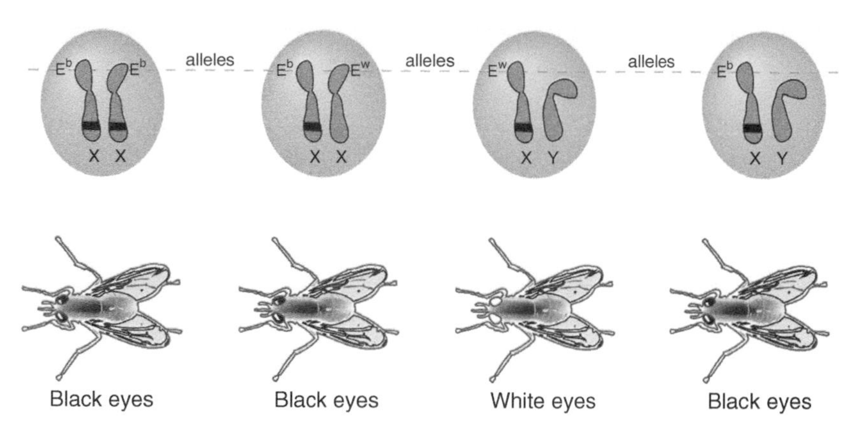

Figure 6.1 An example of alleles. *Source*: Courtesy of National Human Genome Research Institute. For detailed definitions of genetic terms go to: https://www.genome.gov/genetics-glossary.

largely because of their compact shape, whereas Alaskan Malamutes are too large to pull a sled far without overheating (2001). Cats, owing to their shape, size, and sensory abilities, are excellent small rodent hunters. They have the sensory ability to detect and the physical ability to stealthily stalk and kill their prey. Hemmer (1990) noted coat density and body size can inhibit behavior of all types by creating hyperthermia with even minor activity. This is another example of how phenotype may affect behavior and learning.

- One way in which alleles are involved in variations in behaviors is through the differences in the physical shapes of the animals they help to build (Coppinger and Coppinger 2001).

Allelic differences between individuals, breeds, and species allow for differences in the genetic onset, offset, and rate of behaviors; these differences are not in chromosome numbers, shapes, or the placement of genes along the chromosomes (Coppinger and Coppinger 1996, 1998) but instead are differences in non-coding DNA or regulatory DNA within the genetic code. This non-coding DNA was called junk DNA previously as it does not code for proteins (Grandin and Deesing 2014). During a lifetime, genetic modifiers can change related to environmental sources (stress) and these changes can be passed onto offspring (Grandin and Deesing 2014). One of these changes seen in genes is how proteins are attached to DNA (tight or loose) causing genes to be read or not read (Fraga et al. 2005; Poulsen et al. 2007 – twin research, as cited by Grandin and Deesing 2014). Another related epigenetic change is DNA methylation, which when present turns off gene expression (Grandin and Deesing 2014). Some alleles turn on and off genes at different stages of an animal's life, permitting the onset and offset of behaviors during maturation (Trut 1999 – domesticated foxes). Other alleles manage the rate of behavior or the thresholds needed to elicit a behavior. Of course, there are no single alleles or genes that control a specific behavior; behavior is too complex for that. Genes make proteins. Proteins link with other proteins to build the animal's physical and mental characteristics. These characteristics allow behaviors to tend to cluster in individuals that share common genetics and environments.

Besides having a genetic configuration that naturally reinforces a behavior and the correct body shape to allow for a behavior, the gene(s) that allows for that behavior must be turned on before the finished behavior pattern can be produced by the animal. There is no use trying to train an animal for a behavior unless they are capable of learning it. No one would even try to train a neonate to pull a sled. Neonates are not able to perform this behavior; they cannot even walk yet. In time they will be running, but for now, they must pull themselves along by their forelimbs. Later in their ontogeny, they will begin to walk and then run. Once they are running, we can then start teaching them to pull a sled. And if they were well-bred, sled-pulling huskies, they could, with practice, become very good at it. Many behaviors in animals are affected by the onset and offset of genes during ontogeny. Behavior changes throughout an animal's life both because of genetic changes and because of environmental influences (Estep 1996).

- Besides having a genetic configuration that naturally reinforces a behavior and the correct body shape to allow for a behavior, the genes that allow for that behavior must be turned on before the finished behavior pattern can be produced by the animal.

Temperament was found to be a heritable trait in dogs (Scott and Fuller 1965); a dog's temperament is at least in part passed on by its parents. There is evidence that temperaments in cats are also heritable (McCune 1995; Estep 1996). Heritability is only an accurate measure for the group of animals represented in a study. Genes from these animals may or may not be representative of the larger population. The definition of heritability is a shared genome. Consequently, it cannot be assumed that animals outside of the study group share the same genome. Generalization to animal populations at large should be tempered accordingly. Readers are cautioned to keep this in mind when analyzing evidence of heritability in various studies. Although temperament is not a group of specific behaviors, it is a stable way of behaving across time and context. An animal's temperament accounts for its uniqueness (Hall 1941). Temperament includes issues such as emotional reactivity, anxiety, and fearfulness, and it affects learning in various ways.

- Although temperament is not a group of specific behaviors, it is a stable way of behaving across time and context.

Scaring or hurting animals does not help them learn. It contributes to behavioral shut down (learned helplessness) and avoidance of the trainer. In a study using two groups of police dogs (German shepherd dogs), one group was previously trained without using shock but nonetheless using harsh techniques (reported as the use of ". . . prong collars, and that their dogs experienced beatings and other harsh punishments, such as kicks or choke collar corrections"), and the other group was previously trained using shock collars; Schilder and van der Borg (2004) found that dogs trained with shocks exhibited significantly more signs of fear in the presence of their trainers than dogs trained with the same harsh methods without using shock collars. These dogs were not being shocked during the study, yet dogs previously trained with shocks were behaviorally different, exhibiting more fear and stress body language, than the dogs who were never shocked. One of the dogs in the study exhibited the effects of learning with shocks after not being shocked during training for a year and a half. These dogs who were shocked learned an association between the trainers who shocked them and the pain from the shocks. They also made associations between the environment in which they were previously shocked and the shocks, and between the behavioral context when they were previously shocked and the shocks. The dogs exhibited fear, stress, and conflict while in the context of previous shocks (being near the trainer, obedience work, and decoy work). This evidence supports the idea using shock collars to train dogs may cause long-term negative effects on behavior in the given context (see the AVSAB Humane Dog Training position statement for more information on dog training (AVSAB 2021)).

Emotional reactivity is part of an animal's temperament. It is a measure of how much of an emotional reaction an animal has to a stimulus and how long it takes for them to return to homeostasis (normalcy) after being exposed to the stimulus. Emotional reactivity is a heritable trait, and animals with increased emotional reactivity may have more trouble learning specific tasks (Scott and Fuller 1965 – dogs; see the Yerkes-Dodman Law for more information). Although there is evidence of reactivity levels being heritable, the environment exerts a large effect on this measure. A reduction in emotional reactivity can be realized by reduced stress in the mother during pregnancy, allowing normal mother–offspring interactions after parturition, and gentle handling of the neonate by people (Boissy 1998).

- Emotional reactivity is a heritable trait, and animals with increased emotional reactivity may have more trouble learning specific tasks (Scott and Fuller 1965 – dogs).

High reactivity in Rhesus macaques was found to be reduced when affected young monkeys were fostered by nurturing mothers (Suomi 1997). This illustrates how genes and the environment interact to affect reactivity. Rats' deficits, (anxiety, neophobia, and poor performance in learning and spatial memory tasks) because of social isolation, could be reversed using enrichment (Hellemans et al. 2004). Evidence of the effects of fear or overemotionality on learning are found in the study by Fuller and Clark (1966) using chlorpromazine, a tranquilizer, to enable Beagle puppies to learn an attachment to handlers, whereas the puppies not given the tranquilizer were unable to form similar attachments. There is much data to support these parameters. However, many people believe it is best to isolate neonates from human handling or to bottle-raise singleton offspring. Veterinary technicians need to educate animal owners and breeders on these issues to ensure they contribute to creating less reactive animals in the future by promoting the appropriate handling of neonates and by fostering litters on a mother animal or at the very least allowing these neonates access to littermates and adult conspecifics.

- Veterinary technicians need to educate animal owners and breeders on these issues to ensure they contribute to creating less reactive animals in the future by promoting the appropriate handling of neonates and by fostering litters on a mother animal or at the very least allowing these neonates access to littermates and adult conspecifics.

An example of how genes can affect behavior in dog breeds was found in the types of defense behaviors exhibited by three dog breeds. Defense behaviors in dogs can be classified as either active or passive defense. Active defense is characterized as lunging and biting, whereas passive defense is characterized by escape behaviors. Escape behaviors are the flight or freeze seen during sympathetic nervous system arousal. Passive and active defense behavior tendencies in dogs are inherited; however, through breeding studies, the environment was found to influence passive defense more readily than active defense (Krushinskii 1960). Dogs raised in isolation were more likely to exhibit passive defense as long as they were not the product of two dogs with only active defense. German shepherd dogs were more likely to show this trait than were Airedale terriers. Although Airedale terriers were able to be induced into showing passive defense if reared in isolation, they did not show this trait at the same rate as German shepherd dogs did. Doberman Pinschers were not able to be induced into showing passive defense, even when raised in isolation. It is more common today to find Doberman Pinschers that exhibit passive defense, illustrating how heritable behaviors can shift over time because of selective breeding. Another caution while reading this information is to remember breeds are a local phenomenon that may or may not reflect the behaviors seen in breeds of the same type in a different location. For example, Labrador retrievers from England may be calmer than Labrador retrievers from the United States.

- Another caution while reading this information is to remember breeds are a local phenomenon that may or may not reflect the behaviors seen in breeds of the same type in a different location.

Sensory perception is how the animal's brain interprets the sensory input they attend to. There are specific ways in which animals perceive sensations because of the organization of their sensory organs, the brain structures that interpret them, and the environment the animals live in (see Gibson 1958 for a discussion on perception in animals). The effects of sensory perception on learning are large, as it influences how sensory input will be used at the most basic level by setting up parameters for other sensations to be measured against (Goldstone 1998). Wells and Hepper (2006) found that dogs exposed to an odor *in utero* preferred that odor to another or no odor. This supports the hypothesis that even *in utero*, an animal's sensory perception is affecting its learning. Food preferences may also be partially determined *in utero* by sensory input. The chemical composition of the amniotic fluid and the mother's milk includes chemicals from the mother animal's diet (Thorne 1995). This is a mechanism by which animals could learn food preferences from their mother.

In an initially perplexing example, Vervet monkeys were able to use secondary vocal signals to warn about predators but were not able to use secondary visual signals (Cheney and Seyfarth 1992). In this study, monkeys used alarm calls from various bird species to look for predators, but if they saw the physical trail of a python, they did not look for the snake. The explanation given by the authors involved the consistency of the signal being associated with the predator. Alarm calls of birds were associated immediately with the visual image of the predator, whereas the visual signs of the snake were often seen without a snake in proximity. This speaks to the necessary condition for classical conditioning to occur – a conditioned stimulus (python trail) is associated consistently with the conditioned response (fear) for an animal to look for the python when they see a python trail (see Donahoe and Vegas 2004 for more information on the necessary association for classical conditioning to occur).

Attention is a vital aspect of learning. What the animal perceives is affected by the filtering of sensations they are exposed to through the mechanism of attention. Only the stimuli that are noticed can be used for learning purposes. Cats were found to be able to learn a behavior proceeded by a cue; only when that cue was first presented at an intensity level high enough to gain attention could the cats then learn to attend to it at a much less intense level (Bourassa and Weiden 1985). This lower level of intensity did not produce learning if used at the less intense level initially. Although this shows that attention is important for learning to occur, it also shows that attention thresholds can be modified by learning. For example, dogs trained using yelled cues can later be trained to perform behaviors using whispered cues. There is some evidence that attention need not be conscious for learning to occur (Debner and Jacoby 1994 – in humans).

The way in which animals think about the function of stimuli they perceive can also constrain their learning. These constraints of thinking about things are called *affordances*. Affordances were described by Michaels and Carello (1981) as ways in which perceived objects can be used by the perceiver. A hawk seeing a snake may perceive a prey item, whereas a rat seeing a snake may perceive a predator. These different perceptions are both correct, yet they elicit different behaviors. The hawk will dive toward the snake in order to kill and eat it, whereas the rat will jump back and run away from the snake before it can strike.

Humans are often constrained by their perceptions of an object. Riddles take advantage of this tendency using the mainstream perceptions of an object to purposefully misdirect us from the solution. Dogs were shown to be misled by their own affordances when repeatedly trying to reach a goal by a previously functional route. In their minds, that route was the only one that led to the goal, leaving dogs to ignore other possible solutions. These dogs continued for six trials to attempt the unfruitful route without any attempts at alternate routes, and only after they observed another person or dog reach the goal by an alternate route would they attempt it (Pongracz et al. 2001). This study method illustrates behavior modification using social learning.

Paradoxically, learning has a large effect on perception. Perception changes with practice (Gibson 1958). Learning about the environment affects what animals perceive. Animals are able to modify their perception to better assess their specific environment (Goldstone 1998 – humans). With experience, a rat may learn how to kill snakes for a meal, and after being exposed to a riddle's solution, humans are rarely fooled again.

- Learning about the environment affects what animals perceive.

Effect of domestication on learning

Domestication has been defined as the "process by which captive animals adapt to man and the environment he provides" (Price 1998, p. 31). While Ducos (1978, p. 54) defined domestication as, "when living animals are integrated as objects into the socio-economic organization of the human group, in the sense that, while living, those animals are objects for ownership, inheritance, exchange, trade, etc., as are the other objects (or persons) with which human groups have something to do. Living conditions are among the consequences of domestication, not the mark of it." No matter how domestication is defined, it has come to mean animals that live in restricted environments compared to their wild counterparts. The restriction of the environment may be because of the environmental qualities available to the animal as well as the changes to sensory organs of the animals through the process of domestication. These animals depend on humans for artificial selection instead of depending on natural selection as seen in wild animals, and they depend on humans for the satisfaction of their needs.

Domestic animals as a group have common characteristics allowing them to be more easily domesticated than other wild animals. These characteristics include individuals with significantly smaller brain sizes and the ability to reproduce in captive groups; the increase in sexual behavior is accomplished through the stress reduction seen because of the animals' lower reactivity (Hemmer 1990). Lower reactivity and less sensitivity to environmental stimuli are connected. They are the ways in which animals are able to cope with the changes that domestication brings. These changes contribute to the behavioral differences seen between similar wild and domestic animals. Behavioral differences found between domestic and wild animals are largely ones of quantity through changes seen in the thresholds needed to elicit behaviors (Price 1999).

- Domestic animals as a group have common characteristics allowing them to be more easily domesticated than other wild animals.

Increased diversity of appearance in domestic animals is supported through decreased natural selection (relaxed selection) as well as artificial selection for desired traits; this diversity includes size, proportion, color, horns, coat type, and skin type (Hemmer 1990). These variations become abundantly clear when observing the appearance of domestic animals in comparison to their wild counterparts. Changes in appearance can affect behavior and learning through homeostasis along with other mechanisms.

Domestic animals have smaller brains than their nearest wild relatives (Coppinger and Coppinger 2001 – dogs; Hemmer 1990 – dogs and cats; Williams et al. 1993 – cats). The smaller domesticated brain has a smaller neocortex in particular. This reduction in the size of the neocortex causes a reduction in storage capacity and information processing, which is the basis of the lessening of external stimulus reactions observed in domestic animals (Hemmer 1990). This reduction was no longer seen in breeds selected for behavioral specialization. In these breeds, animals' brain sizes increase with the complexity of the task at hand through artificial selection for increased memory and learning ability (Hemmer 1990). Differences in neocortex size between dog breeds and individuals within these breeds likely correlate with the level of social complexity seen in groups of these dogs. Dogs with smaller neocortexes are likely to exhibit less complex social interactions, whereas those with larger neocortexes are likely to exhibit the opposite strategy. Support for this was found in a study by Goodwin et al. (1997), in which they found dog breeds that were morphologically similar to wolves exhibited more complex visual communication patterns than those that were less morphologically similar to wolves. These differences would be especially interesting if we knew external morphological differences represented differences in neocortexes.

- Domestic animals have smaller brains than their nearest wild relatives.

In an ongoing study on domesticating fur foxes, foxes were bred by selecting for tameness. Consequently, other characteristics, physical and neurochemical, were modified (Belyaev 1979). These modifications had even more effect on the animal's behavior through learning. As the foxes were bred to be tamed, it changed their neurochemistry, allowing them to feel more comfortable with people. They solicited people for attention. This behavior was reinforced eliciting more attention-seeking behavior from the foxes. We observe similar behavior patterns in other domesticated species. Domesticated species have longer socialization periods and less reactivity to environmental stimuli because of a change in their hypothalamus–pituitary–adrenal axis resulting from domestication, otherwise known as *selection for the ability to be easily tamed*. Their natural behaviors allow for their easy taming, which then allows for a cascade of learning associated with tame behaviors. In a research by Belyaev (1979), changes in fox visual and auditory signaling to humans due to selection for tame behavior was found to correlate with changes in neurotransmitters. "Selection for behavior can intrinsically change the hormonal status of the breed and this can also have consequences for the ontogenetic development of the animal" (Belyaev 1979 – in foxes). Tame foxes exhibited higher serotonin levels, which inhibit certain types of aggression (Grandin and Deesing 2014). Tame foxes exhibited longer socialization periods extending up to 60 days while wild foxes socialization ends at 45 days; tame foxes developed novel attention-seeking vocal communication with humans; and cortisol levels when interacting with humans were three to four times lower in tame versus wild foxes (Rigterink and Houpt 2014). The most dog-like foxes had white spots/patterns on their heads, drooping ears, and curled tails, generally looking more like dogs than the foxes that still avoided people (Grandin and Deesing 2014). Foxes and dogs with tame versus aggressive and active versus passive response had the same expression on two loci of VVU12; expression of VVU12 depends on interaction with genes related to phenotypes (floppy ears) and on individual parents' genes (Rigterink and Houpt 2014). Wolves were exposed to environmental stimuli that selected for tame behavior causing karyotypic and phenotypic changes in the domestic dog supported by fox farm experiment results (Rigterink and Houpt 2014).

- Domesticated species have longer socialization periods and less reactivity to environmental stimuli because of a change in their hypothalamus–pituitary–adrenal axis resulting from domestication, otherwise known as *selection for the ability to be easily tamed*.

Coat color affects behavior through the common pathway shared by pigments (melanin) and neurotransmitters (catecholamines) (Hemmer 1990). Generally, less pigment corresponds to less behavior. The behaviors affected include activity level, reactivity, and environmental appreciation; corresponding with this information, albino animals generally exhibit lower activity levels and less flight response (Hemmer 1990). A reduction in sensory input (visual and olfactory) in albino animals may cause more fright responses or fearful aggression because their awareness of a stimulus may occur only when it is very close to them. Human interest in the unusual looking animal drove the change from wild-type coat colors to the wide variety of colors found today. Selection for unusual colors was a starting point for domestication and the changes seen in behavior and physiology (Hemmer 1990).

- Coat color affects behavior through the common pathway shared by pigments (melanin) and neurotransmitters (catecholamines) (Hemmer 1990).

Domesticated cats have a reduced brain size when compared to their wild counterparts, and Siamese cats showed an additional reduction in brain size of 5–10% from the average domestic cat (Hemmer 1990). As seen with domesticated dogs, the reduction in genetic variation correlated readily with the reduction in brain size, particularly the neocortex. Hemmer (1990) noted that the predatory behavior of the domestic cat was dissociated by domestication. The cats displayed this dissociation by exhibiting an increase in play behavior paired with a decrease in the killing of prey items along with the behavior of depositing dead uneaten prey animals in conspicuous places for people to find.

The selection for reduced reaction to environmental stimuli, attenuation of behavior, and reduced reactivity are not only correlated to a reduction in brain sizes but also correlated to the reduction in sensitivity of the sensory organs (visual, auditory, and olfactory; Hemmer 1990). This reduced sensitivity seen in domestic animal's sensory organs is likely to accentuate the reduction of brain size by reducing the sensory input the brain receives. In humans, there is evidence of a correlation between sensory and cognitive decline because of aging, but the mechanism and cause for this effect are not yet known (Li and Lindenberger 2003).

The reduced environmental awareness and reactivity of domestic animals enhance their learning ability in controlled situations because they are less distracted by their surroundings than are wild animals (Hemmer 1990). Although Hemmer found wolves to be superior in problem-solving tasks, dogs excelled at trained tasks. Wolves appeared more focused on the goal of the directed activities, whereas dogs seemed more focused on the task itself. Dogs could be taught to persist at tasks when failure rates were high (Figure 6.2), whereas this type of persistence seemed to be inhibited in wolves (Hemmer 1990). There is some evidence that dogs have cognitive abilities wolves and even primates lack. In two different studies, dogs were found to communicate with humans in ways that wolves and primates did not, by following a human gaze or gesture (Hare et al. 2002; Miklósi et al. 2003). Perhaps, domesticated animals do not need large brains to communicate well with people. Instead, large brains may be necessary for cooperative behaviors, hunting strategies, or complex problem solving. For example, although wolves hunt in highly cooperative packs, domesticated dogs mainly scavenge for food (Boitani et al. 1995; Macdonald and Carr 1995).

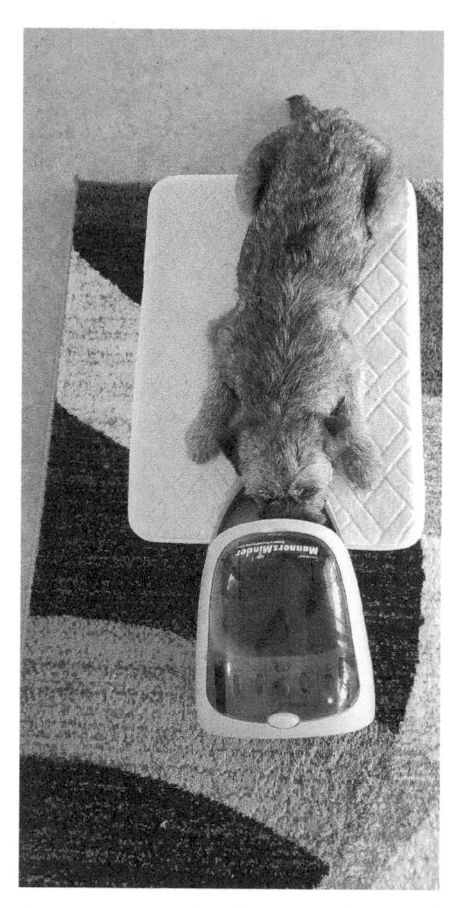

Figure 6.2 An example of persistence, as the dog maintains duration of the position while waiting for reinforcement from a remote treat dispenser.

Wynne discussed how this evidence for dogs having special cognitive abilities for enhanced communication with humans did not include evidence that other species had the same abilities and the effect size was small for dogs exceling in these abilities. He posited that the dogs' abilities were related to the close relationship between dogs and humans, and dogs needed to watch humans closely because they are totally dependent on them (2016).

Because domestic animals bond easily with humans owing to a lengthened socialization period (Scott and McCray 1967 – dogs; Trut 1999 – domesticated foxes), it is more common for them to pay attention to people and learn from them than it is for wild species. Topal et al. (1998) found that dogs formed attachments with people that were similar to the child–parent human relationship by adapting the Ainsworth Strange Situation test for use in dogs. If dogs formed a secure attachment to a person, they were better able to explore and play in the person's presence. The findings using dogs were similar to those found for mothers and toddlers in a research conducted by Ainsworth (1979). In a related study, Topal et al. (2005) found that dogs, but not wolves, formed attachments to humans. These differences were explained by the effects that domestication has had on dogs. An animal's relationship with other animals or people may influence their learning by influencing their attention or application of behaviors.

- An animal's relationship with other animals or people may influence their learning by influencing their attention or application of behaviors.

Although Topal et al. (1997) found dogs that were bonded to a person were less likely to problem-solve without help from that person, they reasoned it had more to do with the relationship between the dog and the person than the dogs being cognitively challenged. These dogs looked to their owner for information to quickly solve problems instead of using trial and error learning analogous to what wolves did (Miklósi et al. 2003). The dog–human partnership helped the dog solve the problem quickly.

In another study, Pongracz et al. (2005) found that a dog learned from a stranger or their owner equally well to find a new route around a barrier. Conversely, Gent (2006) found that dogs learned more effectively when familiar with the person they observed, although familiarity did not affect learning when watching another dog. Pongracz et al. (2008) found that other characteristics in dogs, those that led to differentiated social relationships between dogs, affected whether dogs learned from another dog's behavior. In their study, dogs that were determined to be dominant over other dogs in their home environment (using owner questionnaires) showed significantly less social learning than that exhibited by dogs that were determined to be submissive when the demonstrator was a dog. These differences in learning were not found when a person was the demonstrator. It is not clear how the relationship between a dog and a person affects learning in dogs, but we are starting to collect the clues through these studies. There is little evidence available on how relationships between cats and people affect their learning, but it was established that cats can find food when a person points to its location (Miklósi et al. 2005).

Animals that are less reactive to environmental stimuli have smaller adrenal glands. Now that domestic animals are bred with smaller adrenal glands, they are less reactive to stimuli, but this also means that they cannot respond well to drastic changes in the environment. They are dependent on the environment remaining somewhat consistent through the manipulation of humans for their survival. This is illustrated by the lack of adequate predatory avoidance behavior in most domesticated species (Price 1999). Domestic cats and dogs are frequent prey items for birds of prey as well as wild canids.

- Now that domestic animals are bred with smaller adrenal glands, they are less reactive to stimuli, but this also means that they cannot respond well to drastic changes in the environment. They are dependent on the environment remaining somewhat consistent through the manipulation of humans for their survival.

Effects of nutrition on learning

Nutrition of the fetus and the neonate affects the development of the neurological system, which affects learning at the most basic level. The creation of myelin sheaths on the outside of nerves is affected by the nutrition consumed by the animal. These sheaths affect the speed of neural transmissions throughout the body. Brain and neural growth are also affected by adequate protein and calories. If there are not enough of these nutrients in the diet, the animal will not be able to create the neural framework necessary to carry the nerve impulses quickly and efficiently throughout the body to the brain. When animals are deprived of the needed nutrition, the brain is affected in all regions, with the cerebellum showing the most effect (Wiggins and Fuller 1978).

- When animals are deprived of the needed nutrition, the brain is affected in all regions, with the cerebellum showing the most effect (Wiggins and Fuller 1978).

If the animal starves during the first few weeks of life, during glial cell multiplication (0–14 days in rats) and rapid myelin synthesis (0–20 days in rats), the animal cannot recover these losses even after eating normally for a year (Wiggins and Fuller 1978). Children with these nutritional deficits exhibited reduced exploratory behavior and developmental lags in the following domains: motor, hearing and speech, social–personal, problem solving, eye–hand coordination, categorization, integration of information from different sensory systems, and temporal integration of information (Cravioto and DeLicardie 1975). Communication and language development showed the worst effects and the least recovery after the child began receiving good nutrition. Cravioto and DeLicardie reported in their study about Zimmerman (1973) using monkeys, that the main deficits found were in tasks using attention and observation (1975). Taking this evidence into account, early malnutrition in animals is likely to cause permanent damage to areas of the nervous system that control attention, observation, and the synthesis of information from different sensory systems. Damage to these systems could then cause problems with species-specific and general learning of social and communication behaviors. A lack of proficiencies in these systems could also contribute to an increase in aggression.

- Taking this evidence into account, early malnutrition in animals is likely to cause permanent damage to areas of the nervous system that control attention, observation, and the synthesis of information from different sensory systems.

What an animal eats during its later development will also affect its ability to learn. There are a few pet foods that contain docosahexaenoic acid (DHA), an omega-3 fatty acid in fish oil, which enhances learning in animals (Horrocks and Yeo 1999). Specifically, dogs were found to have enhanced learning when DHA was included in their diet (Reynolds et al. 2005 and Kelley et al. 2004 as cited by Bauer 2006).

A 2018 review article focusing on the effects of the gastrointestinal (GI) microbiome, found that the GI microbiome has an influence on social and affective behaviors through its interactions with the central nervous, endocrine, and immune systems (Sylvia and Demas 2018). Many influences can affect the quality of an animal's GI microbiome and change

CHAPTER 6

the animal's behavior and ability to learn. A few examples of these influences include: early lifetime stressors such as separation from their mother. The use of antibiotics and probiotics. In 2021, Jin et al. found the GI microbiome partially regulated genetic effects on anxiety in mice. These studies help support the idea that maintaining a healthy GI microbiome has a positive effect on an animal's ability to learn and maintain healthy behaviors over their lifetime.

Early environment and learning

The environment in which the animal develops sets up the systems by which they learn. Even the time spent by the fetus *in utero* affects learning. The senses of animals provide the stimuli by which they learn about their environment throughout life. Learning about their environment is a serious business for animals that want to live long enough to reproduce.

- The senses of animals provide the stimuli by which they learn about their environment throughout life.

Tactile stimuli or touch is vital for normal development. Neonates have highly developed tactile sensation systems (Caulfield 2000). They are set up to use tactile stimulations to learn about their environment, and these stimulations affect the development of their nervous systems. Premature human infants were found to have fewer neurological deficits if they received "stimulating" tactile stimulation (Weiss et al. 2004). Animals without normal maternal interactions develop abnormal neurological systems, including increased neural cell death and an increased stress response (Zhang et al. 2002). At least some of the responses that were affected by maternal deprivation can be reversed using tactile stimulus (van Oers et al. 1998 – in rats; Weiss et al. 2004 – in human infants). There is also evidence that handling during a neonates' development will enhance learning ability through the reduction of reactivity (Fox 1970; see Morton 1968 for more information). All this evidence supports the importance of the tactile sense for normal neurological development and learning about the environment.

- Animals without normal maternal interactions develop abnormal neurological systems, including increased neural cell death and an increased stress response (Zhang et al. 2002).

Sounds can affect learning by their ability to orient an animal toward a stimulus. Once the animal focuses on the stimulus, they can learn about it. Animals can also learn about sound. They can make associations with different sounds and can learn to attend to the different characteristics of sound. Changes to an animal's behavior in response to sound can be indications of neural changes in the auditory cortex (Blake et al. 2002 – monkeys). Often, people use auditory cues to elicit behaviors in animals. Animals are able to discriminate between auditory cues but may not be as accurate as we believe they are.

Visual stimuli are likely to affect learning in various ways. Both the dog's and the cat's visual systems are geared toward high visual contrast in low light situations and moving visual stimuli (Miller 2001). Fukuzawa et al. (2005) found that visual cues are important for dogs, and that dogs used these visual cues in combination with the verbal cues used by people. When only the verbal cues were used, the dogs were significantly less likely to perform the cued behavior than when both visual and verbal cues were present. Dogs were found to be sensitive to the gaze of humans when the person was giving a cue for a behavior (Viranyi et al. 2004). This was demonstrated by the dog being significantly more likely to perform a behavior if the person giving the cue was looking at the dog than if the person was looking somewhere else or if they were behind a screen.

Animals learn how to learn by being exposed to different environmental stimuli and by having problems to solve (Overall 2009). When an animal is provided with all its physical needs and its environment remains static, it is less likely to develop the skills necessary to learn efficiently. Animals in barren environments have smaller brains and less versatile neurological systems (Bennett et al. 1964 – rats). These animals can develop stereotypic behaviors (Mason et al. 2007). They may have a reduced or altered appreciation of pain (Melzak and Scott 1957 – dogs). They may also be more difficult to train than animals with a more enriched past. Mice raised in an impoverished environment were slower to learn a maze than those with an enriched environment (Iso et al. 2007). Although there is some evidence, in mice, that being raised in complex social environments predicts complex social skills rather than increased learning ability (D'Andrea et al. 2007). In this study, social learning was not investigated.

The increase of fear responses during the seventh or eighth week of development (Scott and Fuller 1965 – dogs; Karsh 1983 – cats) weakens the animal's curiosity about new experiences, objects, and individuals. The animal now learns and remembers consciously which stimuli are reinforcing and which are punishing. As the learning rate about the environment decreases, the sensitive period called *socialization* slowly comes to a close. The socialization period is one of accelerated learning in which the animal learns much about its relationships with other animals as well as its environment. This is not the only time during an animal's life that they learn about the environment or other animals. This type of learning continues throughout the animal's life; it is the accelerated rate of learning that slows. This explains why animals exposed to a rich social environment when young show increased social abilities throughout their lives (D'Andrea et al. 2007 – mice).

- Animals exposed to a rich social environment when young show increased social abilities throughout their lives.

Habituation and sensitization

Habituation and sensitization are simple forms of nonassociative learning in which an animal learns to either ignore or attend closely to a stimulus. They are not making pairings with a stimulus and behavior. Instead, during habituation, an animal learns that a stimulus is not important and stops noticing it. Habituation occurs after repeated exposures. This is not something someone does to an animal such as the behavior modification technique, desensitization. Instead, this is a way in which an animal learns on its own. The animal figures out over time whether the stimulus is dangerous. Animals habituate to wearing a collar just as humans habituate to wearing a watch.

Sensitization is seen when an animal becomes more aware of a stimulus after repeated exposures. These stimuli may be loud, painful, or frightening in other ways to the animal. Once an animal is sensitized to a stimulus, it is more difficult to desensitize them to it. Animals can become sensitized to thunder as do people. It startles them causing fear. They learn to listen for the scary sound of thunder. They may also learn to associate other stimuli with thunder through higher order conditioning seen in classical conditioning. Through higher order conditioning the animal may learn to fear the increased wind and darkening skies they associate with thunder.

There is an evolutionary basis to nonassociative learning through natural selection. It is adaptive for animals to learn which stimuli are harmful and which are not. It is also adaptive for animals to become used to stimuli that will not harm them. Being in a constant state of fear and hyperarousal is not beneficial to any animal; it is vital they learn through repeated exposures which stimuli are truly dangerous and which are not.

- Being in a constant state of fear and hyperarousal is not beneficial to any animal; it is vital that they learn through repeated exposures which stimuli are truly dangerous and which are not.

For a stimulus to elicit habituation or sensitization, the animal must notice it. The animal's attention on the stimulus is necessary for them to learn about it. The rate of exposure to the stimulus will affect the animal's ability to learn about it. If the stimulus is often present, the animal can learn more quickly about it. Even after habituation has occurred if the animal is not around the stimulus for a long time, the animal may react to it as if it were novel. This is called *spontaneous recovery*. Spontaneous recovery occurs in all types of learning. It is as if everything the animal has learned is stored waiting for the proper time to present itself. If new learning is not used, the animal can revert back to earlier learning.

- Spontaneous recovery: even after habituation has occurred if the stimulus is not presented to the animal for a long time, the animal may react to it as if it were novel.

The intensity of the stimulus will affect the animal's reaction to it. Loud sounds are more likely to cause sensitization than habituation as are any intense stimuli. The more severe the stimulus is the more likely it will cause the animal to become sensitized to it. Habituation is more probable if the stimulus is innocuous or harmless. Of course, this judgment is made from the animal's perspective.

The temperament of an animal affects how they make judgments about the environment surrounding them. If the animal is highly reactive and fearful, it will judge more stimuli to be dangerous and thus will become sensitized to them. Although an animal's temperament is largely present at birth, it can and is modified throughout life by experience. During an animal's socialization period, they can be exposed to many stimuli, creating a broad basis of exposure to many objects, experiences, sounds, and living things. This allows them to have the best chance of being able to habituate to stimuli commonly found in their environment throughout their life.

- Although an animal's temperament is largely present at birth, it can and is modified throughout life by experience.

Operant conditioning

Learning in which a behavior is affected by its consequences is called *operant conditioning* (Box 6.1). This type of learning is seen in animals when they associate performing a specific behavior with some sort of benefit or detriment. Operant conditioning is classified as an associative type of learning (Skinner 1966). When a behavior earns something the animal wants, the behavior will strengthen; conversely, if the behavior earns something the animal fears or dislikes, the behavior will weaken. Weakening of behavior can also be seen when the behavior earns nothing. Operant conditioning is used when training animals to perform behaviors, as it primarily deals with voluntary behaviors. It is the type of learning involved when a behavior is weakened using punishment. This type of learning is not synonymous with positive reinforcement training, as punishment is part of operant conditioning.

BOX 6.1: DIFFERENT TERMS FOR OPERANT CONDITIONING

- Skinnerian learning
- Trial and error learning
- Instrumental learning – some slight differences
- Type 2 conditioning
- Type R conditioning

- Learning in which a behavior is affected by its consequences is called *operant conditioning*.

Teaching an animal to come by giving it some sort of reinforcer each time it comes to you, such as a food treat, is one example of operant conditioning. Another example using punishment is when an animal's behavior of jumping into a bathtub is weakened if the bathtub contains water. The animal would have to dislike being in water for this to weaken the behavior. The stimulus following the behavior does not have to be something a person or other animal does to them. Instead, it can be a natural consequence of the animal's behavior. If an animal walks on a spiny plant, they will be injured, teaching them to avoid that plant in the future. There are other factors that can affect this type of learning. They are discussed later in this section.

Operant conditioning is occurring all the time throughout an animal's life. They learn through operating in their environment which behaviors bring them stimuli that they want and which bring them stimuli they dislike. All types of training use operant conditioning, and animals use operant conditioning when not being trained. The stimuli affecting an animal's behavior can be a variety of food, touches, sounds, activities, and odors. It is up to the individual animal whether a stimulus is reinforcement or punishment. Both reinforcement and punishment must occur contingent on the behavior's performance, during the behavior, or before the performance of another behavior otherwise their effect on the behavior will be weakened tremendously. In laboratory testing Skinner found learning decreased dramatically if the reinforcer occurred two seconds after the behavior (1966).

Animals appearing to look guilty during verbal scolding are likely showing appeasement behaviors in response to anger exhibited by the person scolding them instead of exhibiting knowledge that the behavior was wrong (Horowitz and Horowitz 2009). Animals who did not perform the unwanted behavior will show appeasement behaviors, which supports the hypothesis that when an animal exhibits behavior judged to be guilt by a person, they are no more likely to have committed the unwanted behavior than an animal who does not exhibit these behaviors. Instead of exhibiting knowledge the behavior performed was wrong dogs are responding to the owner's behavior (body language and verbal scolding) (Horowitz and Horowitz 2009).

- It is up to the individual animal whether a stimulus is reinforcement or punishment.

Reinforcement has a functional definition. It must fulfill the function of strengthening the likelihood a behavior will be performed in the future for it to be labeled a reinforcer. All reinforcers are stimuli the animal wants and will work to obtain, but it depends on the animal which stimuli are reinforcers for them. For example, my dog Scarlett finds broccoli extremely reinforcing, whereas my dog Lily does not. Lily is better reinforced using bread. Although both my dogs prefer food reinforcers, other dogs may prefer some sort of touch or play. Reinforcers are the consequences of maintaining behaviors. When a behavior is no longer earning a reinforcer, the behavior will extinguish.

- Reinforcement has a functional definition. It must fulfill the function of strengthening a behavior for it to be labeled a reinforcer. All reinforcers are stimuli the animal wants, but it depends on the animal which stimuli are reinforcers for them.

There are two types of reinforcements used in operant conditioning: negative and positive reinforcement. When you read these terms, you may think negative means bad and positive means good, but in this case that would be incorrect. When referring to these behavior principles think about the mathematical symbols of subtraction (−) for negative and addition (+) for positive (Table 6.1).

Negative reinforcement takes away a stimulus when a behavior happens, causing the behavior to strengthen. Think about the types of things you would work to have removed. You might want someone to stop yelling at you, hitting you, or shocking you. If you performed a behavior and one of these stimuli stopped, your behavior would be reinforced through negative reinforcement.

A common example of negative reinforcement seen in a veterinary hospital is when a person approaches a patient exhibiting aggression. If the animal lunges at the approaching person causing the person to back up, the animal will learn lunging behavior removes the scary person. Consequently, the behavior of lunging at the person will strengthen. The cue for this behavior is the person approaching the cage. Although the cage-aggressive behavior was initially performed in response to fear of the person, over time and repeated performances, the animal might become very confident using this behavior and appear to be confident instead of fearful.

Positive reinforcement involves adding a stimulus the animal wants immediately after or during a behavior they are performing. Adding this stimulus strengthens the behavior that precedes it. You may hear people say they use positive reinforcement training, but if they use any type of punishment during training, they are actually using operant conditioning instead of only positive reinforcement.

If I teach my cat to jump onto a box and give her a food treat when she does so, I am using positive reinforcement to train this behavior. Animals can be taught an almost endless variety of behaviors and

Table 6.1 Reinforcement and punishment.

Effect on behavior	Adding something	Taking something away
The behavior strengthens	Positive (+) reinforcement	Negative (−) reinforcement
Behavior of asking for candy is strengthened	Parent presents candy dish when child asks for candy	Parent squeezes the child's hand until they ask for candy
The behavior weakens	Positive (+) punishment	Negative (−) punishment
Behavior of asking for candy is weakened	Child is spanked for asking for candy	Candy dish is removed when the child asks for candy

complex behavioral chains using positive reinforcement. This type of training is very forgiving. You can make mistakes, and the worst that can happen is you confuse the animal or teach an unwanted behavior. Using this technique, you are more likely to strengthen the bond you have with an animal because through classical conditioning the animal will associate you with the positive reinforcement.

Reinforcers are often primary or unconditioned reinforcers. This means that the animal did not have to learn that these stimuli are good to receive. Examples of primary reinforcers are food, water, and temperature changes that enhance homeostasis. Reinforcers can also be learned through the associations during classical conditioning. These reinforcers are called *secondary or conditioned reinforcers*. They are associated through repeated pairings with a primary reinforcer or they can be associated with a previously associated secondary reinforcer. Examples of secondary reinforcers are toys and praise. Some training techniques use a conditioned reinforcer such as clicker training. The click sound is a secondary or conditioned reinforcer because once taught, that click means a treat is coming; the click is associated with a forthcoming food reward. When clicker training, the click sound is used to communicate to the learner they are performing a wanted behavior now and will earn a positive reinforcer. (See more information about clicker training at www.clickertraining.com.)

Theoretically, if you want to weaken a behavior, you could use punishment. Punishment is also defined functionally. A stimulus is only a punishment if when it is applied immediately after or during a behavior that behavior weakens. No matter how punishing you think a stimulus is, it is not a punishment unless it weakens the behavior it follows. You may come home each day to a dog that greets you by jumping on you. You may yell at this dog each day "no" or "get down," but these are not punishments for your dog because each day he continues to jump on you to greet you. For yelling to be a punishment for this dog, his behavior of jumping to greet you must weaken over time. Honestly, when you observe animals and notice the stimuli they find reinforcing (e.g. dogs eating cat feces), it is no wonder we are baffled at what they find punishing. When working with other species, you must suspend your own preferences and try to imagine the animal's sensory preferences. You can verify your ideas by watching their body language and keeping track of their behavior. Body language denoting pleasure is a likely sign of reinforcement, whereas body language denoting fear or avoidance is a likely sign of punishment. Counting behaviors to assess their strengthening or weakening is a reliable technique for judging whether a stimulus is reinforcement or punishment. Using measurements of behavior increases our accuracy.

- A stimulus is only a punishment if when it is applied immediately after or during a behavior that behavior weakens.

There are two types of punishments mirroring the two types of reinforcements: positive and negative punishment. Positive (+) means we are adding something, and negative (−) means we are removing something.

Positive punishment is being used when a stimulus is added either during or immediately after a behavior is performed, and the behavior is weakened. If the behavior does not weaken, then whatever you are doing is not punishment for that animal. If punishment is going to weaken a behavior, it does so within one or two trials. Continuing to use the same technique after no weakening of the behavior is observed is fruitless and potentially damaging to the human–animal bond. The types of stimuli used as punishment are all things the animal wants to avoid or escape from. Using positive punishment, especially if you are present during the punishment, will cause the animal to associate you with the aversive stimulus. Your presence will become a conditioned punisher. This can undermine any trust you have built with the animal. Other objects in the environment as well as contexts can be associated with punishment. Keep in mind what the animal may learn if you decide to use punishment. If you use loud sounds as punishment, the animal may learn loud sounds are punishing and may generalize that fear to a variety of loud sounds.

- Continuing to use the same technique after no weakening of the behavior is observed is fruitless and potentially damaging to the human–animal bond.

When a stimulus is removed as a consequence of a behavior and the behavior weakens, negative punishment is being used. These stimuli would be something the animal wants. An example of negative punishment is when a person leaves the room when an animal performs an attention-seeking behavior. Because the animal wants attention and attention from the person is removed, as long as the behavior weakens, this would be considered negative punishment.

Animals can learn to associate stimuli with punishment through classical conditioning. When a stimulus is consistently associated with punishment, it becomes a conditioned or secondary punishment. A disapproving look or verbal reprimand can become a conditioned punishment. Even an owner coming home can become a conditioned punishment if coming home is consistently associated with another punishment. Primary or unconditioned punishments cause discomfort or fear. Examples of primary punishments are electric shocks and hitting.

Punishment is difficult to use properly, and even if it is used properly, it does not teach the animal to perform the desired behavior. I may want my dog to greet my friends by sitting. I can punish his jumping to greet behavior for years; it will never teach him to sit to greet people. The animal is left trying to figure out what behavior is wanted. This can cause conflict and frustration. An inconsistent punishment can also be thought of as an intermittent reinforcer because the behavior will sometimes continue to be reinforced. When this happens, the behavior will be strengthened not weakened. Using an intermittent reinforcer also leads to behavior that is the most difficult to extinguish (Skinner 1966). Other techniques that can be used to change behavior are discussed in the section Behavior modification using operant conditioning. See the American Veterinary Society of Animal Behavior's position statement called Position Statement for Humane Dog Training for more information on the effects of using punishment when training (https://avsab.org/?s=Humane+dog+training).

Positive punishment and negative reinforcement are two completely different operant conditioning consequences, although they are often confused. A behavior must be weakened for a consequence to be called a punishment. A behavior is strengthened when using negative reinforcement. There are some common characteristics of these two consequences. Both positive punishment and negative reinforcement involve an adverse stimulus. These aversive stimuli cause fear and/or discomfort for the animal. Positive punishment adds the stimulus, whereas negative reinforcement removes the stimulus. Using these two consequences for behavior, positive punishment and negative reinforcement, can cause some unintended side effects. Side effects can include avoidance, aggression, and behavioral suppression.

Cues, a type of antecedent, are signals that communicate to animals if they perform a specific behavior they will earn a reinforcer. Some cues are intentional, and others are not. Animals may attend to a different cue than which we have intended and they may use multiple cues as a signal for one behavior. For example, a cat may use an owner waking up as a cue to meow, and the owner may reinforce this behavior with food. The owner may not be aware their behavior of waking up is a cue for the meow behavior. They may also not be aware of reinforcing meowing by feeding their cat. Animals learn to perform behaviors associated with a cue. This cue precedes the behavior, and the animal learns that if they perform the behavior after the cue, they are likely to be reinforced for it. A cue is also called a *discriminative stimulus* (D^s). These stimuli help the animal to discriminate when they will be reinforced for a behavior and when they will not. Once the animal reliably performs the behavior on cue, the behavior can be said to be under stimulus control (Box 6.2). The type of cue used can affect the speed of learning. Prichard et al., found that when using functional magnetic resonance imaging (fMRI) on fully awake dogs, dogs showed brain activation indicating that they learned faster using visual and olfactory stimuli than verbal stimuli (2018).

Setting up the environment to support the animal learning a specific behavior is called antecedent arrangements. This is the least stressful effective technique for changing behavior after making sure the animal's needs are being met (Friedman and Fritzler 2019).

BOX 6.2: CHARACTERISTICS OF STIMULUS CONTROL

Characteristics of stimulus control

1. Responds to the cue correctly a minimum of 80% of the time
2. Does not offer the behavior (in training session) without the cue
3. Does not perform a different behavior in response to the cue
4. Does not perform this behavior in response to a different cue

For example, if I want my puppy to learn to keep all four paws on the floor when greeting a person, I can place food on the floor every time he approaches me. If my cat is exhibiting stress when it sees a feral cat outside a window, I can place a film over that window inhibiting the cat from seeing out. By removing the view of the feral cat, my cat will change his behavior. Using antecedent arrangement is sometimes called management or managing a behavior.

Motivation encompasses the individual differences in how animals respond to stimuli in specific contexts. There are many principles that can help us understand why animals are motivated to behave in differing ways even when exposed to the exact same stimuli.

Although animals are afraid of novel items, neophobia, in their environment, they are also fascinated by them, neophilia (Grandin and Deesing 2014). This fascination of animals for new stimuli can be used to teach them to habituate to a variety of objects and manipulations. The use of force when introducing novel items is associated with increased fear, whereas if animals are left alone with a novel item, they will frequently approach it faster (Grandin and Deesing 2014). Instead of restraining an animal and putting the otoscope into their ear, we could let them approach and explore the otoscope on their own terms first. We could reinforce their approach toward the otoscope and even allow them to sniff or touch the otoscope with their nose. While using operant conditioning to reinforce approaching the otoscope we would also be using classical conditioning to make a pleasant association between the otoscope and something the animal likes: a treat or petting. After they are comfortable with it, we could then place it in their ear without incident. All pieces of equipment used on animals in veterinary practices could be introduced in this manner, making the animals more comfortable and making procedures go smoothly.

- Animals should be allowed to explore veterinary equipment on their own terms. The equipment should be associated with something the animal likes. This will help the animal become comfortable and more accepting of the procedures.

Under laboratory conditions, animals were shown to behaviorally conform to the theory of operant conditioning, but once the animals came out into the complexity of the everyday world, instincts or innate behaviors began to show effects on learned behavior. These discrepancies in learning theory were already showing themselves in the autoshaping behavior of pigeons pecking a light for food reinforcements (Brown and Jenkins 1968). It is a normal species-specific behavior that pigeons peck for food. In the study by Brown and Jenkins, they were taught to expect food to appear in a food dish after a light in their enclosure was illuminated. They learned this association quickly. But after many repeated trials, the pigeons began pecking the light when it was lit as if pecking produced the food. They had begun to behave toward the light as if it were food. Along with other innate behaviors, animals have species-specific behaviors affecting food gathering, and these behaviors were shown to affect behaviors learned through operant conditioning (Breland and Breland 1961). Known as *instinctual drift*, this effect modifies learned behaviors to become more analogous to naturally occurring foraging behaviors. The animal begins to associate the learned behavior with the food reinforcer. This association then changes the way they behave when presented with the cue for the learned behavior. In a training scenario for a fair, the Brelands attempted to teach chickens to stand still on a platform to receive a food reinforcer. The chickens did so for a short time but eventually began to scratch at the surface they were standing on as if they were scratching for food. Although this behavior did not earn the chickens a reinforcer, was more difficult, and took more energy than standing still, the chickens persisted with the scratching behavior. This evidence goes against Skinnerian theories on how organisms learn and behave. When training an animal using a food reinforcer, the natural foraging tendencies of the animal must be taken into consideration as they will make associations between the stimuli: signal for food with food causing an innate response toward the signal for food. Although AutoShaping is often considered within operant conditioning, Burgos proposed a neural-network model for learning, which does not recognize a distinction between operant and classical conditioning as these types of learning are based on the idea of a stimulus response association (2007).

- When training an animal, the natural behavioral tendencies of the animal must be taken into consideration.

It seems logical for animals to be motivated to drink when they are thirsty, whereas animals that have just drunk their fill are no longer motivated to do so. It follows logically that food would be a reinforcer for a hungry animal, but what about running being a reinforcer for drinking behavior? If running is a restricted activity for an animal and the animal must drink to be able to run, the behavior of running becomes the reinforcer for drinking. Experiments with rats showed the same animals in different experimental contexts drank water for the opportunity to run and ran for the opportunity to drink (Premack 1962). This paradoxical law of behavior is called the *Premack Principle*. Animals will perform a less profitable behavior to be able to perform a more profitable behavior; they will perform an unrestricted behavior in order to be able to perform a restricted behavior (Premack 1962). The Premack Principle can help us explain why animals seem determined to perform one behavior for the opportunity to perform a restricted behavior. A dog may bolt out of the door for the opportunity to run the neighborhood, whereas a cat may swim across a river for an opportunity to rest in a warm barn. In the dog example, the more restricted the access to the neighborhood is, the harder the dog will work to escape out of the door. Likewise, the cat will work harder to swim the river if a warm resting place is difficult to find.

Animals become accustomed to performing certain behaviors or chains of behaviors to satisfy their needs or wants. These habits of behavior can be assessed according to their strength, which depends on how many times the animal has been reinforced for performing them (Hull 1943). Habit strength affects how long it takes for animals to unlearn behaviors and learn alternate ones. Reinforcement can be manipulated through the use of different reinforcement schedules (Ferster and Skinner 1957) (Table 6.2). These schedules of reinforcement are used in laboratories and have real-life implementations. It is useful to remember animals are affected by the removal of reinforcers. There are two main categories of reinforcement schedules: ratio and interval. Ratio reinforcements reinforce behavior after they are performed a certain number of times, whereas interval reinforcement schedules reinforce a behavior when it is performed after a certain amount of time or when the duration of the behavior has reached a certain time span. Ratio schedules

Table 6.2 Reinforcement schedules and their effect on behavior.

Reinforcement schedule	Effect on behavior	Common usage
Continuous reinforcement (CRF) Fixed ratio 1 (FR1)	Fast acquisition of behavior Easy to extinguish	Teaching new behaviors
Fixed ratio reinforcement: FR2 – reinforce after two behaviors FR3 – reinforce after three behaviors	Behavior weakens after reinforcement is given High rates of behavior worsen this effect Anticipation of reinforcement common	Transitioning an animal from continuous to partial reinforcement
Partial reinforcement (PR) Intermittent reinforcement (IR) Variable ratio (VR)	Steady, strong behavioral response to cue Protects behavior from extinction Reinforcement rate is unknown to animal	Maintenance of a known behavior
Fixed interval 1 reinforcement (FI1)	Fast acquisition of behavior Easy to extinguish	Teaching new repeated behaviors or new behavioral states
Fixed interval reinforcement: FI2 – reinforce after 2 s FI3 – reinforce after 3 s	Behavior weakens after reinforcement is given High intervals of time worsen this effect Anticipation of reinforcement common	Transitioning an animal from continuous to partial reinforcement
Variable interval (VI)	Steady, strong repeated behavior or behavioral state response to cue Protects repeated behavior or behavioral state from extinction Reinforcement interval is unknown to animal	Maintenance of a known repeated behavior or behavioral state

are used when a trainer wants to obtain a good solid performance of a behavioral event, whereas interval schedules are used to obtain behavioral states or repeated behaviors. If a person wanted to train a dog to lie down, they would use ratio schedules, but if they wanted to reinforce lie down and stay, an interval schedule would probably work best.

When a behavior is reinforced each time it is performed, continuous reinforcement (CRF), the animal's performance increases steadily until they are performing it correctly each time. This is the recommended reinforcement schedule for training new behaviors. Behaviors learned using a CRF schedule are receptive to extinction. Because animals perform behaviors to obtain wants and needs, behaviors we want animals to perform should be reinforced in a way the animal appreciates.

The strength of the reinforcers and punishers used in operant conditioning can be manipulated to some degree by changing the reinforcer or the environment surrounding the reinforcer. There is no need to use deprivation to increase their strength, as animals can be motivated without depriving them of their basic needs. In fact, using food deprivation can inhibit learning by causing the animal to be too focused on obtaining the food or in extreme situations by making the animal weak. Instead of deprivation, opportunistic timing can be used. If food reinforcers are being used, arrange to train just before the animal's regular meal. The animal will be ready for food at that time. If the animal has been alone all day, attention and touch can be used as reinforcers (assuming those things are reinforcing to the animal).

- To create motivation, opportunistic timing of reinforcers is preferred over deprivation.

Designating a treat or toy as special and only using it during training sessions while restricting access to it at other times can be extremely effective. No one wants more food after a feast, and no one wants attention after receiving large quantities of attention. There is no benefit to using a reinforcer after a similar substance sates the animal.

Animals compare reinforcers using negative contrast. In this comparison, one reinforcer loses out to the other. If I give my dog steak as a reinforcer, then switch to dry kibble it is probable she will not work as hard after the switch. Dry kibble is not as reinforcing for most dogs as steak. Even steak can become commonplace and boring for animals if it is used too often. Animals can habituate to any reinforcer. It is good practice to vary your reinforcers to allow them to retain their strength. Surprise reinforcers are the best, but it can be difficult to catch animals unaware as their sense of smell is exceptional.

- It is good practice to vary your reinforcers to allow them to retain their strength.

Likewise, punishments can be overused rendering them ineffective through habituation and poor timing. Only the sparing and proper use of punishment can be effective in weakening unwanted behaviors. Inescapable punishments create a condition in animals called *learned helplessness* (Seligman 1972). When an animal does not know how to avoid or escape punishment, they stop responding to it. But instead of ignoring it as in habituation, they become almost zombie-like. They learn that their behavior does not affect what happens to them (Figure 6.3). They stop trying to learn behaviors, as there is no sense in it any longer as their behavior does not cause wanted consequences. This condition was found through research on human depression, and when an animal exhibits learned helplessness, they appear to be depressed. Overmier and Seligman

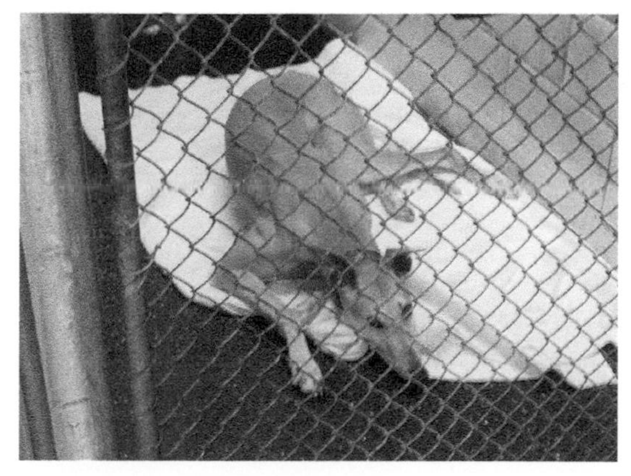

Figure 6.3 A Greyhound, Sancho, showing signs of learned helplessness by not exhibiting any behaviors when approached by a person.

(1967) found dogs exposed to inescapable shock were significantly less likely to try to escape a shock after they were trained how to escape it. Even when they did escape the shock by jumping over a barrier, they were no more likely to try to escape the shock next time it occurred. This suppression of learned behavior is unique to learned helplessness and was contingent on the animal not having control over the occurrence of the punishment. If dogs were able to escape punishment by performing a behavior (negative reinforcement), they did not develop learned helplessness, but if their behavior had no influence on the receipt of the punishment, they were highly predisposed to it.

Another issue related to reinforcement and punishment use is client compliance. Clients would rather use reinforcement when working with their pets. However, people are generally better at noticing undesirable behavior rather than noticing and reinforcing desirable behavior. Punishing behavior (even a verbal reprimand) can be reinforcing to the punisher. It is a better use of our time to teach owners how to use positive reinforcement effectively; changing an owner's focus to notice desirable behavior rather than to punish each misstep. Punishment is a challenge to administer successfully, see Table 6.3 for the criteria for punishment to be successful.

An animal's attention is a powerful tool during training (Figure 6.4). Without their attention, they are not going to learn the behaviors you want them to learn. Having an appropriate reinforcer goes a long way toward gaining and keeping an animal's attention. Other factors that affect attention are the relationship between the trainer and the animal, the environment within which the training is occurring, the environment in which the animal was socialized, the temperament of the animal (anxiety and fear can inhibit learning), and the animal's genetics. Attention is so vital to learning in animals it is often the first behavior taught, "look at me."

Once a behavior is taught in one context, it must be taught in other contexts or the animal will only associate that one context with the behavior. Owners may train an animal to perform a behavior in one context, yet expect them to perform the behavior in a totally different context. Examples of this phenomenon are seen when dogs trained for obedience trials only heel when on rubber mats. They were taught to heel on these mats in dog obedience classes, and the trials are conducted on them as well. The dogs may not understand that heeling is desired from them off rubber mats. Teaching a behavior on a cue in a variety of situations and environments is called *generalization*. A behavior is not truly learned until the animal will perform it in multiple contexts when given the cue.

Table 6.3 Criteria for successful punishment.

Criterion	Comment
Punishment must occur every time the behavior happens	If you cannot be present each time the behavior is performed, you must set up a remote punishment device that punishes every time the behavior is performed Only the unwanted behavior can be punished with this remote device Indiscriminate punishment causes learned helplessness If the punishment does not occur every time the behavior repeats, the animal is likely being reinforced intermittently for the behavior. This makes the behavior resistant to extinction
Punishment must be harsh enough to stop the behavior	Generally, people do not want to use harsh punishments on their animals Animals can habituate to different levels of punishment if you start with a weaker one and slowly increase it
Punishment must occur during the behavior or before any other behavior has been performed	Associative learning drops off sharply after 2 s following a behavior If another behavior is performed before the punishment that is the behavior being punished not the intended one

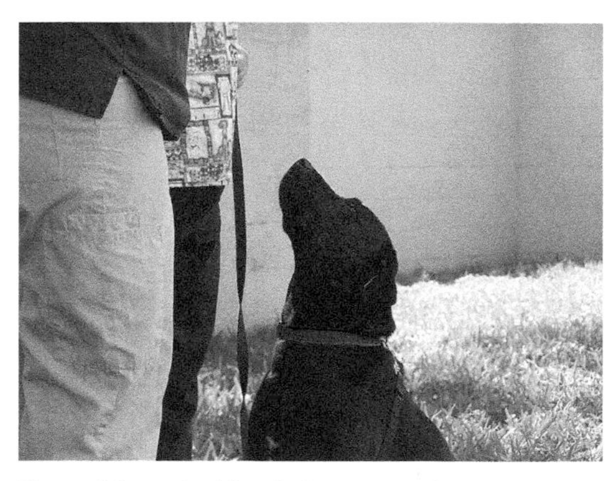

Figure 6.4 A mixed-breed dog, Trixie, showing attention toward one of the kennel technicians, Jessica Rice, and a veterinary technology student, Jeanne Rowe.

Aspects of training a behavior to fluency include precision, duration, distance, latency, speed, and distraction (Luck 2015). Precision is seen when the behavior being performed meets the trainer's criteria for the behavior. Duration or length of the behavior meets the criteria of the trainer. For example, a minute-long sit stay. If the animal can perform the behavior when at a distance from the trainer then the animal's behavior meets the trainer's distance requirements. Latency is how fast the animal begins to perform the behavior after the cue is given, while speed is how fast the entire behavior is performed. Once the behavior is performed reliably in the presence of distractions the behavior meets this criterion for fluency.

When looking at operant conditioning through the lens of Applied Behavior Analysis it contains three parts: the antecedent, the behavior, and the consequences of performing the behavior. These parts can be used to predict whether or not the animal will continue to perform the behavior. The antecedent can be a signal to communicate to the animal they will earn a wanted reinforcer if they perform a specific behavior now. The behavior is the action the animal performs to earn the reinforcer and the consequences are the results of performing the behavior – either a reinforcer or a punisher. When a behavior no longer earns the desired reinforcer it is extinguished.

Behavior modification using operant conditioning

Behavior can be weakened without using punishment. It is more effective to train an animal to perform the behaviors you want rather than punishing each behavioral mistake they make. Using Friedman and Fritzler's Hierarchy of Behavior-Change Procedures Most Positive, Least Intrusive Effective Interventions (Figure 6.5), the best way to start changing behavior is to make sure the animal's physical and mental needs are being met (2019). The next step is using antecedent arrangements; setting up the environmental cues to create a situation where the animal is more likely to perform the wanted behavior instead of the unwanted behavior.

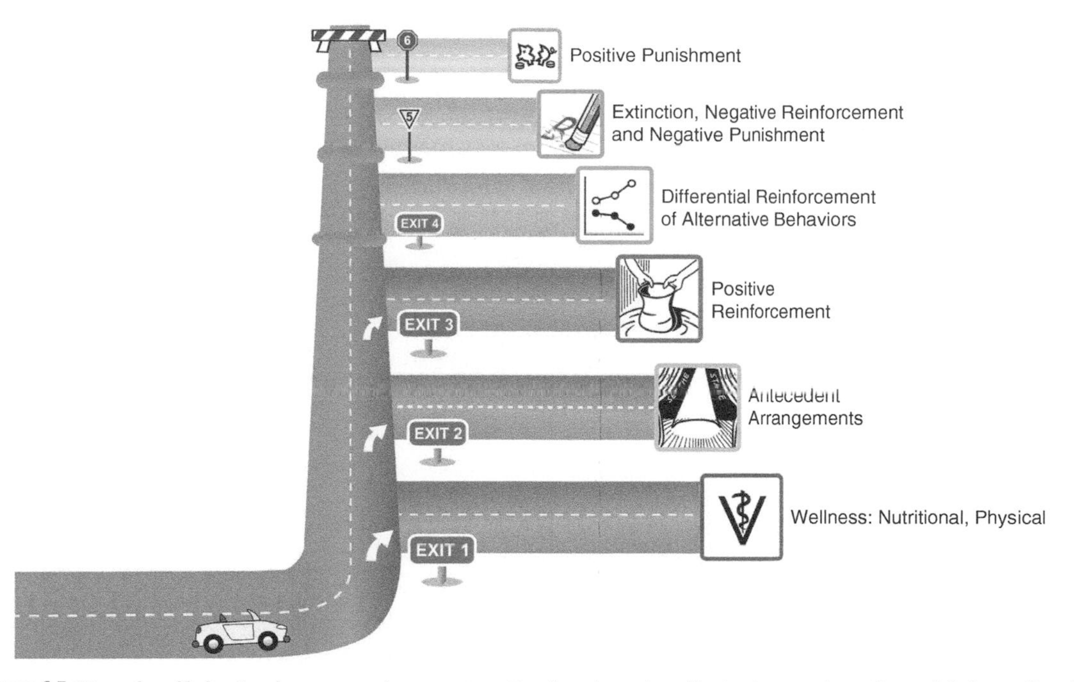

Figure 6.5 Hierarchy of behavior-change procedures most positive, least intrusive effective interventions. *Source*: Friedman, S. and Fritzler, J. 2019. With permission of Friedman, S.

BOX 6.3: BEHAVIOR MODIFICATION USING OPERANT CONDITIONING

- Operant counter conditioning: different terms used
  - Counter conditioning
  - Response substitution
- Operant extinction: different terms used
  - Extinction
  - Removing the reinforcer for the behavior
  - Ignoring or removing attention

Please refer to the two articles at behaviorworks.org for more information about the Hierarchy of Behavior-Change Procedures (see **Additional resources**). When the wanted behavior is performed it is reinforced making the wanted behavior more likely to occur in this context in the future. Another of these behavior modification techniques is called *operant counter conditioning* (Box 6.3). This technique is one in which the animal is taught to perform a wanted behavior in place of the unwanted behavior. When using this technique, the animal can more easily be taught the wanted behavior outside of the situation in which they are performing the unwanted behavior. The behavior must be taught in a relaxed environment for the animal to best be able to learn it. Then, the behavior can be transferred over to the environment where the unwanted behavior is being performed. Notice the cue that elicits the unwanted behavior. Once trained, this cue can be used to elicit the wanted behavior. The animal learns this new, wanted behavior is reinforcing in this situation, whereas the unwanted behavior is not. A selection of reinforcement rules can be used in human psychology and in animal training when using operant counter conditioning. In these situations, the behavior being reinforced is related to the unwanted behavior in a variety of ways (Table 6.4).

This technique of operant counter conditioning can be used in combination with operant extinction. Operant extinction, often called *extinction*, is used to weaken a behavior by removing its reinforcer. It is not a technique in which you only ignore the animal when they perform the behavior because some behaviors are not reinforced by attention. If your dog steals food from a coffee table, you can ignore the behavior forever; however, the dog will never learn to stop stealing the food. This is because obtaining the food is the reinforcer not attention. Sometimes, attention is the reinforcer for the behavior. Attention often reinforces jumping to greet behaviors in dogs. This is why removal of attention when they jump on you and teaching them to sit to greet you instead work so well.

When using extinction, you must first know what is reinforcing the behavior. You can find this out by observing the animal and noting what happens right after they perform the behavior. If you cannot figure out what is reinforcing the behavior or if you cannot remove the reinforcer, then you can still use operant counter conditioning, but you will not be able to use extinction with it. Animals may find performing the behavior reinforcing in itself. This occurs when animals masturbate, and many people believe that it also occurs when dogs bark. If you are

Table 6.4 Various reinforcement options for operant counter conditioning.

Technique	Full name	Description	Comment
DRO	Differential reinforcement of other behaviors	The trainer reinforces any other behavior besides the unwanted behavior	This is used in circumstances in which an animal does not offer many behaviors. We want to increase any behavior besides the unwanted one
DRA	Differential reinforcement of an alternate behavior	The trainer reinforces a behavior the animal cannot perform at the same time as the unwanted behavior	This is used to substitute a wanted behavior for an unwanted one
DRH	Differential reinforcement of high rates of responding	The trainer reinforces a burst of wanted behaviors	This is used to create quick bursts of a wanted behavior
DRL	Differential reinforcement of low rates of responding	The trainer reinforces the behavior only when the behavior occurs after specific timed pauses	This is used to cause pauses between a series of wanted behaviors

able to ascertain the reinforcer and remove it, you can then use extinction.

Extinction has unwanted side effects including what is called an extinction burst. When the reinforcer is removed, the animal will exhibit an extinction burst. This affects the unwanted behavior by making it more intense and variable. The animal may react by becoming frustrated and even behaving aggressively. To reduce the intensity and length of the extinction burst, operant counter conditioning is used. Using both techniques together, the animal learns the unwanted behavior no longer obtains them any reinforcement, but the wanted behavior is now reinforced instead. An even better idea is for the trainer to use operant counter conditioning without using extinction by using antecedent arrangements to make it more likely the animal will perform the wanted behavior than the unwanted behavior. A brilliant example of this is Emily Larlham's video called "STOP Jumping Up!" (2010). Emily places the food treat on the floor as the puppy approaches her causing the puppy to keep all four paws on the floor instead of jumping up. Once this wanted approach behavior occurs it is reinforced strengthening it in the future.

- When designing a behavior modification plan it is important to use the "least intrusive effective intervention" to reduce stress and fear in the learner (Friedman and Fritzler 2019).

Behaviors that are reinforced on an intermittent or partial reinforcement schedule are difficult to extinguish (Skinner 1966). The animal has learned they will not be reinforced for each behavior performed, thus will continue to perform the behavior many times reliably without a reinforcer.

The process of using operant extinction is stressful for the learner. A behavior the animal used to obtain a wanted reinforcer no longer works to obtain it. Instead of using extinction with operant counter conditioning, antecedent arrangement can be used to make it more likely the new wanted behavior will be performed instead of the unwanted behavior. When designing a behavior modification plan it is important to use the "least intrusive effective intervention" to reduce stress and fear in the learner (Friedman and Fritzler 2019).

Classical conditioning

This type of associative learning is one in which an animal associates a novel stimulus with a reaction (Box 6.4). It is the contiguity of the conditioned stimulus and the conditioned response that is the vital aspect for learning the conditioned stimulus is associated with the conditioned response (Donahoe and Vegas 2004). In real-life learning situations, the unconditioned stimulus must be presented to elicit the unconditioned response, but the vital aspect for classical conditioning to occur is for the animal learning that the conditioned stimulus and the unconditioned response/conditioned response are found close together temporally.

After repeated pairings between the conditioned stimulus and the conditioned response, the novel stimulus will also cause this reaction. The paradigm for classical conditioning that produces the strongest and fastest learning is presenting a conditioned stimulus then an unconditioned stimulus, which elicits an unconditioned response. After many pairings, the conditioned stimulus will elicit a conditioned response, which is often indistinguishable from the unconditioned response seen when exposed to the unconditioned stimulus (Table 6.5).

When thinking about all these stimuli and responses, it may help to remember that if a stimulus or response is conditioned, learning had

BOX 6.4: DIFFERENT TERMS USED FOR CLASSICAL CONDITIONING

- Respondent conditioning
- Signal learning
- Pavlovian conditioning
- Type 1 conditioning
- Type S conditioning

Table 6.5 Classical conditioning schematic.

Cat sees food (US)	Becomes excited (UR)	
Cat hears can opener (CS)	Sees food (US)	Becomes excited (UR)
Cat hears can opener (CS)	Becomes excited (CR)	

CR: conditioned response; CS: conditioned stimulus; UR: unconditioned response; US: unconditioned stimulus.

to occur for it to have meaning. If a stimulus is unconditioned, this instead indicates that no learning needs to occur for it to elicit a response. The conditioned stimulus can occur in various temporal relationships to the unconditioned stimulus to elicit the unconditioned response as the animal is learning about the conditioned stimulus in this arrangement. Four types of temporal relationships between the conditioned stimulus and the unconditioned stimulus are labeled as delayed, trace, simultaneous, and backward. Delayed conditioning is being used when the conditioned stimulus precedes and slightly overlaps the beginning of the unconditioned stimulus then the unconditioned response occurs. Trace conditioning is being used when the conditioned stimulus precedes the unconditioned stimulus with a small gap in time between them and then the unconditioned response occurs. Simultaneous conditioning is being used when the conditioned stimulus and the unconditioned stimulus are presented at the same time then the unconditioned response occurs. Backward conditioning is being used when the unconditioned stimulus precedes the conditioned stimulus then the unconditioned response occurs. Each of these temporal arrangements can be useful for learning in different situations with animals. Yin used low-stress techniques where she presented food overlapping the food presentation with a part of a nail trim procedure to change the dog's emotional state related to nail trims. This order of procedures is used to increase safety in hospital when working with a fearful patient. Within all four temporal procedures lies the vital association between the conditioned stimulus and the unconditioned response/conditioned response, which is the basis of classical conditioning (Donahoe and Vegas 2004).

This type of learning was studied by Pavlov in the late 1800s and early 1900s. His experiments with dogs involved the reflex of salivation. Most of the behaviors related to classical conditioning are involuntary; they include reflexes, emotions, and secretions. Classical conditioning is powerful because the learning takes place within the unconscious mind. Learning of this type cannot be set aside by the conscious brain, although it can be mitigated by experience (Krushinskii 1960).

Evidence of classical conditioning is seen when a cat learns that being put in his carrier signifies he is going to the veterinary hospital. When he is placed in the carrier, he now feels what he feels when at the veterinary hospital. In a real way, the carrier has become the veterinary hospital for this cat. We can use classical conditioning to our advantage by teaching animals to associate the hospital and/or the carrier with stimuli they enjoy. Every piece of equipment at the veterinary hospital can be associated with something that individual animal enjoys, making it easier for us to assess our patients. Procedures and individuals can be associated with desired stimuli as well as to facilitate an animal's diagnostics and treatment.

- Every piece of equipment at the veterinary hospital can be associated with something that individual animal enjoys, making it easier for us to assess our patients.

Not only can animals associate one stimulus with another to elicit a response, they can also associate any number of stimuli with each other, creating a huge chain of associations. Evidence of this is seen in every veterinary hospital. A client comes in and remarks how their dog knows he is coming to the veterinary hospital when the owner turns right on a particular road, as the dog becomes fearful when the client turns the car. The dog has associated the turn with being at the hospital, which he associates with something fear or pain producing. Thus, the fear is elicited by the right turn on a road, which is not fear or pain producing at all. This process is called *higher order conditioning*. Because of this phenomenon, animals can associate an entire string of stimuli with a feared stimulus, creating fear responses when exposed to each individual stimulus.

Animals more readily learn some associations than others. This phenomenon is called *preparedness*. In the work by Seligman (1970, 1971) on preparedness, he found that animals exhibited three levels of preparedness to learn specific associations: prepared, unprepared, and contraprepared. When the animal was learning something in the prepared category, they learned it very quickly, often within one trial. Learning something in the unprepared category took many more trials for an animal, and learning something in the contraprepared category took a significant number of trials or it could not be learned. These categories of preparedness seemed tied to the evolution of the animal. Animals seemed to learn some associations easily. For example, the fear of snakes or spiders was learned easily, whereas other associations such as fear of flowers were very difficult if not impossible for them to learn. There are many studies showing this effect. Cook and Mineka (1990) found that primates were more easily trained to associate a snake than a flower with fear after watching videos of monkeys' fearful response to both stimuli.

Overshadowing is present when two conditioned stimuli are conditioned to an unconditioned stimulus together and one stimulus has a stronger connection to the unconditioned stimulus than the other. Blocking is similar, but in blocking, only one of the conditioned stimuli is actually conditioned, whereas the other is not. Both of these principles can be illustrated with one example. When conditioning a clicker, the click sound is often paired with a food treat. If the food treat is located within a crinkling bag, that sound may also be conditioned to the food treat at some level. If the crinkle sound and the click sound are conditioned to the food, but one has a stronger connection, then it is an example of overshadowing. If instead only one of the sounds is associated with the food, then that stimulus has blocked the other from forming an association.

Another factor that affects classical conditioning is potentiation. It appears that some pairings of associations create more powerful responses than others. Associations of various sensory stimuli with the gustatory sense are more potent than other pairings. Somehow the animal brain is wired to make stronger associations when taste is involved. This differs from preparedness in that preparedness is related to the ease of learning fear-producing stimuli, whereas potentiation is related to associations of taste and other sensory information with food and eating.

Interestingly, an animal can associate a stimulus with food so strongly that they treat the stimulus as if it were food. This is seen when an animal, after being conditioned to the clicker, licks a clicker when they hear the click sound. They behave as if the clicker is a food treat instead of behaving as if the click sound is predicting the presentation of food. This type of association is called *autoshaping*. It can affect the behavior of an animal by changing the response to a conditioned cue in unexpected ways. Autoshaping may be the learning that causes instinctual drift when using operant conditioning in animals (Barker 2001). Automaintenance is seen when the behavior learned during autoshaping continues despite an apparent lack of reinforcer. In reality, the autoshaped behavior is reinforced through unconditioned and conditioned reinforcers (Barker 2001).

Animals can learn superstitious behaviors by making associations between stimuli. For example, retired racing Greyhounds are unaccustomed to walking on slick tile floors. The floors at the college where I work have dark-colored tiles along the walls and light-colored tiles in the middle of the floor. When the Greyhounds first come to the building, they walk very close to the walls because they are not confident about walking on the slippery floors. Over time they learn to habituate to walking on the tile flooring, but they also associate the dark-colored tiles close to the wall with safe walking. Thus, they learn to walk only on the dark-colored tiles avoiding the light-colored ones (Figure 6.6).

Behavior modification using classical conditioning

Behavior can be modified by changing the associations learned through classical conditioning (Box 6.5). One type of classical conditioning behavior modification technique is called *classical counter conditioning*, whereby the association is changed by changing the unconditioned response that is being associated with the conditioned stimulus. For practical behavior modification purposes, this will mean changing the unconditioned stimulus that elicits the unconditioned response. Changing the unconditioned stimulus associated with the conditioned stimulus will change the conditioned response (Figure 6.7).

If a dog is afraid of the examination room at a veterinary hospital, it has probably associated a fearful

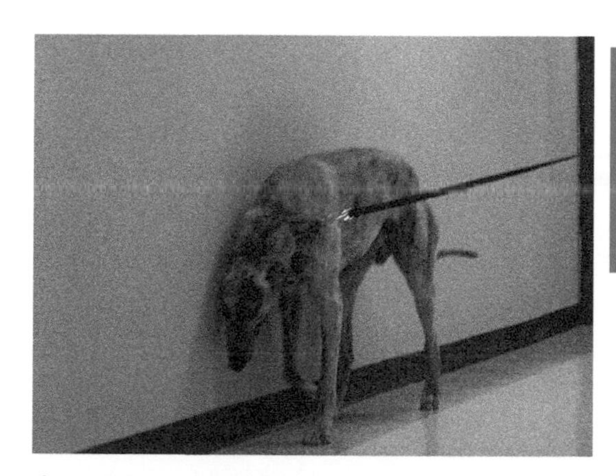

Figure 6.6 A Greyhound, Buck, is showing superstitious behavior by choosing to walk on the dark-colored tiles of the floor. He is afraid of the light-colored tiles.

BOX 6.5: BEHAVIOR MODIFICATION USING CLASSICAL CONDITIONING

- Classical extinction
- Classical counter conditioning
- Flooding
- Desensitization
- Affective conditioning
- Aversion or avoidance conditioning
- Conditioned taste aversion

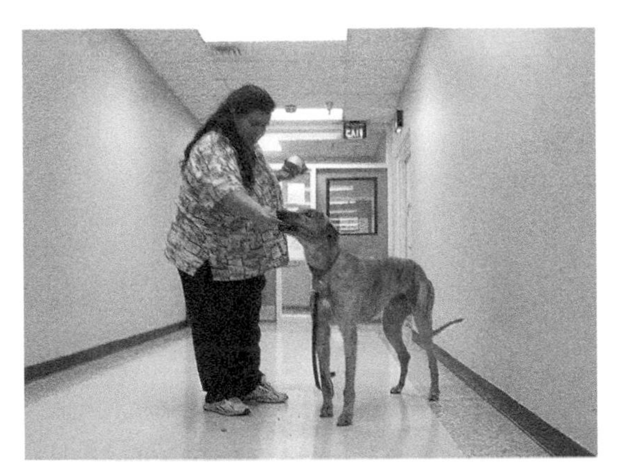

Figure 6.7 A Greyhound, Buck, showing signs of learning through classical counter conditioning that the light-colored tiles are fun to walk on.

or painful stimulus with its presence in the examination room; otherwise, the examination room could be a novel experience that produces fear. Fear can become generalized and associated with contexts, events, people, and other animals. To change the conditioned response from fear to a positive emotion, the examination room would need to become associated with something the dog enjoys. This could be play, petting, happy talk, or a food treat. There must be repeated pairings for the dog to learn the new association (examination room = food treat = happy dog; Table 6.6). The conditioned response does not have to be an emotion. It could be a secretion or a reflex. It is possible to counter condition a blink response or salivation. Amazingly, it is also possible to condition immune suppression and a healthy immune response (Ader and Cohen 1982 – immunosuppression; Ader and Cohen 1993 – immune enhancement).

Table 6.6 Classical counter conditioning schematic.

Dog enters examination room (CS)	Nails are quicked (US)	Feels pain and fear (UR)
Dog enters examination room (CS)	Feels fear (CR)	
Dog enters examination room (CS)	Receives treat (new US)	Feels happy and relaxed (new UR)
Dog enters examination room (CS)	Feels happy and relaxed (new CR)	

CR: conditioned response; CS: conditioned stimulus; UR: unconditioned response; US: unconditioned stimulus.

Although the dog is changing its voluntary behaviors at the same time as changing its conditioned response, these voluntary behaviors are not being classically conditioned. They are conditioned through operant conditioning. Operant and classical conditioning are occurring together all the time.

In the aforementioned example, the dog is learning through classical conditioning to be happy in the examination room, but he may also learn to sit instead of pacing. The sitting or pacing behaviors are learned through operant conditioning and are being reinforced by some stimulus in the room, perhaps actions of the owner and/or the veterinary professionals.

Conditioned responses can also be changed by removing the association between the conditioned stimulus and the unconditioned stimulus. Thus, when the conditioned stimulus occurs, the unconditioned stimulus and unconditioned response will no longer follow. This technique uses classical extinction. Extinction within classical conditioning removes the link between the associated stimuli, which changes the conditioned response.

If a cat is fed using a can opener, they will learn to associate the sound the can opener makes with obtaining a canned food meal, causing them to have a positive emotion. When the can opener no longer opens cans of cat food, the cat then habituates to the sound. They learn the sound no longer causes a positive emotion as the unconditioned stimulus that elicited the required unconditioned response is not present. Their response changes from a positive emotion to nothing. As with operant extinction, the behavior may go through an extinction burst becoming more variable and intense. The animal may become frustrated and stressed while learning the new paradigm.

Besides learning that one stimulus is associated with another, animals can learn that a stimulus means something wanted or unwanted for them through classical conditioning. We can manipulate this type of emotional learning by using affective conditioning. To modify an animal's feelings related to a stimulus, pairings need to be made between the stimulus and something the animal already likes or dislikes. A cat could learn to like getting into her carrier if the cat associated the carrier with other things she likes, such as canned food. Affective conditioning is a type of classical conditioning in which emotions are associated with contexts, objects, or individuals. This technique can be used to create a positive association between an animal and a new baby. The presence of the baby is associated with a positive emotion by presenting stimuli the animal likes in the presence of the baby, whereby the baby consequently elicits a positive emotional response from the animal.

While affective conditioning is a broader type of classical conditioning having to do with the animal's emotions, aversive or avoidance conditioning specifically teaches an animal to avoid a stimulus by making an association between the stimulus and something the animal fears or dislikes. Spray collars triggered by the close proximity of a target use this technique to teach dogs an association between being near an object with a spray in their face. This causes a dog to associate being near that object with being sprayed, thus teaching them the object is bad or to avoid that object. Conditioning of this type can be used to teach a dog to avoid proximity to a cat's litter box or the garbage can. Remember since operant behavior is also happening simultaneously, the act of approaching the object resulting in the consequence of a citronella spray would also be positive punishment if it decreased the behavior of approaching the object in the future. Note the American Veterinary Society of Animal Behavior's (AVSAB) Position Statement on Humane Dog Training discusses how a technique can be effective yet due to its effects on the learner it is not recommended. "Current literature on dog training methods shows a clear advantage of reward-based methods over aversive-based methods with respect to immediate and long-term welfare, training effectiveness, and the dog–human relationship." (AVSAB 2021).

Flooding is a technique that places the animal near the feared stimulus or in the feared situation until they no longer react with fear. This can be a useful technique if the animal is not very afraid of the stimulus or situation and if they quickly pair the feared stimulus with another stimulus causing a positive emotion (relaxation). If the animal is affected greatly by the stimulus, they can become more fearful by using this technique. Flooding can cause intense fear and stress for the animal (Figure 6.8). A great example of flooding is the television show Fear Factor. Contestants are placed so that they cannot escape, then something they fear (rats, spiders, or cockroaches) are put on them. On the show, the contestants rarely feel better about the source of their fear after competing. Similarly, animals can become more fearful of the stimulus after using this technique. Reactions to flooding can include attempting to flee the procedure or behaving aggressively while trying to flee. The animal may even be injured while trying to escape. If they are not exposed to the feared stimulus until the fear is completely gone, they will continue to associate the stimulus with danger. Flooding is not a recommended technique because of its unwanted side effects, increased fear, and because unlike humans, animals cannot opt into the treatment method.

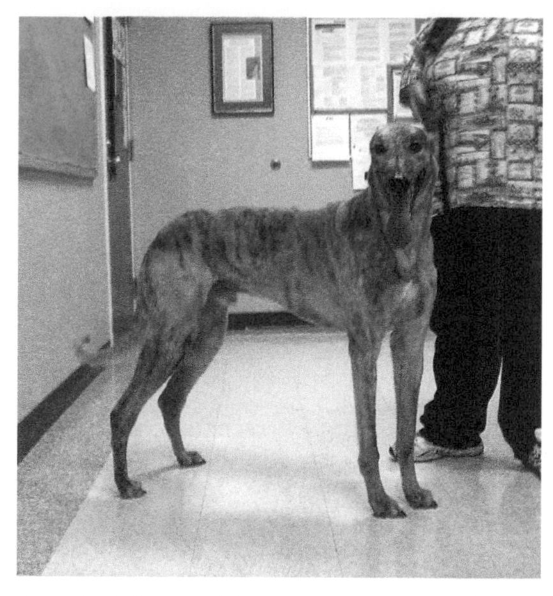

Figure 6.8 A Greyhound, Buck, showing signs of stress because of flooding. He is afraid of the light-colored floor tiles.

Desensitization is another method of using classical conditioning to teach an animal to pair a feared stimulus with relaxation. Box 6.6 provides terms and definitions for human psychological terms for desensitization. These human psychological techniques are

BOX 6.6: PSYCHOLOGICAL TERMS FOR DESENSITIZATION

- *In vitro* desensitization – A person imagines the situation or object of their fear while relaxing. The fear-producing stimuli are put into a list according to their fear-producing properties. The person begins imagining the least feared item and works up to the most feared item.
- *In vivo* desensitization – A person is exposed to the situation or object of their fear while relaxing. All other aspects of this behavior modification technique are the same as *in vitro* desensitization.

modified when working with nonverbal patients like animals. With desensitization, the feared stimulus is broken down into its components and modified to lower its intensity. Then, these components are ranked from the least to the most feared component. A plan is made in which the animal will be exposed to the least feared aspects of the stimulus first beginning at a non-stressful starting point. The animal must be relaxed with the beginning exposures to facilitate them learning to pair the stimulus with relaxation. Over time, and as the animal learns to stop responding to the stimulus with fear at one level, each feared component of the stimulus is presented in turn. With repeated exposure, the animal learns to pair each part of the stimulus with relaxation. Because the components are presented independently and because the intensity is modified to increase the speed of learning, the animal learns quickly to cope with the stimulus without the intense anxiety flooding can elicit.

Using the example of a human's fear of spiders, we can list the frightening components as size, speed of movement, proximity, and hairiness. It would depend on the individual how these components were ranked. Each component can be modified in some way to make the spider initially less scary. For example, we could start off with a very small, bald, dead spider contained in a sealed jar 10 ft away from the subject. This stimulus is small (size), cannot move because of death and is contained (speed of movement), is not hairy, and is far away (proximity). After the subject is relaxed with this stimulus, we could modify one of the characteristics of the spider. We could use a very small, live, bald spider contained in a sealed jar 10 ft away from the subject. We would continue in this way until the subject could pick up a very large, hairy, fast moving, live spider without fear.

Desensitization is almost always used with additional classical counter-conditioning techniques by pairing the feared stimulus with a stimulus the animal wants. This combination of techniques allows the animal to quickly learn a new positive emotional response through classical conditioning by pairing the feared stimulus with relaxation and a stimulus they want.

- Desensitization is almost always used with additional classical counter-conditioning techniques by pairing the feared stimulus with a stimulus the animal wants. This combination of techniques allows the animal to quickly learn a new positive emotional response through classical conditioning by pairing the feared stimulus with relaxation and a stimulus they want.

Attention focusing and relaxation exercises can enhance the results of these techniques. Animals can be taught to focus on another stimulus besides the feared one. However, an animal will not be able to do this when they are very afraid. The relationship the animal has with the person conducting the behavior modification may affect the process. If the animal is able to learn to focus on another stimulus, then they are learning to ignore the feared one. An example of this procedure is when a trainer clicks and treats when a dog looks at another dog they fear. The dog learns over time to look at the dog, they fear, then look at the trainer for their treat. They associate seeing the dog with getting a treat, which changes their emotions associated with seeing the dog. The desensitization portion of this behavior modification plan would involve how the characteristics of the other dog that frighten this dog are modified to keep the dog relaxed and associating the feared dog with relaxation.

Relaxation can be measured by observing behaviors or by measuring physiological parameters (Poppen 1988). Overall updated her Protocol for Relaxation: Behavior Modification Tier 1 in the second edition of her *Manual of Clinical Animal Behavior* and added a Protocol for Teaching Your Dog to Take a Deep Breath and Use Other Biofeedback Methods as Part of Relaxation (2013). Included is new information on how to reinforce biofeedback methods for achieving relaxation in an animal; she focuses on dogs, but these methods can be modified for most animals. Overall's protocols emphasize how behavior modification techniques need to be precise to be effective, the importance of measuring behavior, and how the brain functions related to sensory stimuli and learning (Overall 2013).

Conditioned taste aversion

Classical conditioning contains quite a few specific scenarios for learning, but conditioned taste aversion is so special it has its own category. Taste aversion differs from classical conditioning in that it does not require the two stimuli to be timed closely together. There can be hours separating them. An animal must experience nausea after eating a substance for taste aversion to occur (Rozin and Kalat 1971). Taste, color, and odor are all stimuli that can be used by the animal to predict what will happen after they eat a substance. It does not matter if the nausea is caused by the substance consumed by the animal. The substance could be inert. If the animal is nauseous because of an illness and they consume a substance, taste aversion can occur. Novel substances are even more likely to be associated with the nausea than recognized substances.

Cats with kidney failure are likely cases for taste aversion because of their medical condition causing nausea. If they are fed a novel diet while experiencing nausea, they will not find that diet palatable because of taste aversion conditioning (Kirk et al. 2000). The cat associates the food with feeling ill.

Augmentation of taste aversion is seen when an animal first learns to avoid a substance through one sensory modality, such as taste, then is presented with that modality (taste) along with another (odor). This second association is even stronger than the first. Augmentation is seen when another stimulus becomes a reliable cue for conditioned taste aversion, strengthening the response through a synergistic effect (Batsell and Batson 1999). Through augmentation, an animal can learn a stronger response to a conditioned stimulus.

Behavior modification using taste aversion conditioning

Taste aversion conditioning can be used as an effective behavior modification method for weakening predatory behavior in animals (Gustavson et al. 1982 – in coyotes). If an animal learns to associate eating a specific type of animal with nausea, they will stop eating them. Animals can be made to feel nausea and will vomit with the use of apomorphine or lithium chloride. This method can be extremely effective, as it uses classical conditioning that is very powerful.

For taste aversion to work well, the animal must not notice any difference in taste or odor between the treated and the untreated meat. If a predator can assess which meat is treated, they will eat the untreated meat. They will learn an aversion to the emetic not the meat. In addition, the treated meat must be associated with the live animal in the mind of the predator. If this is not the case, the predator will learn not to eat the meat but will still kill and eat the live animal. Evidence for this was found in a study in which penned coyotes were conditioned through taste aversion to avoid laced mutton, but not live sheep (Burns and Connolly 1980). A similar result was found in huskies in which they became avoidant of the meat, but not the live animal; they also exhibited an increase in inter-dog aggression when lithium chloride was used to produce taste aversion (Hansen et al. 1997). Another study using 10 adult domestic dogs showed that dogs formed a taste aversion to ground meat from a specific animal (sheep, rabbit, or beef), but this aversion only lasted 24 hours (Rathore 1984). Dogs may not develop as strong taste aversions as other species.

Social learning

Social learning is defined as a type of learning using information received by watching another knowledgeable individual or group (Kubinyi et al. 2009). For evidence of learning to occur, the animal must then produce the learned behavior while no longer in the presence of the individual they watched (Kubinyi et al. 2009). The animal watches another animal's behavior, then they also watch what happens as a consequence of performing the behavior. If an animal performs a behavior and they are reinforced, the watching animal may want to perform the behavior as well. If instead the consequence of the behavior is punishment, the watching animal may learn they do not want to perform that behavior. Social learning should not be confused with social facilitation or social influence, which is a tendency for groups of animals to behave in a similar manner when together (Scott and McCray 1967). During this phenomenon, no generalization of operant learning is occurring in terms of the shared behavior. Of course, there will be classical conditioning going on between the emotional response created by the shared behavior and the accompanying animals.

Mechanisms used to measure social learning include focusing attention on a stimulus, focusing attention on a problem that can be solved, and how the problem can be solved (Kubinyi et al. 2009). When a person or another animal spends time near an object or in a particular place, other animals may also want to spend time there. In this situation, the animals are calling attention to an object or location by proximity. At another level, a person or animal may show through their actions that there is something hidden in a location that can be obtained. This can be shown by the person or animal trying to obtain an object from a location. An animal watching these activities may come to the conclusion that there is an advantage in performing similar actions to obtain a hidden object. The final mechanism used to measure social learning is one in which an animal observes how to solve the problem by watching another animal or person solve it. These mechanisms and the terms describing different forms of social learning are still being defined (Kubinyi et al. 2009), as this is a growing area of interest in behavioral research.

A more recent social learning model uses the following labels to describe the concepts within social learning and their relationships with transfer learning (generalization of learning) and associative learning (Table 6.7) (Lind et al. 2019).

In other research, the Family Dog Project located in Budapest, Hungary studied social learning between humans and dogs related to the advantages of using social learning over other associative types of learning for training complex behaviors (see Fugazza and Miklósi 2014a for examples). Through a variety of studies evidence supports the hypothesis that dogs form a different type of mental representation when learning through social learning compared to other associative types of learning,

Table 6.7 Social learning labels and relationships with transfer learning and associative learning.

Descriptive term	Definition	Requires transfer learning	Accounted for by associative learning
Inadvertent coaching	Feedback from experienced animal modifies learner's behaviour	No	Yes
Social facilitation	Presence of experienced animal triggers learner behaviour	No	Yes
Response facilitation	Behaviour of experienced animal triggers similar behaviour in learner	No	Yes
Contextual imitation	Learner copies a familiar action displayed by experienced animal	No	Yes
Stimulus enhancement	Behaviour of experienced animal causes learner to learn about a stimulus	Yes	Yes
Local enhancement	Behaviour of experienced animal causes learner to learn about a location	Yes	Yes
Opportunity providing	Behaviour of experienced animal creates favourable conditions for learning	Yes	Yes
Emulation	Learner uses outcomes of experienced animal's actions to learn, but does not copy actions of experienced animal	Yes	Yes
Observational conditioning	Observations of experienced animal's behaviour change S–S[a] associations in the learner	Yes	Yes
Social enhancement of food preferences	Food preferences are learned from experienced animal	Yes	Yes
Observational S–R[a] and R–S[a] learning	Observations of experienced animal's behaviour change S–R[a] or R–S[a] associations in the learner	Yes	No
Production imitation	Learner copies one or more unfamiliar actions displayed by experienced animal	Yes	No

[a] S stands for stimulus and R for response.

Source: Lind et al. 2019. The Royal Society.

CHAPTER 6

which allows dogs to learn the behavior and generalize it faster than when they learn through shaping using clicker training (Fugazza and Miklósi 2014b). Fugazza et al. found social learning present in eight-week-old dog puppies when the puppies observed a human or a conspecific perform a behavior (2018). The behavioral evidence of learning persisted for at least an hour in the dog puppies tested.

Play facilitates social learning in animals. Much communication and information about the physical ability of conspecifics are learned by the participants. Playful animals are less aggressive, and groups of animals that play together spend more time together (Bekoff 1974). Play enhances the ability of animals to learn from each other socially by increasing the time spent together and by making the participants familiar with each other's signals.

Reader (2003), while writing about innovation in primates and bird species, noted that social species that were "generalists or opportunists" were likely to exhibit innovation as well as social learning (p. 155). Dogs are generalists and opportunists. They show evidence of social learning from conspecifics as well as from humans, and they often live in groups. The use of animal culture as a way to learn new behaviors is an advantage of living in a group. It is evidence for behavioral flexibility and cognition in domestic species. Evidence of social learning is seen in both dogs and cats; they found food equally well using a human pointing gesture for orientation (Miklósi et al. 2005) (Figure 6.9).

Gent (2006) found an effect of social familiarity on observational learning in her study using 60 shelter dogs. The dogs learned tasks significantly faster if they were shown how to perform them by familiar people or dogs than if shown by unfamiliar people, unfamiliar dogs, or if they were taught through operant conditioning methods.

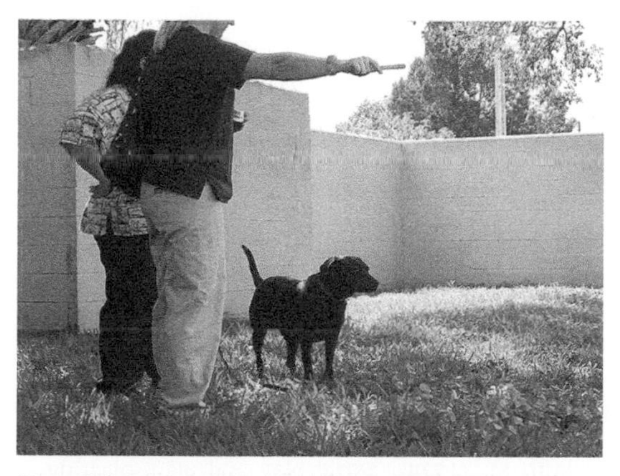

Figure 6.9 Trixie looking where Jeanne Rowe is pointing. This shows dogs look in the direction that humans are pointing.

Evidence was found using humans as the model for the wanted behavior in the studies by Pongracz et al. (2001). Using a detour task and a desired item, the dogs involved in the study had to learn how to obtain the item by going around the fence shaped in a "V." After viewing a person obtaining the item by walking around the fence, the dogs were easily able to do so themselves.

Behavior modification using social learning

Modeling is a technique of behavior modification in which one animal watches another animal or a human perform a behavior, which helps them to learn how to perform that behavior faster and better (Box 6.7). Evidence of this is found in the study by Slabbert and Rasa (1997) using drug-sniffing German shepherd dogs. The dogs were split into four groups: one that stayed with their mothers until six weeks of age and the other that stayed with their mothers until three months of age. Puppies from each of these groups were further divided according to whether they had trained or untrained narcotic sniffing mothers.

The four groups consisted of:

1. puppies with mother until six weeks and mothers were trained narcotic detection dogs;
2. puppies with mother until three months and mothers were trained narcotic detection dogs;
3. puppies with mother until six weeks, untrained mother;
4. puppies with mother until three months, untrained mother.

Puppies that stayed until three months with trained mother dogs learned the task of finding narcotics significantly faster than puppies that were either removed at six weeks or stayed with untrained mother dogs. This illustrates that modeling behaviors can reduce training time in dogs.

BOX 6.7: BEHAVIOR MODIFICATION TECHNIQUES USING SOCIAL LEARNING

Modeling

Conclusion

Learning is complex. There are many variables affecting the ways in which an animal learns. Their genetic code and their environment will affect how and what they learn.

Animals can learn using nonassociative learning such as habituation and sensitization as well as through associative learning such as operant and classical conditioning as well as social learning.

Behavior can be modified using a variety of behavior modification techniques. Generally, counter conditioning of operant or classically conditioned behaviors involves changing the consequences or associations between different learning factors. When using operant conditioning, antecedent arrangement is used to make the wanted behavior more likely to occur. Extinction involves the removal of reinforcement for operant behaviors and of the unconditioned stimulus for classically conditioned behaviors. Extinction is effective but it is not the "... most positive, least intrusive effective intervention" (Friedman and Fritzler 2019).

Social learning has recently seen more interest in the animal behavior domain. Animals are now acknowledged to have emotions and a rudimentary theory of mind as discussed by Horowitz (2011). This allows them to learn through watching others and may even allow them to understand what another animal is thinking or feeling. "In particular, if the animal seems to be operating with regard to some mediating element between others' appearance and their behaviors, this behavior could be described as a rudimentary theory of mind" (Horowitz 2011).

A good foundation in how animals learn is vital to working successfully with animals. Animals can be taught to be participants in their medical diagnostics and treatments instead of being forced into them. Learning about how animals learn can foster empathy for them. If you believe an animal is being stubborn, then force seems justified. While if you know the animal is afraid, a plan can be formed to attempt to change the fear to another emotion in order to facilitate humane medical care. Understanding why animals perform certain behaviors can help people work with the animals through the use of learning or behavior modification techniques. Understanding these techniques can help technicians in all aspects of their work with animals throughout their careers.

CHAPTER 6

- A good foundation in how animals learn is vital to working successfully with animals.

Additional resources

Articles regarding Hierarchy of Behavior-Change Procedures:

- https://behaviorworks.org/files/articles/What's%20Wrong%20With%20this%20Picture-General.pdf
- https://behaviorworks.org/files/articles/Why%20Animals%20Need%20Trainers%20Who%20Adhere%20to%20a%20Procedural%20Hierarchy.pdf

References

Ader, R. and Cohen, N. (1982). Behaviorally conditioned immunosuppression and murine systemic lupus erythematosus. *Science* 214: 1534–1536.

Ader, R. and Cohen, N. (1993). Psychoneuroimmunology: conditioning and stress. *Annual Review of Psychology* 44: 53–85.

Ainsworth, M.D. (1979). Infant–mother attachment. *American Psychologist* 34 (10): 932–937.

Ainsworth, C. (2015). Sex redefined. *Nature* 518: 288–291.

American Veterinary Society of Animal Behavior (2021). Position statement on Humane Dog Training. https://avsab.org/?s=Humane+dog+training (accessed November 3, 2022).

Barker, L.M. (2001). *Learning and Behavior: Biological, Psychological, and Sociocultural Perspectives*, 3e. Upper Saddle River, NJ: Prentice Hall.

Barry, K.J. and Crowell-Davis, S.L. (1999). Gender differences in the social behavior of neutered indoor only domestic cat. *Applied Animal Behaviour Sciences* 64: 193–211.

Batsell, W.R. and Batson, J.D. (1999). Augmentation of taste conditioning by a preconditioned odor. *Journal of Experimental Psychology: Animal Behavior Processes* 25 (3): 374–388.

Bauer, J.E. (2006). Facilitative and functional fats in diets of cats and dogs. *Journal of the American Veterinary Medical Association* 229 (5): 680–684.

Beach, F.A., Buehler, M.G., and Dunbar, I.F. (1982). Competitive behavior in male, female, and pseudohemaphiditic female dogs. *Journal of Comparative and Physiological Psychology* 96 (6): 855–874.

Bekoff, M. (1974). Social play and play-soliciting in infant canids. *American Zoologist* 14: 323–340.

Belyaev, D.K. (1979). Destabilizing selection as a factor in domestication. *Journal of Heredity* 70 (5): 301–307.

Bennett, E.L., Diamond, M.C., Krech, D., and Rosenzweig, M.R. (1964). Chemical and anatomical plasticity of brain: changes in brain through experience, demanded by learning theories, are found in experiments in rats. *Science* 146 (October): 610–619.

Blake, D.T., Strata, F., Churchland, A.K., and Merzenich, M. (2002). Neural correlates of instrumental learning in primary auditory cortexes. *Proceedings of the National Academy of Sciences* 99 (15): 10114–10119.

Boissy, A. (1998). Fear and fearfulness in determining behavior. In: *Genetics and the Behavior of Domestic Animals*, 67–111. San Diego, CA: Academic Press.

Boitani, L., Francisci, F., Ciucd, P., and Andreoli, G. (1995). Population biology and ecology of feral dogs in Central Italy. In: *The Domestic Dog: Its Evolution, Behaviour and Interactions with People*, 217–244. Cambridge: Cambridge University Press.

Bourassa, C.M. and Weiden, T.D. (1985). Orienting response and detection of thalamic stimulation: mechanism of perceptual learning in the cat. *Behavioral Neuroscience* 99 (2): 381–384.

Breland, K. and Breland, M. (1961). The misbehavior of organisms. *American Psychologist* 16: 681–684.

Brown, P.L. and Jenkins, H.M. (1968). Auto-shaping of the pigeon's key-peck. *Journal of the Experimental Analysis of Behavior* 11: 1–8.

Burgos, J.E. (2007). Autoshaping and automaintenance: a neural-network approach. *Journal of the Experimental Analysis of Behavior* 88: 115–130.

Burns, R.J. and Connolly, G.E. (1980). Lithium chloride bait aversion did not influence prey killing by coyotes. In: *Proceedings of the 19th Vertebrate Pest Conference, DigitalCom-mons@University of Nebraska, Lincoln*, 200–204.

Caulfield, R. (2000). Beneficial effects of tactile stimulation on early development. *Early Childhood Education Journal* 27 (4): 255–257.

Cheney, D.L. and Seyfarth, R.M. (1992). Dogs that don't bark in the night: how to investigate the lack of a domain of experience? *Proceedings of the Biennial Meeting of the Philosophy of Science Association*, 1992 2: 92–109.

Cook, M. and Mineka, S. (1990). Selective associations in the observational conditioning of fear in rhesus monkeys. *Journal of Experimental Psychology: Animal Behavioural Processes* 16 (4): 372–389.

Coppinger, R. and Coppinger, L. (1996). Biologic bases of behavior of domestic dog breeds. In: *Readings in Companion Animal Behavior*, 9–18. Trenton, NJ: Veterinary Learning Systems.

Coppinger, R. and Coppinger, L. (1998). Differences in the behavior of dog breeds. In: *Genetics and the Behavior of Domestic Animals*, 167–202. San Diego, CA: Academic Press.

Coppinger, R. and Coppinger, L. (2001). *Dogs: A New Understanding of Canine Origin, Behavior, and Evolution*. Chicago: University of Chicago Press.

Cravioto, J. and DeLicarie, E. (1975). Environmental and learning deprivation in children with learning disabilities. In: *Perceptual and Learning Disabilities in Children*, vol. 2, 3–102. Syracuse, New York: Syracuse University Press.

Crowell-Davis, S.L., Curtis, T.M., and Knowles, R.J. (2004). Social organization in the cat: a modern understanding. *Journal of Feline Medicine and Surgery* 6: 19–28.

D'Andrea, I., Alleva, E., and Branchi, I. (2007). Communal nesting, an early social enrichment, affects social competencies not learning and memory abilities at adulthood. *Behavioral Brain Research* 123: 60–66.

Darwin, C. (1859/2004). *On the Origin of Species*. New York: Barnes & Noble Originally published in 1859.

Debner, J.A. and Jacoby, L.L. (1994). Unconscious perception: attention, awareness, and control. *Journal of Experimental Psychology: Learning, Memory, and Cognition* 20 (2): 304–317.

Donahoe, J.W. and Vegas, R. (2004). Pavlovian conditioning: the CS-UR relation. *Journal of Experimental Psychology: Animal Behavior Processes* 30 (1): 17–33.

Ducos, P. (1978). Domestication defined and methodological approaches to its recognition in the faunal assemblages. In: *Approaches to Faunal Analysis in the Middle East*, 53–56. Cambridge, MA: Peabody Museum Bulletin 2/Peabody Museum of Archaeology and Ethnology/Harvard University Publications Department.

Estep, D.Q. (1996). The ontogeny of behavior. In: *Readings in Companion Animal Behavior*, 19–31. Trenton, New Jersey: Veterinary Learning Systems.

Ferster, C.B. and Skinner, B.F. (1957). *Schedules of Reinforcement*. New York: Appleton-Century-Crofts.

Fox, M.W. (1970). Neurobehavioral development and the genotype–environment interaction. *The Quarterly Review of Biology* 45 (2): 131–147.

Fraga, M.F. Ballestar, E., Paz, M.F. et al. (2005). Epigenetic differences arise during the lifetime of monozygotic twins. *Proceedings of the National Academy of Sciences of the United States of America* 102 (30): 10604–10609. https://doi.org/10.1073/pnas.0500398102.

Friedman, S. and Fritzler, J. (2019). Hierarchy road map. *Behavior Works* https://www.behaviorworks.org/htm/downloads_art.html.

Fugazza, C. and Miklósi, Á. (2014a). Deferred imitation and declarative memory in domestic dogs. *Animal Cognition* 17: 237–247. https://doi.org/10.1007/s10071-013-0656-5.

Fugazza, C. and Miklósi, Á. (2014b). Should old dog trainers learn new tricks? The efficancy of the do as I do method and the shaping/clicker training method to train dogs. *Applied Animal Behaviour Science* 153: 53–61.

Fugazza, C., Moesta, A., Pogány, A. and Miklósi, A. (2018). Social learning from conspecifics and humans in dog puppies. *Scientific Reports* 8:9257 DOI:10.1038/s41598-018-27654-0.

Fukuzawa, M., Mills, D.S., and Cooper, J.J. (2005). More than just a word: non-semantic command variables affect obedience in the domestic dog (*Canis familiaris*). *Applied Animal Behaviour Science* 91: 129–141.

Fuller, J.L. and Clark, L.D. (1966). Genetic and treatment factors modifying the post-isolation syndrome in dogs. *Journal of Comparative and Physiological Psychology* 61 (2): 251–257.

Gent, L.M. (2006). *Social Familiarity as a Predictor of Observational Learning in the Domestic Dog (Canis familiaris).* Unpublished doctoral dissertation. University of Texas at Arlington.

Gibson, J.J. (1958). Visually controlled locomotion and visual orientation in animals. *General Psychology* 49 (3): 182–194.

Goldstone, R.L. (1998). Perceptual learning. *Annual Reviews in Psychology* 49: 585–612.

Goodwin, D., Bradshaw, J.W.S., and Wickens, S.M. (1997). Paedomorphosis affects agonistic visual signals in domestic dogs. *Animal Behaviour* 53 (2): 297–304.

Grandin, T. and Deesing, M.J. (2014). Behavioral genetics and animal science. In: *Genetics and the Behavior of Domestic Animals*, 2e (ed. T. Grandin and M.J. Deesing), 1–40. Waltham, MA: Elsevier.

Gustavson, C.R., Jowsey, J.R., and Milligan, D.N. (1982). A 3-year evaluation of taste aversion control in Saskatchewan. *Journal of Range Management* 35 (1): 57–59.

Hall, C.S. (1941). Temperament: a survey of animal studies. *Psychological Bulletin* 38 (10): 909–943.

Hansen, I., Bakken, M., and Braastad, B.O. (1997). Failure of LiCl-conditioned taste aversion to prevent dogs from attacking sheep. *Applied Animal Behaviour Science* 54: 251–256.

Hare, B., Brown, M., Williamson, C., and Tomasello, M. (2002). The domestication of social cognition in dogs. *Science* 298 (5598): 1634–1637.

Hart, B.L. (1995). Analyzing breed and gender differences in behavior. In: *The Domestic Dog: Its Evolution, Behaviour and Interactions with People*, 66–77. Cambridge: Cambridge University Press.

Hellemans, K.G.C., Benge, L.C., and Olmstead, M.C. (2004). Adolescent enrichment partially reverses the social isolation syndrome. *Developmental Brain Research* 150: 103–115.

Hemmer, H. (1990). *Domestication: The Decline of Environmental Appreciation*. Cambridge: Cambridge University Press.

Horowitz, A. (2011). Theory of mind in dogs? Examining method and concept. *Learning and Behavior* 39: 314–317.

Horowitz, D. and Horowitz, A. (2009). A comparison of dog owner's claims about their pet's guilt with evidence from dog's behavior. *Journal of Veterinary Behavior* 4 (2): 104.

Horrocks, L.A. and Yeo, Y.K. (1999). Health benefits of docosahexaenoic acid (DHA). *Pharmacological Research* 40 (3): 211–225.

Hull, C.L. (1943). *Principles of Behavior*. New York: Appleton.

Ilska, J., Haskell, M.J., Blott, S.C. et al. (2017). Genetic characterization of dog personality traits. *Genetics* 206: 1101–1111.

Iso, H., Simoda, S., and Matsuyama, T. (2007). Environmental change during postnatal development alters behaviour, cognition, and neurogenesis of mice. *Behavioural Brain Research* 179: 90–98.

Jin, X., Zhang, Y., Celniker, S.E. Xia, Y. et al. (2021). Gut microbiome partially mediates and coordinates the effects of genetics on anxiety-like behavior in collaborative cross mice. *Scientific Report* 11: 270. https://doi.org/10.1038/s41598-020-79538-x.

Karsh, E.B. (1983). The effects of early handling on the development of social bonds between cats and people. In: *New Prospective on our Lives with Companion Animals* (ed. A.H. Katcherand and A.M. Beck), 22–28. Philadelphia: University of Pennsylvania Press.

Kirk, C.A., Debraekeleer, J., and Jane, A.P. (2000). Normal cats. In: *Small Animal Clinical Nutrition*, 4e, 291–320. Marceline, Missouri: Mark Morris Institute.

Kockaya, M. and Demirbas, Y.S. (2020). The use of carbetocin in the treatment of maternal cannibalism in dogs. *Journal of Veterinary Behavior* 40: 98–102. https://doi.org/10.1016/j.jveb.2020.10.004.

Krushinskii, L.V. (1960). *Animal Behavior: Its Normal and Abnormal Development. The International Behavioral Sciences Series*. New York: Consultants Bureau.

Kubinyi, E., Pongracz, P., and Miklósi, A. (2009). Dog as a model for studying conspedfics and heterospecific social learning. *Journal of Veterinary Behavior: Clinical Applications and Research* 4 (1): 31–41.

Larlham, E. (2010). STOP jumping up! https://youtu.be/lC_OKgQFgzw [video] (accessed November 3, 2022).

Li, K.Z.H. and Lindenberger, U. (2003). Relations between aging sensory/sensorimotor and cognitive functions. *Neuroscience and Biobehavioral Reviews* 26: 777–783.

Lind, J., Ghirlanda, S., and Enquist, M. (2019). Social learning through associative processes: a computational theory. *R. Soc. Open sci.* 6: 181777. https://doi.org/10.1098/rsos.181777.

Lord, K., Coppinger, L., and Coppinger, R. (2014). Differences in the behavior of landraces and breeds of dogs. In: *Genetics and the Behavior of Domestic Animals*, 2e (ed. T. Grandin and M.J. Deesing), 195–235. Waltham, MA: Elsevier.

Lorenz, K. (1965). *Evolution and Modification of Behavior*. Chicago: University of Chicago Press.

Luck, L. (2015). My dog knows it, he just won't do it! How to achieve fluency. https://www.clickertraining.com/node/4881 (accessed November 3, 2022).

Macdonald, D.W. and Carr, G.M. (1995). Variation in dog society: between resource dispersion and social flux. In: *The Domestic Dog: Its Evolution, Behaviour and Interactions with People*, 199–216. Cambridge: Cambridge University Press.

Mason, G., Clubb, R., Latham, N., and Vickery, S. (2007). Why and how should we use environmental enrichment to tackle stereotypic behaviour? *Applied Animal Behaviour Science* 102: 163–188.

McCune, S. (1995). The impact of paternity and early socialization on the development of cat's behaviour to people and novel objects. *Applied Animal Behaviour Science* 45: 109–124.

Melzak, R. and Scott, T.H. (1957). The effect of early experience on response to pain. *Journal of Comparative and Physiological Psychology* 50 (2): 155–161.

Michaels, C.F. and Carello, C. (1981). *Direct Perception*. Englewood Cliffs, NJ: Prentice Hall.

Miklósi, A., Kubinyi, E., Topal, J. et al. (2003). A simple reason for a big difference: wolves do not look back at humans, but dogs do. *Current Biology* 13: 763–766.

Miklósi, A., Pongracz, P., Lakatos, G. et al. (2005). A comparative study of the use of visual communicative signals in interactions between dogs (*Canis familiaris*) and humans and cats (*Felis catus*) and humans. *Journal of Comparative Psychology* 119 (2): 179–186.

Miller, P.E. (2001). Vision in animals: what do dogs and cats see? *Proceedings of the 25th Annual Waltham/OSU Symposium, Small Animal Ophthalmology* (October 27–28, 2001). https://www.vin.com/apputil/content/defaultadv1.aspx?pId=11132&id=3844144 (accessed November 3, 2022).

Morton, J.R.C. (1968). Effects of early experience "handling and gentlying" in laboratory animals. In: *Abnormal Behavior in Animals* (Chapter 17) (ed. M.W. Fox), 261–292. Philadelphia: MB Sanders.

National Human Genome Research Institute (NHGRI) (n.d.). Allele. Talking glossary of genomic and genetic terms. https://www.genome.gov/genetics-glossary (accessed November 3, 2022).

van Oers, H.J.J., de Kloet, E.R., Whelan, T., and Levine, S. (1998). Maternal deprivation effect on the infant's neural stress markers is reversed by tactile stimulation but not by suppressing corticosterone. *Journal of Neuroscience* 18 (23): 10171–10179.

Overall, K.L. (2009). Canine behavior: a new synthesis of canine humane care. *Proceedings of the North American Veterinary Conference*, Orlando, FL (January 17–21, 2009), 155–159. Gainesville, FL: North American Veterinary Conference.

Overall, K.L. (2013). *Clinical Behavioral Medicine for Small Animals*, 2e. Elsevier.

Overall, K.L. and Arnold, S.E. (2007). Olfactory neuron biopsies in dogs: a feasibility pilot study. *Applied Animal Behaviour Science* 105: 351–357.

Overmier, J.B. and Seligman, M.E.P. (1967). Effects of inescapable shock upon subsequent escape and avoidance responding. *Journal of Comparative and Physiological Psychology* 63 (1): 28–33.

Pongracz, P., Miklósi, A., Kubinyi, E. et al. (2001). Social learning in dogs: the effect of a human demonstrator on the performance of dogs in a detour task. *Animal Behaviour* 62 (6): 1109–1117.

Pongracz, P., Miklósi, A., Vida, V., and Csanyi, V. (2005). The pet dogs' ability for learning from a human demonstrator in a detour task is independent from the breed and age. *Animal Behaviour Science* 90: 309–323.

Pongracz, P., Vida, V., Banhegyi, P., and Miklósi, A. (2008). How does dominance rank status affect individual and social learning performance in the dog (*Canis familiaris*)? *Animal Cognition* 11: 75–82.

Poppen, R. (1988). *Behavioral Relaxation Training and Assessment*. New York: Penguin.

Poulsen, P., Esteller, M., Vaag, A., and Fraga, M.F. (2007). The epigenetic basis of twin discordance in age-related diseases. *Pediatric Research* 61 (5): 38R–42R. https://doi.org/10.1203/pdr.0b013e31803c7b98.

Premack, D. (1962). Reversibility of reinforcement relation. *Science* 136 (3512): 255–257.

Price, E.O. (1998). Behavioral genetics and the process of animal domestication. In: *Genetics and the Behavior of Domestic Animals*, 31–65. San Diego, CA: Academic Press.

Price, E.O. (1999). Behavioral development in animals undergoing domestication. *Applied Animal Behaviour Science* 65: 245–271.

Prichard, A., Chhibber, R., Athanassiades, K. et al. (2018). Fast neural learning in dogs: a multimodal sensory fMRI study. *Scientific Reports* 8: 14614. https://doi.org/10.1038/s41598-018-32990-2.

Rathore, A.K. (1984). Evaluation of lithium chloride taste aversion in penned domestic dogs. *Journal of Wildlife Management* 48 (4): 1424.

Reader, S.M. (2003). Innovation and social learning: individual variation and brain evolution. *Animal Biology* 53 (2): 147–158.

Rigterink, A. and Houpt, K. (2014). Genetics of canine behavior: a review. *World Journal of Medical Genetics* 4 (3): 46–57.

Rozin, P. and Kalat, J.W. (1971). Specific hungers and poison avoidance as adaptive specializations of learning. *Psychological Review* 78 (6): 459–486.

Schilder, M.B.H. and van der Borg, J.A.M. (2004). Training dogs with help of the shock collar: short and long term behavioural effects. *Applied Animal Behavioural Science* 85: 319–334.

Scott, J.P. and Fuller, J.L. (1965). *Genetics and the Social Behavior of the Dog*. Chicago: University of Chicago Press.

Scott, J.P. and McCray, C. (1967). Allelomimetic behavior in dogs: negative effects of competition on social facilitation. *Journal of Comparative Physiological Psychology* 63 (2): 316–319.

Seligman, M.E.P. (1970). On the generality of the laws of learning. *Psychological Review* 77 (5): 406–418.

Seligman, M.E.P. (1971). Phobias and preparedness. *Behavior Therapy* 2: 307–321.

Seligman, M.E.P. (1972). Learned helplessness. *Annual Review of Medicine* 23: 407–412.

Serpell, J.A. and Hsu, Y. (2005). Effects of age, breed and neuter status on trainability in dogs. *Anthrozoos* 18: 196–207.

Seyfarth, R.M., Cheney, D.L., and Marler, P. (1980). Monkey responses to three different alarm calls: evidence of predator classification and semantic communication. *Science* 210 (4417): 801–803.

Skinner, B.F. (1966). *The Behavior of Organisms*. New York: Appleton-Century-Crofts Originally published in 1938.

Slabbert, J.M. and Rasa, O.A.E. (1997). Observational learning of an acquired maternal behaviour pattern by working dog pups: an alternative training method? *Applied Animal Behaviour Science* 53: 309–316.

Smith, B.H. and Mendel, R. (1989). An analysis in variability in the feeding model program of the honey bee: the role of learning in releasing a model action pattern. *Ethology* 82: 68–81.

Suomi, S.J. (1997). Early determinants of behavior: evidence from primate studies. *British Medical Bulletin* 53 (1): 170–184.

Sylvia, K.E. and Demas, G.E. (2018). A gut feeling: microbiome–brain–immune interactions modulate social and affective behaviors. *Hormones and Behavior* 99: 41–49.

Thorne, C. (1995). Feeding behavior of domestic dogs and the role of experience. In: *The Domestic Dog: Its Evolution, Behaviour and Interactions with People*, 104–114. Cambridge: Cambridge University Press.

Tolman, E.C. and Honzik, C.H. (1930). Insight in rats. *University of California Publications in Psychology* 4: 215–232.

Topal, J., Miklósi, A., and Csanyi, V. (1997). Dog-human relationship affects problem solving behavior in dogs. *Anthrozoos* 10 (4): 214–224.

Topal, J., Miklósi, A., Csanyi, V., and Doka, A. (1998). Attachment behavior in dogs (*Canis familiaris*): a new application of Ainsworth's (1969) strange situation test. *Journal of Comparative Psychology* 112 (3): 219–229.

Topal, J., Gacsi, M., Miklósi, A. et al. (2005). Attachment to humans: a comparative study of hand-reared wolves and differentially socialized dog puppies. *Animal Behaviour* 70 (6): 1367–1375.

Trut, L.N. (1999). Early canid domestication: the fox farm experiment. *American Scientist* 87 (March–April): 160–169.

Viranyi, Z., Topal, J., Gacsi, M. et al. (2004). Dogs respond appropriately to cues of humans' attentional focus. *Behavioural Processes* 66: 161–172.

Wallis, L.J., Szabo, D., and Kubinyl, E. (2020). Cross-sectional age differences in canine personality traits; influence of breed, sex, previous trauma, and dog obedience tasks. *Frontiers in Veterinary Science* 6: 1–17. https://doi.org/10.3389/fvets.2019.00493.

Weiss, S.J., Wilson, P., and Morrison, D. (2004). Maternal tactile stimulation and the neurodevelopment of low birth weight infants. *Infancy* 5 (1): 85–107.

Wells, D.L. and Hepper, P.G. (1999). Male and female dogs respond differently to men and women. *Applied Animal Behaviour* 61 (4): 341–349.

Wells, D.L. and Hepper, P.G. (2006). Prenatal olfactory learning in the domestic dog. *Animal Behaviour* 72 (3): 681–686.

Wiggins, R.C. and Fuller, G.M. (1978). Early post natal starvation causes lasting brain hypomyelination. *Journal of Neurochemistry* 30: 1231–1237.

Williams, R.W., Cavada, C., and Reinoso-Suarez, F. (1993). Rapid evolution of the visual system: a cellular assay of the retina and dorsal lateral geniculate nucleus of the Spanish wild cat and the domestic cat. *Journal of Neuroscience* 13 (1): 208–228.

Wynne, C.D.L. (2016). What is special about dog cognition? *Current Directions in Psychological Science* 25 (5): 345–350. https://doi.org/10.1177/0963721416657540.

Zhang, L.-X., Levine, S., Dent, G. et al. (2002). Maternal deprivation increases cell death in the infant rat brain. *Developmental Brain Research* 133 (1): 1–11.

The PowerPoint of figures, appendices, MCQ's are available at www.wiley.com/go/martin/behavior

7 Problem prevention

Debbie Martin[1,2]
[1]TEAM Education in Animal Behavior, LLC, Spicewood, TX, USA
[2]Veterinary Behavior Consultations, LLC, Spicewood, TX, USA

CHAPTER MENU

Canine and Feline Behavior for Veterinary Technicians and Nurses, Second Edition. Edited by Debbie Martin and Julie K. Shaw.

Companion website: www.wiley.com/go/martin/behavior

Introduction

Benjamin Franklin's adage "An ounce of prevention is worth a pound of cure" is especially appropriate when applied to pets. It is much less work for owners to practice prevention than to address a problem that has become established. Although this fact alone should make the topic of problem prevention a high priority for anyone working with pets and owners, there are additional benefits to be achieved.

Each year, thousands of dogs and cats are given up by their owners. The majority of these animals are not bad pets but rather victims of unanticipated circumstances or misinformed owners. Reasons cited for relinquishment can often be traced back to poor choices during the pet selection process, unrealistic owner expectations, and lack of adequate training for the pet. Whatever the cause, the result for many of these animals culminates in the relinquishment of the pet. Programs that focus on prevention, early intervention, and education for owners have the potential to help many of these animals remain in their homes.

The medical community has long recognized the benefits of pet ownership to people. It is an accepted fact that pets enrich lives, improve physical health, and offer emotional encouragement to those around them. Studies have demonstrated that the cognitive development of children can be enhanced through pet ownership (Poresky and Hendrix 1990), as well as a child's level of positive self-esteem (Bergesen 1989). Pet owners also tend to be less fearful of becoming crime victims when walking with or sharing their residence with a dog (Serpell 1991).

In a September 1998 presentation at the 8th International Conference on Human–Animal Interactions, P. Raina, PhD, B. Bonnett, PhD, and D. Waltner-Toews, PhD, cited a research project they conducted within a population of senior citizens living in Canada. Results from this study provided evidence that pet ownership serves as an important coping mechanism. This in turn allows the senior owners to deal with stressful life events without the need for healthcare assistance.

The benefits cited above support the importance of a strong bond between owners and their pets. However, this bond cannot develop and grow without ongoing opportunities for positive interactions between pet and owner. Providing education, counseling, and support to owners through all stages of the relationship is one way to ensure that a positive connection between pet and owner continues, thus strengthening the human–animal bond.

Besides the obvious initial financial benefits to clinics, individuals, and businesses that offer training classes and prepurchase services (pet selection counseling), there are additional, often overlooked, advantages. Satisfied owners share information with friends and family. For veterinary practices, this provides a unique opportunity to gain recognition in the community as experts in the care of the total animal. Counseling and animal behavior services can also help create a relationship of trust between the practice and owners spanning the lifetime of the pet, making it possible to market other, equally important, services.

Employees interested in advancing their skills and ultimately their value to employers, often find the field of owner education and counseling on pet behavior to be a perfect venue. Pet counseling programs present an excellent outlet for veterinary clinics that want to reward technicians and experienced team members with continuing opportunities for professional growth and increased responsibility.

An added advantage of working closely with owners and pets is the ability to build a relationship of trust and improved pet behavior that ultimately results in a cooperative and happy patient.

There are a limitless number of services and programs available that can help owners achieve the goal of problem prevention. A review of common prevention services and topics is covered in this chapter. As discussed in Chapter 1, preventive care "refers to measures taken to prevent the development of behavior problems or disorders rather than treating the symptoms of an existing problem or disorder" whereas intervention care refers to measures taken to improve or alter an existing behavior disorder (psychological or behavioral patterns outside the behavioral norms for the species). Intervention requires a veterinary diagnosis and treatment plan. Chapter 9 will address intervention care.

Ideal characteristics for pet owners

Before discussing prevention and behavior solution strategies, first let's look at the ideal characteristics for pet owners. To be a successful "canine or feline parent," there are some simple rules to follow. (i) Be fair. Understand the pet's perspective. Pets are amoral, opportunistic, constantly learning, curious, enjoy exploration, social, olfactory communicators, and predatory. Dogs are avid chewers, and cats need vertical living space. Understanding builds empathy and results in owners having realistic expectations for their pet. Because they understand the pet's perspective and they are fair, they provide appropriate outlets for typical cat and dog behavior. (ii) Be a good teacher. Control what the pet learns through management and supervision. Guide it to make the right decisions. Rather than focus on what you do not want the pet to do, teach the correct behavior. Set the pet up to succeed. (iii) Clearly communicate to the pet when it is performing the correct behavior. Catch it doing things right and reward them for it. A high occurrence of positive reinforcement will help the pet learn quickly. (iv) Be consistent. Inconsistency and unpredictability cause fear, anxiety, and distrust, which can be a precursor to behavioral disorders. Establish a routine and set the rules of the house and make interactions as predictable, pleasant, and consistent as possible. (v) Advocate for the pet. Dogs and cats cannot speak up for themselves. It is our responsibility to be their advocate. This includes ensuring pleasant and positive learning experiences and avoiding overwhelming the pet.

The importance of consistency is not always well understood. It has been clarified that the relationship between humans and dogs is not one of submission and domination (Bradshaw et al. 2009). However, we have to control the contingencies of the dog's behavior. That means we need to be consistent in regard to which behaviors are reinforced and which are not. The establishment and enforcement of rules is extremely important. If rules are not consistent, the dog can never figure them out, and cannot function within them to achieve success. This situation would be similar to you visiting with friends who play a card game that you do not know. They ask you to participate and explain the rules to you. You go along with it and after some time think you have the winning hand, put your cards down and claim that you have won. Now of course, your friends add another rule. After two or three times of this, you will become frustrated and likely fairly irritated and not want to participate any longer. Frustration can even lead to aggression. This is how our dogs must feel if we have no rules or are constantly changing them. They may either compensate for this by developing survival behaviors that yield short-term predictable consequences (such as aggression), or develop learned helplessness (i.e. they learn that their behavior has no effect on what happens around them). Deciding on the "rules of the house" and adhering to them has nothing to do with dominance, but with giving the dog a chance to operate successfully within the environment and achieve predictable outcomes. Predictability is empowering to an animal. In particular, a highly trainable dog, that is, a dog that is keen on operating in his environment, is in a state of compromised welfare if a consistent rule structure is not maintained. The pet owner is the one who defines the rules of the house. What may be acceptable behavior for my dogs in my house may be unacceptable in someone else's house or vice versa.

- Predictability is empowering to an animal.
- In particular, a highly trainable dog, that is, a dog that is keen on operating in his environment, is in a state of compromised welfare if a consistent rule structure is not maintained.

Desirable behavior should be consistently rewarded (once a behavior is well trained, an intermittent reinforcement schedule or varied reinforcers can be used). Undesirable behavior should be ignored (a behavior that is not rewarded, that is, not successful, will go into extinction). Of course, a behavior that is self-rewarding such as going through the trash or ripping up a kitchen towel does not go into extinction when ignored. Such behavior needs to be prevented by setting up the environment accordingly, or through supervision and redirection to an alternative, appropriate behavior (such as chewing on a chew toy). In the section titled **Behavior Solutions for normal species-specific behavior**, you will learn about other alternatives to address undesirable behaviors in a positive manner but first we will explore prevention and management techniques.

Canine management and prevention techniques

Prevention of problem behaviors is easier than treatment. Many behavior problems and disorders in dogs can be prevented through early appropriate socialization and training.

Understanding dogs and their characteristics

Understanding what motivates the dog, helps us to be better at meeting the dog's needs and preventing issues from arising. In *The Culture Clash*, Jean Donaldson discusses the characteristics of dogs and some of the characteristics identified here are from her book (Donaldson 1996) (Box 7.1).

BOX 7.1: GENERAL CHARACTERISTICS OF DOGS

- Amoral
- Constantly learning
- Opportunistic
- Curious
- Avid chewers
- Complex olfactory communication system
- Social
- Predatory
- It is NOT about dominance

Amoral

Dogs are amoral. Amoral is different from immoral. Amoral simply means they do not have a concept of right or wrong. It does not mean they are deliberately performing behaviors that are considered wrong. Many things that dogs do that we humans consider to be "wrong" are just typical dog behaviors. Dogs are not spiteful, they respond to situations based on their individual genetics and past learning experiences. You may have had clients say to you, "My dog looks guilty; he knows he did wrong!" or you may think that yourself.

Dogs and cats can be sensitive to our moods. The dog may learn that when you come in the room and see a chewed-up piece of paper on the floor, you take a deep breath and expel the air with a harsh sound, as you put your hands on your hips and say in a deep tone, "Who chewed this up?" In response to your exacerbation, your dog gives you appeasement gestures, such as putting his ears down, cowering, turning into a C shape, and approaching you in a tentative manner. We often interpret this as guilt. However, these are polite non-threatening canine gestures to avoid confrontation and are designed to dispel aggression. The dog is responding to the human behavior not showing guilt.

When a pet performs an undesirable behavior only out of sight of the owner, many people consider that evidence that the pet knows right from wrong and is simply being sneaky. It's more likely that the pet has learned "safe" and "unsafe." For example, a dog may learn that it is safe to get into the garbage when people are not around but unsafe if they are present because they fuss at him and scare him.

Recurring situations result in predictive consequences. Thus, animals learn to perform species-typical behaviors when it is safe; in other words, when humans are not around. Similarly, appeasement gestures can start to be given in anticipation of the person's response, seeming to further confirm the idea of "guilt" in our minds. Remember that the dog's behavior is a result of actual or anticipated reactions from us, not knowledge of doing wrong.

Rather than punishing undesired behaviors and potentially teaching the dog to fear humans and perform those behaviors only when we are out of sight, we can help them make the right choices by managing the environment and providing suitable alternatives for natural behaviors. You will learn more about how to do this in upcoming sections of this chapter.

Constantly learning

Dogs are constantly learning, even when we are not actively teaching. Behavior is a combination of genetics, prior experiences, and learning. Learned behaviors may be desirable or undesirable for human counterparts. Evaluate the pet's behavior from a learning perspective.

- Dogs are constantly learning, even when we are not actively teaching.

Opportunistic

Dogs tend to be opportunistic. Following the motto *carpe diem*, they seize the day or moment. Very much like toddlers, they act in the moment without regard for the future. If the dog notices a wonderful-smelling turkey sandwich sitting on the coffee table and it is safe because the owner is out of sight, he might be opportunistic and think about helping himself.

Curious

Dogs are naturally curious resulting in exploratory behavior. Humans search the internet for answers to our questions, and dogs search and explore their world too. Exploratory activities should appeal to our pets' senses, such as sight, sound, smell, taste, and touch. Providing appropriate exploratory activities for our canine friends is enriching both mentally and physically. Food-dispensing toys are an example of an exploratory option.

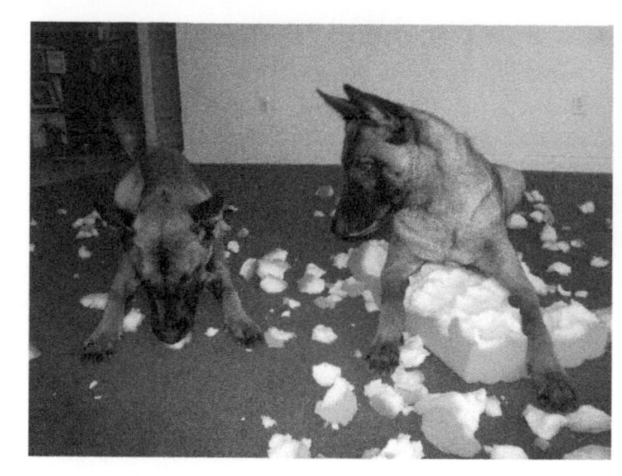

Figure 7.1 Two adolescent Belgian Malinois left unsupervised chewed a therapeutic pillow.

Avid chewer

Dogs explore the world with their mouths. Puppies especially find everything to be a potential chew toy. They do not understand that only certain things come from the pet store and are designed for them. They cannot read the labels! Figure 7.1 demonstrates the result of allowing two adolescent dogs to be unsupervised: "Goodbye, therapeutic pillow!" Managing the environment and providing appropriate outlets for natural behavior is necessary to set dogs up for success and to help them develop more desirable habits.

Complex olfactory communication system

Dogs have a complex olfactory communication system and a far more sensitive sense of smell than humans. Their superior sense of smell is the reason that dogs are often used for a variety of utilitarian services, such as hunting and various types of detection work. Smells can convey to the dog whether something is safe or dangerous. Being able to explore their world by smelling things is a necessary and enriching behavior for dogs.

Social

Dogs have been domesticated for at least 12 000 years. Through domestication they have been selected to remain behaviorally immature compared to their closest ancestors, the gray wolf. Dogs show many behaviors characteristic of wolf pups; they remain playful, enjoy physical contact, are highly social, bark, paw, and nuzzle. Dogs need companions. For the overall well-being of our dogs, it is important for us to meet their social needs.

Predatory

Dogs are predatory. Not all predatory behavior is bad. Predatory behavior is the reason dogs chase and retrieve balls. Predatory behavior in dogs varies from breed to breed, depending on the utilitarian purpose of the breed. Pointing, retrieving, and herding are all based on predatory behaviors.

It is NOT about dominance

Although the concept of dogs being dominant animals is still popular in media and among pet owners, research indicates that dogs do not share a dominance hierarchy with people. Consequently, there is no need to maintain a dominant relationship with pets. It is incorrect to imply that a dominance issue is the reason a patient is showing aggression while at the veterinary hospital or at home with the owner and that the owner needs to apply dominance techniques to correct the behavior. This type of misinformation can be dangerous for the owner and pet and damaging to the human–animal bond.

- It is incorrect to imply that a dominance issue is the reason a patient is showing aggression while at the veterinary hospital or at home with the owner and that the owner needs to apply dominance techniques to correct the behavior. This type of misinformation can be dangerous for the owner and pet and damaging to the human–animal bond.

Always keeping these general canine characteristics in mind allows one to have empathy and to understand why dogs do the things they do. It is not because they are spiteful. Often it is because they are dogs. Those same characteristics that we love about them can also make it challenging to share our homes with them.

Management of the learning history

Managing and controlling what the dog learns is important to prevent the learning of undesirable behaviors. Puppy and dog owners should puppy-proof the house: use baby gates, an exercise pen, and/or a crate to help manage the dog, especially young dogs. The more opportunity the dog has to practice undesirable behavior (in the eyes of the human), the better he will get at it. Habits begin to form. A preference for chewing on chair legs or pillows can develop quickly without good supervision (Figure 7.1).

Problem prevention includes setting the dog up for success, that is, arranging the environment so the dog can only or is more likely to make the desired choices. If the desired behaviors are successful from the beginning, the dog will repeat those behaviors. The environment should be set up in such a way that unwanted behaviors cannot occur or are much more difficult to perform than the desired behaviors. This includes puppy-proofing the house and utilizing appropriate confinement and supervision.

- Problem prevention includes setting the dog up for success, that is, arranging the environment so the dog can only or is more likely to make the desired choices.

Although kitchens are a common place for confinement, they also hold several potential dangers. Garbage cans should be kept safely locked away with child-proof latches on the door or be tall enough and fashioned with a lid to prevent access. If a dog gains access to the garbage, it is usually rewarded by some food product, so it will likely return to it throughout its life if not properly managed. Dangers that lurk in garbage cans include spoiled food, sharp bones, peach and cherry pits, and empty snack bags that can cause suffocation. It is also important to keep all household chemicals safely locked away. Even child-proof caps are no match for a dog's sharp teeth.

Bathrooms provide many temptations for the curious canine. A good rule is to keep bathroom doors closed. Toilet bowl cleaning products, especially the cakes that hang on the inside of the bowl, can be attractive to pets but are highly toxic. Waste-basket items such as feminine hygiene products and disposable razor blades can cause serious medical problems if ingested. Medications must be kept out of reach.

Electric cords should be securely taped to the wall using electrical tape. If this is not possible, they should be treated daily with an antichew product. Toxic household plants should be noted and removed from any pet living areas. Both dogs and cats enjoy ingesting some roughage, which may include houseplants. Other potential common household toxins include rodenticides, insecticides, and antifreeze.

Owners should also be educated on responsible pet ownership and keeping their pet safely confined to their property or walked on leash off the property. Just as important as puppy-proofing the house, the yard will also need to be made safe. Providing clients with a list of potential plant toxins will allow them to evaluate the safety of plants in their yard and house.

Routine

Maintaining a schedule and routine with puppies and adult dogs makes their lives more consistent and predictable. Ideally, all dogs should be meal-fed twice a day (very young or small puppies may require three meals a day initially), walked off the property twice a day for 10–20 minutes, and trained using positive reinforcement twice a day for 5–10 minutes.

- Ideally, all dogs should be meal-fed twice a day (very young or small puppies may require three meals a day initially), walked off the property twice a day for 10–20 minutes, and trained using positive reinforcement twice a day for 5–10 minutes.

The importance of walking a puppy or a dog is often misunderstood and is one of the most important problem-prevention tools. Exercise off the property will satisfy the dog's innate motivation to explore new things, help with exposure and desensitization to stimuli, and facilitate socialization. Walks can also decrease arousal, reactivity, and anxiety. A romp around an enclosed area is no substitute for a relationship-building walk with the owner. The same old yard can also get rather boring whereas the neighborhood environment is ever changing. The walk should be a combination of a controlled training walk by the owner's side and safe exploration. It is helpful to put walking at the owner's side on cue ("Let's go") and also teach a cue to release the dog to go explore ("Go play" or "Go smell"). Walking by the owner's side is not a natural behavior for dogs and will take time to develop. A high rate of reinforcement (a yummy treat every few steps) will be necessary in the beginning. For strong pullers, a head collar or front clip harness may be needed for management initially. These products also help protect the dog from trachea damage due to pulling on a collar. Leashed walks in the neighborhood are an activity that should be a lifelong exercise. They might help prevent behavior disorders such as territorial aggression and fearful and anxious behavior.

An established routine to meet the dog's exploratory, physical, and social needs will help set dogs up to be successful in the home environment and often eliminate undesirable behaviors.

Canine environmental enrichment

Dogs whose exploratory, physical, and social needs are met are better behaved and more enjoyable pets. Many unruly behaviors that clients are concerned about are a result of a pet being under-stimulated. Exercise and play are important for the pet's mental and physical health and social development. Routine walks that allow for "smell" time are just one way to meet these needs. Toys and games are other ways to provide an enriching environment.

Toys

In the home, a variety of toys should be available to the dog and the toys should be rotated, so it appears that there are always "new" toys. Providing appropriate toys will help generate mental and physical stimulation, an important part of early development. Toys are also great tools to intercept and redirect unwanted behaviors.

Food-dispensing toys are designed to act as puzzles. They can be loaded with a variety of treats or the pet's own diet. When physically manipulated using paws, mouth, or muzzle food is dispensed in a variety of ways. Before domestication, animals used a tremendous amount of mental and physical energy to obtain food. Placing food in a bowl provides little if any challenge for the pet. Food-dispensing toys are ideal for redirecting unwanted behaviors including mouthing and destructive chewing. It is best for the client to proactively identify potentially problematic times to occupy the pet with these toys. Many of the more durable varieties can also be used to pacify dogs while adapting to the crate or the owner's absence (Figure 7.2).

Toys designed for chewing purposes are also especially important for puppies that are teething. It is natural for young pets to explore using their mouth. Items such as nylon bones, and hard rubber toys can

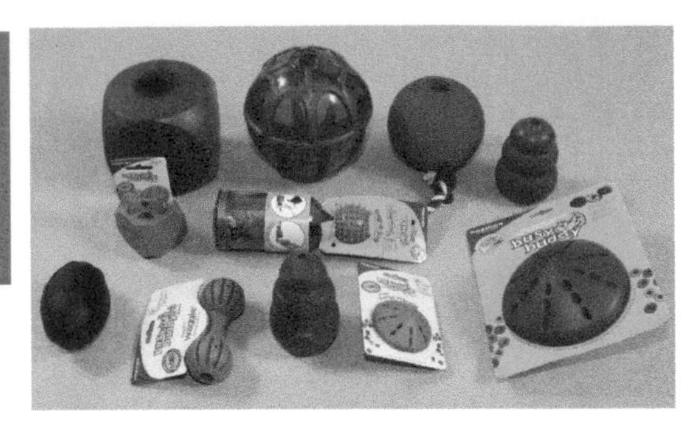

Figure 7.2 Variety of food-dispensing toys.

help satisfy these needs and prevent destructive behaviors. There are numerous commercially available chew toys. Despite manufacturer claims, no toy is indestructible. Dogs can destroy and ingest a toy very quickly. Hard rubber toys are more resistant to destruction. When offering a dog a new toy, monitor it closely. Instruct owners to check their dog's toys daily for damage. Toys will become damaged or worn over time and will need to be replaced periodically. Some chew items might be too hard and pose a risk of dental injury. The Veterinary Oral Health Council (VOHC) provides a list of acceptable products (http://www.vohc.org).

Games

The following are examples of games that can be recommended to clients to help facilitate the human–animal bond. The games are also designed to provide the dog with physical and mental exercise and promote the development of foundation skills such as come, sit, impulse control, take it, and drop it.

Retrieving

Retrieving is an excellent way to combine the use of exercise and foundation training skills. It can be used to teach the cues "take it" and "drop it." Similarly, other cues, such as "sit," "down," and "stay," can be incorporated into retrieving sessions to strengthen those behaviors as well as assist with teaching impulse control to help with over-arousal issues. Even the unmotivated dog owners can exercise their dog while relaxing in a chair. Although some breeds are natural retrievers, most puppies that do not display such tendencies can be taught the behavior. Video 7.1 on the companion website demonstrates the beginning stages of teaching a retrieve with the cues, get it, bring, and out. Notice with the first release of the toy, no cue is given because the treat prompts the release. In the following repetitions the trainer gives the out cue prior to prompting with a treat.

Biscuit hunt or find it

Dogs need an outlet for exploratory or searching behavior. If we do not provide them with a human-approved outlet for this behavior, they will likely find one that is less acceptable to us (digging in the garden, stealing items off the counters or out of the laundry, etc.). The biscuit hunt or find it game is a great game for providing mental stimulation.

When first teaching this game, let the dog see you place the treats about the room. "Hide" the treats in dog-allowed locations (on or near the floor in clear sight initially). Potential locations are on the ledge or the foot of a chair leg or table (not on the table). Avoid locations where human food is placed or any location that you would not want the dog to explore. Place 10 treats about the room while someone holds the dog or it is behind a barrier, watching. Give the cue, "Find it" or "Seek" just before letting it go, explore, and find the treats. Let it find them on its own. It will learn to use its nose! Once the dog understands this game, increase the difficulty level by hiding the treats while the dog is out of sight. Always start the game with your cue word or phrase.

Another self-contained option is using a snuffle mat. Snuffle mats are commercially available and can also be homemade. There are a variety of options available. A washable option is ideal to allow for routine cleaning. Video 7.2 on the companion website shows a senior dog using a snuffle mat.

As simple as this activity sounds, the owner is providing the dog with an outlet to explore and use its sense of smell. It is great mental stimulation. This is a wonderful activity for children to be involved in with adult supervision.

- Dogs need an outlet for exploratory or searching behavior. If we do not provide them with a human-approved outlet for this behavior, they will likely find one that is less acceptable to us.

Hide and seek

This game is an excellent training game and often a favorite among households with children but should always include adults. As one person gently restrains the dog or while the dog is distracted, the other person finds a hiding place. Once hidden, the dog is called and receives a treat when it discovers the person. Meanwhile the other person has hidden and the sequence can be repeated. Make it easy at first, just going around a piece of furniture or around the corner. As the dog becomes more proficient, the game can be made more challenging. Through play, the owner will also be teaching the dog to come when called.

Round robin

Round robin can be played during family television time. When a commercial comes on, family members take turns calling the dog to them, asking for a sit and rewarding the dog with a treat. When the TV show comes back on, a handful of treats can be scattered on the floor to end the game on a positive note. This is another activity that will reinforce coming when called and also helps generalize the behavior among all family members.

Chase the toy

Many dogs are highly motivated to chase things. This game can help direct that motivation to an appropriate outlet, a toy. There are commercially available toys or you can make your own by tying a rope to a toy (Figure 7.3). Initially the owner should stand still and make only the toy move. Give a cue, such as "take it" or "get it," just before presenting the toy. Pulling the toy in a direction away from the dog will encourage him to chase it. To prevent injury, over-arousal, or frustration, keep the toy near the ground rather than lifting it up out of reach. Once the dog catches the toy, engage him for a few seconds with a few light tugs on the toy. Then cue "drop it," or do an exchange with a food treat. Other known cues can be added into the game, such as "sit" or "down." This can help slow down the arousal level. As the dog becomes proficient at the game and is focused on grabbing the toy rather than mouthing pants legs or people, the owner can start to move around during the game. Any attempt to catch the owner should cause the person to freeze. The dog should be redirected to the toy. This game helps teach the dog to control his arousal level and also builds on foundation skills such as "take it," "drop it," "sit," and "down." Similarly, it teaches the dog appropriate things to chase and mouth.

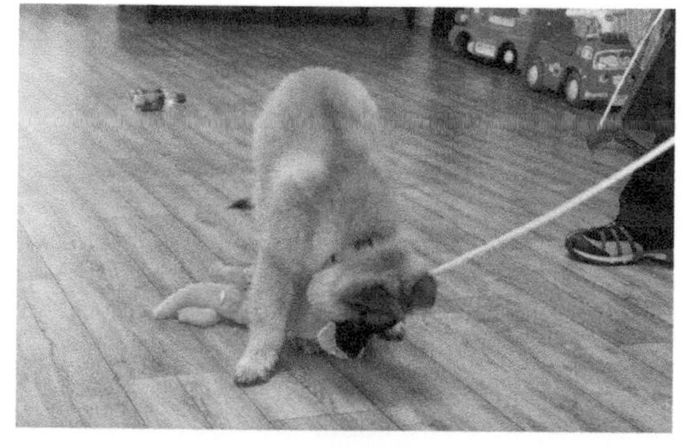

Figure 7.3 Teaching a dog to chase after a toy can provide an appropriate outlet for a dog's natural desire to chase and mouth and be a fun game to play together.

Dog parks and dog daycares

Dog parks generally are an uncontrolled situation, which lack supervision from professionals trained in canine body language and behavior. Owners should be aware that potential negative experiences with dogs at a dog park can have a lasting negative effect on their dog.

Dog daycare can be an appropriate option for some dogs and for busy owners. It can provide dogs with an outlet for exercise, companionship, and mental stimulation. Before recommending any daycare, the animal behavior technician should observe the facility and talk to the staff. Centers that combine many dogs of all age groups in play sessions should be avoided. A good daycare will offer small closely supervised play groups with a balance of down time for the dogs. They will also have an evaluation process and be selective regarding dogs that are accepted into daycare. The staff should be knowledgeable on dog behavior, especially body language. Interactions between staff members and the dogs should always be positive reinforcement based. The veterinary technician should ask the staff how conflicts are managed. Facilities that use squirt bottles and shaker cans to manage dog behavior are not the best options.

Dog parks and dog daycare can be enjoyable for some young and well-socialized adolescent dogs. Even with repetitive exposure, it is normal for a socially mature dog to become less accepting of unfamiliar dogs. It is important for the owner to ensure that their dog truly enjoys the experience. The dog should be relaxed, interested in interacting with the people and other dogs, but not overstimulated in the context. Just because a dog comes home tired from daycare, does not necessarily mean he enjoyed it. Dogs that are uncomfortable in the context will be vigilant and unable to relax all day. So for some dogs it can be a great outlet and other dogs may prefer to stay home.

Canine prevention: effects of neutering

There are medical and behavioral benefits and disadvantages of neutering a dog. Behavioral effects of neutering male dogs and the effect of reducing testosterone levels include decreased sexual interest in female dogs, decreased tendency to roam in 90% of dogs, decreased urine marking in 50% of dogs, decreased mounting in 67% of dogs, decreased competitive aggression between males in 60% of dogs (Hopkins et al. 1976), and a slight increased risk of developing senior-onset cognitive dysfunction syndrome (senility or dementia).

Spaying the female dog correlates to the following behavioral effects as a result of reduction in sex hormones: eliminates the potential for maternal aggression associated with having a litter of puppies or pseudopregnancy and eliminates the potential for estrus-induced inter-dog aggression, and a possible increased risk of developing senior-onset cognitive dysfunction syndrome (senility or dementia).

Research has also shown a correlation between animals that are neutered being at increased risk of certain behavior issues. One of two studies done by Duffy and Serpell (2006) with approximately 1500 breed club dog owners demonstrated a correlation in the following behavior characteristics:

- Spayed females were more aggressive toward both strangers and owners than intact females.
- Spayed females were more fearful and sensitive to touch than intact females.
- Both males and females that were altered were more likely to beg for food and to engage in excessive licking of people or objects.
- Dog-directed fear/aggression varied quite a bit by breed.
- Neutered males were much less likely to mark their territories.

In the second study by Duffy and Serpell, with a sample of more than 3500 dog owners, the following correlations were identified:

- Neutered dogs of both genders were more likely to show dog-directed aggression/fear.
- Neutered dogs of both genders were more likely to show owner-directed aggression.
- Neutered dogs of both genders were also more likely to have touch sensitivity and nonsocial fear.
- Neutered dogs were also likely to be less energetic/active.

So although differences in behavioral characteristics were associated or correlated with reproductive status, the research does not determine a cause and effect relationship. What is evidenced by this research is that neutering is not an effective treatment for aggression in dogs.

Although neutering has some potential medical and behavior benefits, there are also medical and behavioral disadvantages to altering. The veterinary technician should strive to continue to evaluate research findings regarding the effects of neutering.

Canine prevention: socialization

Dogs experience sensitive periods of development. Of particular importance is the socialization period that occurs between 3 and 12 weeks of age. There is some fluidity of the period but the optimal time for socialization is up to about 12 weeks of age. This period is particularly important because what a puppy learns during this time will have a lifelong effect on its personality and reactions to people, other animals, and environments. This is a well-documented stage of development in which puppies can readily learn to become comfortable with novelty and develop appropriate social skills. Lack of exposure is just as detrimental as a negative experience. Socializing a dog is an active process of positive exposure to novel environments, people, and circumstances and it needs to continue throughout the dog's life. Over the past decades, there has been recognition of the importance of early environmental exposure for puppies. However, all exposure is not the same. Positive, proactive exposure is an active process that takes preparation and planning. When most people think about socialization they think about habituation and exposure; get the puppy out and allow him to habituate to the environment. The problem here is that without positive, proactive socialization, the puppy may actually become sensitized to environmental stimuli. Socialization is not simply about habituation; rather, it is about making exposure fun and positive.

- Socialization is not simply about habituation; rather, it is about making exposure fun and positive.

Rather than just a neutral experience or even worse an overwhelming experience, new experiences should be made positive by proactively utilizing desensitization and classical conditioning or classical counter conditioning. Undersocialization can cause or exacerbate behavior problems. Enrolling a 7 to 12-week-old puppy into a good puppy class is the single most important thing in the dog's lifetime that a new puppy owner can do for its behavioral well-being. More information about puppy socialization classes is covered in the section titled **Prevention services**.

Canine prevention: crate training

A crate is a valuable tool for house training and management. Teaching a puppy to be comfortable and relaxed in a crate should be done as early as possible. A dog's crate can be a place for him to get away from the complex human world (Figure 7.4).

There are many benefits if a dog is comfortable spending time in a crate. Crates provide for a safe puppy-proof area. They limit access to potential hazards when the dog is unable to be directly supervised. The crate helps control the dog's learning history (limits opportunity to "get into trouble") and assists with elimination training (house training). It can also be a safe way to manage adult and elderly dogs.

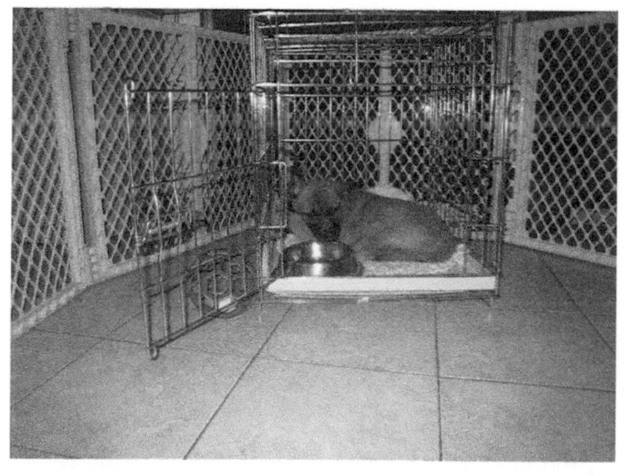

Figure 7.4 A young puppy taking a break in her crate.

An alternative to a crate is an exercise pen. It can prevent destructive behavior while giving the dog a bit more freedom. This is similar to a playpen for toddlers. The crate might be placed within or attached to the exercise pen. Toys and water should be made available in this area. The exercise pen can be used for short periods of time while the owner is home but can also be used if the owner is forced to leave the young puppy (less than four months) for an extended period of time (three to four hours). An elimination area may be placed in the exercise pen, to provide an appropriate location for the young puppy to eliminate. This will allow the puppy to relieve itself without soiling the crate (Figure 7.5).

There are a variety of crates available.

Wire and plastic are the two most common crate types. Fold-up wire crates are easy to transport and allow superior ventilation, but some dogs prefer the closed in, den-like area of plastic crates.

How big should a crate be? That depends. When house training a dog, the crate should be large enough for the dog to get up, stretch, turn around, and lie down. A dog may eliminate in a crate that is too large. Once the dog is house trained, a larger crate is preferred to provide more freedom but still allow for good management.

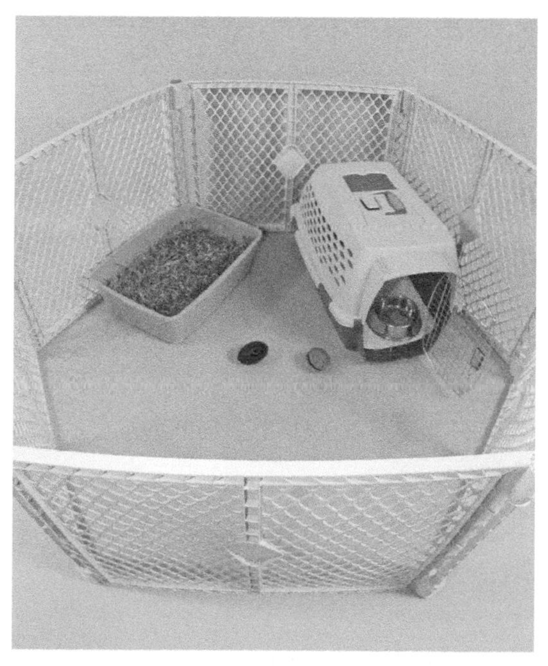

Figure 7.5 An exercise pen, elimination area, crate, and toys provide a safe area for a puppy or dog.

Initially young dogs should be in the crate or exercise pen whenever they are unable to be supervised. While trying to take care of the children, fixing breakfast, getting school supplies together, or talking on the phone, the young dog might be grabbing food off the table, chewing a pair of socks, and basically learning undesirable behavior. The confinement area should be used to help control the dog's learning history.

The crate can be used throughout a dog's life. The amount of time a dog will spend in the crate will decrease as it grows. Plan to use the crate regularly for at least the first few years.

Although confinement in a dog-proof area is recommended for the safety and learning history of young dogs, overuse of confinement can cause excitability issues. It is important to provide ample exploratory, social, and physical exercise when the dog is out of the confinement area. This may be accomplished through scheduled training, play, and walks. Alternatively, a dog can learn to be calm in other parts of the house by using the "umbilical cord method": the dog is on leash and goes with the pet owner from room to room. Using a leash teaches the dog in a controlled manner (it cannot wander off) how to acclimate to the human domestic environment. It also allows the pet owner to notice and reward the dog for desirable behavior.

- Although confinement in a dog-proof area is recommended for the safety and learning history of young dogs, overuse of confinement can cause excitability issues.
- SAFETY warning: the collar should be removed before leaving a dog unattended in a confinement area to prevent accidental strangulation!

For instructions on how to teach a dog to love its crate, see Appendix 23: Acclimatizing a pet to a crate. Video 7.3 on the companion website illustrates introducing a puppy to a crate. The Fear Free Happy Homes website also has a video tutorial available free. The link is provided at the end of this chapter in the Additional resources section.

Canine prevention: elimination training

One of the most common reasons owners relinquish their pet is house soiling (Patronek et al. 1996; Mondelli et al. 2004). Therefore, house training should be discussed at the first and every appointment. House training is a term used to describe teaching a dog a "human-approved" appropriate elimination area. Usually, this location is outdoors on grass, but dogs can be litter box trained or trained to eliminate on other surfaces such as concrete.

A dog's natural preference is to eliminate on porous surfaces (grass, carpet, bedding, etc.), in a place where elimination has previously occurred, and away from his eating and sleeping areas.

- A dog's natural preference is to eliminate on porous surfaces (grass, carpet, bedding, etc.), in a place where elimination has previously occurred, and away from his eating and sleeping areas.

Successful elimination training depends on the pet owners' ability to effectively communicate where they consider it appropriate for the dog to eliminate. This process will not occur overnight. Punishment, including verbal reprimands, only teaches a dog not to eliminate in front of people, making house training very difficult. The prevention of accidents through management and supervision is the key to successful house training!

- The prevention of accidents through management and supervision is the key to successful house training!

Elimination training can be broken into five key steps (Table 7.1).

1. Prevent accidents from occurring: Direct supervision and management, via a confinement area or the umbilical cord technique, are imperative until the desired location has become the dog's preference. Educate puppy owners on physiological constraints based on the puppy's age. A puppy can hold its urine for one hour and its age in months, when not active. The maximum amount of time a two-month-old puppy can be expected to have between elimination is three hours. It may need to eliminate every 30 minutes when active. Maximum duration of urine retention should not routinely exceed eight hours for

Table 7.1 Five steps to successful elimination training.

1. Prevent accidents	Management and supervision
2. Reward elimination in appropriate locations	Specific location and on leash Cue word, "Outside" Praise and treat after completion
3. Anticipate	Keep a log
4. Know what to do when accidents happen	Interrupt in a calm and non-threatening manner, redirect, reward! Avoid punishment
5. Clean soiled areas	Enzymatic cleaners Apply non-toxic, diluted citrus scent

any dog older than seven months of age. Full bladder control may take four to five months to develop, but accidents may occasionally occur up to one year of age. Once the dog starts reliably relieving himself outdoors, the intervals between trips outside can gradually be increased.

Water should be available at all times to prevent excessive consumption at one time and subsequent frequent urination. Feeding a highly digestible diet on a set schedule will limit defecation to set times. Most dogs are like clockwork and will need to defecate within 10–20 minutes after a meal.

2. Reward elimination in appropriate areas: Use a cue phrase, such as, "Let's go outside" or "Outside." Ideally the pet owner should exit from the same door each time and take the dog out on a leash (even if they have a fenced-in yard). Many dogs that do not have experience with eliminating while on leash may be hesitant to do so in the future. This can be problematic in settings away from the yard that require a leash. Designate a specific area of the yard for elimination. Once established, it will become saturated with the dog's pheromones, which will help stimulate the dog to relieve himself. The owner should withhold attention from the dog until it eliminates. This means basically standing like a pole and not even looking at the dog. Allow the dog about five minutes to eliminate; if not successful, take him inside and supervise or confine him and then try again in 10–15 minutes. ***After*** elimination is complete, the owner should praise the dog and offer a treat. If the owner begins to praise the dog while he is still eliminating, he may not complete the void. Wait until just after he has finished. The dog may be let off the leash for playtime once he eliminates, if in a secure area.

It can be helpful for the owner to add a cue, such as "get busy," when the dog relieves himself. As the owner predicts the dog is about to relieve himself by watching its body language, they can add the cue just before the dog begins to eliminate.

3. Anticipate when the dog needs to eliminate: Set the dog up to succeed by anticipating when he will need to eliminate. Keeping a journal or log of activity can prove helpful in determining a dog's individual routine and elimination patterns. Most commonly, the log will serve as reassurance to the owners that their dog is having fewer accidents (see Appendix 24: Elimination training log). The log also allows the owner to track when the dog is full or empty. At first, with a young puppy, it is important to make repeated trips, first thing in the morning, last thing at night, and several times in between. Take a potty break after eating, playing, and sleeping. Puppies are likely to eliminate after finishing one activity and before beginning another. The idea is that initially the owner will happen to have the puppy outside when he has to eliminate, thus allowing the owner to capture elimination in the desired location.

It is helpful to teach the dog a signal to go outside. Owners often believe a dog will clearly signal to them when it needs to eliminate. In reality, dogs usually only show subtle signs of impending elimination such as sniffing the ground, wandering toward the door, circling, or walking slowly. Teaching a dog to ring a bell to indicate the need to eliminate may be useful, especially in busy households. For instructions on how to teach a dog to ring a bell to signal the need to eliminate, see Appendix 25: Shaping plan for teaching a dog to ring a bell to go outside to eliminate.

4. Know what to do when accidents happen: Accidents will happen, so prepare clients on how to react to make it a productive learning experience for the dog. The best course of action if the owner sees the dog starting to eliminate in the house, is to use the cue, "outside," in a non-threatening tone to interrupt the behavior. This may momentarily make him stop and give the owner an opportunity to take him outside and reward him for eliminating in the proper location.

Relieving a full bladder is reinforcing. Yelling at or scolding a dog for eliminating in front of you in the house will make him hesitant to go in front of you outside. This makes house training difficult because the owner then is unable to reward appropriate eliminations. Punishment does not teach the dog where it is appropriate to eliminate, just that it is not safe to do it in front of people. Reprimanding the dog will likely train him to find a quiet place away from people to eliminate. Unfortunately, this might be in the closet, behind the couch, or in the guest room!

5. Clean soiled areas: Because dogs will be drawn to spots where elimination has previously occurred, it is extremely important to thoroughly clean soiled areas to prevent further accidents. Cleaning products that contain ammonia or vinegar are likely to act as an attractant for pets to eliminate in the same spot and therefore should be avoided. Enzymatic cleaners use natural enzymes to break down the waste, odor, and remove the stain. Because enzymes can be deactivated by harsh chemicals, it is advised to not combine other disinfectants when using an enzymatic product because they are likely to neutralize the desired effects of the enzymes.

   To effectively clean an area, first remove as much urine and stool as possible with paper towels. Apply an enzymatic cleaner designed for eliminating pet odors and allow it to dry for 24 hours. Then make the area locally less attractive to the pet as an elimination spot by applying a non-toxic, diluted, citrus scent. Do not use citrus scents on bedding, in areas where the dog is confined, or on objects that may be chewed or ingested (Table 7.1) as they might find the odor unpleasant.

Using these techniques, most dogs can be successfully house trained. To be effective, however, all steps must be followed simultaneously and consistently. See Video 7.4 on the companion website to see an example of house training a puppy.

Besides the lack of training, there are numerous other reasons for inappropriate elimination. When the dog owner fails to make progress or encounters a regression in house training, the dog should be immediately evaluated by a veterinarian. Excessive urination (~10+ times a day) can be caused by a variety of medical conditions, including a urinary tract infection or vaginitis. Excessive water consumption and urination can be a sign of a congenital medical disorder (diabetes insipidus). Limiting water intake is generally not advised with house training. In the case of a medical problem causing excessive water consumption, limiting water could be life threatening.

- When the dog owner fails to make progress or encounters a regression in house training, the dog should be immediately evaluated by a veterinarian.

Urine marking is associated with a perceived threat to the territory and is more common in unneutered male dogs, although neutered males and some females (intact or spayed) might also mark. It is most often an anxiety-related behavior rather than an issue of elimination training. Neutering and/or treating the underlying anxiety are the key to improving this behavior.

Excitement urination is common in young dogs still developing sphincter control. It is unrelated to house training. Prevention, through low-key greetings, is the best solution until the dog develops better muscle control.

Appeasement or fear-related urination is a normal behavior and can occur in dogs at any age. It is a fear reaction to a perceived threat and unrelated to house training. The dog may squat down, turn slightly to the side, or even roll over while urinating. It is attempting to communicate nonthreat and some fear of the situation. The behavior may be related to underdeveloped urinary sphincter tone in puppies. Positive-based training and using food treats boosts confidence and allows for positive associations with people. Any form of punishment is counterproductive. Avoid threatening body language, including direct eye contact and leaning over or reaching for the dog.

Litter/pad training puppies

Another option many dog owners are considering and hospital personnel should be prepared to counsel on is litter box or puppy pad training. Some reasons for clients to choose this option include small breeds of dogs poorly suited for a harsh outdoor climate and it is an option more conducive to apartment or high-rise living, as well as lifestyles that include traveling with their pet. The type of substrate used can vary from incontinence pad placed in a frame to an actual litter box filled with an array of products. There should be close supervision initially due to a dog's natural desire to shred and perhaps ingest the pads or litter. The techniques of training to an indoor-approved elimination area are the same as training a dog to relieve itself outdoors: positive reinforcement for going on the desired surface, supervision, and confinement. As the crate is used for sleeping and eating, the litter box/pad should be located outside of the crate. An exercise pen works quite nicely. Within the exercise pen, a crate area and a separate toileting area provide for a management system that meets all the puppy's needs (Figure 7.5). This system can also be used in the owner's absence.

Canine prevention: independence training

Dogs are social animals; it is not natural for them to be left alone for extended periods of time. Most puppies will show some mild signs of stress when first separated from their mother and littermates. Separation anxiety is a common disorder of dogs manifesting in co-dependence. Dogs with separation anxiety show signs of distress and may panic when separated from their attachment figure. Often the attachment figure is a person, but occasionally it can be another pet. Distress signs may include barking, whining, howling, pacing, drooling, destructive chewing, urinating, or defecating. When associated with separation anxiety, these signs occur when left alone or confined away from people. The diagnosis and treatment of separation anxiety is an intervention service. However, there are preventive steps that can be taken to minimize the risk of the development of separation anxiety (see Table 7.2: Steps to help prevent the development of canine separation anxiety).

- Separation anxiety is a common disorder of dogs manifesting in co-dependence. Dogs with separation anxiety show signs of distress and may panic when separated from their attachment figure.

The first 48 hours that a young puppy is in the client's home can be important for preventing separation issues. The owner should resist the temptation to shower the puppy with attention but instead, simply let the puppy relax in his crate if the dog has already been introduced to a crate and is comfortable and relaxed in a crate. If the dog is not comfortable with crating, allow the puppy to sleep in a cardboard box or other temporary containment area for the first 48 hours before transferring to a crate. The first 48 hours will likely be the most stressful and the puppy will not associate the crate with this stress. The transition may also be made easier by installing a calming pheromone diffuser near the puppy's confinement area. After the first couple of days the puppy can be transitioned to the crate.

The puppy should become acclimated to the owner's normal schedule as soon as possible. In the case of clients who do not routinely leave the home, it is important for them to leave the puppy alone for

Table 7.2 Steps to help prevent the development of canine separation anxiety.

Acclimatize the dog to the confinement area	See Appendix 23: Acclimatizing a pet to a crate
Confine when people are home	Dogs should be confined at times when people are home to prevent an association of being locked away only when people leave the home
Confine for variable periods of time	Confinement for short periods of time (5–10 min) periodically throughout the day prevents confinement being associated with long departures
Calm "hellos" and "goodbyes"	Arrivals and departures to and from the dog should be calm and nonchalant
Teaching a relaxed sit or down stay is an exercise of independence	Teach the dog that people leaving the dog can be a good thing
Reward calm behavior	Dogs often get attention for being excited. Teach clients to catch their dogs being calm and reward this behavior
Provide a routine for interactions with the dog	Providing scheduled routine walks, training, and play will help to meet the dog's needs for social and exploratory interactions and mental and physical exercise
Consider pheromone or music therapy	Dog Appeasing Pheromone (DAP) is a synthetic form of a pheromone that comes from the mammary tissue of the female dog and is available in a diffuser form that can be used in the confinement area to help decrease stress. Music therapy, such as Through a Dog's Ear™, has also been shown to help calm dogs

periods of time during their first few days in the household. Other pet owners may find that their current schedule requires they are away from the dog for longer periods of time. It may be necessary to bring in additional support in the form of dog walkers and daycare facilities. However, there should also be opportunity for the dog to learn to be comfortable alone.

When the owners return, they should avoid scolding or reprimanding the dog regardless of what may have transpired while they were away. Reprimands will not lessen the dog's anxiety or teach him not to do the same behavior in the future. Ideally, dogs should not be let out of their crate or other enclosed area if they are barking or whining, unless the owner suspects the dog needs to urinate or defecate or is having an anxiety or panic attack.

Owners should create departure and arrival routines with no fanfare. They should be unemotional when leaving as well as coming home. Providing a food storage toy in the confinement area can be used to create a positive focus away from the departure of the owner. This should be presented to the dog about 10 minutes before leaving so it does not become a cue for departure.

Dogs that do not respond to the above preventive strategies or that are showing separation issues should be seen by the veterinarian. Very serious separation anxiety requiring pharmaceutical intervention is not unheard of, even in juvenile dogs. Often, medication in these cases is only temporary. If left untreated, the anxiety is likely to escalate and the longer the negative learning history, the more difficult it can be to make improvement. Severe cases of separation anxiety can negatively affect the welfare of the dog, damage the developing human–animal bond, and result in relinquishment or even euthanasia.

- Dogs that do not respond to the above preventive strategies or that are showing separation issues should be seen by the veterinarian. Very serious separation anxiety requiring pharmaceutical intervention is not unheard of, even in juvenile dogs.

Separation anxiety is the most common behavioral disorder of dogs. It may develop at any age. The condition can sometimes be prevented. However, there can be a genetic or learned component to the disorder. A dog showing signs of separation anxiety is past the preventive stage and indicates a need for a behavior intervention service.

Canine prevention: handling and restraint

Handling refers to manipulating or touching parts of the dog's body, such as its ears, mouth, nose, tail, feet, and so on.

To make handling less likely to be an aversive experience, dogs should learn to associate being touched with earning treats. Although many dogs will tolerate being handled, making it a pleasant experience rather than a neutral or an aversive one is necessary to make future experiences less traumatic for the dog. In short, be proactive! (Figures 7.6 and 7.7).

- To make handling less likely to be an aversive experience, dogs should learn to associate being touched with earning treats.

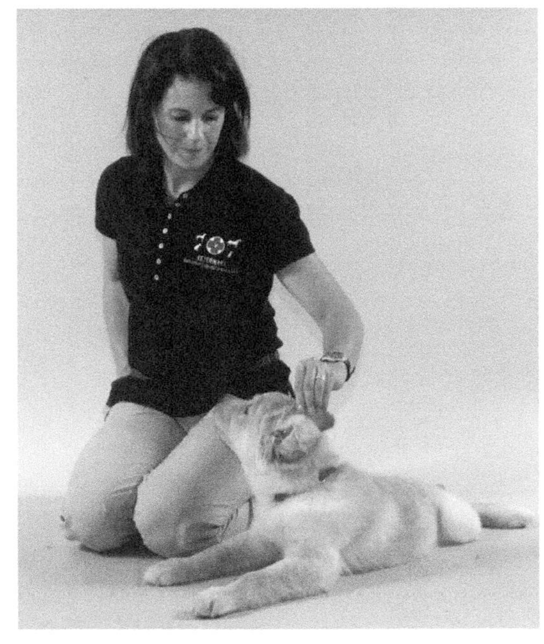

Figure 7.6 Handler touches the ear and clicks with a clicker to mark the event.

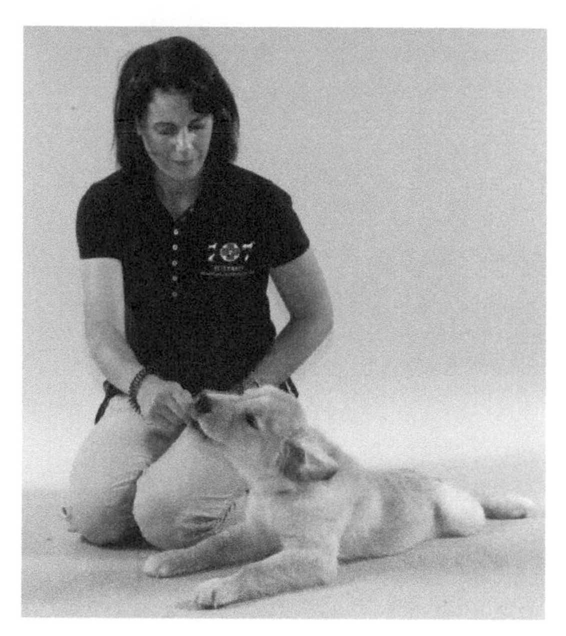

Figure 7.7 The hand is removed and a treat is delivered.

Owners can teach their puppy to enjoy handling by using the puppy's daily food as a training tool. Starting at a neutral location and using a gliding touch, referred to as a Touch Gradient (see Chapter 8), will prevent a startle response and allow the pet owner to assess the dog's response to the touch. Begin by gliding hands toward the collar, then offering a piece of food. Glide a hand to touch one ear, then offer food, touch the other ear and offer food. Glide a hand down the leg and touch a paw, and then offer food. Continue this with all four feet. Open the puppy's mouth and offer food. Touch the puppy on his abdomen, rear end, and private parts and then offer food. Repeat this several times a week. Predictor cues (Chapter 8) can also be incorporated. If the dog shifts or moves away, decrease the touch to where he is accepting and reward.

Restraint refers to physically holding a dog still and is often used during routine veterinary procedures. Dogs learn very quickly that something unpleasant is about to happen when they are restrained. Through experience, they learn that when held still, they may have their nails trimmed, temperature taken, vaccinations given, blood drawn, ears cleaned, or groomed.

Through desensitization and classical and/or counter conditioning, many handling procedures can be performed with little or no restraint. However, there will be times when the veterinary technician or even the pet owner will need the dog to hold completely still. By being proactive, you can teach puppies that being gently restrained is a predictor of good things. Regardless of the age of the pet, it can learn that restraint is nothing to fear. The older the dog, the more likely a negative association with restraint has already developed, unless proactive prevention exercises have previously been implemented. Video 7.5 on the companion website illuminates the process of acclimating a dog to restraint.

Clicker or marker training can be very effective in acclimatizing a dog to being handled and restrained. See Appendix 26: Preventive handling and restraint exercises for instructions on how to implement these exercises.

Another alternative is to teach the patient an operant behavior, such as targeting a specific object. A dog can be taught to place his chin in the owner's cupped hand on cue or rest his head on a towel draped across the owner's lap. This provides a cued stationary behavior for the animal to perform. See Chapter 8 and **Cooperative care and cooperative care training** for more information and videos regarding these techniques.

As a veterinary technician, you will encounter patients that are already concerned about being handled or restrained. Signs a dog has become uncomfortable with handling/restraint exercises include stops taking treats, freezes, ears back and/or tail tucked, wants to get away. In this situation, stop and do not escalate any further. Maintain the current level and offer treats until the dog relaxes and begins to take them again. Once the dog is taking treats, release or let go. As discussed earlier, this is for mild fear or resistance. If aggression or extreme fear or anxiety is being displayed, abort the exercise completely and recognize that the dog is not in a preventive stage of learning; behavioral intervention services are indicated. For detailed information about handling for veterinary and husbandry care, refer to Chapter 8.

- Signs a dog has become uncomfortable with handling/restraint exercises include stops taking treats, freezes, ears back and/or tail tucked, wants to get away.

Canine prevention: safety around the food bowl and relinquishing objects

It is natural for a dog, or person for that matter, in possession of a high-value item to want to keep it. If a dog considers people as a potential threat (often due to previous learning experiences) to a high-value item, serious problems can arise. Educating owners on proper etiquette and implementing prevention exercises in puppyhood will help to prevent future issues with resources. Food, the food bowl, toys, and food-based items (long-lasting high-value treats, food-storage toys) are considered high-value items for most dogs. "Stolen" items, such as socks, paper towels, or the remote control, can also become high-value items depending on the human's response. To a certain extent, guarding is a normal behavior in dogs. In multiple-pet households, it is imperative to manage resources to prevent competition and consequently, aggression over items between resident animals. It is especially problematic when the guarding of resources becomes a trigger for human-directed aggression.

- Educating owners on proper etiquette and implementing prevention exercises in puppyhood will help to prevent future issues with resources.

Most dogs guard objects because they are afraid the object will be taken away. The foundation for preventing this behavior is to teach the dog to trust you and that leaving an object is frequently more rewarding than picking up the object. Certain exercises such as "leave it" and "drop it" if taught correctly can prevent a bite from occurring.

As the food bowl is a common area of tension for many dogs, preventive training is imperative. Review Box 7.2 for management recommendations for minimizing tension at feeding time. There are several valuable exercises puppy owners can do with their new puppy while the puppy is eating, to associate people near the food bowl as a welcome thing. The first is to simply walk past the puppy while he is eating a regular meal and drop a really tasty treat, chicken or cheese, into the bowl (see Figure 7.8). This will teach puppies to eagerly anticipate the approach of humans while eating. Provided

BOX 7.2: FOOD BOWL RECOMMENDATIONS

- Offer food at a set time at least twice a day. Allow up to 20 minutes for the dog to eat.
- If any food is left, call the dog away and pick up the bowl when he is out of sight.
- Place the food bowl in a low-traffic location to avoid the dog being startled. The confinement area or crate is the ideal location.
- In multiple-pet households, avoid competition over food by having separate bowls and locations for feeding.
- People should always be the giver of food, not the taker of food. Pulling a food bowl away from a dog while he is eating only teaches him that people are unpredictable and they might try to steal the food bowl.
- Dogs do not enjoy being touched or petted while eating. (People do not either.) Although this might be a useful skill to teach, to utilize distraction techniques with food while providing veterinary and home care (Chapter 8).

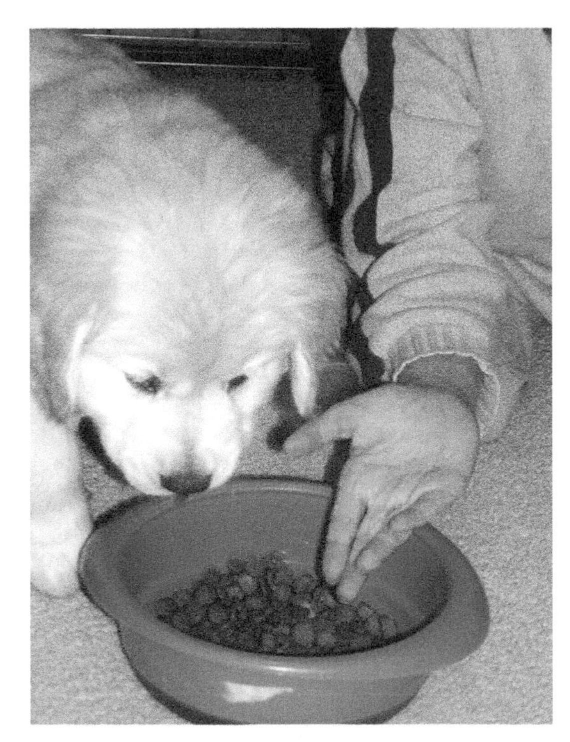

Figure 7.8 A young puppy learning that human hands near the food bowl mean a special treat!

the puppy is comfortable with the approach and there is no body posturing over the bowl, exercises can continue. See Appendix 27 for a detailed process on implementing preventive food bowl training exercises. Video 7.6 on the companion website details playing the food bowl game with a young puppy.

If there is any sign a dog is uncomfortable with the food bowl exercises, such as stiffening, suddenly freezing over the bowl, or eating more quickly, a behavior consultation should be scheduled. It is important to note that aggression toward people over food in puppies is a red flag predicting human-directed aggression later in life. The puppy is not going through a phase and is unlikely to just grow out of the behavior. Immediate behavior counseling should be provided if a puppy or dog is showing aggression toward people over food.

- Aggression toward people over food in puppies is a red flag predicting human-directed aggression later in life.

Because dogs explore the world with their mouths, they are likely to pick up things that for their own safety or due to the nature of the item, their owner will want them to release. In the section titled **Behavior solutions for typical canine behaviors**, strategies for addressing the immediate concern of obtaining an item from the dog will be addressed. However, preventive exercises to teach the dog appropriate items to play with and also relinquishing them to their owner should be implemented.

When the dog is chewing on an appropriate item, the owner approaches and drops a tasty treat; like the food bowl exercise, it teaches the dog to enjoy people approaching. The owner can also do a trade by taking the toy away briefly, giving the puppy a special treat, then returning the item to the puppy. Video 7.7 on the companion website demonstrates approaching a dog while it has an object and giving the dog a treat. You will notice the dog initially tenses up. After several repetitions the dog is anticipating getting a treat and keeping the "toy."

Caution should be given to those fastidious dog owners who want to take everything out of the puppy's mouth. Puppies are exploring with their mouths and if every little thing is taken away from them, there is potential to create a guarding problem. Instead, owners should be instructed to give the puppy a treat for relinquishing the item, examine the item in question but return the object to the puppy if it is determined to be safe. Instructing owners on teaching "take it" and "drop it" with positive reinforcement training can provide a way to communicate effectively with the dog and prevent conflict over items.

The purpose of "drop it" is to teach the dog to drop an object it may have. Again, the goal is for the dog to not fear giving a person an object in its possession but to instead look forward to releasing the object. Never punish the dog once he has an object; it is far too late. It will only associate having the object and your presence with "danger." The dog learns it is "unsafe" to have things in its mouth when people are nearby. Some dogs may then try to hide with the object or be placed in a motivational conflict. For example, wanting the object but fearing your response. Instead, if the dog is always rewarded for relinquishing the object, there will be no conflict. If the dog continues to acquire inappropriate objects, the pet owner's management plan for avoiding these situations should be reviewed.

Tug can be an interactive, energetic, and appropriate game to play with a dog. Play fosters a social relationship between people and their dog. Teaching dogs to enjoy playing tug with their owners allows the tug to become a useful tool for motivation and reward. When taught correctly, it allows you to contain and control the dog's arousal (impulse control) and can aid in teaching the dog to enjoy relinquishing a toy (or other item) to the owner.

Teaching a dog to play tug will not make him aggressive. Tug can be a physical and mental outlet for energetic dogs. However, it is not recommended to play tug with dogs that guard objects and/or display aggression in certain context because previous learning history potentially could make the game unsafe or over-arouse the dog. Caution should be taken with children playing tug with any dog and it may be safer to make it an adult-only game, because the excitement level may be more difficult to control with children. See Appendix 28 for specific instructions on teaching tug.

There may be certain items some dogs should never have. Really high-value items are animal-based products such as real bones, rawhides, and pig ears. Some dogs just cannot resist the urge to guard these high-value items, almost a primal reaction.

In addition, trying to find something of higher value to trade with the dog may be difficult. If a dog only guards a rawhide and truly only guards a rawhide, then simply never offering those objects to the dog is a viable management option.

Households with small children should be extra aware of guarding issues. A dog with a tendency to guard items in a household with children can be a dangerous situation. No management is 100% effective. Implementation of early prevention exercises is even more vital in households with children to minimize the chance of aggression over resources from developing.

- A dog with a tendency to guard items in a household with children can be a dangerous situation.

Feline management and prevention techniques

As in dogs, early prevention exercises and training in cats can have a profound impact on the success of their integration into the human household.

Understanding cats and their characteristics

A large part of prevention is educating cat owners about typical behavioral tendencies and characteristics of cats. By developing empathy for the cat's natural tendencies, the cat owner can funnel those desires to appropriate outlets. Box 7.3 depicts general characteristics of domestic cats.

BOX 7.3: GENERAL CHARACTERISTICS OF CATS

- Amoral
- Constantly learning
- Opportunistic
- Curious
- Complex olfactory communication system
- Social
- Predatory
- Vertical living space is important
- It is NOT about being a "prey" species

As you learned in Chapter 3, friendliness is largely genetic and early experiences play a role in the cat's ability to adapt to changes in the environment. Cats are social animals, and they develop a communal smell which identifies members of the group and the territory. One of the cat's most influential forms of communication seems to be olfactory; however, visual and vocal communication also plays an important role.

Like dogs, cats are amoral, constantly learning, opportunistic, curious, have a complex olfactory communication system, social, and predatory. The wild ancestor of the cat was solitary, yet domestic cats are largely social animals under specific living conditions. The sociability and friendliness of cats and dogs varies, just as it does with many species of animals, including humans. Individuals have different preferences and personalities, but in general, domestic cats are a social species.

Unlike dogs, though some cats chew things, they are not usually avid chewers. A characteristic specific to cats is the importance of vertical living space. Anyone who has lived with a cat knows that they are agile climbers. Increasing vertical living space through platforms, shelves, and cat trees provides for increased territory. It is like adding square feet to your house. A cat will utilize approximately 360 square feet of living space. Increasing vertical living space in multi-pet households helps to avoid confrontation and dispel conflict between pets. Social stress in multi-pet households can be greatly reduced by providing numerous resources in various locations and increasing vertical living. Vertical space can also provide safety for a cat who lives with an exuberant dog or children. A cat resting on an elevated surface is less likely to be stepped on and is better able to visualize his surroundings, thus providing for comfort and security. Vertical space also allows for exploration of a larger area. Some cats find hiding spaces such as under a bed or in a cubby hole to be a quiet and safe place to relax. Cat owners need to provide appropriate vertical living space and hiding spots for their cats. If they prefer the cat to not be on the counters, they need to provide alternatives. In the veterinary hospital you can provide perches and hiding spots in the housing area and exam rooms to provide cats with appropriate outlets to feel safe and secure (Figure 7.9).

An interesting trend has been to explain cat behavior based on the perception they are not only a predatory but also prey. In fact, this author, Debbie Martin, used to teach that very concept to others. However,

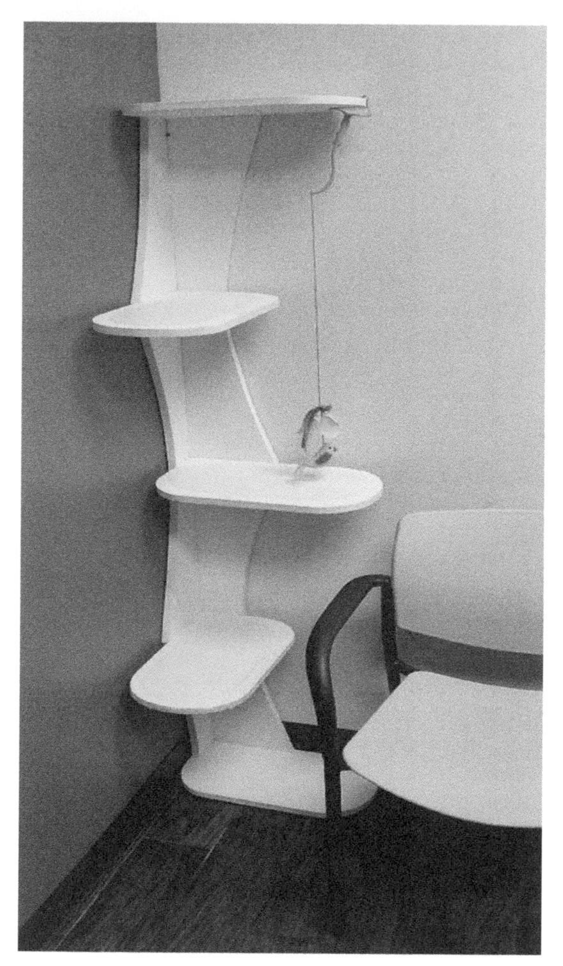

Figure 7.9 An example of perching stations for cats that can easily be cleaned in an exam room. *Source*: Picture taken at Bigger Road Veterinary Center in Springboro, OH.

since cats are predators, why were we also considering them a prey species, when pretty much everything can become preyed upon, whether prey or predator? It appears behaviors reported as being associated with being a prey species include things such as seeking elevated surfaces, hiding, fear of novel items, unfamiliar environments and/or animals, as well as general hypervigilance. In reality most of these behaviors are more likely associated with fear and under-socialization. Seeking elevated surfaces could be associated with fear but it could also be that cats learn that being up high allows them to avoid being stepped on! Why is it important to make a distinction between these behaviors being associated with fear and under-socialization versus being a "prey species"? When we attribute the behavior to being a prey species, we imply it is normal and there is nothing that can be done to help. If your dog hid under the bed for hours when you had guests in your house, you would be concerned and think it was abnormal, but many people dismiss this behavior in cats as just part of their genetic makeup. And what about our adventure cats (cats who go camping, hiking, and on adventures with their owners)? Did they miss out on the prey species behaviors or perhaps they inherited adventure traits and had proper socialization!

Feline management recommendations

Feline management recommendations include preventing potentially stress-inducing or dangerous situations and developing a consistent routine.

Special inspection should be given to homes adding a small kitten to the household. A frightened kitten will often seek out a small hiding area. Places such as behind appliances, sump pumps, and cabinets should be blocked off. Kitten-proofing the house is as important as puppy-proofing it. Kittens are notorious for playing with yarn and string of all sorts. However, if ingested, they can cause potentially fatal intestinal disorders. Just as with puppies, everyday household items have the potential to be dangerous if appropriate management and supervision are not initiated.

Because cats are territorial, threats to the territory by outsiders can cause stress and anxiety. The indoor-only cat that is exposed to the sight, sound, or smell of other cats approaching the house will often display behaviors associated with agitation or stress. Exposure to cats approaching the territory may stimulate urine marking as well as irritation and aggression toward people or other cats in the household. For the comfort of the indoor cat, owners should prevent exposure to outside cats. Some options include blocking visual access out of windows, avoiding feeding outside cats near the house, or deterring the outside cats through the use of a motion detection sprinkler.

- Because cats are territorial, threats to the territory by outsiders can cause stress and anxiety. The indoor-only cat that is exposed to the sight, sound, or smell of other cats approaching the house will often display behaviors associated with agitation or stress.

In regard to territorial ranges, male cats have on average three times more territory than female cats. In the indoor setting, the male cat's average range was 4–5 rooms whereas the female cat's range was 3–3.6 rooms (Liberg et al. 2000; Bernstein and Strack 1996). In multiple-cat households, providing abundant resources/provisions spaced throughout the entire house, minimizes competition between cats over resources. Provisions refer to feeding areas, water stations, resting areas, and litter boxes. By providing access to resources in several locations, resident cats can avoid conflict over the use of the resource at the same time. Similarly, increasing vertical living space through platforms, shelves, and cat trees can avoid confrontation and potential conflict. The increased living space allows for increased territory. Social stress in multiple-cat households can be greatly reduced by providing numerous resources in various locations and increasing vertical living space.

Good management in the feline household not only involves setting the environment up to allow for success, it also includes having a consistent routine of interaction with the cat. Set times to train and play each day will ensure the cat's social, exploratory, and physical needs are met.

Feline environmental enrichment

The majority of cats in the United States are kept as indoor pets, which can cause a severe lack of mental stimulation and exercise. The animal behavior technician can assist cat owners in creating a household setting that provides the cat with an enriched environment, thereby helping to prevent potential behavior problems.

In the United Kingdom, the common belief is that cats should have access to the outdoors. Outside access allows for natural outlets for exploration, mental stimulation, exercise, and hunting. Having access to the outdoors can decrease obesity and possibly prevent some behavior disorders in cats.

The accepted position from most pet-care professionals in the United States is that cats should be kept as indoor pets. By doing so, owners can prevent injuries such as being hit by a car, poisoning, bite wounds from other cats, and attacks by predators. Indoor cats will be at less risk of contracting diseases such as FIV (feline immunodeficiency disease), FeLV (feline leukemia virus), and FIP (feline infectious peritonitis), or parasites.

Environmental enrichment provides outlets for normal feline behaviors and allows the pet owner to provide for the cat's mental and physical well-being. This is especially important for the indoor-only cat because the human domestic environment is often void of opportunities for normal feline exploratory behavior.

- Environmental enrichment provides outlets for normal feline behaviors and allows the pet owner to provide for the cat's mental and physical well-being.

Feeding, toys, and play

Kittens, like puppies, benefit from toys that deliver food and/or treats. In the wild, cats eat numerous small meals each day and spend a great part of their day hunting. Providing food-searching activities and food-dispensing toys is mentally and physically enriching. There are feeding systems that put the hunt back into eating for cats and provide them with much needed exploration. Cats are natural grazers and designed to eat small amounts of food at frequent intervals. Food puzzle toys can help to prevent obesity in cats as there is more activity involved in the feeding process and they provide great mental stimulation. Although there are many commercial products available, homemade items such as holes cut out of storage boxes filled with food can be recommended (puzzle feeder) (Figure 7.10).

Hiding food and treats around the house in small dishes or cups will promote exploratory behavior and appease the cat's natural desire to search for food. Although not a toy, some cats enjoy the option of having indoor grass available. Most of them are easily grown indoors and are made up of either wheat or oat grasses. Offering fresh grass can prevent them eating house plants while adding roughage to their diet.

Providing exploratory outlets through a variety of interactive toys will help to appease the cat's curiosity. Interactive homemade toys can provide cats with hours of entertainment. A cardboard box with holes for the cat's paws and toys dangling from sisal rope is an easy-to-make homemade toy that most cats will appreciate. Sisal rope is a durable rope made from plant fiber. It is often used for scratching posts for cats (Figures 7.11 and 7.12). These toys can be inexpensively made to entertain boarding felines and sent home with the owners at pick up.

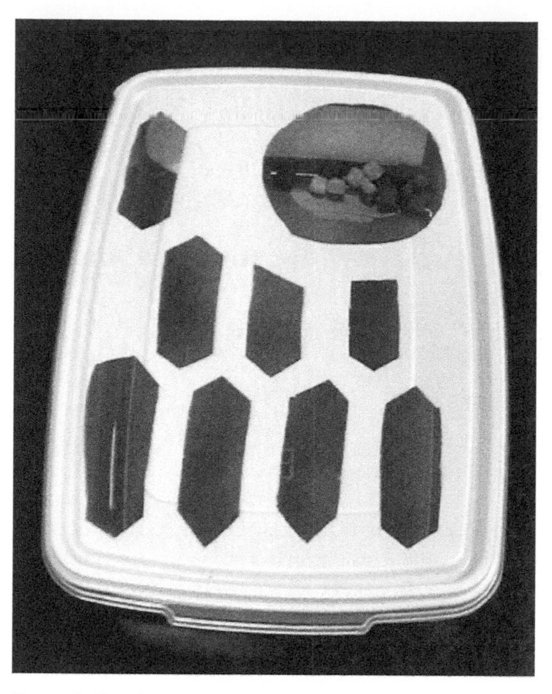

Figure 7.10 A homemade "puzzle feeder" for cats. The round hole is made large enough for the cat to stick his head in the box and the slats allow the cat to paw the food to the large feeding hole.

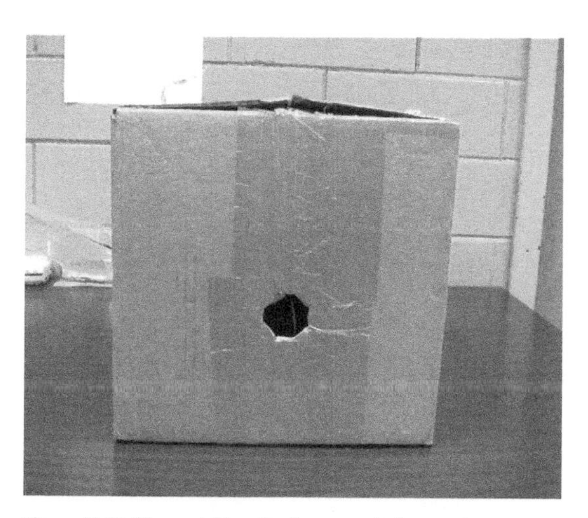

Figure 7.11 The outside of a homemade interactive cat toy. Numerous openings can be cut around the box to allow for multiple exploration ports for the paws.

A set time for play sessions with the owner in the morning and evening is ideal because cats tend to be more active at these times. Cats enjoy playing with

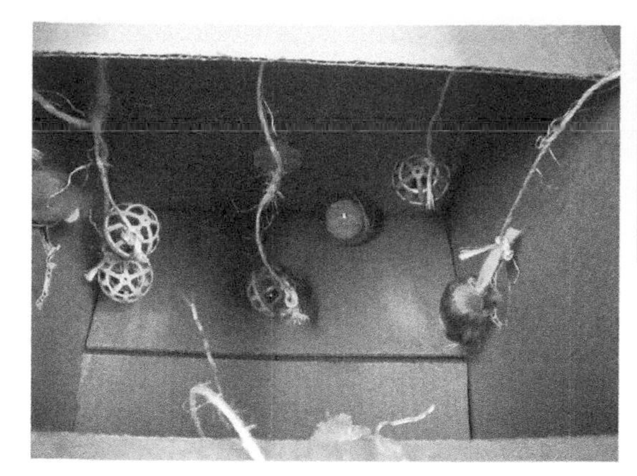

Figure 7.12 The inside of the same homemade toy. Toys dangling from sisal rope and also a loose ball to bat around.

toys that encourage pouncing and stalking (predatory sequence). Feather toys on the end of a pole, small stuffed toys, and balls encourage exercise and positive interactions with the owners. Any type of direct play with human hands should be avoided as it can promote inappropriate play and result in potential injury to humans through accidental scratches and bites.

Vertical space and places to hide

Vertical space is important not only for management but also environmental enrichment. Vertical space creates areas for exploration and additional hiding places. Cat trees, perches, shelves, and elevated hiding places are great options for creating vertical space for cats. Tunnels, boxes, and paper bags can be used at lower levels.

In the veterinary setting, a cardboard box or paper bag placed in a cage with a feline patient can allow the cat a safe place to hide in the novel environment.

Outdoor exposure

Secure outdoor enclosures and fences are available to allow cats to have exposure to the outdoor environment within a confined area. Most are designed to not only keep the pet cat in the yard but also prevent other feline intruders from entering the yard. For safety, supervision by the owner is recommended during controlled outdoor exposure. Acclimatizing a kitten to wearing a cat harness can also allow the owner to manage the cat outside, thus allowing for more exploration. Adult cats that have not had previous exposure to the outside may never be comfortable or enjoy being outside, regardless of the owners' best efforts. Instead, the owner can focus on making indoors as enriching as possible.

Training

Most people believe cats are not as trainable as dogs. Perhaps this has to do with the lack of expectation to do formal training with cats. Most dog owners recognize they need to do early training and foster training interactions almost immediately upon acquisition. The dog learns quickly they can access rewards by responding to learned cues or prompts. Cats often learn how to access rewards from their people but without any formal training. Many cats vocalize and run to the cupboard around feeding time, and their owners feed them. Providing formal positive training interactions can not only improve communication between cats and people and enhance the relationship, it also can provide for physical, social, and mental enrichment. Not to mention some fun tricks to show off to your friends.

Success with training is dependent on finding the right rewards or motivators for the individual learner. The more reinforcers you have in your toolkit, the better. Having a variety of reinforcers such as food, play, touch, access to a desired activity, scent, or social companion, is advantageous as it provides options for reinforcement in a variety of contexts. Some cats may prefer human social interaction over food and other reinforcers (Vitale Shreve et al. 2017).

Determine the individual cat's preferences but realize preferences can be enhanced through learning. A cat might not have learned to take food from a person, with a learning history of only receiving food in a bowl.

Video 7.8 on the companion website illustrates how quickly a cat can be trained even during a behavior consultation. Both cats were being seen for a behavior consultation while this training took place.

Feline prevention: effects of neutering

Neutering the male cat can decrease inter-male aggression (testosterone-driven aggression); however, it does not increase amicable behavior or decrease other forms of aggression (nontestosterone driven) (Crowell-Davis et al. 1997; Neville and Remfry 1984). In female cats, no significant behavioral changes were noted associated with ovariohysterectomy, with the exception of the cessation of behavior patterns associated with estrus (Stubbs et al. 1996). In contrast, neutering of the male and female cat significantly reduces urine marking, 90% in males and 95% in females (Hart and Cooper 1984).

Feline prevention: socialization

Although the socialization period (two to seven weeks) is usually over by the time the kitten goes to a new home, continued positive exposure to novelty is still important. The cat can be taken on car rides and given a special meal or treat. Treats and play can be utilized while visiting a friend's house or the veterinary hospital to make a positive association with the environment. Friends can be encouraged to come to the house and play with the kitten and give it treats. This may help prevent the fear and hiding often displayed by house cats when a visitor arrives. Kitten classes and fun visits to the veterinary hospital should be encouraged with young cats. Kitten classes and fun visits will be discussed in more detail in the **Preventive services** section of this chapter.

- Although the socialization period (two to seven weeks) is usually over by the time the kitten goes to a new home, continued positive exposure to novelty is still important.

Feline prevention: litter-box training

Kittens usually enter their new homes ready to use a litter box, unlike puppies which are not always ready to eliminate outdoors. However, as litter box problems are the number one behavior problem seen in cats, it is important to set cats and cat owners up for success.

The rule regarding the number of litter boxes is to provide as many litter boxes as there are cats and one extra box. If the home is multilevel, there should be at least one box on each floor the cat has access to. This is especially important for younger kittens and geriatric cats. In either instance, the need to void may be urgent and youngsters and arthritic seniors may not be able to travel far. The locations should be variable throughout the home as cats tend to prefer to urinate in one location and defecate in another. Litter boxes in numerous locations are particularly important if there are multiple cats as one cat may block the other cat's access to a box. Other pets or small children also may inadvertently block a cat's access to a litter box. All locations should be in low-traffic areas. Many cats have been startled while using a box in the basement or utility room if the furnace happened to kick on or the washing machine suddenly whirled into spin mode while the cat was in the box. These frightening events can easily be associated with the use of the litter box and many cats will not return to the area, choosing to eliminate elsewhere instead.

Cats generally prefer unscented, clumping litter as the substrate in the litter box (Neilson 2001). Their ancestors would have been using sand for elimination, so this type of litter may be the closest option to what they seek. Preferences for elimination substrates are developed at an early age and are based on exposure to the substrate during the first few weeks and months of life. Consequently, cats will have individual preferences. Providing a cafeteria of litter-box types and litters may help identify a preference with a new feline companion. Good recommendations when first providing substrate options to cats are to use 2–3 inches of a fine, unscented clumping litter in an uncovered litter box with no liner. This is preferred by many cats. Cats prefer larger (1.5 times the length of their body is suggested), uncovered boxes (Neilson 2008). Most commercial cat litter pans are too small for the average adult cat so it is best to start with a cement mixing pan, an under-the-bed storage Tupperware bin, or a dog litter box. Young kittens should have litter boxes low enough for them to easily step into. Older cats with less mobility may also need lower sided boxes. Being fastidious creatures, cats will be more willing to use a litter box that is kept clean. Scooping at least once daily is recommended.

- Providing a cafeteria of litter-box types and litters may help identify a preference with a new feline companion. Good recommendations when first providing substrate options to cats are to use 2–3 inches of a fine, unscented clumping litter in an uncovered litter box with no liner.

Prevention of inappropriate elimination is always easier on everyone involved. Kitten classes are a great platform for educating owners regarding litter box preferences. Fielding questions using a pre-exam questionnaire (see Appendices 13–18 for life stage questionnaires) can identify potential problems. Questions should be included regarding litter box habits. For example, how many litter boxes are in the home? Where are they located? What type of litter is used? Unscented or scented? Liners? Covered or uncovered? How often are they scooped? These questions may open the door toward thwarting a potential problem.

The number one reason for inappropriate elimination is due to medical problems. It is imperative that medical reasons for elimination cases be ruled out before a behavioral diagnosis is explored. There are many medical etiologies for both inappropriate urination and defecation, including bladder stones, urinary tract infections, interstitial cystitis, irritable bowel disease, constipation, osteoarthritis, and hyperthyroidism. If these conditions are allowed to progress, they can be painful for the animal, may cause more serious health issues, and create or exacerbate a behavioral problem. Pain from an underlying medical condition can create an aversion to the litter box.

Behavioral reasons for inappropriate elimination generally fall into one of two categories: house training (aversion to the box or preference for another surface) or urine marking (anxiety related). Inappropriate elimination can be a multifaceted issue including medical, house training, and marking components. Cats displaying inappropriate elimination need a thorough medical and behavioral work up to determine an appropriate treatment plan.

- Inappropriate elimination can be a multifaceted issue including medical, house training, and marking components.
- Cats displaying inappropriate elimination need a thorough medical and behavioral work up to determine an appropriate treatment plan.

Feline prevention: crate training

Generally, the carrier comes out in most cat houses for one reason, a trip to the veterinarian. Cats can quickly associate the presence of the carrier with a trip to the doctor, which is not always a pleasant experience for all cats. Cat owners may call to cancel their appointment because they are unable to find the cat or get the cat out from under the bed. Taking some preventive measures early on can alleviate this problem from developing in the first place.

Cat carriers are commonly available in two different materials, plastic or a combination of canvas and mesh. As with puppies, proper introduction is important. Kittens should have the option to go in and out by choice. They will be easily enticed with toys, treats, and comfortable bedding. Clicker training is also an excellent tool for teaching kittens to enter the crate.

Having a cat that is comfortable in a carrier or even a larger cat cage can provide for easy management in multicat households, with introductions to new pets, with convalescence, and also with travel. Commercially available cat cages are large enough to accommodate a litter box, bed, and bowls. They also have several different levels with perches to allow for vertical living space (Figure 7.13). By acclimating cats to various confinement methods, it allows for safe management without creating stress, such as when needing to travel, during a move, or when acclimating cats to new situations or pets.

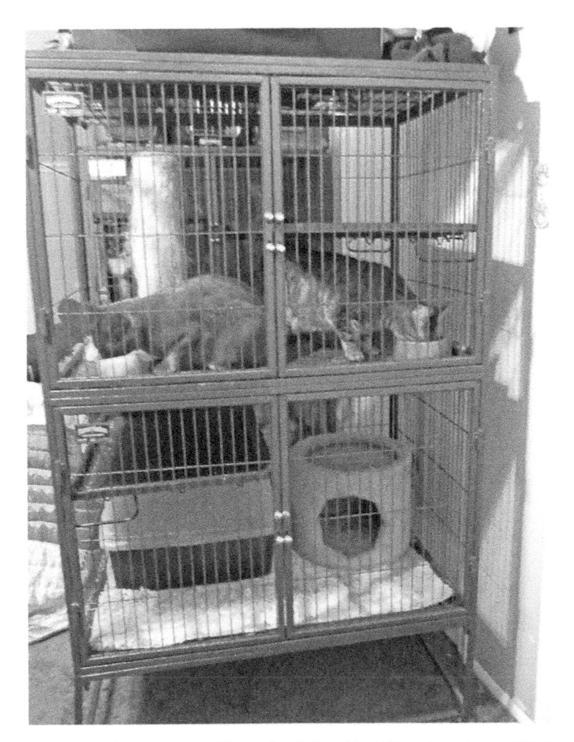

Figure 7.13 Cat cage with multiple levels. A litter box is provided in the lower level and food in the upper level.

Feline prevention: handling and restraint

Prevention is very important. Teaching the cat to tolerate restraint and handling at an early age is much easier than treating a cat that is defensively aggressive with handling. Like dogs, cats quickly figure out that being held still or manipulated usually means something unpleasant is about to happen. Canned cat food smeared on the exam room table or delivered on a spoon can be used to facilitate a positive association (classical conditioning) to handling. If the cat becomes frightened and aggressive, avoid punishment. Verbally reprimanding the cat may inhibit her behavior, but it does not make the situation any more pleasant for the cat, or client.

Minimal restraint is generally better tolerated by cats. Towels can be used to aid in the restraint of cats, providing safety and security for some cats and the veterinary team. Sophia Yin's book, *Low Stress Handling, Restraint and Behavior Modification of Dogs & Cats*, is a thorough resource for appropriate handling techniques in the veterinary hospital. For more information on handling and restraint techniques, see Chapter 8.

- With cats, the less the restraint that is used, generally, the more the acceptance.

Prevention (canine and feline): introducing a new pet

When bringing a new pet into the household, a few preventive steps should be recommended. Being proactive can sometimes be the difference between successful integration of a new pet versus rejection.

Introductions: dog to dog

Introducing a new puppy or adult dog to resident pets can be of great concern to the owners. Introducing a new puppy to an adult dog that has been well socialized should be relatively smooth. If there is doubt how the interaction will go, neutral territory is best. Adult dogs tend to be less accepting of other adult dogs and the first introduction should be made on neutral territory. It may even be advisable to take the resident dog to the breeder's home or the shelter for the first introduction. Parks and other open areas can also be used. The owner should be relaxed and make all interactions positive ones, using plenty of food treats to reward positive interactions. Sniffing and play bows are good interactions but keep them very brief at first. Any signs of tension should be calmly interrupted and then redirected by cuing a known cue such as come. Once the interactions are going smoothly, they can be moved into the home, repeating the same process.

The resident dog should learn to associate good things with the presence of the new dog. Think of all the activities the resident dog enjoys, such as walks, play, and training. These activities should be performed along with the new dog. Reinforce appropriate behavior with treats.

It is normal for interactions to include corrections to the puppy from the older dog. This is helping the puppy to learn about dog body language and setting limits on the puppy's interactions. Short of injury or prolonged, excessive reprimands, these communications should be allowed between the two dogs. Owners should resist the temptation to interfere as this can complicate relations.

Separate feeding areas should be established for good management. Food bowl guarding is a normal behavior and can be a site of aggression. Chances are they will be on different diets and the separation will prevent them from eating each other's food.

A safe haven should also be established for both the resident dog and the new dog. These areas can be used to give them both a break and allow for alone time. The safe havens should be made as pleasant as possible, using beds and chew toys. Fear Free Happy Homes provides a video tutorial on tips for introducing two dogs; https://www.fearfreehappyhomes.com/video/a-fear-free-approach-to-introducing-your-dog-to-a-new-dog.

A resident dog that has poor social skills or limited experience with other dogs should be referred for behavior intervention services before the client obtains another dog.

Introductions: cat to cat

Integrating a new cat to a multi-cat household can be stressful for the new cat as well as the resident cats. To ensure the most harmonious integration, it is best to take a proactive approach and systematically provide a gradual introduction. Although the process may seem tedious, it often can progress quickly. However, if owners decide to "just see what happens," a negative initial introduction could result in a much longer acclimation process or even worse, an inability for the cats to cohabit.

Introductions to resident cats should be gradual. For the first few days, the new cat should be kept confined in a room. The room should have all necessary resources, including a litter box, scratching station, food, water, bedding, and toys. Although the litter box should be accessible, it should not be in immediate proximity to the rest of the items. It is also a good idea to include a large multilevel cat cage (Figure 7.13). Confining the new cat to a room will give the resident cats the opportunity to become accustomed to the new cat's scent through a closed door. The procedure can be helped along by exchanging bedding between the animals. The scents of the cats can also be mixed by allowing the new cat to explore other parts of the house while confining the resident cats to a room. Another way to mix the scents of the cats is called artificial allomarking: pet each cat with a few small towels, so the cat's scent is on the towel. Mix each cat's individual towels together, for example Cat A towel and Cat B towel are placed together in a neutral location in each cat's living area. This allows the cats to choose to investigate the towels. There will be the familiar scent of the individual cat but also the other cat's scented towel. Treats can be placed around or between the towels to encourage exploration and positive associations. This helps to "mix" their odors and develops a communal scent between the cats. If any of the cats show continued negative reactions to the scent of the other cat's towel or bedding, discontinue this process.

Ideally the resident cats and the new cat should become acclimated to their own individual multilevel cat cage and voluntarily and eagerly enter them. This will aid in the visual introductions of the cats and provide the greatest amount of safety. All cats should be managed in their multilevel cage for a special mealtime twice a day. Alternatives to the multilevel cat cage are the use of baby gates or screens, a travel carrier, or a harness and leash. If using a cat cage, carrier, or harness and leash, all the cats must be comfortable with the confinement method or harness prior to starting the introduction process. They must voluntarily enter the area and not show signs of fear or distress. If using baby gates or screens, it is imperative the cats can be redirected away from the barrier in a positive manner by the owner, should the cats want to approach too quickly.

We will explore one option for systematically acclimating the cats to each other. However, adaptations to the process may be necessary depending on the individual cats and their responses, such as the types of reinforcers or confinement you use. Some cats might do better with calm play or grooming as a distraction and positive activity during the sessions instead of a special meal. It is imperative the cat owners are able to recognize subtle signs of fear and anxiety in cats before starting these exercises. With the cats confined, start at a distance at which the cats can see each other but are not dissuaded from eating their special meal (the furthest distance possible for the layout of the house is best). Closely monitor for any signs of increasing stress. If the cats remain relaxed and enjoying the session, the cages can be moved a foot closer during the next session, until they can be about 5–10 ft away from each other while eating. Once this has been accomplished, if the resident cats are not overly interested in the new cat, the owner may consider keeping the new cat in the cat cage for supervised periods of time (only if using the multilevel cat cage) while allowing the resident cats to be loose in the room. This should only be done if the owner is actively monitoring for any changes in body language and ready to redirect the cats if needed. The owner needs to be able to monitor the new cat's body language closely as well. An extra baby gate or exercise pen can be placed around the multilevel cat cage to prevent the resident cats from coming too close to the cage. This can help to facilitate habituation to the presence of each other without the cats being able to directly interact with each other. The next step might be to allow the new cat to be loose in the room and the resident cats to be confined to their multilevel cage or carrier. Once it is determined that the cats behave amicably and are relaxed in each other's presence, allow supervised periods of time loose together. Introducing favorite toys or items for exploration when bringing the cats to a communal area can help minimize over interest in each other. They can focus on exploring a box or favorite toy rather than focus on the other cat.

If owners observe cat behavior such as direct staring, hissing, growling, or other threats, they should place a towel over the cage to interrupt the threat and separate the cats. In the event of aggressive reactions, wait 24 to 48 hours before attempting introductions again. With the next session increase the distance between the cats and progress more gradually. Ideally, avoid all negative experiences while introducing the cats. Slower is actually faster because negative experiences will be remembered and will take time to overcome. Calming feline pheromone products can also be useful to prevent and alleviate stress with the process. The entire process may take two to six weeks to accomplish depending on the individual cats. A quick progression of the same techniques can be used when reintroducing cats after one of the household cats has had a visit to the veterinary clinic or groomer. The cat who remained home will often reject the returning cat because the cat may smell or look unfamiliar. Simply mixing their scents and doing a controlled special mealtime and gradual introduction over a few hours or days (depending on the returning cat's medical status) can be effective in preventing a long-lasting negative reintroduction.

Introductions interspecies

An introduction between a resident dog and a new cat is normally less stressful for both pets than cat-to-cat introductions. The exception to this would be an adult cat that is unfamiliar with dogs or a dog that views the new cat as prey. Before adding a new cat to the household, foundation training is recommended. The dog should be trained to settle on a dog bed or mat so he has an alternative behavior that is not conducive with chasing. In addition, a "look at that" cue (meaning look at an object or animal away from the owner) and a "watch me" cue (look at the owner) should be taught. These opposite cues can allow the owner to make a game of looking at things and looking at the owner, ping-ponging back and forth between these two cues. These cues should first be taught in a nondistracting environment with familiar items before incorporating into a session with a new cat in the house. When a new cat is coming into the home, set up a sanctuary room for the cat and allow it to settle in and become comfortable with her new people for at least a few days prior to introducing the cat to other resident pets.

To assess the cat's and dog's reactions to each other, the first interaction should occur with the cat in a multilevel cat cage or elevated travel carrier and the dog on leash. The dog should be rewarded with high-value treats for being able to settle on a mat and play the "look at that-watch me" game. If the dog is intently focused on the cat, the dog should be redirected with a food treat if possible and moved further away from the cat. Once the dog is reliably able to respond to cues and is offering calm behaviors around the cat, gradually allow the cat to have time out of the cat cage with the dog either on leash with the owner or confined to a kennel. The owner continues to reward the dog for calm behavior and response to cues. Eventually, with supervision, the dog can drag the leash (in case redirection is necessary to prevent injury) as the pets become accustomed to each other. If there is any concern about the dog's reaction to the cat, a referral for a behavior consultation should be made and further safety recommendations, such as a basket muzzle, may be necessary. Supervision of both pets is essential during initial introductions.

Care should be taken when introducing a puppy to a household with cats. Many times, this relationship will work out naturally as cats and dogs can be great companions, sometimes better than with their own species. Trouble spots can occur, however, with an overzealous puppy and a cat who is startled or frightened. Puppies love to chase things but we do not want the cat to be one of them. Attempts can be managed through the use of a leash and redirection to an appropriate toy. Calm behavior while both pets are in the room should be rewarded. Both pets involved need to have safe havens established. For the puppy, this simply means a crate, exercise pen, or a puppy-proofed room. For the cats, this would mean plenty of vertical space and areas they can escape to that are off limits to the puppy. These areas can be set up with cat doors too small for the puppy to get through or areas gated off but off the ground, enough for a cat to slip under.

The cats' food stations, resting areas, and litter boxes should be inaccessible to the puppy and located in the cats' safe area. Establishing these areas will decrease the cats' stress associated with living with a new puppy.

Prevention (canine and feline): children and pets

A pet in a child's life can provide endless hours of companionship and fun. If properly planned, it can be a meaningful and powerful relationship. Pets can be instrumental in teaching a child responsibility, compassion, and empathy.

Some parents may start out thinking they want a dog as a pet for their children but through planning they may discover their lifestyle is more conducive to cat ownership or even a guinea pig. Education can prevent parents from choosing the wrong pet, which may result in relinquishment or, worse yet, injury to the child. Both of these situations can be traumatic for the child and are not a positive learning experience. The experience should be one that promotes responsible pet ownership and the human–animal bond. The pet's well-being should not be solely the child's responsibility. Pet care should always be shared or supervised by all family members to ensure success.

It should be noted that kids and dogs are both egocentric, therefore both do what works best for them. Good kids and good dogs are likely to have misunderstandings every day. Consequently, children and dogs should never be left without adult guidance and direct supervision.

The majority of dog bites involve young children and interactions with a familiar or a family dog. The prevalence of dog bites in children is 2.2% and is double when compared to the general population (Kahn et al. 2004). The majority of children suffer from facial injuries as the result of dog bites (Kahn et al. 2003; Bernardo et al. 2002; Schalomon et al. 2006). The average age of children is five years, with boys more commonly bitten than girls. A dog well socialized to children is less likely to bite out of fear. Early appropriate socialization is important for the prevention of future dog bites to adults and children. Predictive factors of aggressive behavior, particularly toward children, include lack of training, little or no socialization with children, aggression over food toys and/or places, being overly sensitive to touch or fearful of people, a history of preying on small animals, or aggression to family members (Lindsay 2001; Xavier et al. 2008).

Every dog has the potential to bite or show aggression. Even a dog that has been well socialized can still escalate to aggression, depending on the circumstances. Behaviorally normal dogs will get up and walk away in order to avoid confrontation. Children do not always understand the message and parents should be present to intervene and teach their child what is appropriate. It is unrealistic to believe that all dogs should tolerate inappropriate behavior from children. If parents fail to advocate for the dog, unsuccessful attempts to avoid the situation can evolve into aggression. Prevention does not stop with the dog; it also involves teaching children appropriate ways to interact with dogs.

The old adage, "let sleeping dogs lie," is a good rule to follow. Children should be taught to leave dogs alone when the dog is resting, sleeping, eliminating, eating, drinking, hiding, or chewing on a bone or toy. Children should avoid approaching any dog behind a barrier such as a fence, baby gate, or in a kennel. They should be taught to ask for permission to approach and pet an unfamiliar dog. Behaviors from children that have the potential to elicit aggression from a dog include rough play or handling, running after or chasing a dog, hugging, kissing, or crawling on a dog, reaching to pet an unfamiliar or neighborhood dog, teasing, taunting, or barking at a dog, and reprimanding a dog. Children should learn that if a dog is chasing them, they should stop and "be a tree." Movement is often a trigger for the chase and freezing is the safest course of action. Face-to-face interactions between children and all dogs, whether in their own household or elsewhere, should be prevented. Not only may this be perceived as a threat by the dog, but the child's face is in a very vulnerable position. Parents should be quick to interrupt and redirect undesirable interactions and reinforce appropriate ones by the dog or child.

All households with children should include a safe haven for the dog. This area is "off limits" to the children. The dog-only zone can be the crate, an exercise pen, a room that can be closed off, or a combination. Another possibility is circling the dog's mat area with a jump rope and teaching the children they are to stay on their side of the boundary. This dog-only zone should not be a place of punishment but should be made as appealing as possible to the dog. A soft bed and chew toys should be included. The dog's meals can be given here.

The board game Doggone Crazy!™ is intended to introduce the tools children and parents/guardians can use to help reduce the risk of occurrence of a dog bite (Figure 7.14). The board game helps children decide whether a dog is safe or dangerous to approach and teaches children appropriate and inappropriate interactions with a dog. Doggone safe (www.doggonesafe.com) is a nonprofit organization dedicated to dog bite prevention through education and dog bite victim support. They provide educational opportunities for veterinary professionals and the general public.

Cats represent ~10% of bites treated annually in the United States and Canada (dogs 80–85%). The average age of a human for a cat bite is 19–20 years (while for dog bites, the average age is 13) and

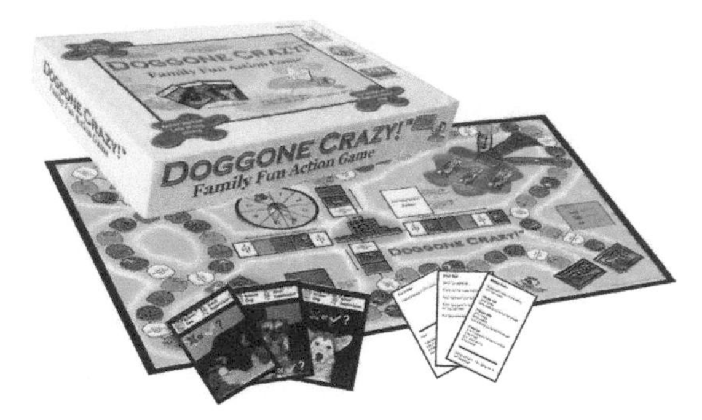

Figure 7.14 Doggone Crazy!™ board game. Courtesy of Doggone Crazy. Permission granted by Joan Orr.

women are more likely than men to be bitten by a cat. Most cat bites occur on the hands and arms and have a high incidence of infection. Often the bites are associated with a person trying to pick up or pet the cat. Bites are more commonly from stray or feral cats (80%) (Barrett et al. 2016). In the human domestic household, it is usually easy for a cat to evade an approaching child because cats use vertical living space. However, just as with dogs, adults need to teach children appropriate ways to interact with the cat and remain the cat's advocate. Cat-only areas of the house should be designed to allow the cat a safe haven.

For additional resources for children and pets see the Additional resources section at the end of this chapter.

- Good kids and good dogs are likely to have misunderstandings every day.

Behavior solutions for normal species-specific behavior

We have discussed preventive and management techniques with dogs and cats to set them up for success in the human domestic household. Even with the implementation of these techniques, there are bound to be times that the pet owner will encounter normal behaviors for the species that he/she finds undesirable. This section will explore a general model to help address these behaviors in a positive manner and then apply the model to a variety of normal dog and cat behaviors.

Always, first help the owner decide if the behavior is actually an undesirable behavior. Many owners have read or heard that "Dogs should not be allowed on furniture, sleep in the bed, or eat before you." Consequently, they might believe this to be true. What is acceptable behavior for the pet owner will vary from person to person. Some owners enjoy having their cat on the counters, and their dog jump on them, get on furniture, and sleep in the bed; others do not. As long as the behavior is not harmful to the pet, the owner, or other people or animals, it should be the owners who define their expectations for their pet. The animal behavior technician can help owners set realistic expectations and facilitate a harmonious relationship with their pets through consistent and predictable expectations and interactions.

- What is acceptable behavior for the pet owner will vary from person to person. Some owners enjoy having their cat on the counters, and their dog jump on them, get on furniture, and sleep in the bed; others do not. As long as the behavior is not harmful to the pet, the owner, or other people or animals, it should be the owners who define their expectations for their pet.

General behavior solutions model

Once you have identified with the owner that this is a behavior that is normal yet undesirable for the owner, it is time to apply the behavior solution model. Although addressing normal undesirable behaviors should be individualized to the particular situation, providing a step-by-step approach can help you keep on track when providing guidance. No two pets or owners are the same and providing a cookbook approach to addressing pet owners' concerns should be avoided because it does not necessarily allow for two-way communication to occur. This behavior solution model will allow you to break down behavior and seek positive solutions for addressing everyday canine and feline challenges (it works with people too). This model has been adapted from *Puppy Start Right: Foundation Training for the Companion Dog* by Martin and Martin (2011) (Table 7.3).

Table 7.3 Behavior solutions model.

Identify the ABCs	**A**ntecedent, **b**ehavior, **c**onsequence
Hypothesize motivation	Socially motivated? Self-reinforcing? Both?
Prevention or management	Prevent practicing of the behavior Proactively reward appropriate behavior Provide appropriate outlets Prevention/management does not change the behavior; it controls the learning history
Solve it!	Ignore/Avoid reinforcing Response substitution

The behavior solutions model is a four-step process for addressing or changing behavior in the pet: First, identify the ABCs (antecedent, behavior, consequence); second, hypothesize the motivation; third, utilize prevention and/or management techniques to minimize the practicing of the undesirable behavior and funnel the behavior to an appropriate outlet; and fourth, if prevention and management have failed, solve it by using pet-friendly techniques to address the behavior and promote desired learning.

The first step is to identify the ABCs. The **A**ntecedent: Antecedents are what precede and/or prompt the behavior and set the occasion for the behavior to occur. Examples include the pet being loose in the house, doorbells, the rattle of a food bag, the whirr of a can opener, or a cue, such as "sit." The antecedent may be related to a social interaction (human or another animal), a sound, or an inanimate object. Multiple stimuli may be identified and the antecedent may be context-specific. Ask yourself, what is the specific situation in which the behavior occurs? At times, the antecedent is not identifiable and may be related to the pet's internal motivation or needs. For example, your dog may have a full urinary bladder and need to void. When analyzing antecedents think of the 4 Ws: **Who** is present? Does it happen only when the male or female pet owner is home? **Where** does the behavior occur? Does it happen inside the house, and if so, where? Does it happen outside? If so, is it on or off the property? **When** does the behavior occur? Does it happen only in the morning or evening? Is it every time the owner leaves the home? **What** specific actions induce the behavior? Is it when a person stares at the cat? Does it happen when the other cat in the house approaches?

The **B**ehavior: Defining the behavior is a small part of developing solutions. What is the undesirable behavior? Looking at the pet's body language and having an understanding of normal and abnormal behavior is helpful. The actual behavior might give insight to the antecedent, especially when it is related to an internal motivation. The behavior is only a small piece of the puzzle and not that relevant, although for the pet owners it is. Behavior changes when antecedents and consequences are adjusted, and alternate behaviors are taught.

The **C**onsequence: The consequence refers to what happens immediately after or during the behavior. The consequence should be viewed from the pet's perspective. Initially, ask yourself, what did the pet get out of the situation? For example, a dog who barks at the mail person might perceive that the mail person's departure is the consequence of his barking. Consequences affect future behavior. If the behavior persists or increases in frequency, then it has been reinforced. The dog who barked at the mail person may find the mail carrier leaving to be a desirable consequence, and thus the behavior persists because it is being negatively reinforced by the person's departure. If in the future the behavior decreases in frequency, then either extinction or punishment has occurred.

The second step is to hypothesize the motivation. Identifying the ABCs will often give insight into the possible motivation. Remember, cats and dogs are amoral and opportunistic. They do what cats and dogs do, and they do not have a concept of right versus wrong. They are not spiteful or malicious. When postulating a motivation, try to keep it as simple as possible. Motivation can be considered to be either socially motivated (seeking human interaction) or self-reinforcing (not associated with seeking human attention). Self-reinforcing behaviors offer an immediate benefit to the pet. For example, a full bladder is emptied, and the dog or cat feels better. Behaviors can be both socially motivated and self-reinforcing through learning and experience. For example, knocking items off a counter might start as a self-reinforcing exploratory behavior by a kitten. However, part of the consequence of the behavior is that the owner comes over and picks the item up, looks at the kitten, and pets her. This behavior could develop into a way to get the owner's attention when the kitten desires social interactions. The reason it is important to determine the motivation or motivations for a behavior are so that possible prevention and management options can be identified and to provide an appropriate response to future displays of the behavior.

Once the ABCs and motivation have been determined, the ability to prevent or manage the behavior should be explored. Step 3 is to determine if the behavior can be prevented or managed in a humane way. Management and prevention include proactively reinforcing desired behaviors, controlling antecedents, and supervision. Management and avoidance may not actually change a behavior, but they can prevent it, and sometimes that is enough of an answer for the pet owner. Proactively reinforce desired behaviors: catch the cat or dog performing desired behaviors. It is best to be proactive instead of reactive. When pets are reinforced for desired behaviors rather than owners reacting to undesirable behaviors, the cat and dog learn more quickly which behaviors the owner desires. This takes some training of the person because in general people are more likely to react than to act. Controlling antecedents: managing and controlling what pets learn through antecedent arrangement is important to prevent them from learning undesirable behaviors. Pet owners should implement the canine and feline management recommendations explored earlier in this chapter, such as kitten- and puppy-proofing the house, and using baby gates, an exercise pen, and/or a crate. Supervision: close supervision, especially with kittens and puppies, is necessary to help guide their learning and set them up for success. When cat and dog behaviors become problematic for the pet owner, make sure a routine has been established that includes enriching activities to meet the pet's exploratory, physical, and social needs. If those needs are not being met, troublesome behaviors can occur from the lack of physical and mental stimulation.

If the behavior cannot be prevented or managed (or the management system has failed), then proceed to step 4: Solve it! There are two options depending on the motivation: Ignore the behavior or response substitution. If the motivation and consequence are socially motivated for human attention, the owner should ignore the behavior if possible. Behaviors that are not self-reinforcing or rewarding to the pet will cease to occur if ignored (no reinforcement is provided). If the reward for the behavior is human attention – for instance, the dog jumps on a person and is pushed away, the dog nudges the person and is petted, the cat meows and is fed – it is likely that ignoring the pet in these situations will cause the learned behavior to cease. Ignoring means not looking at, talking to, or touching the pet at these times. Initially, the attention-getting behavior will worsen because in the past it has resulted in a desired consequence, but if the pet continues to be ignored, theoretically the behavior should extinguish. However, implementing extinction can be difficult for owners and can produce stress or frustration for the animal. Ignoring (avoiding reinforcing) generally works best if it is not a long-established behavior. It is also important to recognize that the emergence of numerous undesirable behaviors may reflect a lack of adequate social, physical, and exploratory outlets for the pet. Rather than using extinction, the owner can proactively (before the pet does the undesirable behavior) direct the pet to perform a desired behavior that can be reinforced.

Self-reinforcing behaviors cannot be ignored. The dog barking at the mail person at the door makes the mail person leave, and it works every time. Some socially motivated behaviors may also not be able to be ignored and allowed to extinguish. For these behaviors it may be necessary to use response substitution: interrupt, redirect, reinforce. **Interrupt** the behavior by getting the pet's attention. Softly clap the hands, pat a leg, or call the pet's name in an upbeat tone of voice. The interruption should not be frightening, an indicator of impending punishment, or delivered in a negative tone. Avoid the use of "Ah-Ah" or "No." **Redirect** by giving the pet a cue for an alternate appropriate behavior that has been previously taught with positive-reinforcement training. The alternate behavior should be incompatible with the undesirable one. For example, if the dog is barking at the mail person, the owner can softly clap her hands or call the dog's name (using an upbeat, calm tone), and ask him to come and sit. Gently prompt the appropriate behavior with a flat collar and leash if necessary. Ideally the owner should be proactive by getting the pet's attention before the undesirable behavior is already in full swing. **Reinforce** the pet for the appropriate behavior with a food treat or other high-value reinforcer. Keep the pet busy with a food-stuffed toy or practice of different behaviors such as sits and downs or redirect the pet to an appropriate activity. It is best to avoid reprimands or punishment when addressing behavior concerns with pets.

It is important to realize that pets also need to communicate information to us. There will be times the pet will be asking for you to meet a specific need through attention-seeking behaviors. The dog that needs to urinate might come to you and then run to the door. He is trying to tell you he needs to eliminate. Respond to this request. Equally as important to ignoring undesirable behavior is making sure that the exploratory, social, and physical needs of the pet are being met (prevention). Providing adequate outlets through routine potty breaks, walks, play, and positive training will often drastically decrease the frequency of undesirable attention-seeking behaviors.

- Providing adequate outlets through routine potty breaks, walks, play, and positive training will often drastically decrease the frequency of undesirable attention-seeking behaviors.

Problems with aversive training techniques and equipment

You may have noticed that the behavior solutions model focuses on identifying desirable behavior and rewarding the pet. There is no need to communicate to the pet what you do not want or what they did "wrong." Verbal or physical reprimands are often used because the pet owner feels the pet needs to know "he did wrong." Shouting "No" or "Ahh" has a negative association, is positive punishment, or a predictor of positive punishment. A verbal or physical reprimand may suppress behavior, but it does not teach or tell the pet to perform an appropriate behavior in any given situation. Instead teach owners to focus on what they want their pet to do and reward them for those behaviors. Making the pet successful through management and training will enhance the human–animal bond.

There are numerous problems with utilizing aversives to try to effect behavior change in pets. Aversives inhibit learning and reduce creativity and all behavior. Being afraid of having the wrong answer makes learning difficult and stressful. Punishment does not teach the animal what to do. Aversives can induce fear, anxiety, or conflict, which can create behavior disorders.

Punishment-based training collars such as pinch collars, choke chains, and electric collars are aversive and meant to induce pain/discomfort. The use of these techniques may lead to the development of fear, anxiety, and/or aggressive behavior.

Although aversive techniques often do inhibit behavior, they are riddled with problems and therefore should not be recommended. The effects of coercive or aversive training include the following:

- It damages the human–animal bond.
- Not only does it inhibit the pet at the moment but it also inhibits learning and all behavior. If the pet is worried about being reprimanded it is difficult to try to learn something new. Aversive training can induce learned helplessness.
- It induces anxiety, fear of the handler, or of the environmental situation. One cannot control the pet's perceived association that is going to be made when the aversive is applied. A dog may become aggressive with other dogs because of an association of the correction on a pinch collar and the approach of other dogs. The handler may have intended to correct the dog for pulling to visit the other dogs but may inadvertently create a serious behavior issue.
- It can induce aggression toward humans and other animals.
- It does not change the motivation for the behavior. Nor does it teach the pet what is appropriate in the context or appease the pet's desire to perform the behavior. Important warning signs or communication may be inhibited by correction, thus creating a pet that is less likely to give warning and consequently is more dangerous.
- Although aversive techniques often do inhibit behavior, they are riddled with problems and therefore should not be recommended.

Alternatives to correction-based collars are head halters and front clip harnesses. They can aid an owner who has difficulty controlling the dog. If properly introduced, most dogs tolerate them well. However, some dogs will find them restrictive or perhaps even a little irritating, thus causing frustration. The key is that head collars and harnesses are not designed to inflict pain; instead they provide a leverage perspective which makes it more difficult for the dog to pull forward. They are appropriate and sometimes necessary tools for management with some dogs until the desired behavior has been taught. However, happy acceptance and a desire to wear the equipment is a necessary prerequisite to their use.

Behavior solutions for typical canine behaviors

Even after setting up an ideal environment for learning with appropriate management and a consistent routine, there will still be normal behaviors that a canine will exhibit that may be problematic for the pet owner. Let us apply the behavior solutions model to several normal behaviors of dogs such as mouthing/play biting, chewing, taking items, jumping on people, digging, and barking.

Mouthing and play biting

Mouthing is a normal social behavior in dogs. Puppies learn to control the pressure of their bite from playing with other puppies. When one puppy bites too hard, the other puppy yelps and stops playing. This ends the play, teaching the puppy bite inhibition. Although mouthing is normal in canine social circles, it can be problematic when directed at humans. Puppies need to learn that mouthing or biting people is not the way to prompt people to play.

The antecedent is the presence of people and the desire to interact with them. The behavior itself may involve mouthing the hands, grabbing clothes or nipping at the person's legs in a playful manner. The consequence is generally some form of reaction from the person or a fun game of tug on the person's clothes. The motivation for mouthing is a social one; the dog is seeking a friendly interaction with the person. However, it can potentially be self-reinforcing as mouthing hands, feet, and clothing feels good to the dog.

Owners can be advised to avoid playing with puppies with their hands, clothes, or shoes. They can also teach their puppy to play with toys or a tug for an appropriate outlet for this behavior. Meeting the social, physical, and exploratory needs through routine and environmental enrichment will help to minimize mouthing and play biting. When unable to address the problem, the dog should be managed safely in his confinement area to prevent the perpetuation of the undesirable behavior.

Often puppies will exhibit increased mouthing during certain times of the day, which usually correspond with increased level of activity. Many puppy owners report that when the family attempts to settle down for the evening is a common time for increased activity and mouthing. Behaviors such as running laps (zoomies), jumping on people and furniture, along with or without the mouthing are commonly described. This is normal behavior in puppies that is designed to expel excess energy that usually occurs in the evening or another predictable time. Sometimes this behavior can be intercepted by a walk prior to the normal time of onset or by teaching the dog to settle on a mat with food-dispensing toys.

As it is a solicitation for play and interaction, the owner should immediately withdraw attention to

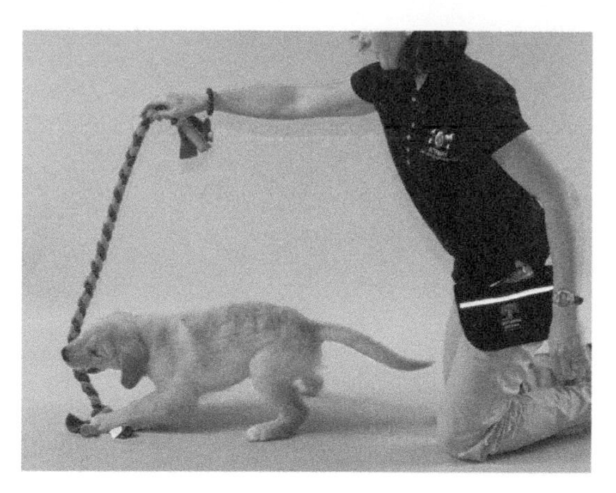

Figure 7.15 Person playing with a puppy with a long tug toy to encourage mouthing of the toy rather than her hands, arms, or legs.

avoid reinforcing the behavior. The instant the puppy's teeth touch human skin or clothes, the person should freeze for a second. If the puppy has stopped nipping, an appropriate toy should be offered to provide an outlet for mouthing. The owner should interact with the puppy with the toy instead (Figure 7.15). When the behavior persists or results in torn clothing or physical injury, it may not be possible to just ignore the behavior. In this case, the puppy owner can redirect and reward an alternate appropriate response (response substitution). The person should calmly and quietly withdraw attention for two to three seconds. Then they can redirect the puppy to sit or perform any alternate behavior other than mouthing and then reward by offering a treat or toy (Table 7.4). To channel the behavior in an appropriate direction, the owner may teach the dog to find a toy. A toy in the mouth prevents human extremities or clothing being in the mouth.

Caution owners to resist the urge to do any type of physical or verbal corrections. Any infliction of fear, pain, or discomfort must be avoided. This includes methods such as verbal reprimands, grabbing the muzzle, pinching the tongue, biting the puppy back, or pushing a fist into the puppy's mouth. Any such methods will serve to make the puppy fearful or defensive, both of which can promote aggression. They do not teach the puppy an acceptable way to play with the owner and can result in a dog that becomes head or hand shy.

Placing the puppy in its crate is helpful when the owner needs a break. Puppies can become overtired and overly aroused. If the owners become frustrated

Table 7.4 Canine mouthing and play biting.

Identify the ABCs	• Antecedent: People present and normal natural social behavior of dogs (especially puppies) • Behavior: Bites or mouths hands/legs or clothes of people • Consequence: Usually some type of social interaction from people
Hypothesize motivation	Generally, socially motivated but can also be self-reinforcing
Prevention or management	• Avoid play with hands or clothes • Teach the dog to play with toys or tugs • Use confinement if unable to address at the time • Meet the dogs social, physical, and exploratory needs through routine and enrichment
Solve it!	• Ignore: freeze or remove attention to avoid reinforcing • Redirect to an appropriate toy to mouth when the dog is not mouthing the person • Response substitution when unable to ignore

with the puppy, they may lose their temper and punish the dog. At those times it is better to put the puppy in its crate with a safe exploratory food puzzle toy, rather than allow it to continue to learn the wrong things.

There are simply times when a puppy becomes overly stimulated and does not have the ability to calm down, similar to an overtired child. During these times, placing the puppy in the crate or other area of confinement provides the needed opportunity to relax. Confinement can be used to manage the situation but should not be used to punish the behavior. The puppy should be rewarded for going to the confinement area. This technique is not designed to teach the dog appropriate or inappropriate behavior but instead to provide relief to the owner and help calm the dog down. Often, after a few minutes, the puppy will fall asleep.

Video 7.9 on the companion website demonstrates the veterinary nurse and trainer using appropriate techniques to address a puppy biting her pant legs. She purposely overstimulates the puppy to get the video footage.

Chewing

Chewing is a normal exploratory behavior of puppies and adolescent dogs. It is comparable to a human one-year-old child who places objects in its mouth because it is both exploring its environment and teething. Chewing may be associated with teething or a recreational exploration of the world with the mouth. It is important to note that chewing is also an anxiety reliever. Although considered a normal behavior, if it becomes excessive, it could be a symptom of a larger problem. If the chewing is excessive or only associated with the owner's departure, this could be a sign of an underlying anxiety disorder.

The antecedent is the access to items to chew and a normal desire to explore the environment. It could also be associated with the discomfort of teething. The exact behavior will be defined by what items the dog is chewing, although all are nonhuman-approved items for chewing. The consequence is the desire to explore and chew has been satisfied. The motivation for chewing is self-reinforcing!

Management and supervision are extremely important to prevent dogs from developing undesirable chewing habits. A puppy-proofed confinement area should be utilized when the young dog is unable to be directly supervised. Access to the dog's favorite inappropriate chew items should be blocked. A lack of stimulation may lead to excessive chewing; ensure all the social, physical, and exploratory needs are being met through routine enrichment activities. The owner should be encouraged to reward and encourage chewing on appropriate objects; catch the dog getting it right! To prevent a preference for items that have human scent, avoid offering objects to chew that are concentrated with human scent, such as old shoes, socks, or shirts. The dog will not know the difference between an old or new pair of shoes. Similarly, provide a variety of appropriate chew toys.

Chewing cannot be ignored because the behavior is self-reinforcing. The owner will need to use response substitution, call the dog's name in an upbeat tone or clap hands to get the dog's attention, call him to you, and provide an appropriate chew toy. It is best to be proactive. If the owner sees the dog ready to chew on a chair leg, redirect him to an appropriate hard chew toy before he makes the undesirable choice (Table 7.5).

Verbal or physical reprimands will only teach the dog that it is unsafe to chew the chair when people are around. He will instead do it in your absence. Make chewing on appropriate objects more rewarding. If unable to block access to inappropriate objects, it may be necessary to make these objects taste unpleasant through the use of a commercially available taste deterrent. These products need to be applied daily as they do lose their potency and they only seem to work in about 50% of patients. Good chewing habits will be developed through management, supervision, and providing appropriate chewing alternatives.

Table 7.5 Canine chewing.

Identify the ABCs	• Antecedent: Access to items to chew and a natural desire to explore • Behavior: Chewing of nonhuman-approved items • Consequence: Desire for exploration and chewing has been fulfilled
Hypothesize motivation	Self-reinforcing!
Prevention or management	• Manage access • Supervision • Provide a variety of appropriate chew toys • Reward appropriate chewing • Meet the dog's social, physical, and exploratory needs through routine and enrichment
Solve it!	• Response substitution; interrupt, redirect, reinforce

Stealing objects

Stealing is another common concern of clients and one that is easily reinforced by family members. It should be noted, from the puppy's perspective there is no such thing as "stealing." They are amoral creatures and stealing is a human rationalized statement. Some puppies enjoy being chased and will quickly catch on to the game. Over time the puppy may become anxious when chased and develop guarding issues.

Dogs are opportunistic and they have a great sense of smell. Dogs are also curious and explore their world with their mouth. You can see how a piece of pizza left on the counter might go missing. Dogs are likely to check out the kitchen counter, trash cans, or coffee table at some point. What they learn when this happens will set the precedent for future behavior.

The antecedent is items within reach and normal exploratory behavior. The behavior itself may involve taking food or nonfood-based items found in the house and ingesting or chewing them. From the dog's perspective the consequence can be ingestion of yummy food, exploration with a novel chew item, or a fun game of chase while the owners try to retrieve the item.

The motivation can be exploratory or appetitive (self-reinforcing). It can also develop into an attention-seeking behavior (socially motivated). If the dog learns that taking an object in front of people gets a reaction, he is likely to repeat it. Conversely, many dogs will check the counters, trash can, and tables because they smell food. If this behavior pays off on occasion, this will make for a very strong behavior resistant to extinction. It is just like playing the slot machine: sometimes you hit the jackpot. Typical consequences that perpetuate counter surfing and object stealing may include finding food, a game of chase, a verbal reprimand (this is attention), physical contact, or any combination of the above.

Preventing this behavior involves good management by all family members. Keeping items picked up and floors free of socks and other temptations will help the dog be successful. It may be necessary to block access to the problem areas with the use of baby gates or an exercise pen. Keep the counters clean and place the trash can in a cupboard or closet. Many covered trash cans designed to make it difficult for a dog to access the contents are commercially available. Proactively, teach the dog to settle on a dog bed located outside of the kitchen or away from the table. Resting on his bed is the place to be when people are in the kitchen or sitting at the table (Figure 7.16). While the process of "settle on a bed" behavior is being taught, the dog should be crated or confined to an area during mealtimes to prevent the practicing of undesirable behavior. A frozen food storage device (toy) will help occupy the dog on his bed or in his confinement area. Advise owners to only offer treats and food outside of the kitchen so the area is not associated with obtaining food. It is important that the dog is provided appropriate opportunities to appease his exploratory motivation through games suggested in the section titled **Canine environmental enrichment**.

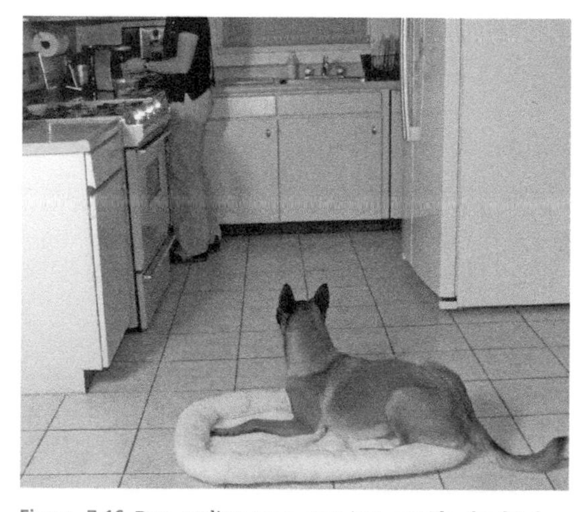

Figure 7.16 Dog settling on a mat just outside the kitchen while the owner prepares food.

There are a variety of possible scenarios with this behavior and the response will vary depending on the circumstances.

Scenario 1: Dog checks out the counter or coffee table but there is nothing he can get. It is best to just ignore this behavior. Exploration is normal and if it does not pay off (with food or human attention) it will decrease in frequency.

Scenario 2: The dog is checking the counters and there are items in reach, but the dog has not obtained an item yet. The best course of action is to use response substitution; gently interrupt/distract by clapping your hands to get the dog's attention, give him a previously taught cue ("Leave it," "Place," "Sit," "Come"), and reward him for the alternate behavior. Video 7.10 on the companion website highlights the beginning stages of teaching the cue "Leave it." The trainer chooses an object the dog is not interested in putting in his mouth. She initially places the object on the ground and then begins to drop it on the ground. After it hits the ground the trainer says, "Leave it," in a calm and non-threatening tone. She marks and treats the dog for remaining still.

Scenario 3: The dog has an item. It is important that owners avoid chasing the dog because this just makes for a fun game of "keep away" and increases the dog's perceived value of the object. It can also lead to guarding of objects.

- If it is a low value object (i.e. a paper towel, tissue) that will not harm the dog, it is best for owners to ignore the situation. They should not look at or say anything to the dog; instead they can leave the room. The dog may follow. Any reaction from the owner will increase the value of the item and risks reinforcing the behavior as a way to get the owner's attention. The dog likely will grow bored of the item on his own and walk away. Owners should reevaluate their prevention and management system, to avoid continued opportunities for the behavior.

- If the dog obtains a high-value object or one that may cause him harm (i.e. cell phone, wallet, candy bar), the owner has three options:
  1. Response substitution: If the dog knows a release cue, the owner can prompt the release and reward for complying.
  2. Distraction: If the dog does not yet know a release cue, the owner can create a distraction by such means as ringing the doorbell, crinkling cellophane or giving another pet or person a hug or acting silly and running out of the room with the dog's favorite toy. This distraction will likely cause the dog to drop the item to investigate. The item can be picked up while the dog's focus is elsewhere.
  3. Exchange: If the dog is not dissuaded by the distraction, then the owner can use a special treat such as a piece of cheese, hotdog, or sandwich meat, to prompt the dog to release the item. The dog can be led away from the object by giving it several treats. Once he is in another room or outside, the owner can return to pick up the object without having the dog underfoot. The distraction and exchange should not substitute for appropriate management and teaching the dog to willingly relinquish objects (Table 7.6).
  4. Another option is to distract the dog with the "Counting Game." The counting game, popularized by animal trainer and behavioral professional, Chirag Patel, can be helpful for managing and preventing negative associations with the removal of resources in the dog's possession. At a distance from the dog, the person places one treat after another on the ground while they count. Once the dog approaches to eat the treats, the person moves to another location and repeats. Watch Video 7.11 on the companion website demonstrating the counting game. Notice how the person moves away once the dog approaches. This removes any social pressure of the person lingering over the dog while he is eating. The dog is also learning to move away from an object and come to the person on the cue, "One, two, three. . . ." This game can be used in a variety of contexts, even as an icebreaker when getting to know a dog for the first time.

Owners should be advised when a dog retreats under a bed or table and hunkers down over an item, the dog should NOT BE CONFRONTED. If it is necessary to get the item from the dog, safely distract the dog out of hiding using a toy or special treat in exchange for the object. Guarding as a young puppy can be the first sign that the puppy is not comfortable or is in conflict and should be investigated more fully.

Verbal or physical reprimands are not advised as they will only teach a dog to explore and take items when people are not around and ultimately can lead to a serious guarding issue.

Commercial pet deterrents are available, but they should not be used as a first option. Gadgets and gizmos are never a substitute for teaching an appropriate response, and they can have unpleasant side effects, eliciting fear and anxiety in the dog.

Table 7.6 Stealing objects.

Identify the ABCs	• Antecedent: Access to items and a desire to explore/chew • Behavior: Takes or investigates nonhuman-approved items • Consequence: Game of chase and/or desire to explore and chew has been met
Hypothesize motivation	Self-reinforcing but can also become socially motivated
Prevention or management	• Block access, keep items out of reach • Teach to settle on a mat • Meet the dogs social, physical, and exploratory needs through routine and enrichment
Solve it!	• Ignore • Response substitution • Distract • Exchange • Counting game

Jumping on people

Jumping is a normal and friendly greeting behavior of dogs. Puppies learn to solicit attention and feeding through jumping and licking the commissure of their mother's lips and muzzle. Dogs jump on people in an attempt to show affection and it is usually intended as a friendly gesture. Some people like their dogs to jump on them. As long as it does not create a safety or welfare issue for the owner, the dog, or others, it is not necessarily an issue that needs to be addressed. It is often more tolerated in small dogs compared to large dogs, simply due to the difference in the experience and safety for the people. If the pet owners do not want their dog to jump when greeting them or others, then it will be necessary to teach the dog an alternate greeting behavior.

The antecedent for jumping is the presence of people and a natural greeting behavior of dogs. The behavior can be defined as jumping on a person in friendly greeting. The context (arrival home after a long or short departure) and the target of the jumping (familiar versus unfamiliar people) may vary from case to case. The consequence generally involves some type of social interaction from people.

The motivation for the behavior is excitement and social interaction. Because dogs are social, typical human responses that perpetuate jumping may include an eye glance, a verbal reprimand, physical contact, such as pushing the dog off, or any combination of the above.

Prevention and management techniques should be geared toward rewarding an alternate behavior and managing the learning history to set the dog up to be successful from the beginning. Proactively provide ample exploratory, social, and physical exercise with at least two short walks off the property daily, two short training sessions daily and other exploration opportunities to make sure the dog's social needs are being met. Owners should initially make their social interactions and greetings very calm. The higher the excitement level, the more likely the dog will jump. To prevent the escalation of jumping, owners should avoid encouraging the puppy to jump on them. However, because many owners actually enjoy it when their dog jumps on them, an alternative is to teach the dog to jump when cued. To help prevent others from reinforcing the dog for jumping, a leash can be utilized to prevent the behavior. Expecting a sit may be too much at first with young puppies or over-exuberant greeters. Owners should be encouraged to catch their dog with four feet on the floor and reward the dog for not jumping.

Alternatively, telling the dog what to do before it makes the undesirable choice of jumping will help it learn faster. The owner should also reward the dog often for sitting. The dog will learn that sitting, rather than jumping, results in people turning, looking at, talking to, and petting it. Thus, the act of sitting becomes an appropriate greeting behavior (see Figure 7.17).

A release cue, such as "make a friend," can teach the dog when it is time to visit and greet guests. Combined with "settle on a mat," the dog is rewarded for going to his mat while the guest enters the home and then calmly released to "make a friend" if appropriate in the context.

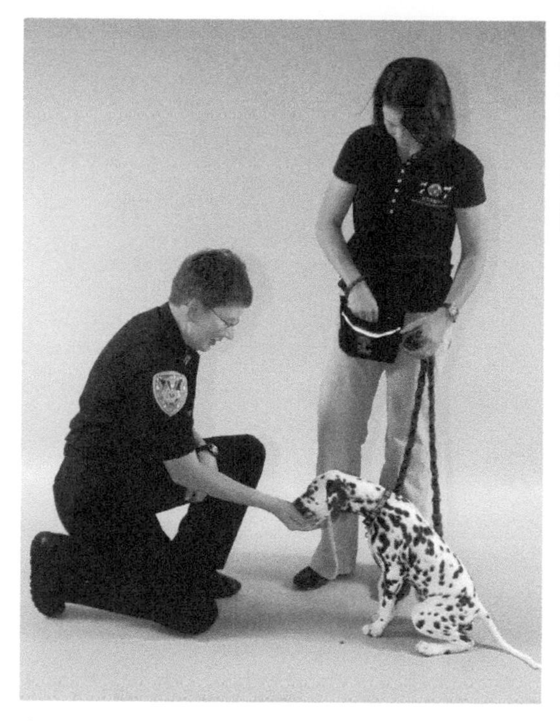

Figure 7.17 A puppy being rewarded with treats and attention for a calm greeting.

Regardless of how well a preventive system is implemented, there are likely to be times that jumping will still occur. Counseling owners on how to respond to jumping should promote a positive learning experience for the dog. Remember, we are teaching them a human-approved appropriate greeting that is not a natural greeting behavior in their repertoire. If the dog jumps, the owner should avoid reinforcing it with any form of attention (eye contact, talking, or even reprimanding). The best response is no response at all. It might be necessary for the person to step back or away to avoid the initial contact and protect himself/herself. If the person is sitting, he/she can calmly and quietly stand up and look away. When the dog is not jumping, it can then be rewarded with calm attention and even better, a treat placed on the ground or close to the ground.

There are times when trying to ignore the behavior of an over-exuberant dog is not possible because it hurts or the dog simply continues to jump. Likely just making any contact with the person, even without any social interaction, can act to reinforce

Table 7.7 Jumping on people.

Identify the ABCs	• Antecedent: Presence of people and natural greeting behavior • Behavior: Jumps on person • Consequence: Tactile contact and attention
Hypothesize motivation	Socially motivated
Prevention or management	• Calm greetings • Reward four feet on the floor • Use a leash if needed • Reward sitting often • Teach "settle on mat" and "make a friend" cues • Meet the dog's social, physical, and exploratory needs through routine and enrichment
Solve it!	• Ignore/avoid reinforcing • Response substitution if necessary

the behavior. If the behavior cannot be ignored, response substitution can be used:

1. Calmly and quietly withdraw attention for two to three seconds.
2. Redirect the dog to sit, down, or any behavior incompatible with jumping.
3. Reward the alternate behavior with a treat and calm attention. Over-exuberant praise is likely to result in more jumping (Table 7.7).

It is important to emphasize to owners that verbal and physical reprimands should be avoided. Shouting "NO," swatting, pushing, or kneeing the dog in the chest, may inhibit the jumping, but they are counterproductive techniques that can often result in dogs becoming afraid of people. It would be analogous to introducing yourself to a person by reaching to shake his/her hand and the person yells at you or slaps you. Punishment for jumping does not teach a dog how to interact appropriately and may cause or directly contribute to the development of serious aggression toward the owners or others.

Video 7.12 on the companion website depicts proactively reinforcing a puppy for not jumping.

Digging

Some breeds of dogs are more likely to dig than others. Terriers are notorious for being diggers. Terrier comes from the Latin word, "Terra" meaning "of the earth." Many terrier and some hound breeds have been selectively bred to dig and chase vermin underground. Regardless of the dog's breeding, all dogs have the potential to dig.

Antecedents for digging can include access to digging areas, normal exploratory behavior, and potentially escape behavior. Sometimes the behavior will involve digging holes in flower beds or in the middle of the yard. If the digging occurs along a fence line it could be an attempt to escape the confinement. Digging can have a variety of consequences such as finding things, a cool/warm spot to rest, or escape.

The motivation for digging is self-reinforcing. Digging can occur for a multitude of reasons. The motivation can include the following:

1. Thermoregulation: To keep warm or cool when outside for prolonged periods of time.
2. Hunting: Insects or other animals. Dogs can smell and hear animals in the ground.
3. Burying: Hiding a treasured item to be recovered later.
4. Escape or anxiety: This usually involves digging along a fence line. For example, a dog may become panicked by a thunderstorm or an intact male dog may be motivated to roam the neighborhood.

Supervision will play a role in preventing this behavior from starting in the first place. If a dog that enjoys digging is left unattended in a suitable digging location, it will do what is natural for it. Blocking access to these areas can remove the temptation for the dog. Lack of stimulation may lead to excessive digging. Routine scheduled walks, play time, and training are important. Time in the backyard alone should not be a substitute for human-initiated exercise and interactions.

To provide the dog with an appropriate place to dig, owners may decide to give the dog a digging box. Similar to a sand box for a child, a digging box for the dog can provide it with hours of appropriate digging entertainment (Figure 7.18). The digging

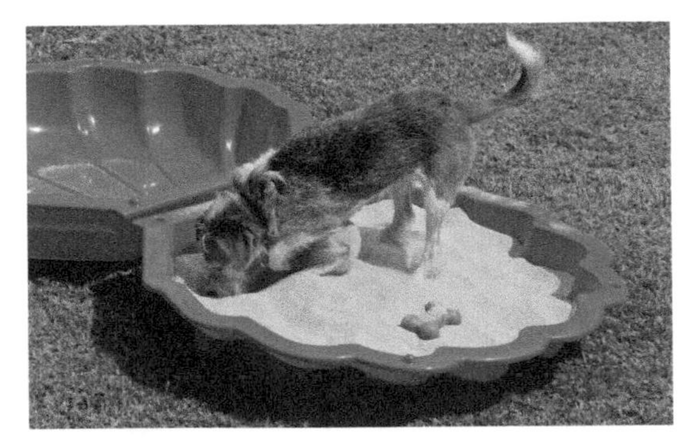

Figure 7.18 Example of providing a digging box for the dog to provide an appropriate outlet for this exploratory behavior.

box can be made enticing to the dog by hiding treats in the substrate and rewarding the dog for showing interest in the digging spot. There are also commercially available indoor mobile digging stations which provide a great alternative for dogs who like to dig on rugs or furniture in the house or for pet owners who do not have space for an outside digging box.

What should the owners do if they catch their dog digging in an inappropriate location? Verbal or physical reprimands will teach the dog it is unsafe to dig in front of people, consequently the dog will learn to do it when it is safe; no people around. Digging cannot be ignored because the behavior is self-reinforcing. The owner will need to use response substitution.

1. In an upbeat tone, call the dog's name or clap your hands to get his attention.
2. Call him to you.
3. Redirect him to an appropriate digging area, a short game of play, or other incompatible behavior, and reward (Table 7.8).

Advise owners to be proactive. If they see their dog getting ready to dig, redirect him before it makes the undesirable choice.

Placing the dog's feces in the unwanted digging spot will make that area unattractive. However, without supervision, management, and appropriate alternatives, the dog may find a new location to dig.

Barking

Some breeds of dogs are genetically predisposed to barking. The ability to vocalize was an important feature required for some dogs to do a job. Classic examples are some of the herding breeds, such as shelties and corgis, which depended on barking to move livestock on a farm. Barking is also a method for dogs to communicate within their own species and with humans. Different pitches in barking can mean different things. There can be multiple antecedents and consequences for barking, therefore identifying the ABCs of this behavior will be important.

Table 7.8 Digging.

Identify the ABCs	• Antecedent: Access to digging areas, exploration, escape, anxiety • Behavior: Digs in yard or flower beds • Consequence: Finds things, makes a comfortable resting spot, escapes
Hypothesize motivation	Self-rewarding
Prevention or management	• Direct supervision • Block access • Provide digging location • If applicable, address underlying anxiety • Meet the dog's social, physical, and exploratory needs through routine and enrichment
Solve it!	• Response substitution

Possible triggers or antecedents for barking include desire for human attention, physical and mental needs (hunger, elimination, social contact), a sound (car door, doorbell), or presentation of a feared stimulus. The behavior will vary in the pitch of the barking and the accompanying body language of the dog depending on the trigger/antecedent that started it. High-pitched barking is generally a distance-decreasing signal (come closer), while low-pitched barking is a distance-increasing signal (go away). The consequence of the behavior will also be variable. Consequences that typically perpetuate barking include human responses in the case of barking triggered by social or physical needs and cessation of the sound or stimulus in the latter example.

The motivation for the behavior will vary. It can be self-reinforcing and it can also be socially motivated. The antecedents and consequences will make the distinction in motivation.

Prevention of excessive barking often relies on the owners being able to meet the physical, exploratory, and social needs of their companion. Some dogs have more needs than others. Early and continued proper socialization can help curb the development of stimuli or sound-induced barking.

Blocking visual or auditory access to the dog's triggers will inhibit the practicing of the barking behavior. This can be accomplished by blocking access out of the front windows or gates with window film, blinds, or screens. A white noise machine or classical music can be utilized to minimize outside sounds. Classical music has been shown to have a calming effect on dogs in the shelter setting (Wells et al. 2002).

The important foundation skill of settling on a mat should be trained early and incorporated with times that might induce high arousal and consequently barking. The owner can proactively redirect the dog to settle in his kennel or mat when the owner is preparing food or answering the door. It is much easier to ignore a quiet dog than it is to ignore a barking one. Counseling owners to recognize and reward their dogs when they are quiet and calm can also be helpful in preventing unwanted barking.

Table 7.9 Barking.

Identify the ABCs	• Antecedent: Social interaction, physical or mental needs, response to a sound or other stimuli • Behavior: Variety of forms of barking depending on the trigger • Consequence: Attention, needs met, stimuli goes away
Hypothesize motivation	Can be socially motivated or self-reinforcing
Prevention or management	• Meet the dog's social, physical, and exploratory needs through routine and enrichment • Proper early and continued socialization • Block access to stimuli • Reward quiet and calm behavior • Teach "settle on a mat"
Solve it!	• Ignore or • Response substitution

Depending on the circumstances barking can either be ignored or response substitution can be applied. Attention and communication barking, if undesirable to the owner, should be ignored. However, it is important to educate owners that frequent attention barking is usually a sign that the dog's exploratory, physical, and social needs are not being met. Ignoring the barking will prevent owner reinforcement of the behavior but does not address the underlying issue. If the dog is barking at a stimulus, response substitution (interrupt, cue an alternate behavior, reinforce) can alleviate the situation at the moment (Table 7.9).

Dogs bark; this is normal. However, excessive barking or reactivity can be a sign of underlying fear and/or anxiety. Behavioral intervention services may be warranted.

Behavior solutions for typical feline behaviors

Feline behavior concerns that are normal behaviors for cats include play biting and/or scratching, scratching that causes damage to property, and climbing on surfaces. The same behavior solutions model can be used to analyze and create positive solutions for these natural behaviors.

Play biting and scratching

Play biting and scratching is a normal behavior of cats. Cats will bite and scratch in other contexts not associated with play but here we are specifically addressing a play behavior. They interact and explore their world with their feet and mouth. Cat bites and scratches have the potential to cause severe infections so should not be taken lightly. On average, 80% of cat bites caused by punctures will become infected. It is important to address feline play biting and scratching of humans because it can become a dangerous problem in the human household. The antecedent for this particular behavior is the presence of people and the cat's desire to play. The behavior itself may involve the cat stalking the owner and ambushing her as she walks down a hallway or it could be associated with the cat turning and mouthing a hand and grabbing the person's forearm with the front feet and kicking with the back legs while being petted. The consequence of the behavior is generally some kind of reaction from the human. The motivation for this particular type of biting and scratching is socially motivated.

To prevent this behavior, owners should be advised to only play with their cat with toys. Playing with the cat with their hands can create a problem that can be very damaging to the human–animal bond. Providing environmental enrichment and a set routine for play time and training can funnel this desire to appropriate outlets. Although not recommended with puppies, obtaining two kittens at the same time is advantageous, especially in regard to providing an interactive playmate. To minimize over-stimulation followed by mouthing and scratching, provide short petting sessions with touch being centered on the head and ears rather than down the back. Having a safe bell collar on the cat can help prevent surprise attacks.

If preventive measures fail and the cat is play biting or scratching, the recommended treatment involves a combination of ignoring and response substitution. Owners should be instructed to immediately freeze and withdraw any attention, the moment the cat begins to mouth or scratch them. If the cat knows a stationing cue (go to a perch or cat tree) or a sit cue, the owner can cue that after withdrawing attention for a few seconds. If no cues are known, then the cat should simply be ignored for a few seconds while the owner remains still. In both scenarios the cat should be redirected to an appropriate toy (wand-type chase toys) to play with the owner (Table 7.10). To funnel the behavior in an appropriate direction, teach the cat to get a toy on cue. A toy in the mouth prevents human extremities there.

Table 7.10 Feline play biting and scratching.

Identify the ABCs	• Antecedent: People present and normal, natural social behavior of cats (especially kittens) • Behavior: Bites or scratches hands/legs of people • Consequence: Usually some type of social interaction from people
Hypothesize motivation	Generally, socially motivated
Prevention or management	• Avoid play with hands • Play with cat with appropriate toys, teach get a toy • Obtain two kittens at the same time • Meet the cat's social, physical, and exploratory needs through routine and enrichment
Solve it!	• Ignore: Freeze or remove attention to avoid reinforcing • Redirect to an appropriate toy to mouth when the cat is not biting or scratching the person • Response substitution if the cat knows a stationing or sit cue

As with dogs, positive punishment (squirt bottles, verbal reprimands) should be avoided because it creates fear and distrust and can lead to more serious aggression. Positive punishment does not appease the cat's motivation for friendly play nor does it teach the cat an appropriate way to interact with people.

Destructive scratching

Scratching surfaces with the front claws is a normal behavior of cats. Approximately 60% of house cats will scratch furniture without the presence of any underlying behavioral problem (Morgan and Houpt 1990). The potential problem of scratching should be considered before obtaining a cat. Because the behavior is normal, it is not realistic to eliminate the behavior completely. Scratching objects serves to remove dead cells from their nails. Scratching is also used as a form of territorial communication or marking. It leaves both a visual and chemical scent on the object. Pheromones secreted from the scent glands between the pads of the feet are left on the surface. The antecedent for scratching items is access to items that stimulate the behavior in the cat as well as an innate desire to scratch. The behavior is more common in multi-cat households where there is social tension among cats. In solitary cat households, the presence of other cats outside the home may be a trigger. While some cats seem to prefer to scratch on vertical surfaces, other cats will choose to scratch horizontal ones. The behavior will vary depending on the individual cat's preferences. The motivation for this behavior is self-reinforcing and consequently, it will not go away if ignored. Because the behavior is normal, it is not realistic to expect to eliminate the behavior completely. The goal should be to teach the cat to use specific scratching areas.

Owners should attempt to prevent the undesirable scratching by providing an appropriate outlet. Keeping the cat's nails trimmed may also decrease the need to scratch. The cat's preferred location and surface attributes (position-vertical/horizontal, height, type of material) should be noted. A scratching post or board that mimics the preferred attributes should be provided near the object the cat is likely to scratch. This provides a human-approved alternative. All cat owners should provide their cat with multiple scratching posts/boards. Most commercially available scratching posts/boards will be covered with sisal, fabric, carpet, or corrugated cardboard. Favored locations for scratching seem to be near sleeping areas and in other prominent areas of the home which the cat chooses to frequent. Reinforce the cat for interest in and use of the appropriate scratching posts. Catnip and the dispersion of toys near or on the scratching post/board may make it more intriguing. Temporarily blocking the cat's access to certain items as well as supervision will be necessary while directing scratching to a preferred location. If unable to block access, consider using a feline cheek-marking pheromone spray such as Feliway Classic to induce cheek marking rather than scratching in undesired areas.

If preventive techniques have failed and the cat is scratching an inappropriate object, the owner should use response substitution: gently interrupt the behavior, call the cat away, redirect to an appropriate scratching area, and reinforce. Reinforce the cat with verbal encouragement and possibly treats for scratching the desired item (Table 7.11). Avoid punishment in the form of verbal reprimands or squirting the cat with water; these actions create fear, anxiety, and distrust and teach the cat to perform the behavior only when the owner is not present. Punishment does not satisfy the cat's motivation for using her claws to scratch or teach her an appropriate location for scratching, but it does teach her to avoid the owner.

Table 7.11 Feline destructive scratching.

Identify the ABCs	• Antecedent: Innate behavior of cats • Behavior: Scratches nonhuman-approved objects causing destruction • Consequence: Pacifies innate desire
Hypothesize motivation	Self-reinforcing
Prevention or management	• Avoid access to objects or make them less attractive • Feliway® to promote cheek marking • Reward appropriate scratching • Meet the cat's social, physical, and exploratory needs through routine and provide appropriate scratching areas
Solve it!	• Response substitution and redirect to appropriate scratching location

Table 7.12 Feline climbing on surfaces.

Identify the ABCs	• Antecedent: Access to vertical surfaces, innate desire to explore • Behavior: Exploring vertical surfaces of the home • Consequence: Comfort and safety
Hypothesize motivation	Generally, self-reinforcing but could also be socially motivated
Prevention or management	• Environmental enrichment and routine • Appropriate outlets for climbing • Reward appropriate climbing • Block access and supervision • Teach go to place or stationing
Solve it!	• Response substitution and redirect to appropriate climbing location

Excessive scratching can be a sign of anxiety and may warrant behavioral intervention services to address the underlying anxiety issue.

Climbing on surfaces

As discussed earlier, cats like to use vertical surfaces! Some owners do not mind if their cats are on the counters and furniture. Other owners may prefer the cat to avoid kitchen counters or particular pieces of furniture in the house. It only becomes an issue when the owner's desires are not the same as the cat's.

The antecedent for climbing is access to items that stimulate the behavior in the cat as well as an innate desire to explore and use vertical space. The behavior itself is simply the cat exploring the vertical surfaces of the home. Consequences for cats performing the behavior without human intervention are likely the enjoyment of exploring the area and finding a comfortable and safe location for resting.

The motivation for this behavior is self-reinforcing and consequently it will not go away if ignored. Some cats may learn that climbing or jumping on certain things gets attention from the owner, so it could also be a socially motivated behavior.

If there are "off-limit" areas where the cat should not climb, owners should attempt to prevent the undesirable climbing by ensuring that the cat's exploratory needs are met by environmental enrichment and a routine. It is also important to provide appropriate outlets for climbing, such as multiple perching areas in lived-in areas of the home. Make sure cat perches are sturdy, non-slip, and comfortable. Attract the cat to the area by feeding special meals on the perches, hiding treats there, or placing catnip in the area to promote interest. When cats climb in appropriate locations, owners should reinforce them with a small food treat or praise. Blocking access and using supervision are necessary to prevent undesired climbing and allow for redirecting the cat to an appropriate alternative. Teaching a cat to go to a place or station such as a cat tree can allow for easy proactive redirection before the cat jumps on an "off-limits" surface.

If preventive techniques have failed and the cat is climbing onto an inappropriate area, the owner should use response substitution: gently interrupt the behavior by calling the cat away, redirect to an appropriate area and reinforce with a small food treat or petting and praise (Table 7.12). Do not use reprimands and aversives, which create fear, distrust, and avoidance, and teach the cat to perform the behavior when the owner is not present. Punishment also does not teach the cat an appropriate location for climbing.

Prevention services

The behavior technician should take the lead to provide prevention services within the hospital. Because prevention services do not require a diagnosis and treatment plan from a veterinarian, this is an amenity the technician can provide without the need for direct supervision by the veterinarian. Not only will vital experiences and information be shared but also the high achieving technician can manage and supervise these services, adding to job satisfaction.

This section explores several prevention services, including pet selection counseling, puppy and kitten classes, juvenile, adolescent, and adult dog classes, fun visits and formal training for veterinary experiences, private training lessons, and special topic seminars or classes.

Pet selection counseling

Pet selection counseling is one of the most valuable, yet under-utilized, services available to owners. Also referred to as *pre-adoption* or *prepurchase counseling,* this type of service provides guidance prior to the acquisition of a pet. It can decrease the possibility of mismatches by ensuring that owners have the information necessary to make educated decisions before bringing a new pet into the home.

- Pet selection counseling is one of the most valuable, yet under-utilized, services available to owners.

A well-planned program encourages clients to consider whether this is the appropriate time to acquire a new pet and whether the pet they are interested in is suited to their lifestyle. This is also an opportunity to assess expectations of the entire household toward a new pet and instill realistic expectations about the responsibility associated with pet ownership.

There are several components present in every successful selection service. They are keys to having a program that achieves the desired results.

Although knowledgeable counselors can advise and guide clients in their selection of an appropriate pet, they should not be expected to choose the specific breed, age, or sex of the pet for the owner. Counselors should possess and demonstrate a working knowledge of the breed or species-specific traits for many of the animals commonly considered as household pets. This includes the normal growth and developmental stages. Species-specific and breed-specific behavior refers to those behaviors commonly engaged in by members of a species or breed within a species.

A good example of species-specific behavior is the inherent desire felines have to scratch. This trait serves multiple purposes. Scratching allows cats to expend excess energy, stretch their bodies, flex their feet, and tone muscles, mark their territory both visually and with scent, and remove the dead sheaths from their claws. All domestic cats, including those that are declawed, exhibit this behavior in some form or another. A knowledgeable counselor, aware that this behavior is not something owners can prevent, will instead educate owners on a variety of ways to redirect scratching toward appropriate objects.

Breed-specific behavior is often readily observed. For instance, while scent hounds, like Beagles, tend to pursue their prey with their noses to the ground, sight hounds such as Greyhounds generally run with their head up, looking toward the object of their pursuit.

Singing canaries have no distinguishing physical characteristics, but they do have their own behavior traits.

Roller Canaries sing with their beaks closed and have lower, softer, more rolling melodies to their songs. Chopper Canaries sing with fully open beaks and produce louder, vibrant, choppier musical notes that some people might consider too shrill.

It is important that counselors learn about behavior traits and the reasons they exist. This enables them to direct owners toward a pet with traits they are seeking. Counselors who understand the importance of species- and breed-specific behavior can provide accurate explanations of why one pet may be better suited to a home than another animal that the client may be considering.

Although a veterinary degree is not necessary, pet selection counselors should be familiar with common genetic disorders within a breed. This allows them to make valuable recommendations of pets that would fit into a specific home.

The English Bulldog breed serves as a good example. This dog was listed sixth in the 2021 American Kennel Club list of most popular breeds. It tends to be a favored sports mascot and is one of the most recognized breed of dogs in the United States. Many people consider English Bulldogs to be tolerant, family-friendly pets. They are also predisposed to several genetic disorders, including hip dysplasia, brachycephalic airway obstruction syndrome (BAOS), keratoconjunctivitis sicca (KCS), and pulmonic stenosis. An English Bulldog would not be the best choice for an active individual seeking a dog to accompany them in rigorous outdoor activities or for people living in hot, humid climates.

Families also benefit from information about the care and maintenance requirement for various types and breeds of pets. This topic is often the first thing potential owners think of. They want to know how much and what type of food a pet eats, its housing and space requirements, whether an animal sheds excessively, needs frequent professional grooming, and yearly vaccinations. The counselor must be prepared to provide answers to these and other similar questions.

In situations where clients are interested in pets that counselors are unfamiliar with, it is beneficial to research and gather information about the animal prior to making any recommendations. Counselors can use the opportunity to collect information and develop a comprehensive library listing common physical and behavioral traits, normal developmental stages, care and husbandry. Creating a list with the pros and cons of ownership on each animal being researched and links to reliable websites that provide additional detailed information will increase the client's confidence in a counselor's ability.

Knowledge about animals alone does not guarantee a successful counseling session. An equally important trait that counselors should possess is the ability to communicate meaningfully with clients. This entails the skill of listening to, processing, and correctly interpreting what the client is saying and the aptitude to clearly and concisely communicate suggestions back in a manner that is conducive to reaching the best decision possible. Tactfulness and diplomacy are the standard trademarks of good counselors. Additionally, counselors should strive to be nonjudgmental and avoid interjecting their own personal feelings into the session.

Counseling sessions

Pre-adoption counseling can be provided in several different formats. Each one has its own set of advantages and disadvantages.

Counselors who work privately with people during one-on-one sessions can establish themselves as important mentors. This personalized relationship has the potential to increase client receptivity and compliance with alternative suggestions. Individualized sessions are usually scheduled as appointments. This allows them to fit into the daily routine of the clinic or business while still meeting the needs of each client. Counselors are able to tailor the information presented to the individual situation. In some cases counselors can arrange to accompany the clients and evaluate the pet prior to the owner making a final decision. Additionally, preselection counseling offers an opportunity to schedule a follow-up visit once a new pet is decided upon and opens the door to a lasting relationship with the clients.

In-home counseling offers the same advantages as individual sessions done in the office. However, there are additional benefits associated with home visits. Technicians can schedule visits for evenings or weekends when the clinic may be closed, but the client is available. As a bonus, technicians are provided with an inside view to the home environment. This information is handy when educating clients on setting up the home for a new arrival.

There are several possible disadvantages to doing private counseling sessions. They can be extremely time intensive in the preparation work. Private preselection appointments may require a time commitment or initial cost that some clients are not willing or able to make. In-home visits involve travel time to and from the client's home, in addition to the time spent during the sessions.

Besides private sessions, another option is group sessions. One obvious benefit of group counseling class is the ability to schedule the session months in advance. This provides opportunities for marketing the service throughout the community, which can attract a large group of participants. Additionally, people not actively seeking a pet one month, may decide to later, and these classes will be available for them at that time. Group classes allow people to share stories, ask questions, and learn from each other, with the counselor serving the role of both facilitator and educator. Group sessions are generally less costly than private counseling, something that may encourage otherwise reluctant clients.

Drawbacks to group pet selection classes include the obvious inability to provide the same amount of personalized attention to the needs of individuals as private counseling. Some of the information covered may not be pertinent to all of those in attendance. Additionally, there is no guarantee that the group in attendance would be large enough to justify the time and energy involved in preparing for the session. People may be reluctant to fully participate or ask questions in a group setting and would benefit more from private sessions.

There are additional considerations when developing preselection counseling sessions. For instance, who will attend the sessions. One excellent predictor of how successful counseling will be is the number of family members involved in the process. Ideally, everyone in the family will participate in the counseling session. This includes all adults and children old enough to understand and express themselves. Doing this allows everyone to have input into the decision and will assist the counselor in making suggestions. Although not everyone will experience the same amount of attachment to a new pet, involvement of the entire household can help ensure that all family members are comfortable living with the pet.

Counseling forms

Pet selection forms are meant to provide the counselor with insight into the client's preconceived expectations of a pet. They can also identify potential areas in which the client may require further education. There are a variety of forms and handouts available, which can be personalized or adapted to meet the needs of each individual user, or counselors can develop their own form from scratch. See Appendix 19 for an example of a pet selection form to be completed by the client. Regardless of the origin of the form selected, there are essential pieces of information that should be included in every counseling session.

- Pet selection forms are meant to provide the counselor with insight into the client's preconceived expectations of a pet. They can also identify potential areas in which the client may require further education.

Household composition

The personal information section allows clients to provide basic data about family members, such as the number of adults and children residing in the home and whether anyone suffers from allergies or other medical conditions that could be affected by a pet. If there are small children, individuals with allergies, or elders in the residence, the counselor can help to direct clients toward pets that may be more appropriate for the entire family. As an example, a bird that produces large amounts of feather dust (Cockatoo, African Grey, and Cockatiel) is not the best choice for a home where a family member has asthma or allergies.

Previous pets

Counselors often also ask for the history of the family's current and past pets. Some animals do not necessarily make good first-time pets. It is useful to examine why any former pets are no longer owned by the individuals. If the reasons were related to anything other than illness or old age, the counselor should inquire further about what has changed in the household to make owning a pet successful this time. Clients who have not owned a pet in a number of years may also need to be brought up to date with modern training techniques and philosophies.

Household logistics and dynamics

Other considerations are the size, location, and type of home, whether there is a yard, the size of the yard, and, if the yard is fenced, the type of fence. The size and location of the home do not directly preclude owning a pet, but it can influence the final selection. Families living in apartments or homes where residences are bunched close together would have a better chance of success with a small bird, like a budgie, cockatiel, finch, or canary, rather than larger parrots such as a cockatoo, macaw, or conure. The latter birds are capable of ear-piercing screams and can result in complaints from nearby neighbors. When there is no yard, or a small, unfenced yard, clients need to carefully evaluate the exercise needs of the pet that they decide upon. High-energy dogs like Border Collies are not usually good candidates for apartment living, unless owners are able to provide adequate daily mental and physical exercise, perhaps in the form of agility, herding or flyball.

As today's families are busier than ever, it is important that any new pet fits into the household's daily routine. Counselors should inquire about how many vacations, business trips, and other types of travel the family takes regularly. If owners are frequently on the road, what type of accommodations are they prepared to make for the pet's care during their absence? One option can be family and friends who enjoy pets and are willing to perform pet-sitting duty in their home or the owner's home during trips. Dogs and cats may not be the best pet if the owners anticipate frequent use of boarding kennels.

In many households, family members are engaged in nonstop activities every day. This can include lengthy commutes back and forth to work, accompanied by long days spent on the job. Children may spend all day in school with evenings and weekends devoted to extracurricular activities. It then becomes important to determine how much time will realistically be available for pet care and interaction. While there is not a set amount of time owners must spend with their pets on a daily basis, puppies and kittens will always require more time than adult dogs and cats. Will someone be available to provide the dog with opportunities to exercise and relieve itself during the day? The amount of time each pet needs will vary according to the individual animal.

Visitors to the home add another dimension in the area of lifestyle. Active households where there are a variety of people frequently coming and going each day may prefer a pet that is friendly and outgoing. An animal that is quiet and reserved may adapt better to a calmer, more sedate environment. Pets often react differently to adult visitors than to teenagers or toddlers.

Are there any major changes on the horizon for the household, or have there been any major changes within the past six months? This includes, but is not limited to, marriage, an adjustment in living arrangements, relocation, pregnancy, or a new baby, children moving away or moving back home, or a change in work status or hours. If the answer to any of these questions is yes, careful consideration should be given to the timing of bringing in a new pet.

One related question involves why the decision was made to acquire a new pet at this time. The answer to this question can provide much insight for counselors. Did they watch a new movie or read a book starring a specific animal? Did they just purchase a new home? Do they feel that their children are now old enough to care for a pet?

Anticipated responsibilities

Families often make erroneous assumptions about who will assume responsibility for various pet-related duties. Therefore, this topic is one that should be discussed with everyone in the family. There should be a clear idea about who in the family will feed, walk, train, and clean-up after the pet. Parents who bring a pet into their home as a way to teach children responsibility should understand that, in most cases, children cannot be reliably expected to perform these duties. This means that parents must be prepared to assume animal-care duties when necessary.

Living arrangements

Is the pet expected to spend life outside, inside, or a combination? If indoors, will the pet have free access to the entire house, including being allowed on furniture, or restricted to a specific area? What arrangements are owners willing to make in order to safeguard the pet and the home when the pet is left alone? How much time will the pet spend alone each day? These topics can easily cause dissension in a household. One family member may have an entirely different view of what is acceptable and anticipated from another family member.

Financial considerations

The first connection most people make when financial investments of pet ownership are mentioned involves the initial purchase price of the pet. Breeders may charge hundreds or thousands of dollars for a purebred dog or cat. Shelter adoption fees are generally less and many pets are advertised as "free to a good home" in local papers and websites. However, even a free pet has associated costs. All counseling forms should contain questions asking owners about their understanding of expenses related to regular and emergency medical treatment, spaying or neutering, food, treats, toys, and training. This is where veterinary clinics can provide realistic guidance about yearly medical procedures and costs for food.

Husbandry considerations

Some pets require regular grooming sessions where they are bathed and their coat is clipped. Frequent brushing is important for longhaired pets to prevent matted hair from developing. Almost all dogs and cats shed, which is something to remind families about during counseling. Birds shed feathers regularly, and some produce a very fine powder-like feather dust that can leave residue on furniture and cause respiratory problems for some people. Clients should be counseled on the potential husbandry needs of pets they are considering.

Management and training considerations

Not every owner has the willingness or ability to deal with challenging behaviors new pets may demonstrate. First-time owners and people who have not lived with a pet for an extended period of time may be unaware of, or have forgotten, the realities of owning a pet. In this section, the counselor can list behaviors commonly reported as troubling for owners and discuss whether the clients feel confident about dealing with them. Behaviors cited for dogs and cats should include vocalization (barking/meowing), destructive chewing, house-training issues, scratching furniture, exploratory behavior, mouthing or nipping, and other similar issues. When talking with individuals interested in birds and exotics, it is important to counsel about screaming, biting, aggression, and the impact diet and husbandry can have on behavior.

Adopting multiple pets at the same time

People sometimes believe it is best to acquire two pets at the same time. There are some advantages to this situation. Working owners may find multiple animals provide each other with companionship and entertainment during the owner's absence. Caring for two pets may or may not require a significant amount of extra work. As an example, the additional time spent on the care and maintenance of two kittens may be almost negligible. However, if the two pets are puppies, it often takes considerable more time and effort.

Bringing two new animals into a house together presents additional challenges. Training two animals at the same time can be a difficult task. When raised together, animals may bond more closely to each other than their human companions. Anxiety and separation issues can become apparent if the two animals must be separated later in life. Undesirable behaviors can easily be transferred from one pet to the other.

If the client is insistent about owning two dogs, the technician could recommend acquiring only one. Once that dog is trained and understands the household rules, then bring in another one. The resident dog can then serve as a model for the new one.

Personal preferences

An area of the session where all members of the family can have a great deal of input is the section where they discuss their personal preferences for a new pet. One exercise that promotes participation and feedback from everyone is to provide a separate sheet of paper to all family members and ask them each to write down three activities they visualize themselves doing with a new pet. Possible answers may include hunting, lap warmer, companion for themselves, their children or other family pets, competition prospect, jogging partner, and protection. In some cases, the variety of answers from members of the same family can be an eye-opening experience. This often opens the door to further discussion and a better understanding among family members.

Other areas where there can be differences of opinion involve the size, weight, age, and coat length of the pet. Where one family member prefers a puppy or kitten, adult dog or cat, others may look forward to a bird that talks, sings, or does tricks. Still others in the family may dream of living with an unusual or exotic pet, such as a reptile or amphibian.

The last section of a pet selection form can request that clients create a list with the top three to five types or breeds of animals they are considering, as well as any questions or concerns that were not mentioned on the form.

Pet selection reports

Although counselors may have handouts and information available during the session, clients may find it even more helpful to receive a list of magazines, websites, videos, and books they can use for additional referencing during their search. Counselors are positioned to direct owners to materials that provide reliable, scientifically accurate information in an easy-to-follow format. This will prevent owners accessing information of questionable quality.

After everyone has had an opportunity to review all the information provided, there are several possible outcomes. The counselor may recommend one or more of the pets that initially interested the client. Sometimes the animals suggested are not part of the owner's original list of candidates. However, if the counselor has carefully guided clients through the selection process, the recommended animals will not be unexpected. If the clients have indicated a specific breed or species in their consultation, it is important those animals be incorporated into the pet selection report. The counselor may indicate potential issues with those choices but should not exclude them from the report. Completely excluding or negating those possibilities could alienate the client. See Appendix 31 for an example of a pet selection report.

So that there is time to research unusual or unfamiliar types of pets, the counselor may set up another meeting, via an in-person appointment, phone or video call, or email report, in order to provide the client with more specific suggestions.

A client may decide, based upon solid, logical advice from the counselor, that this is not the right time or circumstances for a new pet to join the family. Even though it may cause initial disappointment, tactful counselors can turn the experience into a positive experience by helping owners understand how changes in lifestyle could make pet ownership possible in the future. Counselors can also offer to assist these clients when they are more prepared to select a pet.

Finding a source for obtaining the pet

Often families will take the information provided and begin to search for a pet on their own. The counselor can assist by providing various resources to aid in the search. A good suggestion can be to visit a dog or cat show and talk to competitors that have the breeds they are interested in. Counselors can format a list of breeders known to produce healthy problem-free litters. This client should interview the breeder, asking specific questions and be knowledgeable of acceptable answers. Speaking to breeders can be intimidating for a client. Instructing and empowering clients with a list of questions will help them be more confident during breeder interviews (see Appendix 20 for a Breeder interview questions form). Kennel clubs and feline associations often publish registries of breed rescues and breed associations. Specialty organizations for support and therapy dogs may have animals unsuitable for their purposes, but that would otherwise make an excellent pet.

Animal shelters and breed rescue can also be a source for the public. Adopting a pet can help save a life and provide owners with a feeling of self-satisfaction. However, there are some cautions for clients. Avoid facilities where there are obvious signs of overcrowding or lack of adequate medical treatment. Many shelters observe and assess adult dogs and cats for health, sociability, fear, and level of activity. This may help people to identify a pet that will be well suited to their lifestyle and needs.

Rescues often specialize in one type of purebred dog or cat, but there are rescues for special needs animals such as senior dogs and cats or small-size dogs. Many of these groups lack a physical shelter, and instead rely upon a network of trained members to "foster" animals in their homes. The pet receives individual attention and training while in the home. Additionally, information on how the animal interacts with children and other animals can be easily observed and relayed to the adopter. Potential adopters should anticipate both written and in-person interviews, and several meetings with the pet before the rescue will approve placement. Many rescues also require an in-home visit before finalizing any adoption paperwork. Groups that attempt to talk people into adopting a pet, lack up-to-date medical records, or refuse to allow a potential adopter into the facility, should be avoided.

Clients should be advised to avoid pet shops, puppy mills, and breeding farms. Animals from these locations are usually the by-product of mass breeding, poor husbandry practices, and inadequate management techniques.

- Clients should be advised to avoid pet shops, puppy mills, and breeding farms. Animals from these locations are usually the by-product of mass breeding, poor husbandry practices, and inadequate management techniques.

Other services can be included as part of the pet selection sessions. Counselors may offer to accompany clients who have located a potential new pet and assist in evaluating interactions with the animal. Veterinary clinics may offer a short post-purchase office visit where owners receive behavior counseling and set up follow-up medical care for their new pet.

Pet selection counseling is the first step in problem prevention and encourages creation of a strong human–animal bond. Pet selection counseling results in the selection of a more suitable pet, better educated owners, and establishment of a positive ongoing relationship between the client and the veterinary clinic that will carry through for the life of the pet and beyond.

- Pet selection counseling results in the selection of a more suitable pet, better educated owners, and establishment of a positive ongoing relationship between the client and the veterinary clinic that will carry through for the life of the pet and beyond.

Puppy socialization classes

For many years, little attention was given to any type of classes targeting young puppies. Most training was reserved for dogs six months of age or older and concentrated on skills for people interested in obedience competition. This attitude has changed as studies have increased our understanding of the impact early socialization and training can have on behavior.

In 1998, the National Council on Pet Population Study and Policy conducted a study exploring factors leading to behavior-related surrenders of dogs and cats. The owners of 1984 dogs that were surrendered to 12 shelters across the United States were asked to list up to five reasons why they were relinquishing their pets. Not surprisingly, behavior problems were listed as a reason for canine relinquishment more than any other single category.

Additionally, approximately 96% of all the dog owners reported that their dogs lacked any type of training. Owners who taught their canine companions at least some basic training skills were less likely to surrender them due to behavior problems.

Although this study was not directed at training, it helped provide some insight into the importance of training by suggesting that owners who work with their dogs to teach them even a few basic foundation skills and cues are less likely to give them up due to (mis)behavior.

In the July 2003 issue of the *Journal of the American Veterinary Medical Association*, a study was published that evaluated the association between retention of dogs in their adoptive homes, attendance at puppy socialization classes, and several other factors. The study involved 248 adult dogs that were adopted as puppies from a humane society. Owners were asked to complete a questionnaire regarding demographics, retention of the dogs in the homes, and the dogs' early learning events.

Dogs that participated in puppy socialization classes, wore head collars as puppies, responded to their owners' cues, and lived in homes without young children had higher retention rates. Analysis of the answers suggested several practices that veterinarians may recommend to enhance the likelihood that puppies will remain in their first homes. First on the list was enrolling 7 to 12-week-old puppies in early learning and socialization classes. Additionally, the lower retention rate of dogs in homes with children further emphasized the vital role technicians can play by helping owners develop realistic expectations and effective tools necessary to manage daily interactions between their children and dogs.

- Dogs that participated in puppy socialization classes, wore head collars as puppies, responded to their owners' cues, and lived in homes without young children had higher retention rates.

These studies highlight the significance of a well-run puppy class in providing multiple opportunities to educate owners on problem prevention, behavior management and, if necessary, modification techniques.

Experts in canine behavior now recommend that owners take advantage of the optimum periods of learning and enroll puppies in classes as early as eight weeks of age.

Puppy classes can provide benefits to the veterinary practice by promoting a successful union between clients and their pets early in the relationship. Handling and socialization skills introduced in puppy classes may help create a more cooperative and relaxed patient for examinations. When classes are held inside the veterinary clinic, they can become an excellent practice builder, and provide opportunities to recommend additional products and services beneficial both to the pet and the clinic. Similarly, puppy classes that are held in the veterinary practice can help develop a symbiotic relationship between the clinic and the instructor, regardless of whether that person is an employee of the clinic or teaches classes independently.

All animals that attend class must be healthy and remain current on all vaccinations, which results in pet owners returning to the practice for updated exams and preventive medical treatments. Conversely, the clinic provides a constant source of referrals for the instructor. Not only can puppy classes provide veterinary technicians with a supplementary source of income, but they can also provide a much needed stress relief from the life and death situations encountered every day in the veterinary hospital. The veterinary technicians involved in puppy socialization classes will experience a boost in their own morale. Puppy class is about enhancing the bond between a puppy and its owners at a time when the owners are usually still excited with the new puppy.

Logistics

There are multiple key components involved in developing and implementing a puppy class, including the logistics of a puppy class. The logistics of a puppy class involve deciding on a location for class, identifying competent instructors, selecting criteria for canine and human participants, deciding on a class style, and implementing strategies to minimize health risks.

Location

The ideal location should be climate-controlled, easy to sanitize, puppy- and escape-proof, easily dividable, and free of interruptions.

An indoor, climate-controlled facility is preferred because outdoor locations will cause delays in class sessions due to weather. As the goal is for the class to be completed during a short window of time (the socialization period), delays in class would be problematic.

Similarly, outdoor locations can be difficult to sanitize properly. Porous surfaces such as grass, dirt, mulch, or carpet cannot be effectively sanitized, whereas nonporous surfaces are easily disinfected. If other dogs have been in the facility, then the puppy class location should be disinfected prior to class. Accidents (urine or stool) during class should be cleaned with disposable towels and a parvocidal disinfectant to minimize contamination.

In a puppy socialization class there may be one or two short off-leash play sessions. Classes need to be held in a facility or room that can be secured so as to prevent accidental escapes. Either the doors to the facility should be locked or the room should be secured with sturdy gates (Figure 7.19).

With large classes (more than six puppies) the ability to divide the room provides the instructor with the ability to maintain an appropriate setting for puppy class. Barriers and divisions reduce the risk of overstimulation of the puppies. Gates, exercise pens, and other barriers can be used to divide the room and group the puppies appropriately.

Instructors should be able to see the clients and puppies easily. The space should provide enough seating for all human participants. There will need to be enough room for exploration areas, a play area, and an exercise pen.

The novelty of the environment, people, and other puppies will prove to be highly distracting to the puppies and their human counterparts as well. All

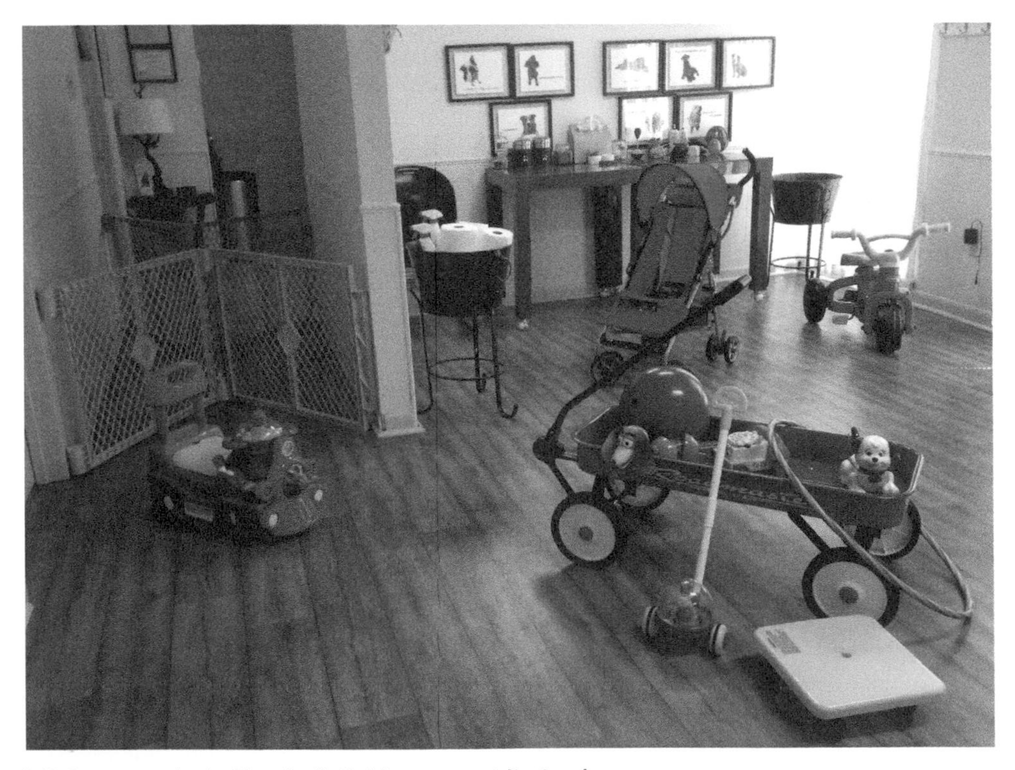

Figure 7.19 Secure area that is able to be divided for puppy socialization class.

other distractions should be minimized. A location that is free of disruptions during the class time is imperative. In a training facility, other classes should not be held in the same area simultaneously. In a veterinary hospital, puppy classes can be offered after hours or in a nonactive area of the hospital.

Instructor characteristics

Competent, knowledgeable instructors are one of the most important requirements for class. Instructors should have a strong understanding of learning theory, canine body language, and puppy growth and development. They must also possess excellent communication skills.

Instructors should demonstrate a well-versed understanding of learning theory. Although it may not be important for clients to have an extensive vocabulary of official terminology, instructors must be able to explain the basic concepts in an easy to understand format. This means it is imperative for technicians to be well informed on the differences between classical conditioning (learning by association) and operant conditioning (learning by consequences) (see Chapter 6).

Dogs communicate with each other predominantly through movement and body postures. Primates (including humans) rely primarily on vocalization as a way of communication. This difference in styles is one reason for the misunderstanding that commonly occurs in owner-pet interactions. A puppy class instructor should be knowledgeable about canine body language and be able to teach pet owners how to interpret dog communication. An instructor who is familiar with basic canine body postures is able to help owners recognize potential emotional signs of stress and fear.

Understanding the growth and developmental stages of puppies allows instructors to structure classes that make the greatest impact in the shortest amount of time. Science has recognized that there are multiple sensitive periods that puppies pass through as they mature. The most significant of these periods occurs between 3 and 12 weeks of age. During this period, puppies learn behaviors that allow them to communicate as adult dogs and are developmentally ready to meet and interact with other species, including people. Puppies exposed to increasingly complex enrichment during this period tend to adapt better to changes as they mature.

An appropriate instructor to puppy ratio should also be considered. Ideally, puppy classes should have one instructor or assistant per three or four puppies. This allows for individual guidance during exploration and exposure activities in class.

Owners, as a group, have very diverse needs that dictate what they are willing and able to do when training their dogs. Each has different physical abilities and learning styles that must be considered.

Physical factors that affect an owner's ability to perform training exercises include age, health, and physical limitations. Classes should be structured to meet the needs of all students. This may entail using an elevated platform to teach "sits" and "downs" for owners who are in wheelchairs or unable to get down on the floor with their dogs.

Individuals tend to rely upon specific approaches when learning. Visual learners retain information best by observation. Auditory learners rely upon hearing what is said. Tactile/kinesthetic learners learn through moving, doing, and touching. The best classes incorporate all the above methods in each session.

It is important to adopt teaching methods that provide owners with a variety of opportunities to learn, practice, and perfect their skills. As a rule of thumb, a well-structured class is one where individuals are encouraged to use their preferred learning styles, instructional activities are designed to appeal to a variety of different learning styles, and evaluation of successful owner education takes into account the different learning styles.

Participant characteristics

When developing a puppy socialization class, guidelines for the participants, canine and human, are necessary to provide an environment conducive to socialization.

What puppies will be accepted into classes? What is the minimum and maximum age for a class? What vaccinations will be required for each puppy prior to starting class? What safeguards will be implemented to verify the health of new puppies entering classes and protect the health of puppies currently attending classes?

There is much discussion about the safest age for a puppy to begin class. However, in an open letter, the late R.K. Anderson DVM, Diplomate ACVB and ACVPM, Professor and Director Emeritus, Animal Behavior Clinic and Center to Study Human/Animal Relationships and Environments University of Minnesota, encouraged veterinarians and puppy owners to make socialization in class a first priority, beginning about eight weeks of age and continuing through 12 weeks. See Appendices 32 and 33 for letters from Purdue University and Dr. R.K. Anderson regarding the recommendations for early puppy socialization classes.

Both letters noted above address concerns about health issues. Dr. Anderson's letter states, "Experience and epidemiologic data support the relative safety and lack of transmission of disease in these puppy socialization classes over the past 10 years in many parts of the United States." He further states that the risk of a puppy dying from distemper or parvovirus disease is much less than the risk of euthanasia due to a behavior problem. Similarly, studies indicate healthy puppies are at low risk of contracting infectious disease with proper socialization if they are actively engaged in a vaccination program and born from healthy and properly vaccinated mothers (De Cramer et al. 2011; Stepida et al. 2013). In one multicenter study, puppies ≤16 weeks that attended socialization classes were at no greater risk of contracting parvovirus than those that did not attend classes (Stepida et al. 2013).

- Dr. Anderson's letter states, "Experience and epidemiologic data support the relative safety and lack of transmission of disease in these puppy socialization classes over the past 10 years in many parts of the United States." He further states that the risk of a puppy dying from distemper or parvovirus disease is much less than the risk of euthanasia due to a behavior problem.

Based upon current available information, many classes use the following guidelines for accepting puppies into class: Puppies are required to be at least eight weeks of age and have had a minimum set of Distemper–Adenovirus 2–Parvo and Bordatella vaccinations prior to attending class. Furthermore, owners must provide proof of ongoing preventive veterinary care throughout the class.

Puppies who attend class should be in their socialization period (between 7 and 12 weeks when starting class). The puppies need to have recently been examined by a veterinarian, in an active vaccine protocol, and considered healthy for puppy class. Ideally the puppy should have been in its current home for a minimum of 10 days prior to starting class. Ten days is the incubation period for many viruses. If the puppy had exposure before being obtained by their current owners, signs of illness should be evident within 10 days.

Puppy classes focus on the socialization of young puppies and the education of new puppy parents. Consequently, there are some limitations associated with a puppy socialization class. The tendency to allow older puppies (older than 12 weeks when starting the class) into a socialization class can negatively affect the older puppy and other participants. However, the information provided in a puppy socialization class can be valuable for all dog owners, regardless of the dog's age. The instructor may consider allowing the owners to audit the class (attend without the puppy). Another option would be to have them attend with the puppy (should be under 4.5 months old), but during off-leash play time the puppy is managed in another area. This option would depend on the individual puppy and whether the owners are able to successfully manage the puppy in class.

Puppy classes are not designed to address abnormal behaviors, including profound fears, phobias, aggression, or excessive reactivity. A puppy showing signs of a behavior disorder can still benefit from attendance in a puppy socialization class, as long as the puppy can be managed in a way that is not disruptive to the class and does not negatively affect the experience of the other puppies in the class. "Problem puppies" should also be enjoying the class and have positive experiences. If a puppy is in its socialization period and is showing profound signs of fear, failing to acclimate to the situation, excessively reactive or disruptive, then the puppy is not in an appropriate setting for learning nor is the puppy enjoying the class. A referral for intervention services would be indicated.

In regard to the human participants in puppy class, the entire family should be encouraged to attend. It is recommended that anyone under 18 years of age be accompanied by an adult and children under 8 should have two adults present (one to supervise the children and one to supervise the puppy).

Class style

Although some basic cues are taught during puppy classes, the emphasis at this point is not on training skills, but on the crucial skills of socialization, problem prevention, and behavior solutions.

Conventional series-style puppy classes are the most common and easiest to manage. They have a definite beginning and end date. However, owners who miss the start of a session must wait until the next one begins, which may result in loss of important socialization time. Additionally, puppies are generally in class with the same puppies throughout the entire session and do not have the advantage of socializing with new puppies entering the class.

A rotational style of class has become increasingly popular and is better able to meet the needs of this time-sensitive experience. Open enrollment classes offer flexibility as puppies can enter the classes at any time but require excellent organizational skills to keep track of student progress. As puppies can begin at any time, new puppies are constantly being introduced to the group, which provides the greatest impact.

Disease prevention

Minimizing the risk of infection is crucial for the safety of the puppies. Besides the health and vaccine requirements previously recommended, as each puppy arrives for class, the instructors should take a brief moment to greet the puppy and owner. While interacting with the puppy, the instructor should note the following:

- Mental state: bright, alert, responsive, and active.
- Mucous membranes: gums and tongue are pink.
- Eyes, ears, nose, throat (airway): free from mucopurulent eye or nasal discharge and not sneezing or coughing.
- Tail and rear end: coat free of fecal staining (possibly from diarrhea).
- Skin and coat: no evidence of hair loss, free of crusty skin lesions, or external parasites (fleas/ticks).

In addition to a brief examination of each puppy upon arrival, the following guidelines will minimize the risk of contamination:

- Veterinary staff who have been working with healthy or ill animals all day should change clothes and shoes before class.
- Disinfect surface areas before and after each class with an appropriate disinfectant which is effective against parvovirus. This is especially important if other dog activities occur in the facility, or it is a veterinary hospital. An accelerated hydrogen peroxide product is preferred as they have low odor, are effective germicides, and are generally considered safer than many other disinfectants.
- Wash any food storage items after each use (dishwasher-safe items should be run through a dishwasher cycle if possible). Better yet, use disposable food storage toys (such as yogurt cups, cottage cheese containers, or empty syringe casings) and dispose of them after use.
- Properly clean up puppy accidents (stool or urine).
  - Remove solid waste and spray with disinfectant and wipe up with disposable or washable towels.

By following the above guidelines, the risk of spreading infectious diseases is minimized.

Puppy socialization class format

A high-quality puppy socialization class will have many components, including a people-only orientation class, short play sessions, positive exposure to sights, sounds, and novelty, preventive exercises, puppy parenting tips, and introduction to positive reinforcement training.

- A high-quality puppy socialization class will have many components, including a people-only orientation class, short play sessions, positive exposure to sights, sounds, and novelty, preventive exercises, puppy parenting tips, and introduction to positive reinforcement training.

Orientation

Providing a mandatory orientation prior to attendance in socialization classes will minimize any surprises for the owner as well as the instructor. Orientation prepares the puppy parent for class and should be a prerequisite to attending socialization classes. It allows for the human participants to learn about what to expect in puppy class. Because orientation is a human-only class (puppies stay home), puppy parents can learn without the distraction of their puppy (Figure 7.20). Providing an online orientation class or a recorded video orientation for clients to complete prior to their first class, can save the instructor time and add convenience for the client.

Puppy play sessions

Controlled, off-leash short play sessions (five minutes or less) with other puppies in a secure environment allow young puppies to familiarize themselves with a variety of different breeds of dogs. Well-organized group play is the benchmark of a good puppy class. It provides a situation where puppies learn how to properly interact with other puppies and begin to learn the vital skill of bite

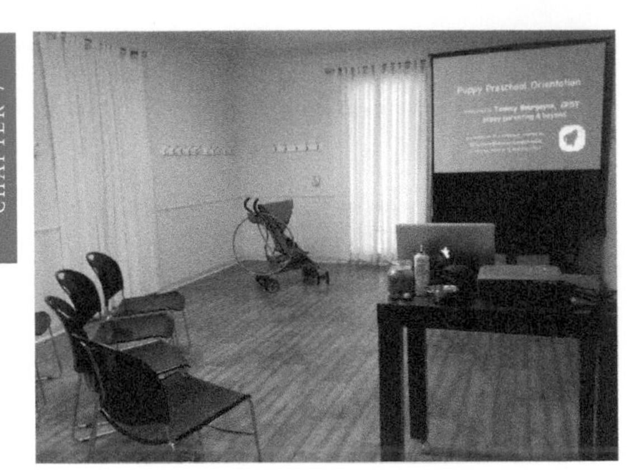

Figure 7.20 Weekly puppy class orientation.

inhibition. In some instances, it is possible to observe giant-size puppies, toy breeds, and many sizes in between playfully interacting together. However, it is usually suggested to divide very small and larger breed puppies to prevent risk of injury. Instructors take advantage of the play time to help owners understand how to interpret what the puppies body postures signify.

Puppies teach each other about bite inhibition and the value of appropriate play behavior. Owners often call their puppies away from play to give them a treat and then release them back to play. In this way the puppy learns that play does not always end when called by the owner.

Play sessions are not intended to be a free-for-all. First-time puppies often hang back during play sessions and some may even attempt to hide. Instructors should strive to help new puppies become comfortable. Puppies showing signs of fear and prolonged reluctance may be placed in a separate play group where they acclimate to the environment slowly. An alternate suggestion is to partition off a small area using dividers or exercise pens. The shy puppy can then observe and interact with the group more slowly (Box 7.4).

BOX 7.4: COMPONENTS OF NORMAL PLAY

- Role reversal.
  - Puppies take turns being chased or chasing, being on the bottom and being on top.
  - It is not just one puppy "winning" all the time.
- Asking for more.
  - When there is a break in the play, the puppy that was on the bottom or being chased asks for more by trying to re-engage the other puppy.
- Play can be rough and vocal.
  - They might tumble around and bite at each other's legs or neck.
  - Some puppies are vocal while playing and will bark and growl.
- High-pitched yips or screams are a sign of pain or fear and can be normal communication.
- Look at the body language of the puppy.
  - Is the body relaxed or tense?
  - Are all participants having fun?
- Self-regulated.
  - Puppies are able to adjust the play on their own.
  - Ebb and flow of activity level.
- Some running/chasing or wrestling.
- Followed by a short break and a role reversal.

Source: From the course *Puppy Start Right for Instructors* with permission from Kenneth Martin, DVM, DACVB, and Debbie Martin, RVT, VTS (Behavior).

Occasionally you will encounter puppies in the socialization period that lack appropriate communication skills or the ability to self-regulate play. This could be due to lack of play during primary socialization, early removal from the litter, genetic predisposition, or learning.

With puppies in their socialization period, it is best to let them learn how to communicate with each other on their own. Exposure to a variety of play styles and breeds of dogs during the socialization period is important for puppies to learn that not all puppies play the same. Allowing a puppy to appropriately communicate (with conflict/calming signals or even a little reprimand – i.e. show of teeth, yip, grumble) to another puppy that its play style is not appropriate is a life skill that should be developed during this time. Ideally, puppy class instructors should try to let the puppies handle it on their own and should avoid frequent interventions.

However, there will be times when the instructor should intervene. According to *Puppy Start Right for Instructors* (Martin and Martin 2012), puppy play should be interrupted when the following conditions occur:

- The target puppy is fearful, does not recover and begin to solicit play, or keeps trying to escape or hide.
- The instigator of play does not reciprocate the message from the target puppy.

- Other puppies are showing signs of fear even when not involved in the play. Perhaps the play is vocal or involves chase and the observer puppies are concerned and not recovering.
- The instructor is unsure if all the puppies are enjoying the play because role reversal has not happened for a while and the "underdog" might or might not be having fun.
- Puppies are having trouble self-regulating; they are having fun but there is no slow-down period.

Just as important, or even more important, is how play is interrupted. The goal with an interruption in play is to promote learning and decrease tension. The recommended technique is using distraction. A treat or squeaky toy can be placed in front of the instigator's nose to get his attention. He can then be lured away from the other puppy and rewarded with a food treat. The puppy should be allowed to return to play. The goal is to distract the puppies in a non-confrontational manner in order to calm down the play session.

- The goal with an interruption in play is to promote learning and decrease tension.

Interruption techniques that should be avoided include verbal reprimands, grabbing the puppy's collar or picking it up. These techniques do not provide a positive learning experience for the puppies.

Verbal reprimands such as an "Ahh" or "No" will only add tension to the situation and can cause a negative association with play. All the puppies (even the ones not involved) learn, "When I interact with other puppies, humans fuss. Therefore, other dogs are not fun."

Grabbing the puppy by the collar will increase tension and frustration, and should be avoided even if the collar grab is followed with a treat. This method could work if the puppy had a long learning history (several months) outside of the play context that collar grabs are great. This will not be the case in a puppy class because the puppies are only two to three months old.

Picking the puppy up to interrupt play should be discouraged because when it is used repetitively to interrupt play, this can be a negative learning experience associated with people. Puppies may learn to avoid people in order to avoid being picked up. Picking the puppy up is likely to increase tension and frustration and could potentially reinforce an unwanted emotional response, such as fear or aggression. People providing "back up" will not teach the puppy how to interact appropriately in these contexts. The exception to this rule is if there is truly abnormal behavior occurring and there is concern about injury to a puppy. Video 7.13 on the companion website demonstrates appropriate ways to interrupt play between young puppies.

If after attempting to interrupt the play between two puppies, the puppies return to inappropriate play again right away, it will be necessary to implement some management. Using an exercise pen for the instigator of the play will allow the target (other) puppy to engage in play with the other puppies in class. To make the exercise pen a positive experience for the puppy, the owner or an assistant should stand next to the pen and hand the puppy a small treat every few seconds (especially when other puppies come near).

Exploration and exposure

A large part of puppy class should be devoted to teaching owners how to provide exposure to a variety of novel environments, people, objects, surfaces, and sounds in a fun and positive manner.

Instructors should teach clients to utilize desensitization by gradually exposing their puppy to novelty in combination with positive reinforcement, through the liberal use of treats, to facilitate pleasant conditioned emotional responses. The puppy should be acclimated to a new environment by staying clear of the "action" when first arriving. Owners need to be proactive; they should assume the puppy could be afraid of a new person, object, or environment and use treats liberally to prevent a fear response and make a positive association from the start. Similarly, the owner should control what the puppy learns and keep experiences positive. This is accomplished by teaching owners how to read their puppy's body language and be the puppy's advocate.

Setting up exploration and exposure stations in puppy class allows the instructor to coach the client in developing these skills (Figure 7.21). Video 7.14 illustrates exploration of novel items during puppy class. Puppy owners learn to work at their dog's pace, attend to body language indicators of fear or apprehension, and proactively increase distance before adding something like sound or movement.

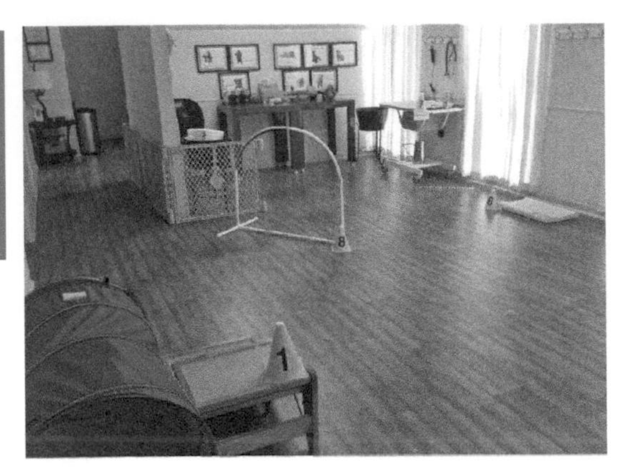

Figure 7.21 Exploration stations set up for a puppy socialization class.

Preventive exercises

The importance of preventive exercises has already been discussed in detail in an earlier section of this chapter. Preventive exercises to be taught and practiced in a puppy socialization class should include crate training and independence exercises, food bowl prevention, how to play with people, and handling and restraint exercises, including the collar game (Figure 7.22). Video 7.15 on the companion website shows a quick progression of the steps in teaching the collar game. Video 7.16 illustrates working on handling and restraint with a puppy during puppy class. The trainer does the handling, marks with a click, and the owner brings a treat to the dog.

Puppy parenting tips

Puppy class should help to educate owners on normal canine body language, learning, and positive behavior solutions. Typical topics to be covered would include play biting and mouthing, elimination training, digging, stealing items, chewing, and jumping.

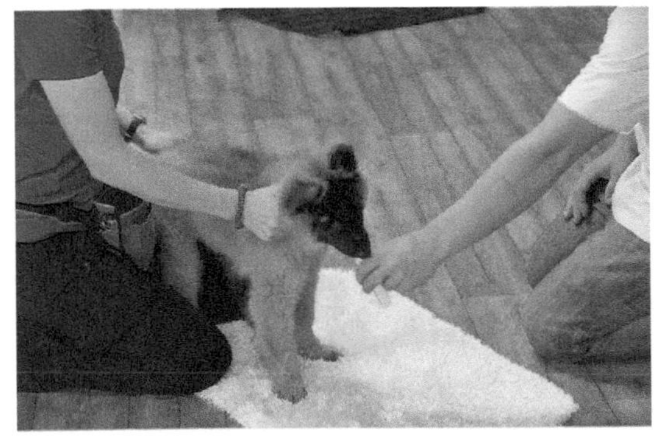

Figure 7.22 A puppy receiving treats from its owner while the instructor demonstrates gently holding the puppy's collar.

Introduction to positive reinforcement training

Although not a training class, puppy socialization class should introduce owners to positive reinforcement training techniques. Beginning to teach attention (eye contact), targeting, sit, come when called, and leash manners with clicker training gets puppies and owners prepped for developing these skills further with additional classes.

For an example of a curriculum for a five-week puppy socialization class, see Appendix 34: Sample puppy socialization class curriculum.

Kitten classes

Veterinarians and owners have long recognized the many advantages of attending classes with puppies. However, it has become equally accepted that there is a similar benefit for kittens enrolled in classes.

Kittens that are handled by humans early in life tend to become easier to handle as adults. When kittens also receive ongoing socialization to people, dogs, and other animals (including other cats), they are able to grow into well-adjusted felines and may become very social family members. Kitten classes provide many of the same benefits as puppy classes. Owners learn important aspects of how to raise a healthy kitten, including how to prevent undesired behaviors, understanding what is normal behavior, and how to redirect unwanted behaviors in an acceptable direction. Single kittens or kittens that are hand-raised have an opportunity to interact with other kittens of their own age. Classes also help kittens learn that travel in the cat carrier is not always a bad thing. The ultimate goal of all these classes is to strengthen the human–animal bond through education and training. Additionally, socialization classes help promote a positive relationship between the veterinary clinic and the cat, which results in a more relaxed and compliant patient during future visits.

The time period during which kittens most benefit from socialization and learning is shorter than that of puppies. In his article "Developmental behaviour in kittens and puppies; puppy and kitten classes for problem prevention," Peter F. Neville DHc BSc (Hons), states "With a kitten, the time available for providing adequate psychological development in terms of producing a friendly pet is even shorter. Though evolved to be a solitary predator, a home bred kitten is destined to transfer the social bond it has with its mother to form a lifelong strong social tie with its new owners. If kittens aren't handled by at least four people in their maternal home before they reach the age of eight weeks, the chances of being able to transfer that bond reduce almost with every day. The critical difference for kitten owners is that if their kitten has not been raised in the right environment, it may be too late by the time they take on their pet at 12 weeks of age, while the puppy owner will still have a chance up to about 20 weeks to make up for any shortfalls in the early environment."

Studies have demonstrated that kittens held and lightly stroked during the first few weeks of life experience greater behavior and physical development than littermates not handled. Attending a kitten class during the early part of their lives takes advantage of their adaptability.

Classes for kittens are not structured in the same way as puppy classes. Kitten classes generally only last two or three weeks and most experts agree that the kittens in class should never be older than 14 weeks of age. After kittens reach 14 weeks of age, they are more likely to fight than play. It is advisable to encourage owners with kittens older than 14 weeks of age to attend the class, but without bringing their kitten.

Based upon current available information, many classes use the following guidelines for accepting kittens into class: kittens are required to be at least eight weeks of age, have lived in the home for a minimum of seven days and have written proof of FVRCP vaccine (feline rhinotracheitis virus, calicivirus, and panleukopenia) ≥10 days prior to first class. They must also be free of all internal and external parasites and have no signs of upper respiratory infection.

Just as with puppies, kitten owners must provide proof of ongoing preventive veterinary care throughout the class. Although there is no way to give a 100% guarantee of health, these requirements provide the best possibility of ensuring only healthy kittens attend class. Additionally, most experts agree that pets are more likely to lose their homes due to behavior problems, than become ill at a kitten class.

Other considerations include where will kitten classes be held? Many classes are held in the veterinary clinic so that kittens can associate a visit to the doctor as a positive experience. However, classes can be held in any secure area. Rooms should be large enough to place equipment and comfortably seat owners, yet small enough so instructors are able to restrict the kittens' movements. The classroom area must be easily cleaned and disinfected between sessions. A variety of small easy-to-transport supplies are essential for classes. Many can be bought ready to use, or with a little imagination can be created from everyday items around the house. They include the following:

- scratching posts – vertical and horizontal
- empty cardboard boxes stacked so that kittens can hide inside or jump onto during play
- a variety of toys (PVC piping or other tubing that can be used as a tunnel, readymade cat tunnels, etc.)
- ping-pong balls inside a shallow tub
- fishing pole-type toys
- interactive toys such as Cat Tracks, food-stuffed Kong toys
- cat baskets or kennels (various types and sizes)
- litter boxes with a variety of different litter.

Additionally, it is wise for instructors to provide a synthetic calming pheromone spray or diffuser in the room.

Classes usually accommodate three to five kittens per session so there are adequate opportunities for instructors to observe and manage the kittens. The size can be increased if there are additional assistants but should still be limited to no more than 10.

Although some basic skills are taught, the main emphasis of this class is to teach owners. Actual training should be limited to short, two-to-four-minute increments with rest and play in between each session. Patience and consistency are the elements to successful learning as each kitten has its own individual rate of learning new skills.

During the weekly kitten classes, instructors typically include play sessions, body handling, name recognition, introduction to other pets, introduction to a harness and leash, clicker training basic behaviors, walking on leash, and teaching owners how to play with the kitten. Discussions about the importance of environmental enrichment at home, basic behavior, and behavior solutions can be incorporated into the class, but if owners report out-of-the-ordinary or severe challenges, it is important to refer them to a qualified behavior specialist for a consultation. For a sample of a two-week kitten class curriculum see Appendix 35.

Juvenile/adolescent/adult canine classes

Socialization and exposure are active and lifelong processes. If a puppy parent were to stop socializing a puppy at three months of age, the puppy would be more likely to become fearful as an adolescent dog. It is much more difficult to socialize a puppy after three months of age without early positive foundation memories. As the puppy developmentally becomes more suspicious of novelty, positive exposure is probably equally important as during the socialization period. Even the well-socialized young puppy might regress if positive exposure does not continue into adolescence. After completion of a puppy socialization class, young dogs should enroll in a class designed for juvenile and adolescent dogs.

- Even the well-socialized young puppy might regress if positive exposure does not continue into adolescence.

The juvenile stage in a dog's development is from about three to six months of age. The adolescence stage is from approximately six months to two years of age. This timing can vary with individual dogs. The adolescence period is the most trying time behaviorally for dog owners. It is also an important time to offer clients additional support to keep these dogs mentally and physically stimulated. Offering adolescent dog training classes is a vital service that can prevent owners from relinquishing their pet during this difficult stage. Veterinary behavior technicians can play an important part in designing and teaching adolescent dog training classes.

Technicians and other staff members who are interested in teaching classes will want to acquire the proper knowledge, skills, and experience from reputable organizations (see Chapter 1).

Clinics offering classes will need to have ample space with secure flooring. Some may have an appropriate area on the premises. If a room is not available, renting space elsewhere in the community should be considered. Church halls, community recreation halls, and picnic shelters are a few options that could be considered. The clinic will need to provide a certificate of insurance when offering classes outside the facility.

When designing a program the family pet and average owner should be kept in mind. The class format should be loaded with practical and easy-to-accomplish exercises. Real-life role playing is valuable to help owners visualize what they should be doing at home. The juvenile/adolescent/adult dog classes should continue to provide exploration and exposure opportunities to novelty, incorporate problem prevention and behavior solutions exercises, and build on the foundation training skills that have been started in puppy socialization class. The following foundation skills are important for a young dog to learn to help owners communicate effectively with the adolescent canine:

- Attention (look at the owner): A high rate of reinforcement for paying attention to the owner will make this a favorite activity for the dog. Building in the ability to focus on the handler even in the face of distractions requires a detailed training plan designed to gradually introduce distraction while keeping the dog successful. Video 7.17 on the companion website shows a puppy learning about the clicker and also learning that offering eye contact will earn him a treat. This is the beginning stage of teaching an attention or eye contact cue.
- Look (look at something in the environment but no need to explore it): It is unrealistic to think that dogs can tune out every little distraction. People are unable to do this. We hear a sound or see someone coming into the training class and it is natural for us to attend to it. Dogs are no different. The more the owners try to make their dog ignore everything, the more likely that conflict and frustration between the owner and dog will develop. By creating a cue that is the opposite of attention, the owner is able to flip-flop back and forth from attention and look, thus, in the end, making for a more attentive dog and a less frustrated owner. Video 7.18 on the companion website illustrates teaching the Look (at that) cue.
- Settle on a mat: This foundation behavior has many uses. Once the behavior has been taught, the dog can be cued to settle on his mat while the owner is cooking, eating, or watching TV, and when visitors arrive at the door: any time the owners need the dog to be at a distance from them. This cue provides an alternative to jumping on people, bolting out the door, begging, or stealing food off the counter.
- Target: Teaching the dog to touch its nose to the owner's hand when cued provides for a way to quickly teach a "come when called." By providing a specific target behavior (touch the owner's hand), the dog is clear about what is expected.

This behavior is first taught up close and gradually the owner cues the behavior from further away. A nose touch to hand target behavior can also be used to refocus or direct the dog in the face of distractions. Targeting can be a quick way to jump start a new behavior such as teaching a spin, over or under an object, or even to walk by the owner's side. Video 7.19 on the companion website shows teaching this behavior, adding a verbal cue, and using the behavior out on a walk.

- Loose leash walking: This is a valuable skill that does not come naturally to dogs. The importance of routine walks for mental and physical stimulation has been discussed earlier in this chapter. If walking the dog is unbearable because it pulls, the owner is less likely to take it for routine walks. Juvenile and adolescent classes should focus on making this a fun and enjoyable behavior for the dog and the owner. A management tool, such as a front clip harness or head collar, may be necessary initially for some dogs while the owner works on making the loose leash walking more reliable. Video 7.20 on the companion website demonstrates a puppy learning about loose leash walking. Notice the high rate of reinforcement (one step = one treat) at the beginning. After several repetitions, the trainer starts to take a few steps before marking and treating. She takes mini breaks by running backward and having the puppy follow her before resetting for another repetition.
- Greeting behaviors and door manners: As discussed in the problem prevention section, dogs naturally want to greet people by jumping up toward their face. This is an innate behavior that is often reinforced. Juvenile and adolescent dog classes should help provide owners with the skills to teach appropriate alternatives to jumping. Skills that could be taught include teaching the dog that the sound of a doorbell or knock is the cue to settle on its bed and training the dog that sitting (instead of jumping) is reinforced. Exercises to practice these skills with a variety of people in the class allows for further socialization at the same time.

The clicker is the ideal training tool when teaching new behaviors or improving an existing behavior. Many dogs are simply confused by their owner's erratic way of communicating. People use their voices for many things, where the clicker is reserved only for the dog. The precision of the clicker to mark a behavior allows for clear communication between the dog and the owner. Clicker training is discussed in more detail in Chapter 9.

The class format could be either a traditional linear series with clients signing up for a set of classes that has a start and end date, or a modular format with an open enrollment that provides for more flexibility.

For the linear series, specific exercises are introduced and practiced each week. Each consecutive class builds on the exercises from the previous week. The same students and dogs complete the class together, usually over a six- to eight-week period.

Modular classes take more planning and organization, but they allow for client convenience and flexibility. The client prepays for a set number of classes; the more they buy the cheaper the per-class cost. Weekly classes are designed around skills (coming when called, loose leash walking, manners at the door, etc.) and the clients can choose which classes they take. Some trainers will have a beginner, intermediate, and advanced level for each skill (i.e. beginner level "come when called" is on Monday at 7 p.m., intermediate level "come when called" is on Monday at 8 p.m.). However, to maximize class size, offering the skill and combining all levels in one class has some advantages for the client as well. The beginner students see the advanced dogs working and it inspires them to train their own dog. The advanced dogs are provided with the distraction of the more unruly beginner dogs. With this type of modular class, stations are set up with specific exercises including beginner, intermediate, and advanced instructions. The clients work at their dog's level and the instructor provides guidance and feedback. During the class they rotate through the various stations to work on several different exercises associated with the skill.

Instructor to student ratio is very important in adolescent and adult dog training. The dogs tend to be more excitable and easily distracted. Many dogs also experience a social regression during adolescence, which can pose some difficulties. Instructors and assistants must be prepared to provide some individual attention if a student is having difficulty mastering the exercises. Having barriers and dividers provides an environment that is conducive to learning because distractions can be minimized (Figure 7.23). Three students per instructor/assistant is ideal.

Whether teaching modular classes or linear classes, the first session should be an orientation

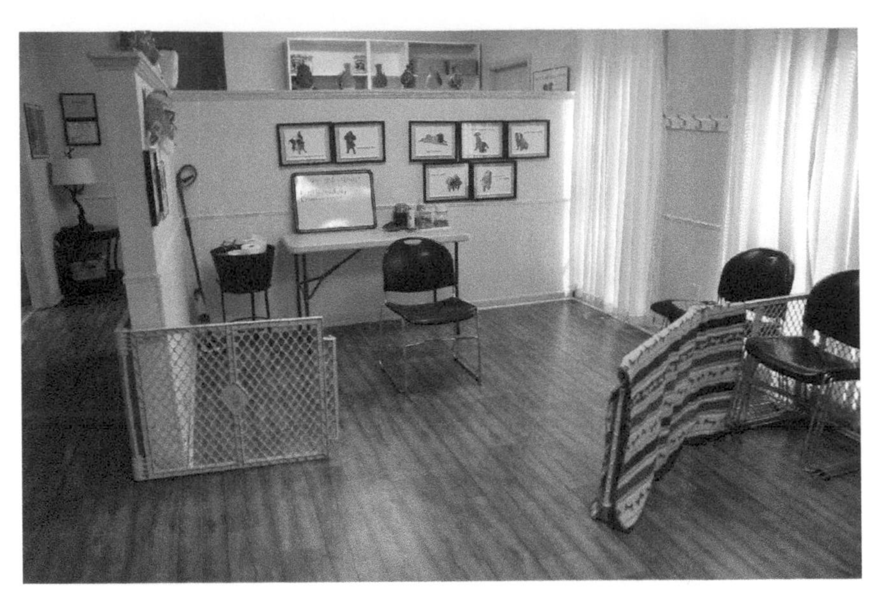

Figure 7.23 Separate training station and barriers to help minimize distraction in a group class.

without the dogs. This prerequisite may have been met with attending a puppy socialization orientation and completing a socialization series. New clients will need to be provided with general instructions and learn their own training skill basics without the distraction of the dogs being present.

Class dynamics need to be carefully managed in adolescent and adult dog classes. Dogs may range from well-socialized alumni of a puppy program to dogs who are in the group environment for the first time. Both situations pose different challenges.

Senior/geriatric canine classes

The aging dog can benefit from group classes as well. A class full of young active dogs learning foundation skills is less likely to meet the needs of a senior or geriatric dog and his owner. The behavior technician can be instrumental in designing and providing classes that take into consideration the difference in activity level of the senior dog. Many dogs develop arthritis as they age and engaging in a training class that requires frequent sitting or mobile activities could be uncomfortable for the older dog. However, mental stimulation, social interactions, and moderate physical activity are important to prevent cognitive and physical decline in older dogs. A senior/geriatric class can be centered around teaching clients how to massage their dogs, provide puzzle-type toys for mental stimulation (see Video 7.2), teaching the dogs to "stretch" on cue, and also educate owners regarding clinical signs for canine cognitive dysfunction syndrome (DISHAAL: **D**isorientation, **I**nteraction changes, **S**leep–wake cycle changes, **H**ouse soiling, **A**ctivity changes, **A**nxiety, **L**earning and memory).

Fun visits and formal training sessions for veterinary experiences

Another behavioral service the veterinary technician can be instrumental in implementing is teaching pets to be relaxed and calm with veterinary care. Providing this service in your veterinary hospital, applies the training in the very context veterinary care will take place for the pet. There are many benefits to offering fun visits and formal training sessions for veterinary experiences (Box 7.5). A fun visit, also sometimes referred to as a happy visit, refers to the pet visiting your hospital just for fun. No veterinary procedures are performed. Kitten and puppy classes in the veterinary hospital could be considered a type of fun visits. However, once the dog/cat has graduated from the class, it is equally as important that they continue to return to the veterinary hospital for good experiences. This helps build a positive emotional response and memories with the facility. Fun visits are usually informal and does not require an appointment with the specially trained team member. During a fun visit, the pet should get treats in areas of the hospital such as the lobby, on the scale, or in an exam room and plays with the owner and possibly veterinary team members. See Appendix 21 and 22 for handouts from Fear Free Pets, LLC providing clients with guidance on how to successfully navigate a fun visit with their dog or cat. The species-specific scavenger hunt cards include an explanation of the purpose of fun visits and provides specific instructions to make the visit a Fear Free® experience for the pet (see Chapter 8). The scavenger hunt card can also serve to educate clients about the Fear Free techniques you have implemented in your hospital, such as a non-slip surface on the scale, aromatherapy, acoustic therapy, special lighting, or scrub colors. Send home the card with kitten and puppy owners at the first visit and encourage them to complete the card prior to the next scheduled visit. For an extra incentive, have clients submit completed cards to be entered into a monthly or quarterly drawing for a discount on a service or product you offer at your hospital. You might collaborate with a distributor to offer a free product in the drawing.

BOX 7.5: SOME OF THE MANY BENEFITS OF OFFERING FUN AND VICTORY VISITS IN THE VETERINARY HOSPITAL

- They can help prevent or decrease fear, anxiety, and stress in patients coming to your hospital.
- Your clients and their pets become bonded to your hospital and your team members.
- Fun and victory visits can be a direct or indirect revenue source. If you are charging for victory visits, they will become an additional revenue source. Even fun visits have the potential to increase revenue, as the client may purchase something while visiting the hospital.
- Long term, if the pet is more comfortable coming to your hospital, the owners will visit more often for care.
- Last but not least, your job is easier because you have happy patients and clients.

In contrast, formal training for veterinary experiences visits, also known as victory visits or cooperative care visits, are scheduled sessions that will involve a qualified team member. These sessions might be set up as short private sessions. To maximize efficiency, they could be scheduled during a

Table 7.13 Comparison of fun versus victory visits.

Fun visits	Victory visits
Less structured	Structured
Preventive service	Preventive and/or intervention service
Unscheduled	Scheduled
No charge	Charged
	Private, semi-private, or group sessions

block of time each week. For example, every Tuesday from 12 to 2 p.m. a victory visit is available every 20 minutes. Or they can be offered as a group class provided after hours that focuses on preparing patients for veterinary visits.

With victory visits, the focus is not just on making the environment a good place but also acclimating the pet to gentle control/restraint/stabilization and veterinary equipment. Victory visits can be a preventive service to work on conditioning to veterinary procedures and manipulations or more of an intervention service for a pet that has established fear, anxiety, and stress associated with the veterinary hospital. If working as an intervention service, usually there has been a previous negative experience and memories that the pet will need to overcome. Trust and positive associations can take several repeated visits to establish. You should charge for this service as it requires a trained team member to implement the techniques effectively. Many clients will be willing to pay for this service so the pet will be more comfortable coming to your hospital, and they will learn how to provide care at home. Consider offering package discounts for repeated visits. Table 7.13 compares the differences between fun and victory visits.

To better understand what a victory visit may look like, watch Video 7.21 on the companion website. The video depicts part of a victory visit with a trainer and veterinary assistant with Fear Free certification who are working together to help a dog feel more comfortable with handling for a blood draw. In the past, this dog has shown severe signs of fear, anxiety, and stress, including aggression, with such handling.

Private in-home or in-clinic prevention/training appointments

The private in-home instruction option is becoming increasingly more popular among both dog owners and instructors. This is another area in which veterinary technicians can play a role while adding to their income.

There are many advantages to such a program. Training the dog in a low-stress environment will speed up the learning process. Adolescent dogs are highly distractible, and they are likely to be better focused in their own home. Owners are most concerned about their dog's behaviors at home during the daily routine. Specific behaviors can be identified and modified where they are most problematic. When designing an in-home program, the instructor can also take into consideration the household dynamics such as behavior of family members.

In-home private training should be a customized program that is initiated with an interview session. In addition to contact information, other areas of information should include household members, their ages, and schedules. The family's history of previous dog ownership, details of why and where the dog was acquired, as well as early environmental history can be beneficial. During the interview process, the technician can observe the dog and inquire about any learning history, including past training experience. Together the client and technician can develop clear training goals for the dog and owner.

Problem behaviors may be identified. With training issues, these can be addressed in the training program. The technician may determine an issue is no longer in the preventive stage and therefore needs to be attended by a veterinarian. Owners may request assistance with a dog barking when guests come to the door but the veterinary technicians may determine the dog is in a high level of arousal with the potential to bite. Owners may not realize when a situation is no longer simply a lack of training but has become a behavior disorder.

In-clinic private training appointments with the behavior technician can be utilized for teaching owners how to fit a head collar or front clip harness. These private lessons could also be used to work on one specific skill such as walking on a loose leash.

Special prevention topic seminars or classes

The behavior technician can be assigned to develop public interest seminars on a variety of prevention topics for the hospital staff, clientele, and general public. For example, a technician with exceptional knowledge of avian or exotic pets may design a seminar for pet owners regarding handling, husbandry, environmental enrichment, and nutrition for the particular species. Other ideal prevention topics include pets and children, such as preparing for a newborn in a house with pets or managing a house with a toddler and pets.

Prevention seminars provide clients with a deeper understanding of their pets, can prevent the development of serious problems, and consequently decrease relinquishment rates.

Integrating behavior wellness into the veterinary hospital

A behavior wellness exam is an opportunity to check up on a pet's behavioral health and answer any related questions a client may have. Behavior wellness exams can be offered in conjunction with a routine physical exam or as a separate service.

Owners may be embarrassed to bring up behavior concerns to their veterinarian, because they often feel they are the cause of their pet's problems. Staff members can set the client at ease by bringing up the subject and providing them with a form to complete that will identify potential medical and behavioral concerns. Behavioral wellness visits are another ideal niche for the veterinary behavior technician.

A behavior check list/questionnaire should be used to obtain a general behavioral and physical health overview. In Appendices 13–18 there are samples of questionnaires for cats and dogs at different life stages. The adult form can be used with adolescent and adult examinations. This check list should become part of the pet's permanent file.

Puppy and kitten visits

The entire hospital staff should play a role in the counseling of new puppy and kitten owners. The staff can make the biggest impact when the new pet is novel and endearing as a puppy or kitten. This makes it the ideal time to educate clients on being successful pet owners. How clients and their new puppies and kittens are handled and counseled in the clinic on their first visit can help guarantee a satisfied client and development of a strong human–animal bond.

The entire clinic staff should be knowledgeable in what will be discussed with clients. The veterinary behavior technician can be the ideal person to educate clinic staff on behavior and coordinate the roles of each team member who interacts with owners.

Regular staff meetings or seminars provide an excellent opportunity to educate the staff, answer questions, share concerns, and offer suggestions. This process ensures the consistency of information given out and promotes a team-oriented approach to behavior education.

The behavior team, including a veterinarian, should decide on appropriate literature to be included in the puppy and kitten packets. Most packets will include information on preventive medicine, such as recommended vaccine protocols, heartworm and other parasite preventives, as well as resources on the prevention of problems and handouts for positive solutions to normal puppy and kitten behaviors. Other pet-care professionals in the community recommended by the hospital may also be invited to provide brochures and business cards to be included in the packet.

The best way to organize behavior resources for new puppy and kitten owners is in a three-ring binder. The handouts can have holes punched in them and be included in the binder along with vaccination records and other veterinary informational handouts. The binder with a clear sleeve on the front cover will accommodate a page with the hospital logo and other contact information.

Utilizing a questionnaire, such as the New Puppy (less than four months) Questionnaire or the New Kitten (less than three months) Questionnaire in Appendices 13–18, ensures all vital information is obtained during the first puppy and kitten appointments. The questionnaire could be texted or e-mailed to the client prior to the appointment or provided at check-in.

As discussed earlier in the chapter, techniques for preventing fear of the veterinary clinic should be implemented with all appointments, but is of particular importance with the new puppy or kitten.

Puppies and kittens displaying signs of fear

Puppies and kittens displaying significant signs of fear with a prolonged recovery, should be identified and treated as soon as possible. Although fear is genetically influenced, early experiences also play a role. The best chance of modifying fearful behaviors is when the pets are still within their sensitive socialization period. If the behavior is dismissed, it is sure to escalate as they mature and could lead to aggression. It is the veterinarian's and the veterinary behavior technician's responsibility to emphasize the importance of early intervention.

In the case of a new puppy or kitten that is still in its socialization period and showing mild fear, a technician can be of great assistance. Owners left on their own can cause further damage by overwhelming their pet. Through the appropriate implementation of positive reinforcement training and desensitization, mild fears can usually be addressed quickly.

A young pet with severe fear and/or anxiety should be referred to a veterinary behaviorist. It has been hypothesized that anxiolytic medication used early may assist in extending the socialization period (direct communication with Dr. Andrew Luescher, Purdue University's Animal Behavior Clinic).

High-risk puppies

Research has shown (Guy et al. 2001) certain factors may predispose a puppy to developing conflict-related aggression (aggression toward family members) (Table 7.14). These puppies may seem more fearful and anxious in general and may demonstrate handling issues or may show guarding behaviors around the food bowl or toys. Conflict behaviors may be observed in these and other situations (see Chapter 2 for a description of conflict behaviors). Puppies that have suffered a serious illness before four months of age are at a higher risk then puppies that have not had a serious physical illness. High-risk puppies are often hyperexcitable and have difficulty calming and may lack impulse control.

Table 7.14 High-risk factors for puppies to develop conflict-related aggression (aggression toward family members).

Increased fear and anxiety	Including early handling and/or guarding issues
Had a serious illness under 4 months of age	Including parasite infestation, skin disorders and other serious physical stressors
Hyperexcitable	May show an inability to calm and lack impulse control
Not walked off the property routinely	That is, lack of mental stimulation, which also contributes to hyperexcitability
Anthropomorphic owners	Increases inconsistency and unpredictability in the environment
Lack of training or harsh, aversive training	Punishment is rarely administered appropriately but rather inconsistently and unpredictably, causing an increase in anxiety

Source: Adapted from Guy et al. 2001.

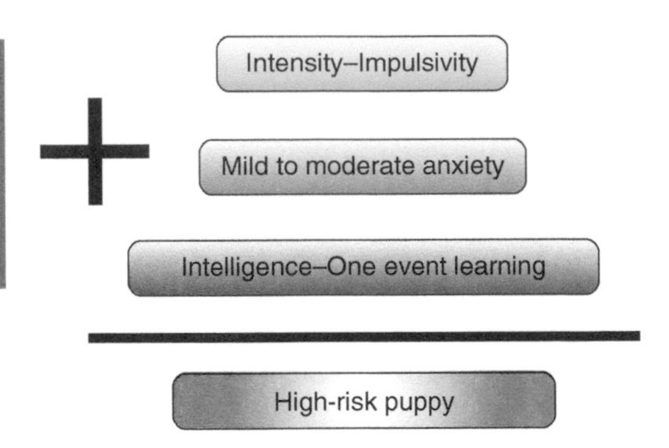

Figure 7.24 High-risk puppy paradigm.

The research also showed a correlation between canine aggression toward owners with first-time owners and owners interacting with a high level of anthropomorphism. The risk increases if there is a lack of training or if harsh training techniques are used (including the use of training tools such as choke, pinch or shock collars). Confrontational "domination" techniques are also likely to increase anxiety and aggression. High-risk puppies often form negative associations quickly, even after only one event. Puppies at high risk or that are demonstrating early signs of conflict-related aggression should be diagnosed and treated by a veterinarian or veterinary behaviorist as early as possible (Figure 7.24).

The adolescent behavior wellness examination

Consideration should be given toward scheduling a specific behavior wellness exam for every adolescent dog and cat between 9 and 12 months of age. Scheduling the session for 30–60 minutes is ideal.

Adolescence is the most trying time in pet ownership. Although dogs and cats may appear fully grown physically, they are not yet socially mature. During this difficult time, there is often no physical reason for a veterinary visit. Vaccination protocols were completed by four to six months of age, just as they are entering adolescence. Adolescence is the time that most dogs and cats are relinquished. By scheduling a behavior wellness exam, technicians can provide an opportunity for the client to learn about this difficult stage and assist clients with positive solutions for normal behavior.

Offering products related to behavior health such as head halters, front clip harnesses, and food storage toys will increase revenue. It also provides staff members with the opportunity to educate clients on proper use and fitting of these items. When offered as a separate service, the behavior wellness exam also provides an opportunity to review other recommendations such as flea and heartworm prevention.

A behavior wellness exam may also identify actions that can potentially lead to a severe behavior problem if left untreated. Many owners are unaware of the warning signs that veterinary behavior technicians see as potential red flags for developing issues. Pet owners may not see the dog that hides behind the owner or barks at incoming guests as potential signs of aggression. It is unfortunate that many do not recognize the warning signs as being problematic until a bite has occurred. By that time the prognosis is much worse. By identifying signs early, bites may be prevented, the human–animal bond maintained, and the animal's life saved. The best way to identify these signs is with a behavior wellness exam.

Another goal of the adolescent behavior wellness exam is to educate clients when they are given poor or outdated advice. The media and internet are filled with unproven, unscientific, and potentially dangerous recommendations. Neighbors and friends are quick to give advice in all areas of pet care but are largely uneducated. Dog trainers may present themselves as experts in behavior. This is a highly unregulated field and although some advice may be beneficial, there are many unknowing dog trainers who can contribute to or even create behavior problems. A behavior wellness exam can help provide clients with appropriate recommendations and resources.

The canine and feline management and enrichment previously discussed in this chapter will be crucial information for the veterinary technician to be fluent with and communicate to the client.

Discussions on training should be included in a behavior wellness exam. All pets benefit from mental stimulation. Training is a great way to enrich the lives of pets and can create a set of positive behaviors in place of less desirable behaviors. It is likely the most troublesome dogs are also the most intelligent. Veterinary staff members need to quickly identify training issues and come up with positive solutions that will fit into the lifestyle of the client and meet the pet's needs.

Training recommendations may be made, including qualified trainers (see Chapter 1 for recommendations of choosing a trainer and Appendix 6 Trainer assessment form) and whether group, private or in-home classes would be the most beneficial.

Some behavioral issues pertaining to lack of stimulation are not evident in kittens but can become increasingly important in adulthood. A noted weight gain is another important reason to stress more exploratory and physical stimulation in the adult cat.

Pointed questions on changes in the environment should be included. As cats are influenced greatly by their surroundings, any changes should be as stress free as possible. It is also important that the client understands how cats show signs of stress. The average cat owner would likely place an anthropomorphic label such as "spite" or "getting back at them" when a cat eliminates outside of a litter box or sprays. Making them aware of the motivating factor behind a behavior will help them become more proactive with solutions for problem behavior.

The adult behavior wellness examination

Feline and canine adult behavior wellness exams can be incorporated into the annual or semi-annual exams. Obtaining an updated questionnaire at each visit will allow the staff to recognize any changes in the physical and behavioral health from previous visits. If we do not ask, the client many not ask for help until they are at their "wits end." When the bond between the owner and pet has been damaged to this point, it can be much more difficult to reconcile (see Chapters 4 and 5). Early intervention is always best. Routine questions designed to uncover potential problems early are key.

The senior and geriatric behavior wellness examination

An important time for practices to include a behavioral exam is when a pet becomes a senior. This timing is going to vary greatly between species as well as individual breeds of dogs. Many giant breed dogs can be considered geriatric as early as six or seven years of age. Smaller breed dogs and cats tend to have a longer life span and therefore may not show signs of aging until 11 or 12 years of age. Other effects on the aging process may include long-standing health problems, the environment, diet, and general care received throughout their lives. When the veterinary staff see signs of a pet becoming aged, they should always question the owners about behavioral changes. This can be a topic owners fail to bring up on their own as they feel it is normal or it is an area that they do not realize veterinary staff are well versed in. It is extra important in this stage of a pet's life to ask about behavioral changes as there is no other time when physical and behavioral problems are more closely linked together. It can also be a time when an owner's bond is the greatest with the pet.

Any behavioral changes in geriatric pets should be followed up with a full medical work up. A physical examination should be performed along with a complete blood count (CBC), blood chemistries, thyroid levels, urinalysis, and a neurological exam. In many cases, the first sign of disease in pets is changes in their personality and activity level. You can also have a physically healthy pet showing signs of cognitive loss through changes in behavior. This is where being well versed in management, nutrition, pharmacology, and behavior modification is important. By offering support to the client in these areas you may be prolonging the pet's life span as well as improving the quality of life.

Common behavioral changes seen in senior and geriatric pets center around house soiling, anxiety, and aggression. Because medical factors are often the causative factor, a combination approach to treatment (medical and behavioral) will be necessary.

Cognitive dysfunction can occur in both dogs and cats. It is by definition an impairment of memory and learning. The DISHAAL signs are often used as a screening tool.

Disorientation
Interaction changes
Sleep–wake cycle changes
House soiling
Activity level changes
Anxiety
Learning and memory impaired

Common symptoms of cognitive dysfunction syndrome include loss of house training, excess vocalization, abnormal sleep–wake cycles, failure to recognize familiar people, standing in corners or going to the hinged side of the door, and abnormal motility such as circling and pacing. Although no cure is available, the progression of the disease can be slowed through pharmaceutical, dietary, and environmental and behavior modification.

Behavior wellness conclusion

If behavior wellness is not a top priority of veterinary practices, valuable information on behavior problem prevention, along with potential medical problems, may go undetected. It is the responsibility of the veterinary team to meet the needs of their client's pets both physically and behaviorally.

Conclusion

A behavior problem is a behavior that is a problem for the pet owner, which can be due to lack of training or conditioned unwanted behaviors. The goal is to prevent "behavior problems" and to certainly prevent them from becoming a "behavioral disorder," which usually has an emotional foundation. Most behavior problems are much easier to prevent than they are to treat. The veterinary clinic is the ideal location to educate owners before problem behaviors become well established. This is a valuable role for the behavior technician to fill in veterinary practice. Prevention and enrichment from puppy and kitten to the geriatric dog and cat is a position in which the veterinary technician can excel and make an impact on the welfare of numerous pets and their owners.

Additional resources

Crate training: https://www.fearfreehappyhomes.com/video/what-you-need-to-know-about-crates-and-your-dog

Introducing two dogs: https://www.fearfreehappyhomes.com/video/a-fear-free-approach-to-introducing-your-dog-to-a-new-dog

Family paws resources: https://www.familypaws.com/resources

The DOGS & KIDS course written by Emily Levine, DVM, DACVB: https://onlineschool.instinctdogtraining.com/course/kids-and-dogs

Pooch Parenting by Michele Stern – online courses and membership: https://poochparenting.net

Puppy Start Right: www.puppystartright.com

Stop the 77: https://www.thefamilydog.com/stop-the-77

Veterinary Oral Health Council (VOHC): http://www.vohc.org

Video 7.1 This video demonstrates the beginning stages of teaching a retrieve with the cues, get it, bring, and out. Notice with the first release of the toy, no cue is given because the treat prompts the release. In the following repetitions the trainer gives the out cue prior to prompting with a treat.

Video 7.2 This video shows a senior dog using a snuffle mat. Notice the mat has been placed on an elevated surface to accommodate this dog's arthritis and make the exploratory activity more comfortable for him.

Video 7.3 This video illustrates introducing a puppy to a crate.

Video 7.4 This video depicts using management and supervised time outside to teach elimination training with a puppy.

Video 7.5 This video illuminates the process of acclimating a dog to restraint.

Video 7.6 This video details playing the food bowl game with a young puppy.

Video 7.7 This video demonstrates approaching a dog while it has an object and giving the dog a treat. You will notice the dog initially tenses up. After several repetitions the dog is anticipating getting a treat and keeping the "toy."

Video 7.8 This video illustrates how quickly cat can be trained even during a behavior consultation. Both cats were being seen for a behavior consultation while this training took place.

Video 7.9 This video demonstrates the veterinary nurse and trainer using appropriate techniques to address a puppy biting her pant legs. She purposely overstimulates the puppy to get the video footage.

Video 7.10 This video highlights the beginning stages of teaching the cue, Leave it. The trainer chooses an object the dog is not interested in putting in his mouth. She initially places the object on the ground and then begins to drop it on the ground. After it hits the ground the trainer says, "Leave it," in a calm and non-threatening tone. She marks and treats the dog for remaining still.

Video 7.11 This video demonstrates the counting game. Notice how the person moves away once the dog approaches. This removes any social pressure of the person lingering over the dog while he is eating. The dog is also learning to move away from an object and come to the person on the cue, "One, two, three. . . ." This game can be used in a variety of contexts, even as an icebreaker when getting to know a dog for the first time.

Video 7.12 This video depicts proactively reinforcing a puppy for not jumping.

Video 7.13 This video demonstrates appropriate ways to interrupt play between young puppies.

Video 7.14 This video illustrates exploration of novel items during puppy class. Puppy owners learn to work at their dog's pace, attend to body language indicators of fear or apprehension, and proactively increase distance before adding something like sound or movement.

Video 7.15 This video shows a quick progression of the steps in teaching the collar game.

Video 7.16 This video illustrates working on handling and restraint with a puppy during puppy class. The trainer does the handling, marks with a click, and the owner brings a treat to the dog.

Video 7.17 This video shows a puppy learning about the clicker and also learning that offering eye contact will earn him a treat. This is the beginning stage of teaching an attention or eye contact cue.

Video 7.18 This video illustrates teaching the Look (at that) cue.

Video 7.19 This video shows teaching the nose touch to hand targeting behavior, adding a verbal cue (touch), and using the behavior out on a walk.

Video 7.20 This video demonstrates a puppy learning about loose leash walking. Notice the high rate of reinforcement (one step = one treat) at the beginning. After several repetitions, the trainer starts to take a few steps before marking and treating. She takes mini breaks by running backward and having the puppy follow her before resetting for another repetition.

Video 7.21 This video depicts part of a victory visit with a trainer and veterinary assistant with Fear Free certification who are working together to help a dog feel more comfortable with handling for a blood draw. In the past, this dog has shown severe signs of fear, anxiety, and stress, including aggression, with such handling. Note that for the animal's safety, some hospitals have a policy requiring a dog on a table to wear a leash loosely held by a person or that a person's hand be on the dog at all times. This is to prevent a dog from becoming startled and jumping off the table. Video courtesy of Mikkel Becker, Lead Animal Trainer for Fear Free Pets, CBCC-KA, CDBC, KPA CTP, CPDT-KA, CTC, Fear Free Cert, BA Comm, co-author of *From Fearful to Fear Free*, and Sarah Pfarr, FFCP (Trainer).

Acknowledgement

The author acknowledges the contribution of Linda M. Campbell and Marcia R. Ritchie to the first edition chapter.

References

Barrett, J., Frey, R., and Thomson, G. (2016). Animal bite infections. In: *The Gale Encyclopedia of Children's Health: Infancy through Adolescence*, 3e. (eBook). https://www.gale.com/ebooks/9781410332745/the-gale-encyclopedia-of-childrens-health-infancy-through-adolescence.

Bergesen, F.J. (1989). The effects of pet facilitated therapy on the self-esteem and socialization of primary school children. In: *Paper Presented at Monaco'89, the 5th International Conference on the Relationship Between Humans and Animals*.

Bernardo, L., Gardner, M., Rosenfield, R. et al. (2002). A comparison of dog bite injuries in younger and older children treated in a pediatric emergency department. *Pediatric Emergency Care* 18 (3): 247–249.

Bernstein, P.L. and Strack, M. (1996). A game of cat and house: spatial patterns andbehavior of 14 cats *(Felis catus)* in the home. *Anthrozoös* 9: 25–39.

Bradshaw, J.W.S., Blackwell, E.J., and Casey, R.A. (2009). Dominance in domestic dogs – useful construct or bad habit? *Journal of Veterinary Behavior: Clinical Applications and Research* 4 (3): 135–144.

Crowell-Davis, S.L., Barry, K., and Wolfe, R. (1997). Social behavior and aggression problems of cats. *The Veterinary Clinics of North America. Small Animal Practice* 27 (3): 549–568.

De Cramer, K.G.M., Stylianides, E., and van Vuuren, M. (2011). Efficacy of vaccination at 4 and 6 weeks in the control of canine parvovirus. *Veterinary Microbiology* 149 (1–2): 126–132.

Donaldson, J. (1996). *The Culture Clash*. Berkeley, California, USA: James and Kenneth Publishers.

Duffy, D.L. and Serpell, J.A. (2006). Non-reproductive effects of spaying and neutering on behavior in dogs. In: *Proceedings of the Third International Symposium on Non-Surgical Contraceptive Methods for Pet Population Control, Center for the Interaction of Animals and Society, School of Veterinary Medicine, University of Pennsylvania, Alexandria, Virginia, USA*.

Guy, N.C., Luescher, U.A., Dohoo, S.E. et al. (2001). Demographic and aggressive characteristics of dogs in a general veterinary caseload. *Applied Animal Behaviour Science* 74 (1): 15–28.

Hart, B.L. and Cooper, L. (1984). Factors relating to urine spraying and fighting in prepubertally gonadectomized cats. *Journal of the American Veterinary Medical Association* 184 (10): 1255–1258.

Hopkins, S.G., Schubert, T.A., and Hart, B.L. (1976). Castration of adult male dogs: effects on roaming, aggression, urine marking, and mounting. *Journal of the American Veterinary Medical Association* 168: 1108–1110.

Kahn, A., Bauche, P., and Lamoureux, J. and the Members of the Dog Bites Research Team(2003). Child victims of dog bites treated in emergency departments. *European Journal of Pediatrics* 162: 254–258.

Kahn, A., Robert, E., Piette, D. et al. (2004). Prevalence of dog bites in children. A telephone survey. *European Journal of Pediatrics* 163: 424.

Liberg, O., Sandell, M., Pontier, D. et al. (2000). Density, spatial organization and reproducive tactics in the domestic cat and other felids. In: *The Domestic Cat: The Biology of its Behavior*, 2e (ed. D.V. Turner and P. Bateson), 119–147. Cambridge, England: Cambridge University Press.

Lindsay, S.R. (2001). *Handbook of Applied Dog Behavior and Training*, vol. 2. Ames: Iowa State University Press.

Martin, K. and Martin, D. (2011). *Puppy Start Right: Foundation Training for the Companion Dog*. Waltham, MA: Sunshine Books.

Martin K. and Martin D. (2012). Puppy Start Right for Instructors. Online course. https://karenpryoracademy.com/courses/puppy-start-right/ (accessed November 16, 2022).

Mondelli, F., Prato Previde, E., Verga, M. et al. (2004). The bond that never developed: adoption and relinquishment of dogs in a rescue shelter. *Journal of Applied Animal Welfare Science* 7 (4): 253–266.

Morgan, M. and Houpt, K.A. (1990). Feline behaviour problems: the influence of declawing. *Antrozoos* 3: 50–53.

Neilson, J.C. (2001). Pearl vs. clumping: litter preference in a population of shelter cats. In: *Proceedings*, 14. American Veterinary Society of Animal Behavior.

Neilson, J.C. (2008). Is bigger better? Litterbox size preference test. *Proceedings of the American College of Veterinary Behaviorists/American Veterinary Society of Animal Behavior*, New Orleans, LA (July 18, 2008), 46–49.

Neville, P.F. and Remfry, J. (1984). Effect of neutering on two groups of feral cats. *Veterinary Record* 114 (5): 447–450.

Patronek, G.J., Glickman, L.T., Beck, A.M. et al. (1996). Risk factors for relinquishment of dogs to an animal shelter. *Journal of the American Veterinary Medical Association* 209 (3): 572–581.

Poresky, R.H. and Hendrix, C. (1990). Differential effects of pet presence and pet-bonding on young children. *Psychological Reports* 67: 51–54.

Schalomon, J., Ainoedhofer, H., Singer, G. et al. (2006). Analysis of dog bites in children who are younger than 17 years. *The Journal of Pediatrics* 117 (3): 374–379.

Serpell, J. (1991). Beneficial effects of pet ownership on some aspects of human health & behaviour. *Journal of Royal Science of Medicine* 84.

Stepida, M.E., Bain, M.J., and Kass, P.H. (2013). Frequency of CPV infection in vaccinated puppies that attended puppy socialization classes. *Journal of the American Animal Hospital Association* 49 (2): 95–100.

Stubbs, W.P., Bloomberg, M.S., Scruggs, S.L. et al. (1996). Effects of perpubertal gonadectomy on physical and behavioral development of cats. *Journal of the American Veterinary Medical Association* 209 (11): 1864–1871.

Vitale Shreve, K., Mehrkam, L., and Udell, M. (2017). Social interaction, food, scent or toys? A formal assessment of domestic pet and shelter cat (Felis silvestris catus) preferences. *Behavioural Processes* 141: 322–328. https://doi.org/10.1016/j.beproc.2017.03.016.

Wells, D.L., Graham, L., and Hepper, P.G. (2002). The influence of auditory stimulation on the behaviour of dogs housed in a rescue shelter. *Animal Welfare* 11: 385–393.

Xavier, M., Fatjo, J., Amat, M., and Mariotti, V. (2008). Preventing canine aggression: what works and what doesn't. In: *Proceeding of the SEVC Southern European Veterinary Conference. October 17–19, 2008 – Barcelona, Spain*.

The PowerPoint of figures, appendices, MCQ's, cited videos are available at www.wiley.com/go/martin/behavior

8 Husbandry and veterinary care

Debbie Martin[1,2] and Rachel M. Lees[3]
[1]*TEAM Education in Animal Behavior, LLC, Spicewood, TX, USA*
[2]*Veterinary Behavior Consultations, LLC, Spicewood, TX, USA*
[3]*University of Tennessee College of Veterinary Medicine, Knoxville, TN, USA*

CHAPTER MENU

Introduction

Veterinary medicine is constantly evolving. There was a time when we did not routinely provide prophylactic analgesics to patients for even things like surgery! The behavioral health and emotional well-being of pets has slowly become a focal point in veterinary medicine.

Over the years veterinary behaviorists and veterinary technician specialists in behavior have facilitated education about the importance of behavior health to veterinary organizations and general practitioners. This has resulted in the inclusion of behavioral health in practice guidelines including the AAHA Canine Life Stage Guidelines and the AAFP/AAHA Feline Life Stage Guidelines. Similarly, the American Animal Hospital Association published Canine and Feline Behavior Management Guidelines.

The late Dr. Sophia Yin's passion for spreading the word on low-stress handling and care, not only sparked many veterinary professional's interest but also give them the knowledge and tools to apply it directly in their daily routine. The creation of Fear Free® Pets by Dr. Marty Becker has resulted in a growing community of animal professionals,

Canine and Feline Behavior for Veterinary Technicians and Nurses, Second Edition. Edited by Debbie Martin and Julie K. Shaw.

Companion website: www.wiley.com/go/martin/behavior

including veterinary professionals, who are invested in protecting not only the physical well-being of pets but also their emotional well-being.

How we provide care to animals is paramount to their acceptance or reluctance for care in the future.

Many dogs and cats may accept handling and restraint at the veterinary hospital. However, some patients become so frightened that they fear for their lives, often resulting in aggression. Regardless of whether the patient is accepting or afraid, it is necessary to proactively attempt to make the veterinary hospital experience as pleasant as possible for all patients. This does not necessarily involve a large amount of time. It involves identifying and modifying potential stressors in the veterinary setting. This might involve a change in protocol with check-in or check-out to avoid congestion in the lobby or creating a calm and relaxing spa-like environment throughout the hospital to promote relaxation in patients, clients, and veterinary team members.

- How we provide care to animals is paramount to their acceptance or reluctance for care in the future.

The few seconds or minutes taken initially to allow a patient to relax and become comfortable may not only save the staff hours in the long run (not to mention decreased risk of injury) but may also save the pet's life. Negative experiences in the veterinary hospital can result in long-lasting aggression issues with handling and routine care from the owner or veterinary team, as well as fear and aggression toward strangers (Yin 2009).

- The few seconds or minutes taken initially to allow a patient to relax and become comfortable may not only save the staff hours in the long run (not to mention decreased risk of injury) but may also save the pet's life.

Proactively providing positive, rather than neutral or, even worse, negative experiences throughout every veterinary event, facilitates pleasant memories of the veterinary hospital, the team, and care. Because the authors of this chapter are both contributors to educational content associated with Fear Free Pets and Fear Free Happy Homes, much of the information and terminology provided within this chapter will be based on Fear Free content.

General core concepts

The mission of Fear Free® is to prevent and alleviate fear, anxiety, and stress (FAS) in pets by inspiring and educating the people who care for them. Some of the general core concepts within the veterinary field to achieve a reduction in FAS are assessing patient FAS, using Considerate Approach, Touch Gradient, and Gentle Control techniques, as well as providing good communication with clients, patients, and veterinary team members.

Assessing FAS

Fear Free suggests utilizing a scale for grading FAS (Figure 8.1). The scale, developed by board-certified veterinary behaviorist Kenneth Martin, and veterinary technician specialist in behavior Debbie Martin, has three categories of FAS: low, moderate, and high, with six numeric scores, from zero through five. The three categories are green for go, yellow for caution or pause, and red for stop.

This guideline helps team members communicate clearly about an animal's experiences in the veterinary clinic and provides guidance on how to proceed. The goal is to use behavior indicators based on the context to infer the possible emotional state of the animal and make decisions on how to proceed in order to protect the animal's emotional well-being. Uniform scoring of FAS is a way that the team can communicate about patients. This scale can also be used as a guide for animal trainers and pet owners while working on husbandry care or providing at-home medical care.

Here is a general overview of the different levels:

Level 0 describes animals with no signs of FAS. Pets display relaxed body language and solicit interactions with the veterinary team.

Level 1 describes animals displaying one to two mild signs of FAS such as lip licking, avoiding eye contact, looking away without moving away, raising a paw, partial pupil dilation, and a dog panting with the commissure of the lips relaxed. These signs occur four times or fewer per minute. The animal is interested in reinforcers such as treats, play, and attention, and chooses to interact with the veterinary team. Even with

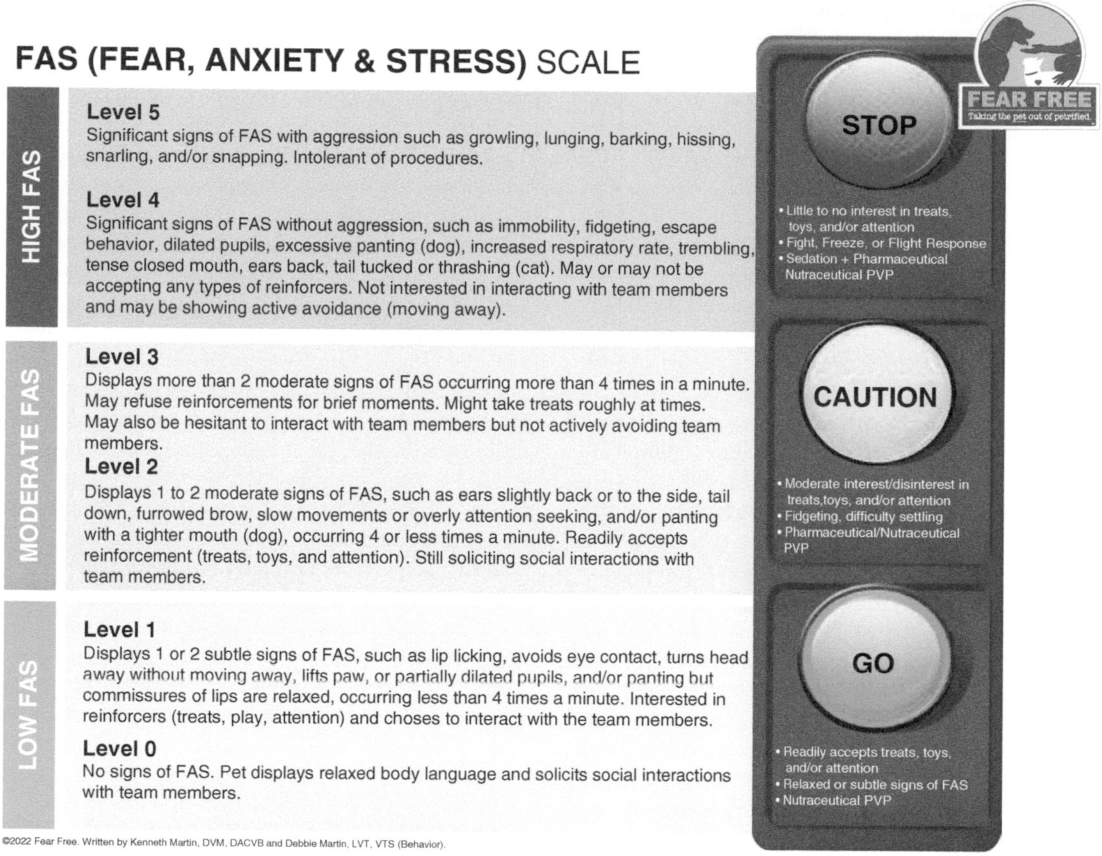

FAS (FEAR, ANXIETY & STRESS) SCALE

FEAR FREE
Taking the pet out of petrified.

HIGH FAS

Level 5
Significant signs of FAS with aggression such as growling, lunging, barking, hissing, snarling, and/or snapping. Intolerant of procedures.

Level 4
Significant signs of FAS without aggression, such as immobility, fidgeting, escape behavior, dilated pupils, excessive panting (dog), increased respiratory rate, trembling, tense closed mouth, ears back, tail tucked or thrashing (cat). May or may not be accepting any types of reinforcers. Not interested in interacting with team members and may be showing active avoidance (moving away).

STOP
- Little to no interest in treats, toys, and/or attention
- Fight, Freeze, or Flight Response
- Sedation + Pharmaceutical Nutraceutical PVP

MODERATE FAS

Level 3
Displays more than 2 moderate signs of FAS occurring more than 4 times in a minute. May refuse reinforcements for brief moments. Might take treats roughly at times. May also be hesitant to interact with team members but not actively avoiding team members.

Level 2
Displays 1 to 2 moderate signs of FAS, such as ears slightly back or to the side, tail down, furrowed brow, slow movements or overly attention seeking, and/or panting with a tighter mouth (dog), occurring 4 or less times a minute. Readily accepts reinforcement (treats, toys, and attention). Still soliciting social interactions with team members.

CAUTION
- Moderate interest/disinterest in treats,toys, and/or attention
- Fidgeting, difficulty settling
- Pharmaceutical/Nutraceutical PVP

LOW FAS

Level 1
Displays 1 or 2 subtle signs of FAS, such as lip licking, avoids eye contact, turns head away without moving away, lifts paw, or partially dilated pupils, and/or panting but commissures of lips are relaxed, occurring less than 4 times a minute. Interested in reinforcers (treats, play, attention) and choses to interact with the team members.

Level 0
No signs of FAS. Pet displays relaxed body language and solicits social interactions with team members.

GO
- Readily accepts treats, toys, and/or attention
- Relaxed or subtle signs of FAS
- Nutraceutical PVP

Figure 8.1 Fear, Anxiety, and Stress Scale. *Source*: FAS Scale/Fear Free, LLC.

Level 0 and 1 FAS patients, the veterinary team might consider medical management of FAS with preventive use of nutraceuticals or pharmaceuticals, especially if a procedure is scheduled that is likely to result in FAS, such as surgery, dental cleaning, extended time in the veterinary hospital away from the owner, or diagnostic imaging. The goal is to keep the pet's association with the hospital a pleasant one!

Level 2 describes animals showing one to two signs of moderate FAS such as ears held slightly back, lowered tail, slowed movements, seeking attention from the owner, or a dog panting with tight lip commissures. These signs are seen four times or fewer per minute. These pets still choose to interact with the veterinary team and readily accept their preferred treats, toys, and attention.

Level 3 describes animals displaying more than two signs of moderate FAS occurring more than four times per minute. They may show intermittent interest in reinforcers, sometimes refusing treats briefly. They may take treats roughly. These animals may interact with team members or may be hesitant to do so, but they are not actively avoiding interaction. Patients who routinely exhibit level 2 and 3 FAS may benefit from pre-visit pharmaceuticals (PVP) and nutraceuticals for future care to prevent escalation of FAS and alleviate the current level of stress.

Level 4 describes animals experiencing severe FAS without overt aggression. These signs include hiding or immobility, fidgeting, attempting to escape, trembling, increased respiratory rate or effort, a tense, closed mouth, dilated pupils, ears held back or flat, tail tucked tightly or cats thrashing the tail. These pets may or may not be interested in reinforcers such as food, toys, or attention, do not choose to interact with team members, and generally avoid team members by moving away.

Level 5 describes animals experiencing severe FAS with aggression such as stiff body with direct staring, growling, lunging, barking, snarling, snapping, swatting, and more. These animals are too afraid to allow handling or procedures. Medical treatment of FAS is imperative with patients experiencing level 4 or 5 FAS.

Rarely will a pet have a single FAS level during a visit to the veterinary hospital. Assessments are taken throughout the entire veterinary experience and most pets will have a range of FAS levels. For example, a dog might eagerly enter the lobby with relaxed body language and accepting treats (FAS 0). While the veterinary nurse is taking a history in the exam room, the dog solicits attention and petting, but shows some mild signs of stress such as panting (lips relaxed), licking lips, and an occasional yawn (FAS 1). During examination, some moderate signs of FAS are observed including furrowed brow, tail down, ears slightly to the side but the dog is still seeking attention from the veterinary team and taking treats (FAS 2). During venipuncture, the dog briefly freezes and refuses the treats (FAS 3) but within a second or two returns to the food. Notes in the emotional record would provide more details but the FAS range for the visit would be FAS 0–3.

Similar to the FAS scale, *Cooperative Veterinary Care, 1st edition* written by Alicea Howell BS, RVT, VTS (Behavior), KPA CTP and Monique Feyrecilde BA, LVT, VTS (Behavior) categorizes patients as Level 1 (green – go ahead with treatments), Level 2 (yellow – proceed with caution), or Level 3 (red – STOP!) (Howell and Feyrecilde 2018).

Considerate Approach

As defined in the Fear Free® Veterinary Certification program, "Considerate Approach(CA) encompasses the interactions between the veterinary team and the patients and inputs from the environment while veterinary care is being administered."

This includes interactions with the patient, creating a physical environment considerate of the animal's senses and perception, as well as interactions with the client and veterinary team members.

When creating an environment that is considerate of animals and clients, think about creating a "Spa-w"-like setting. Avoid noise and smell pollution. Most pets have a greater sense of smell and wider auditory range than humans. Consider using calming pheromones for pets and extremely dilute aromatherapy for owners. Acoustic or music therapy can create a serene setting. There are many choices for music, including species-specific music, reggae, soft rock, harp, classical piano, and audiobooks. For animals to feel safe, we must provide them with non-slip surfaces, such as rubber mats. Having a variety of high-value treats available takes into consideration individual pet preferences. Treats help form a positive association and act as a distraction or reinforcer for the pet. Replace fluorescent lighting with LED lightening. Box 8.1 provides tips on how to use a considerate approach while greeting and interacting patients.

Taking into consideration potential stressors in the veterinary environment and minimizing or avoiding them, makes for a less stressful experience for the pet and the entire team. Additional tips on providing a Considerate Approach in all areas of the veterinary hospital will be covered in more detail in

BOX 8.1: TIPS FOR USING A CONSIDERATE APPROACH WHILE INTERACTING WITH PATIENTS

- Turn sideways to appear less threatening.
- Avoid direct eye contact. Eye contact for more than a second or two from someone you do not have a relationship with is uncomfortable for people and animals.
- Move smoothly and calmly to avoid startling the pet.
- Talk slowly and softly. This will help calm the pet and the owner.
- Allow the pet to approach. When using a considerate approach to interact with patients, the best thing you can do is play a little "hard to get." Let the dog or cat make the first move. Even if the pet is eager to greet you, an overenthusiastic human greeting can overwhelm the pet and heighten FAS.
- Use treats if medically appropriate. To avoid placing the pet in a motivational conflict of wanting the food but also wanting to stay at a distance from you, start by tossing the treat rather than reaching out to hand the treat to the pet.
- Avoid using scents that might be aversive or overwhelming to the sensitive noses of patients. Instead use calming scents such as calming pheromones.

this chapter under the section titled **Creating pleasant experiences throughout the veterinary visit**.

- Taking into consideration potential stressors in the veterinary environment and minimizing or avoiding them, makes for a less stressful experience for the pet and the entire team.

Touch Gradient

Touch Gradient is a term used by Fear Free® to describe how to touch patients to minimize FAS during procedures. Touch Gradient encompasses both Gentle Control and Considerate Approach.

Touch Gradient has two components:

1. It begins by maintaining continual hands-on physical contact with a patient throughout the entire procedure or examination whenever possible and appropriate.
2. It includes acclimating a patient to an increasing level of touch intensity, while continuously measuring the patient's acceptance and comfort.

By keeping contact once touch is initiated, we can avoid surprising the pet and make touch more predictable and easier to understand from the pet's point of view. Using a gliding touch to transfer between body areas and choosing to perform treatments in order starting with those least likely to cause FAS to those most likely to do so allows constant assessment of the patient's comfort level with touch.

Touch Gradient sets up a great basic guideline for standard operating procedures for most animals. However, some animals may become more sensitive to touch and the gliding hands might be met with avoidance. Monitor the patient's response and adjust as needed.

Record individual preferences about touch in the emotional medical record (EMR) so future treatments go smoothly.

Pets and people have touch receptors all over their body. Some areas of the body have an increased density of these receptors. For example, the face, hands, and feet tend to be more sensitive than the leg, torso, or arm. If you stub your toe or finger, it creates an intense sensation that you remember. However, if you bruise your leg or arm, sometimes you cannot recall what caused it because the sensation was not intense. Although we all have touch receptors, our perception of touch varies. Some people find a foot massage to be very relaxing and enjoyable. In fact, they are willing to pay money to receive one. Other people find a foot massage to be extremely unpleasant and would avoid one at all costs (and might even use physical force). This variation in perception of touch holds true with our patients as well. For example, some pets find handling of their paws extremely unpleasant. Think of those patients as being more ticklish or sensitive to paw touching.

Frequently assessing the patient's level of FAS and response to touch throughout procedures will help pets to relax and keep veterinary teams safe. If a certain location, sensation, or type of touch causes increased FAS, pause and assess yourself, the patient and the situation. There could be an underlying medical or emotional cause for the increase in FAS, or something in the environment changed (i.e. the cat hears a door close or a dog bark) and caused the pet to feel uncomfortable.

- Frequently assessing the patient's level of FAS and response to touch throughout procedures will help pets to relax and keep veterinary teams safe. If a certain location, sensation, or type of touch causes increased FAS, pause and assess yourself, the patient and the situation.

Gentle Control

Gentle Control is how the veterinary team comfortably and **safely** positions the patient to allow the administration of veterinary care.

- Many times, it is the restraint that is frightening to our patients, not the actual procedure.

Many times, it is the restraint that is frightening to our patients, not the actual procedure. Most patients do not find injections to be extremely uncomfortable. However, being held still or immobilized by unfamiliar people can quickly escalate a patient's FAS level. When possible, attempt to minimize the amount of restraint, but SAFETY for everyone (the pet, owners, and veterinary team) is of utmost importance. Often, less is more when it comes to restraint.

CHAPTER 8

If we think of handling and restraint more as stabilization of the patient, our attitude and focus change. Instead of focusing on restraint to keep the pet still, focus on stabilizing the patient to provide for more comfortable care. When we pick up a leg on a pet to draw blood or trim a nail, this can put them off balance. When patients are stabilized, they feel more secure. The veterinary assistant or nurse can redirect the patient's body or head as needed to keep the team safe. Gentle control tools such as basket muzzles or towels, when acclimated properly, can allow for added safety and comfort for the patient and veterinary team. Box 8.2 details alternatives to the use of traditional restraint methods, which relied on physically overpowering and immobilizing the pet for care.

- If we think of handling and restraint more as stabilization of the patient, our attitude and focus change. Instead of focusing on restraint to keep the pet still, focus on stabilizing the patient to provide for more comfortable care.

Communication

Communication is key to facilitating a pleasant veterinary experience. This includes communication with our patients and hearing what they are saying. It also involves clear communication with the veterinary team as well as with the client.

Creating and maintaining an EMR for each pet makes implementation a breeze. The patient's preferences, past successes, FAS levels throughout a visit or stay at the hospital, and recommended plans are noted so all team members are informed and can be prepared.

BOX 8.2: ALTERNATIVES TO TRADITIONAL RESTRAINT

- Distraction in the form of treats, petting, brushing, talking, or toys. Distractions the pet enjoys can help create a pleasant association with veterinary care.
- Desensitization and counter-conditioning training.
- Toweling techniques can allow for hiding, swaddling, and minimizing manual restraint.
- Cooperative care training.
- Sedation protocols for patients experiencing or expected to experience moderate to severe levels of FAS from a procedure.

Gentle control techniques will be explored in more detail later in this chapter.

The core concepts, assessing FAS, utilizing Considerate Approach, Touch Gradient, and Gentle Control techniques, and emphasizing good communication with the entire team, when implemented routinely, provide for a better veterinary experience for everyone.

Creating pleasant experiences throughout the veterinary visit

There are a variety of different sights, sounds, smells, tastes, and even potential substrates that may indicate to the patient that a veterinary visit may be on the horizon. It is important to create positive experiences and associations with these environmental stimuli, so they are not predictive of potentially frightening experiences. Veterinary technicians can educate owners of these potential stimuli and focus on changing the meaning of these prompts ahead of time to make veterinary visits as comfortable as possible for the patient, owner, and veterinary team.

Home preparation

The veterinary visit occurs before the animal steps into the practice. The client service representative (CSR) is often the main communicator regarding pre-visit preparation. However, the veterinarian and the veterinary technicians/assistants may also be involved with planning pre-visit recommendations with the client for future visits. The CSR should review the EMR of the patient prior to contacting the client to confirm the scheduled appointment. Any special accommodations that have been noted in the record should be reviewed with the client. For example, if the veterinarian prescribed PVPs or suggested the client call the front desk from the parking lot to notify the hospital of their arrival, the CSR will remind the client of the recommendations and ask them to contact the hospital if they have any questions. Other general pre-visit suggestions that can help to reduce fear, anxiety, and stress associated with travel to the veterinary hospital can be posted on the hospital website or sent in an email reminder prior to an appointment. Some general recommendations include:

- Acclimate and train the pet for transport (carrier, crate, seatbelt) – a qualified professional trainer may need to assist the client with this training.
- Provide non-slip surfaces during transport to prevent sliding.
- Utilize aroma and acoustic therapy to create a calm environment.

- Cool or heat the vehicle to a comfortable temperature before putting the pet in the vehicle.
- Drive smoothly and cautiously; try to avoid abrupt changes in speed and sharp turns.
- If medically and behaviorally warranted, bring a hungry pet and the pet's favorite treats.
- Bring familiar objects from home, such as a bed or toy. Something with the smells of home, brings familiarity to a novel situation.

For both canines and felines, travel does not always indicate a pleasurable experience. In some instances, car rides only take place for veterinary-related visits. Despite our best efforts, these visits typically involve the veterinary team touching, poking, and manipulating patients to determine their overall medical well-being. Just as with humans, pets can also have motion sickness during vehicular travel. Therefore, riding in the vehicle has been paired with nausea and an upset stomach. This creates a predictable pattern that leaving the home and traveling in a vehicle can result in stressful experiences. Screening for motion sickness and treating can help ameliorate FAS resulting from nausea.

Harnesses, leashes, carriers, crates, and vehicles should be paired with positive events and outcomes because these objects can become predictors that the pet is leaving the home. By pairing these stimuli with things the pet finds reinforcing, the experiences can then be strengthened and paired with each other. Placing a harness on the pet and then taking them on a ride to get a whipped cream treat from the client's favorite coffee shop may be a good start. This example can create a positive behavior chain if whipped cream and meeting new people are something that this pet enjoys doing. It pairs the harness and the vehicle and leaving the home environment with travel, treats, and people.

Especially for felines, placing carriers in common areas of the client's home is beneficial. If the carrier is only brought out prior to a veterinary visit, and the pet is stressed, fearful, and anxious the carrier will be the first prompt that a non-pleasurable experience is about to occur. Regardless of species, using a carrier with a removable top is recommended so the veterinary team can easily, safely, and quickly remove a pet from this area with minimal amount of stress. Placing treats, toys, and spraying calming pheromones inside the carrier or in the car a few times per week can be an ideal way to create positive associations with the carrier or car and to also not always pair it with traveling to an unknown destination. Calming pheromones can also be used on bandanas, anxiety wraps, towels, blankets, and car seats prior to any type of travel. Because calming pheromone sprays are alcohol based, they should be sprayed in the area and allowed to dry for a minimum of 15 minutes before the pet has exposure to the area. The spray will last for up to four hours and then should be reapplied.

If the pet is displaying so much FAS that they are hiding when the carrier is in sight or if they need to be pulled, picked up, or physically carried to the car because they are refusing to move in that direction, prevention is unfortunately off the table. In these situations, the veterinary technician can create a desensitization and counter-conditioning plan to change the way the pet feels about each step in the process (Table 8.1).

Scheduling the veterinary appointment

A knowledgeable reception team is one of the first steps to making the visit as pleasurable as possible. It is important that each case be scheduled with enough time to ensure the veterinary team can examine the patient at a pace appropriate for the individual. Scheduling additional time for the first appointment allows the pet to acclimatize to the environment, while the technician provides

Table 8.1 DS-CC plan car travel.

Step 1:	M/T seeing car
Step 2:	M/T weight shifting toward car
Step 3:	M/T movement toward car
Step 4:	M/T for nose touching car
Step 5:	M/T for paw touching car
Step 6:	M/T for jumping into car
Step 7:	M/T for duration of time in the car with the door open (vary time length)
Step 8:	M/T for duration of time in the car with the door closed (vary time length)
Step 9:	M/T for owner sitting in car with pet
Step 10:	M/T for owner sitting in front seat with pet in back seat
Step 11:	M/T for quiet/relaxed/calm behavior in the car
Step 12:	M/T for turning ignition
Step 13:	M/T for 5 seconds of car movement while pet is in the vehicle
Step 14:	M/T for 10 seconds of car movement while pet is in the vehicle
Step 15:	M/T for 30 seconds of car movement while pet is in the vehicle
Step 16:	M/T for 1 minute of car movement while pet is in the vehicle
Step 17:	M/T for 3 minutes of car movement while pet is in the vehicle

DS: desensitization; CC: counter conditioning; M/T: mark and then treat.

CHAPTER 8

guidance regarding preventive medical and behavior care. With new adult patients, the reception team should inquire regarding previous experiences at the veterinary hospital. How has their pet responded in the past to being examined by the veterinarian? Providing a quick questionnaire designed for different life stages of development for the pet owner to complete at each visit will assist the veterinary staff to avoid overlooking vital information (see Appendices 13–18 Puppy, Adult dog, Senior/geriatric dog, Kitten, Adult cat, and Senior/geriatric cat questionnaires). Not only will the client leave better educated about their pet, but they likely will also become more bonded to the practice.

The reception team can set the veterinary examination up for success. They are the first line of defense in battling FAS in the veterinary hospital. The reception team should remind owners to give any PVP ahead of time and to bring their pet fasted, if appropriate. This will ensure that the patient will be hungry for high-value food items so the veterinary team can do their best to create a positive experience. In multiple-pet homes, it is recommended to bring in only one pet per visit to reduce social pressure and to ensure the veterinary team can monitor and treat FAS as thoroughly as possible. Owners should be reminded that cats should come in their own separate carriers to prevent any potential for aggression to each other post visit.

The reception team member should watch for any alerts in the medical record indicating special needs of the pet they are scheduling. For example, the EMR may state that a specific patient has displayed aggression toward other dogs and should be managed to avoid contact with other patients. This means that this pet should be scheduled for a slower time so the veterinary team can manage this dog's FAS as much as possible by clearing hallways and having an examination room ready as soon as possible to prevent exposure to any other animals in the lobby. Consider instructing the client to call the reception team as soon as they arrive at the hospital. The reception team can alert the technician and the technician can go to the car or call the client to discuss the needs of the patient and create a plan to minimize as much stress during entry as possible.

Arrival at the veterinary hospital

The hospital's role of producing a pleasant experience for the pet begins as soon as the patient arrives in the parking lot. The landscaping and approach to the building can even be designed to minimize stress for the patient. Through natural barriers such as bushes or flower beds and wide open walkways, the walk to the front door of the hospital can be a nonthreatening experience for the pet. When possible, provide entrances and exits to the building that minimize congestion. Doorways that provide visualization into and out of the building will allow the pet owner to avoid close encounters with other pets. Safe and secure doors that are easy to manipulate and maneuver reduce the risk of an unpleasant and possibly painful experience. A door that springs shut quickly might start the dog's experience at the hospital with a pinched tail or toes. When possible, have a separate entrance and exit for clients and their pets. This will avert accidental encounters at doorways and avoid crowding because it allows for a smooth flow. Consider offering remote check-in for an appointment from the client's car to allow the pet and owner to remain in the comfort of their vehicle until an examination room is available.

General hospital recommendations

Some general concepts to incorporate throughout the entire hospital to create an environment that is calming and inviting (i.e. utilizes a Considerate Approach) include: providing non-slip surfaces for patients to have good footing, using aroma and acoustic therapy, providing all team members, who are versed on proper treat use, with treat bags for easy access to reinforcers for patients, and integrating a considerate approach when interacting with patients. To avoid overwhelming our patients, it is best to allow them to approach you. Turn sideways and avoid direct eye contact. This makes you appear more approachable. Talk slowly and softly to facilitate a relaxing environment. Move smoothly and calmly and avoid aversive scents and instead use calming ones.

The waiting room/lobby

Proper management of the waiting room will also help keep things running smoothly and ensure the best experience for the pet. It is crucial to have a skilled and properly trained reception team to help in minimizing each pet's fear, anxiety, and stress. Pets can be easily overwhelmed with a kind-hearted person's best intentions in greeting a patient in a happy or excited fashion. Each reception team member should be trained to evaluate patients based on body language.

Positive interactions might be initiated by the receptionist by offering treats to healthy, low FAS patients. (Note that although treats would be used to help treat aggression in the veterinary hospital, only specially trained staff should interact with a patient displaying aggression.)

The reception team should direct the owner to an appropriate space for the patient while they are waiting to be placed in an examination room. The reception team should also monitor the lobby and assure no inappropriate interactions between dogs, cats, or owners occur. Be the patient's advocate! If needed, it should be communicated to the veterinary team that a patient is having a more challenging time, and an exam room should be made available as soon as possible or other recommendations should be made such as having the client walk the dog (if appropriate) outside of the clinic (Figure 8.2), offering remote check-in via text or phone, and having client paperwork completed prior to the appointment via online form submission.

Ideally, patients should be moved to a quiet examination room as soon as possible. Alternatively, providing visual barriers and cornered seating areas away from the doors will decrease stimuli and allow pet owners to safely manage their pet. A stable elevated surface for owners to place their cat or small dog carrier prevents these animals being approached on the floor by passing dogs. Using natural or incandescent lighting can also facilitate a more relaxing environment for clients and pets. A 2015 study (Mariti et al. 2015) was conducted on the welfare of dogs in the waiting room of a veterinary clinic. This study indicated in 28.9% of cases, the stress level of the dog was high. During these displays, the owners did not recognize the signs of FAS their pet had been expressing. The results of this study conclude that the welfare of dogs in a lobby or waiting room of a veterinary hospital is impaired. Moving each patient into a private examination room is the best practice possible in reducing stress and anxiety for the patient.

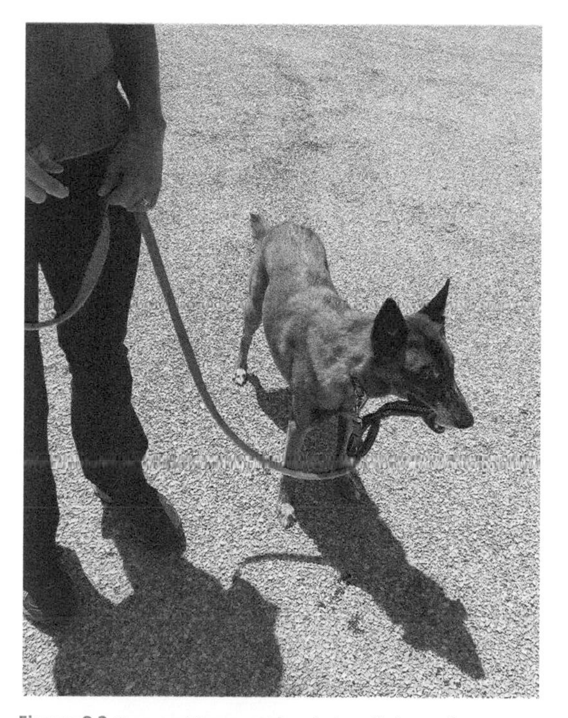

Figure 8.2 Dog waiting outside of the clinic until an exam room is ready. This helps minimize this dog's FAS associated with being in the lobby.

Most clients have become familiar with a curbside check-in process instituted during the COVID-19 pandemic. Modifying client check-ins to occur via text or phone from the comfort of the client's vehicle can prevent the potential of FAS due to waiting in the lobby for an open examination room. Although it may take a minute or two longer to relocate the client into the examination room from the parking lot versus the lobby, avoiding the escalation of FAS will make for a smoother and more accepted exam experience for the pet, which translates to less time and fewer team members involved. The pet's fuse of tolerance has not been used up with environmental triggers encountered in the lobby.

Approach and behavior of veterinary team members

The veterinarian team can change their behavior to prevent a patient from becoming frightened. Direct eye contact or a direct approach is considered a threat, regardless of our intentions. As humans we often smile, look directly at a pet, and walk straight toward them. As discussed in Chapter 2, all of these behaviors signal confrontation. Although many pets have perhaps learned to understand our inappropriate body language toward them, by simply taking a few easy steps we can put our patients at ease. Polite, non-threatening communication includes the following: approach the pet on a curve; avoid maintaining direct eye contact (look and then look away); allow the pet to approach you initially (the pet's choice); turn sideways or squat down to appear less menacing; toss treats to the pet rather than reaching toward the pet. By incorporating these techniques, you will quickly put many patients immediately at ease. See Chapter 9 for techniques to approach a dog displaying body language indicating fear.

- The veterinarian team can change their behavior to prevent a patient from becoming frightened.

Recognizing the subtle signs of fear as detailed in Chapter 2 (Table 2.2 and Figure 2.1 Canine stress ladder) and adapting our interaction with the patient to make the experience more pleasant, when possible, allow for two-way communication to occur (Table 8.2).

Treats should be used whenever possible to promote a positive association. However, ill or fasted patients should not be given treats. Incorporate all other techniques.

Table 8.2 Techniques to prevent negative experiences in the veterinary hospital.

Parking lot and approach to building	Open space with natural barriers, if possible provide separate entrance and exit
Waiting room	Seating area away from the door, barriers or partitions to minimize visual exposure, elevated surface to place cat or small dog carriers, escort to a room as soon as possible, receptionist might provide treats to healthy, low FAS patients
Scale	Treats![a] Non-slip surface
Exam room	Calming pheromone diffusers. Treats should be given when the patient enters the room, on the exam table, and during the physical exam![a] Place a non-slip surface on exam tables or on floors
Non-threatening body language	Approach the pet on a curve, avoid maintaining direct eye contact (look and then look away), allow the pet to approach you initially (the pet's choice), turn sideways or squat down to appear less menacing, toss treats to the pet rather than reaching toward the pet

[a] Recognize signs of fear and modify interaction when possible.

The scale

The scale bears special mention as the pet owners' or team members' attempts to obtain a weight on the pet, often results in fear, anxiety, and stress if special considerations are not made. Ideally, the scale should be stable, with a non-slip surface, and in an open area to avoid the dog having to walk into a corner to get on it. Rather than pulling or forcing the dog to get on the scale, use a treat trail and/or motion to encourage the dog to make the choice to step on the scale. Oftentimes the more we try to force the issue, the more fearful the dog becomes and the more he/she wants to get away. In the end taking a few seconds and a few treats will save you a lot of time and stress. Go to the companion website to view a video that demonstrates using a treat trail to encourage a dog to get on the scale on their own. Using movement and guiding the dog with your body position is also beneficial. Most dogs will naturally follow the direction your feet and shoulders are pointing. Notice in the video how the technician turns her body parallel to the scale as the dog approaches and walks onto the scale (Video 8.1).

The scale should be placed in an open area to eliminate any patient's fear of being confined or unable to escape. Ideally, the scale should be flush with the floor to prevent the animal from needing to step up onto a new substrate.

Small, readily consumed treats or other forms of reinforcement such as toys or scent lures should be provided to the patients as they are allowed to voluntarily walk onto the scale. Keeping reinforcement items near the scale (on shelving units above) can be useful and can assist in coaching the clients and other team members to use these items. Providing a non-slip surface on the scale and examination table will help to put canine and feline patients at ease (Figure 8.3).

The examination room

Creating a stress-free examination room can be crucial to setting the tone for the patient's entire physical examination. Ideally, have patients in species-specific rooms (dogs–dogs and cats–cats). If this cannot be accomplished successfully, the rooms should be cleaned and sanitized well with an enzymatic cleaner to eliminate the scent from other patients that were previously seen in that room. Another option is to have select days and hours for non-emergency feline patients, such as morning appointments twice a week. Offering feline

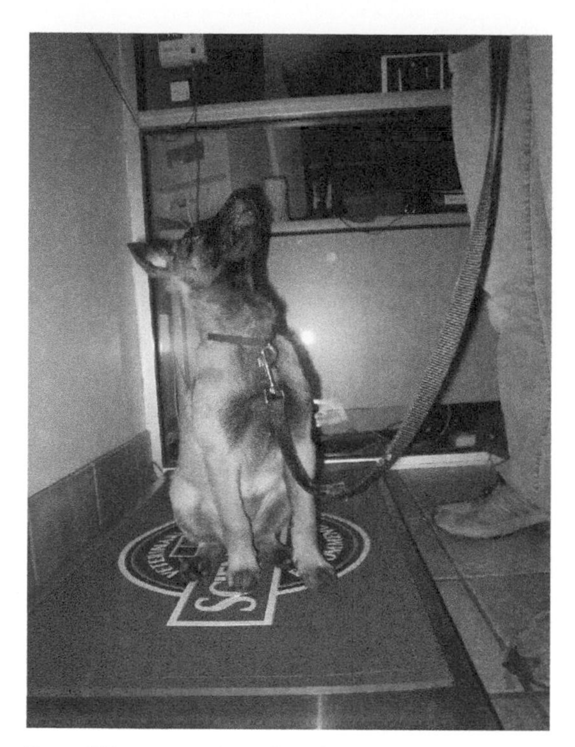

Figure 8.3 Puppy on the scale with a non-slip surface while receiving several small treats.

appointments in the morning minimizes the smell of canine patients in the area.

Select furniture that has a closed bottom to eliminate the potential for cats or small animals to become trapped in a small space. Hiding can be a way to eliminate stress for the patient and appropriate outlets for hiding should be provided in the examination room, such as allowing a cat to remain in their carrier, draping a towel over the pet, using cardboard boxes or elevated cat cubes. Providing a non-slip surface on the exam table or on the floor where the pet is being examined can also be useful to prevent slipping and paw/body contact with a cold surface, helping the pet to feel safe and comfortable. Each exam room should be stocked with a variety of treats and toys. A water bowl should be provided for each patient. Travel to the hospital and treats can make for a thirsty pet. Cats should be provided with access to a litter box to allow them an opportunity for relief.

Allowing time for acclimation to the new environment is especially beneficial. It can take 5–10 minutes for a pet to become comfortable and feel safe in a new environment. Go to the companion website to view a video showing a dog responding to known cues while waiting in the exam room. The room has a large non-slip area and the owner has brought the dog's "Treat-Ment" station from home. There is also species-specific calming music playing. Note the cue "Aboie" is French for bark (Video 8.2). While the technician is collecting the history, if safe to do so, opening the carrier door and/or having the client drop their pet's leash can give the pet an opportunity to explore the space. During this time, the technician can begin to assess the patient's body language and food acceptance. The technician's observations of the pet's emotional state should be recorded and communicated to the veterinarian. Keep zip ties in each examination room to reassemble carriers as needed should the bolts be removed to take the lid off a carrier but then not be able to be secured again.

Minimizing the number of staff arrivals and departures from the room will help to maintain a calmer pet. Sudden environmental changes (people exiting and entering the room), can escalate FAS and alertness in the patient. It is also distracting for the client. It is best to anticipate and have all supplies in the room prior to escorting the client and pet into the room. During the veterinary exam it is important to educate and communicate with the owner and the veterinarian throughout the examination. Creating client compliance with the owner is crucial in teaching pets to become comfortable with the type of handling needed to keep them healthy and well groomed throughout their lives. Monitoring and describing body language seen during the visit can be an invaluable tool for the veterinary technician. Describing and discussing body language can raise the bar and help the owner to understand how their pet may be feeling during the visit. This open communication can make procedures run smoothly and save staff time by creating a relaxed and cooperative patient in the clinic. If fear, anxiety, and stress are noted, this can be addressed at that time so there are no surprises in the future if the patient's behavior progresses over time. The first puppy/kitten appointment is the ideal time to prepare puppies and kittens for physical exams, venipuncture, teeth cleaning, ear cleaning, and pedicures. It is vital that technicians avoid mishandling patients regardless of their age or behavior. The goal should always be to create a positive association with the examination process that can follow the pet through the rest of its life. Rough or forceful handling methods teach fear and mistrust and often result in a difficult-to-handle adult pet. It also sets a poor example for owners to follow and could be considered malpractice. The veterinary team should do their best to match any touching with food reinforcement when able (Figure 8.4). Handling and restraint techniques are discussed in further detail in the upcoming section: **Gentle Control techniques**.

- The goal should always be to create a positive association with the examination process that can follow the pet through the rest of its life. Rough or forceful handling methods teach fear and mistrust and often result in a difficult-to-handle adult pet. It also sets a poor example for owners to follow and could be considered malpractice.

Ideally, once the pet has acclimated to the room, it is best to bring the procedures to the pet whenever possible. This allows the pet to stay in an area that is safe and comfortable and with the owner. If an owner is uncomfortable being in the room during procedures, you may ask them to step out into the reception area for a moment.

Treatment and procedure areas

Treatment areas are essential spaces to the veterinary medical team as they house a large amount of equipment, provide more space to work with patients, and so on. Unfortunately, taking patients away from the owner can cause unnecessary stress for the patient and the client. If it is necessary to take the patient to the treatment area, first reconnaissance your route without the pet. Inform other team members of your intent to bring the patient to the treatment area and make accommodations to avoid or minimize potentially frightening stimuli. Have all supplies prepared for the treatment prior to bringing the patient into the area. This will minimize the amount of time the pet has to be in the unfamiliar area. Utilize barriers as the pet is transported to the treatment area and while in the treatment area to decrease exposure to potentially frightening stimuli.

The treatment area is usually one of the busiest and nosiest locations in the hospital. This space houses unwell patients for close monitoring, has a large amount of loud sounds such as vacuums and clippers suddenly being turned on, beeping from fluid pumps and monitoring equipment, cage doors opening and closing, team members discussing cases (which increases the amount of foot traffic in this location), and so on. It is in the pet's best interest to complete as much of the examination and procedures as possible in the examination room with the owners. In some cases, animals may appear to behave better without their owner's presence. This effect is typically caused more by learned helplessness rather than true comfort. Assess if the pet is able to eat away from the owner and evaluate the patient's body language to fully evaluate if the FAS

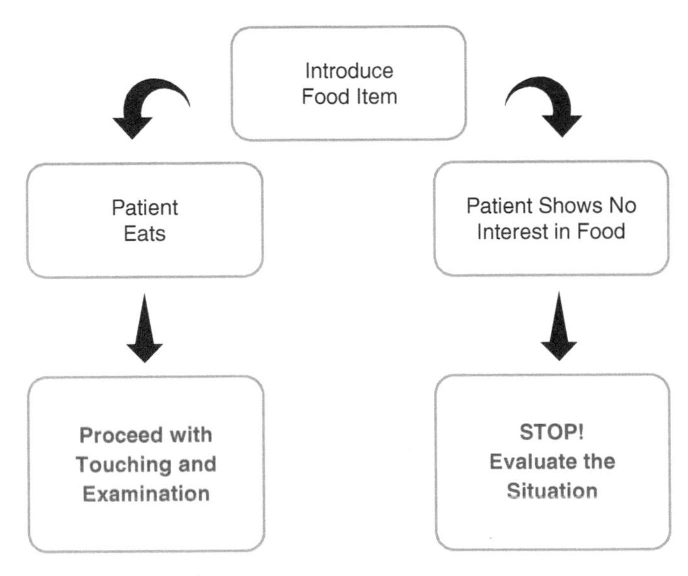

Figure 8.4 Flow chart: food use during physical examination.

level is truly reduced without the owner's presence. The veterinarian, technicians, assistants, and other team members will be the primary advocates for the pets in the treatment room. Continue to assess the patient's emotional well-being and make notes in the EMR as warranted.

- The veterinarian, technicians, assistants, and other team members will be the primary advocates for the pets in the treatment room. Continue to assess the patient's emotional well-being and make notes in the emotional medical record as warranted.

Housing areas and wards

The housing area is often the area in which other team members, such as the pet care specialists or kennel attendants, will be responsible for being the advocate for the pets. Technicians/assistants and the veterinarian will also play an accessory role in this area. The kennel team will be responsible for recognizing fear, anxiety, and stress in patients and recording and communicating this information to others.

In housing areas, it is most important to control the number of stimuli that can increase stress and anxiety. When bringing a pet back to stay at the hospital, it is important to have the kennel or cage space set up ahead of time. Place non-slip mats and blankets to prevent the pet from slipping. Visual barriers such as blankets/towels over the front of the kennel to reduce visual stimuli of other pets and people passing by the space might be necessary and appropriate for some patients. Each species should be separated as much as possible. If the ward area of the hospital is smaller and this cannot be accomplished, visual barriers will be beneficial. Spray calming pheromones on the blankets before use. If the animal does not need to be fasted, use food enrichment toys to give the patient an appropriate outlet for their mouth to prevent as much vocalization as possible. In dog wards, providing sound-reducing acoustic measures such as baffled tiles, acoustic membranes, and acoustic muffling ceiling tiles can be used. For felines, prepare the cage with a non-slip mat, blanket, litter box, and a small place to hide. This can be something as simple as a cardboard box, canvas shopping bags, cat condos, or even the bottom half of a carrier. Visual barriers are crucial in reducing stress and anxiety for feline patients. Use towels and blankets at the front of the cage as mentioned above.

For pets requiring an extended (more than 24 hours) stay in the hospital, providing appropriate enrichment opportunities are necessary to promote mental and physical well-being. The lack of enrichment can result in additional stress and consequently immune suppression and slower healing. What one pet finds enriching another pet might find frightening. Monitoring the pet's FAS level before, during, and after enrichment will help fine-tune appropriate activities for the pet. Because these pets are being treated for medical conditions, enrichment activities should be approved by the attending veterinarian. Some options include, food puzzle toys, gentle petting by a team member, exploratory activity in a quiet room that incorporates pleasant sights, sounds, smells, taste, and touch. Pets should not be left unsupervised with enrichment items as they could ingest them or become entangled in them. Use safety, supervision, and your observations skills. For more information about canine enrichment consider the following online course, Fear Free®: A Close Look at Canine Enrichment.

Appropriate placement of patients should also be considered. Cats generally prefer to be up high. The dog that gets overly aroused when people or dogs walk past, should be placed in an area of lower traffic. Whenever possible, use Considerate Approach when removing the pet from a cage or kennel and close kennel doors quietly. Conversations should be quiet and soft voices should be utilized to maintain a calm and relaxing environment. Use your "spa" tone.

Moving between areas of the hospital

Moving patients through the hospital in a low-stress manner can be an essential way to aid in reducing stress and anxiety when the patient needs to be moved from the examination room or from the housing area while staying in hospital. Cattle Dog Publishing's Low Stress Handling® Certification Course thoroughly demonstrates how to move effectively throughout the hospital. Some key points to remember when moving canine patients:

- The handler should face the direction they want the dog to walk.
- Use clear communication with team members to find whether hallways and rooms are clear and safe for patient movement. Using communication channels such as Slack, may be a good way to

communicate from an examination room to the front desk reception team or to the treatment room.
- Keep a relaxed "U" with the leash between the handler and patient.
- When medically appropriate, pair moving into the new environment with treats by offering high-value food items when entering new spaces.
- When moving cat carriers, always hold the carrier by placing one hand on the bottom of the carrier and one hand holding the top. This will help to keep the carrier stable during movement.

Return home

The return home should also be a fear-free event for the pet and other pets in the home. The same transport considerations as noted in the section **Home preparations** should be applied. Many clients have multi-pet households. To avoid relationship issues between housemates, it is imperative that we educate owners on how to reintroduce their pets. Some pets will give the "returnee" the cold shoulder, acting as if they do not know him. Worse, they may react negatively, even aggressively. That is because the pet may smell or look different (especially if they have been shaved or had a surgical procedure), causing fear and anxiety in the pets who remained home. Here are some tips to help prevent a negative reintroduction when returning home with a pet.

Assume it might not go well and set the pets up for success. A negative reintroduction results in a long-lasting negative memory. There have been cases of cats no longer being able to live together after a reunion went badly. The time and financial commitment sometimes required to repair the relationship between pets can be prohibitive for some.

Take a walk. If appropriate, take the dogs for a walk together. The distraction of doing a normal activity together on neutral territory can help re-establish their familiarity with each other. Ideally, each dog should be walked by a different person.

Cats can be distracted with a play session or special meal for each cat at a distance from each other. Dogs can be distracted by asking for known cues or tricks and reinforcing those with small treats.

Manage the situation by controlling the reintroduction. Control the reintroduction by managing the other pets on leash, restricting them to another room, or keeping them behind a baby gate or exercise pen or inside their crate (if the pets are crate trained). This prevents the other pets from rushing up to the returning pet.

The three-second rule. It is normal for your other pets to want to smell the returning pet, who is bringing back unique odors. Prolonged sniffing can make your pet uncomfortable. Introduce and enforce the three-second rule. If sniffing last for more than three seconds, calmly get your pets' attention by gently clapping your hands or saying their names in an upbeat tone. Keep it calm and avoid creating tension. Call them away to get a toy or follow you to the treat jar.

Provide a safe haven. If the pet was sedated or had any procedures performed that may not make him feel 100%, provide him with a safe and comfortable place to relax without the other pets around. This might be in a crate, exercise pen, or special room. Once he is back to himself, a controlled reintroduction to the household can be implemented.

If you notice excessive interest in the returning pet or body language indicators of fear, anxiety, or stress, such as freezing, walking slowly, hiding, lifted lip, growling, or hissing, to name just a few, separate the pets and work on a more gradual introduction.

Mix their scents. Smell is so important to our pets. Cats, especially, seem to recognize each other by scent. Cats and dogs can be sensitive to unfamiliar smells such as antiseptics or grooming products. Work to familiarize them with each other's scents by allowing them to sniff each other through the space beneath a closed door. You can also artificially mix their scents; to do this, take a dry face cloth and allow the cat or dog to rub on it or pet them with it gently. Repeat with a new cloth for all pets in the house. Leave the cloths out in the environment with treats around them to let them get used to each other's scents.

Calming pheromones may also be helpful in promoting a harmonious reintroduction.

How quickly the reintroduction takes depends on the individual animals and the circumstances. Some pets take just a few minutes to resume a normal relationship. Others might take hours or even a day or two to become comfortable with each other again.

For more information on introducing pets refer to Chapter 7, Prevention (canine and feline): introducing a new pet.

Gentle control techniques

Traditionally, physical restraint has been used to hold animals still while veterinary procedures are performed, because many of the procedures performed in the veterinary hospital require the animal to remain relatively still. The work of the late Dr. Sophia Yin (Low Stress Handling®) and Fear Free® teaches veterinary professionals other options or techniques to minimize the amount of physical restraint or manipulation needed to keep the animal and veterinary team comfortable and safe.

We will discuss two main categories of techniques that we have labeled distraction techniques and touch then reinforce techniques. Cooperative care training and potential gentle control tools will also be examined.

Distraction techniques

Dogs and cats should be encouraged to lick canned cheese, canned dog/cat food or meat-based (onion-free) baby food from the table or a food dispenser (lick mat, cup, or syringe casing) while being examined. Frequently, a complete physical exam can be performed while the patient is licking the treat from the table or from a syringe case held by the owner (Figure 8.5). A treat can be placed in the patient's mouth as the teeth are examined. A patient that is leery of medical instruments such as the stethoscope or otoscope can be allowed to lick a treat from the instrument's surface. Mild restraint, such as a position that mimics drawing a blood sample, can be practiced while the patient is distracted by the treat. The pet is cooperative because it is focused on the treat but at the same time it may develop a positive association with mildly uncomfortable handling. An animal that struggles, growls, or even tries to bite during an examination is not displaying "dominance" but is instead frightened or unsure. Rough handling using "domination techniques" (forcing on the side "until it submits" or grabbing the muzzle) or physically or verbally reprimanding (yelling "No!") will only increase fear and can be permanently damaging to the pet. Should a patient show any sign of apprehension or fearfulness, specifically, if it stops taking treats, the process should be slowed or decreased until it begins taking treats again. If the patient wiggles or pauses from the treat distraction, use the three second/three tries rule for dogs and two second/two tries rule for cats. If the pet refuses the distraction or attempts to move away pause what you are doing to allow the pet to relax again. If the pet continues to refuse the distraction or wiggles for three seconds (dogs)/two seconds (cats), decrease what you are doing or stop completely and come up with a new plan. Three well-tolerated attempts for dogs and two well-tolerated attempts for cats should be the maximum times to try to complete the procedure. If the FAS level cannot be brought back down to a two, other options should be explored, such as giving the pet a break, rescheduling, giving pre-visit medications to decrease FAS, or sedation. Continuing to restrain a panicked animal until he gives up will not teach the pet to enjoy being restrained and is likely to escalate to aggression in future encounters. A pet that has an extreme reaction to restraint or handling indicates the need for a recommendation for intervention behavior services and treatment with desensitization and counter conditioning.

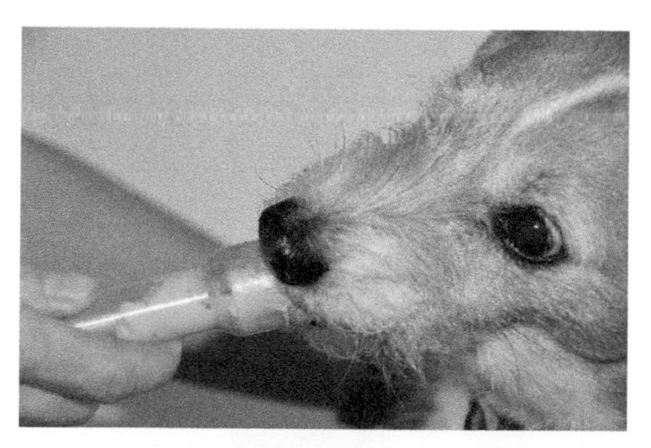

Figure 8.5 An adult dog licking canned cheese from a 12-cc syringe case.

- Should a patient show any sign of apprehension or fearfulness, specifically, if it stops taking treats, the process should be slowed or decreased until it begins taking treats again.

- Continuing to restrain a panicked animal until he gives up will not teach the pet to enjoy being restrained and is likely to escalate to aggression in future encounters.

Initially when Debbie Martin, the co-author of this chapter, heard others talking about the concept of using treats to distract an animal during veterinary care, she thought "NO way! That will not create a conditioned emotional response and you can poison the presentation of the food. How inefficient and ineffective! I used to do that until I learned better." However, there can be a time and place for using these procedures. Veterinary behavior colleagues in general practice indicated that many animals do not find veterinary procedures that aversive. It is often the restraint they dislike the most not the needle sticks or examination (there are exceptions). While giving a vaccination, if you create a yummy distraction (such as a plate of canned dog food) with a pet, who does not have body sensitivity issues, often the pet will happily eat up the food and not even notice getting a vaccine. Although not an efficient way to pair being touched by the veterinarian or getting vaccines with good things, being in the exam room and the veterinary technician are likely to be paired with good things (e.g. dog goes into the room/technician in room and canned food is presented). For perhaps 75% (no data on this just an estimation after speaking with colleagues) of veterinary patients, this strategy will work for procedures that do not have to be repeated often (i.e. only a few times a year) and the animal does not find the procedure aversive.

Distraction techniques are exactly as they sound, distract the animal while care is being provided, i.e. constant feeding. There are a lot more stipulations to it in order to attempt to create a pleasant situation for the animal. The distraction must be something the pet LIKES! Tapping on the cat's head or making a loud noise to startle or distract the animal might work (NOT recommended) but the goal of these techniques should be to make a pleasant experience; something the animal would look forward to in the future. The most common distraction used is food but other things like petting, brushing, smelling something interesting, toys, or talk are potentially other pleasant distractors for some animals.

- The distraction must be something the pet LIKES! Tapping on the cat's head or making a loud noise to startle or distract the animal might work (NOT recommended) but the goal of these techniques should be to make a pleasant experience; something the animal would look forward to in the future.

Here are two scenarios of what distraction might look like while a handling procedure is being performed. TG refers to using a touch gradient (Figures 8.6 and 8.7).

In the first example (Figure 8.6), the basic distraction technique begins with offering a distraction to the pet and the pet becoming involved with the distraction. The distraction could be licking food off a plate, leaning into the hand for petting or brushing, smelling an intriguing odor, or taking a favorite ball in the mouth. Once the animal is engaged in the distraction, handling begins utilizing a touch gradient. The patient is constantly assessed for increasing levels of FAS. The procedure continues if the FAS level remains at a FAS 3 or lower. If the pet pauses from the distraction, the procedure should be paused. Once the procedure and handling end, the distraction can end as well. Please note when the handling and distraction are stopped, there would be a brief pause before starting back at the beginning again. If ending the session or done with the procedure, give several small treats and encourage the learner to do another fun activity such as play with a toy or do a cued behavior. The goal is to prevent the animal from being frustrated or disappointed that the "handling

Distraction Begins
Handling with TG During Distraction
Stop Handling & Distraction

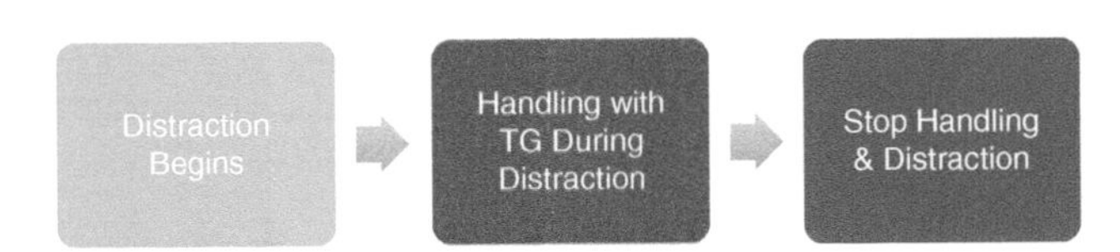

Figure 8.6 Basic distraction technique.

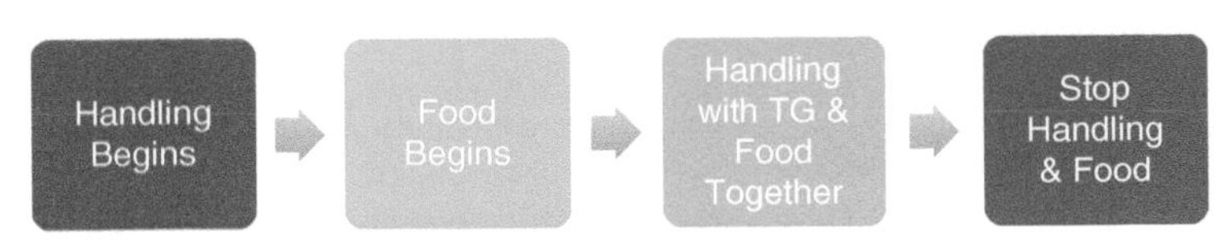

Figure 8.7 Modified distraction technique.

game" is ending. On the companion website Video 8.3 demonstrates the basic distraction technique. A thorough EMR is available on this dog. She is a 7.5-year-old, spayed female, Belgian Malinois named Jazmin and she has only ever exhibited a hard look (stare) and avoidance (moving away) with handling, FAS 4. She has never attempted to bite while being restrained or handled in the 7.5 years she has been owned by the same people. She loves toys and soft, lickable food treats. Precautionary statements: If working with a new patient that you do not have a good emotional record or relationship with already, gentle control tools and safety precautions, such as acclimating to a basket muzzle, may be warranted. In the video a touch gradient is utilized throughout. If the dog stops eating, the procedure is paused. Depending on the dog, the handling may need to be decreased rather than just paused. If the dog pauses for more than three seconds, the technician moves her hands away to allow the dog to relax further. Without the emotional record and previous learning history with the technician, the stares from the dog would be of more concern and a safety issue. Remember if you are feeling uncomfortable with a patient, do not have a good emotional record, or established relationship, do not hesitate to acclimate him/her to a gentle control tool, such as a basket muzzle, prior to attempting gentle control techniques. Notice how when the dog stops eating, the technician stops and avoids eye contact with the dog. The dog is being given the power to tell the technician to slow down. When the dog resumes eating, the technician continues (Video 8.3).

In the second scenario (Figure 8.7), the modified version of the distraction technique starts with the pet being touched in a neutral location THEN the distraction begins. While the handling/procedure proceed the distraction continues. When the handling/procedure are stopped or complete, the distraction stops. If ending the session, transition the pet to another fun activity. Video 8.4 on the companion website demonstrates a version of the modified distraction technique. The technician cues the assistant to bring in the food by saying, "Food," and then to remove the food when she says, "Done." The dog in the video is a nine-year-old spayed female Belgian Malinois named Iliana and she has shown FAS 4 escape behavior with handling but she has not escalated to aggression. Because the dog had arthritis in her legs, she was more comfortable with less contact with the legs, thus the reason that a touch gradient from the shoulder to the foot was not used (Video 8.4).

Distraction can be easy, quick, and successful for animals with low levels of FAS (FAS 2 or lower or Level 1 from Cooperative Veterinary Care) and who are comfortable with the husbandry procedure being performed. Often the pet owner can be coached on how to deliver the food throughout the handling or a food-holding device can be used. Learning how to do this can help the owner treat their pet at home with minimal stress. Owners who reprimanded their pets for refusing care at home were more likely to have animals who would display aggression toward veterinary professionals in the veterinary setting (Mariti et al. 2016).

Distraction can also be a starting point for progressing to other behavior modification and training procedures. When starting a desensitization and counter conditioning plan, you might start with some distraction techniques to prevent any unnecessary behaviors from the animal. By having the animal focus on a treat in hand, the pet is less likely to shift in weight or turn the head toward the hand reaching to touch the animal. Many animals are not showing avoidance in this context but just looking at the touching hand because perhaps they think they are supposed to target the hand. By changing the animals focus to the treat target in the hand, we can avoid the unnecessary behaviors and have a clean repetition to start. Once they see the "picture," then start to switch to another procedure which would involve a delay in the reinforcer. Think of distraction technique as a lure and if you do not want to be dependent on the lure, a plan should be made to fade it out.

Although at first glance the distraction procedure seems simple; give food and do the handling; there is more to it and distraction can be executed well or poorly. When using distraction techniques, it is imperative to continuously monitor the FAS level of the animal and adjust the handling accordingly to maintain low levels of FAS. If the animal stops eating or changes how they are eating (FAS 3–4), stop/pause, wait for consent to proceed. If there is a two- or three-second pause, decrease what you are doing.

- When using distraction techniques, it is imperative to continuously monitor the FAS level of the animal and adjust the handling accordingly to maintain low levels of FAS. If the animal stops eating or changes how they are eating (FAS 3–4), stop/pause, wait for consent to proceed. If there is a two- or three-second pause, decrease what you are doing.

Table 8.3 Pros and cons of distraction techniques.

Pros	Cons
Quick way to minimize stress with handling	Not a good long-term solution for routine procedures
Less physical restraint needed	If not careful, could result in the animal refusing food in the context
Prevent negative experiences	The anxiety level might be masked
Fairly easy for non-trainer to implement	Not safe to use with a pet with resource-guarding tendencies
	Additional people needed for food delivery

Potential disadvantages of using distraction techniques include the animal beginning to refuse food in the context, the food masking the pet's anxiety level about the situation, and potential food guarding (resource guarding) issues especially with dogs (Table 8.3). The refusal of food or "poisoning" of the context is much more likely to occur if we do not use care in monitoring the FAS level of the pet and if we do not adjust what we are doing based on their response. A pet who is leaning away and is roughly snatching the food from the food dispenser is displaying FAS level 3–4 and is likely in a motivational conflict (he wants the food but does not like the handling).

Distraction is not usually a good long-term solution for routine procedures that could potentially be uncomfortable or aversive to the pet (the individual decides this!). Because of the constant feeding of food, logistically it can be difficult for one person to perform unless using a stable food-dispensing device.

Using this technique makes it difficult to create a positive association with the handling procedure because the handling is not predictive of the rewards. However, it can make for a more pleasant experience for many animals, decrease the amount of physical restraint needed, and potentially prevent a negative experience.

Touch then reinforce techniques

To create a clearer pairing with handling/stabilization and "good things," we suggest combining a desensitization procedure and a reinforcer. This model incorporates presenting the reinforcer ***after*** a step in the handling. Because classical (reflexive and emotional) and operant (voluntary and observable) behaviors are happening all the time, this technique capitalizes on pairing good things, like treats, with being touched (classical conditioning) and also reinforcing specific observable behavior, such as relaxed body language, remaining still, or performing a trained behavior (operant conditioning).

Incorporating a positive event marker (details about marker and clicker training are provided in Chapter 9) with this technique, concisely pinpoints the reinforceable moment and bridges the slight delay in treat/reinforcer delivery. Sometimes the positive event marker also acts to prompt a helper to deliver the treat/reinforcer. Just a reminder that classical and operant conditioning are always happening simultaneously. As Dr. Susan Schneider would say, "the whole system is churning" (Schneider 2012).

Whether using a positive event marker or not, there will be behavioral indicators that tell the learner he is about to get a treat/reinforcer (e.g. moving the treat hand) and that will become the marker. However, a precise event marker will be more efficient and effective at communicating the precise behavior you are reinforcing. If choosing to use a clicker as the event marker, the learner should have a sufficient learning history with clicker training and have a strong positive conditioned emotional response to the click before using with handling or other desensitization processes. The dog must be clicker savvy before using a clicker with behavior modification.

One technique is to mark the animal remaining relaxed during the handling, then remove or pause the hands on the animal and bring the treat/reinforcer to the animal (Figure 8.8). Another option is to mark the continuation of an operant behavior (such as chin rest) after completion of the husbandry care or approximation of the husbandry care. They are both valuable procedures with a slightly different focus. So, if using a clicker as the event marker, the click might happen during or after the handling. With this technique it is important to *wait* for the learner to finish the treat/food *before* starting the next repetition.

Because the treat is not happening constantly throughout the handling, this can sometimes be easier to perform if only one person is available. With this technique, it is less likely that the high-value food will mask FAS in the learner. However, some learners might choose to stay in the situation because they want the food even if they are not

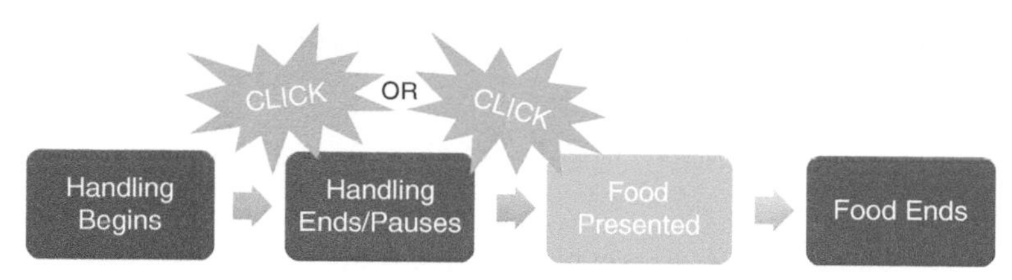

Figure 8.8 Touch then reinforce techniques.

comfortable with the handling. Always continue to monitor the patient's FAS level. Although this procedure might be more likely to create a stronger positive conditioned emotional response with the handling, it can be more difficult for the learner because there is a delay from the handling and the presentation of the food. It can also be more difficult for the pet owner to time correctly (Table 8.4).

Video 8.5 on the companion website demonstrates the touch then reinforce technique with Jazmin the Belgian Malinois you saw having her ears cleaned using the basic distraction technique. In this example, the technician cues the helper to bring a treat to the dog by saying, "treat." Once the word "treat" is spoken the technician removes her hands while the helper delivers the treat. The dog is allowed to eat the treat before the next repetition begins. Notice that this dog is more comfortable with this technique than the basic distraction technique. She still shows some signs of FAS but recovers quickly. Because this is a training situation the technician decides to start at the beginning after each repetition. This could be modified, and the technician could keep her hands on the dog as the treat is delivered and progress from the previous stop point.

Table 8.4 Pros and cons of touch then reinforce techniques.

Pros	Cons
Easier for one person	Delay from handling to food can be challenging for some patients
Less likely to mask anxiety	More difficult for non-trainer to implement
Create a stronger positive conditioned emotional response with handling	
Avoid conflict with eating and being touched	

The second part of this video demonstrates using a clicker, rather than the word "treat," to mark the acceptance of being touched and imminent treat delivery. If using this method, the clicker should have a strong reinforcement history with the individual animal prior to using with gentle control techniques. If this dog had been more uncomfortable with being reached over, the technician could have avoided reaching over the dog's head to access the left ear by moving to the other side of the dog (Video 8.5).

Cooperative care and cooperative care training

Cooperative care is a term used to describe a variety of different procedures. Here is a definition used in the Fear Free® Animal Trainer course: "Cooperative care is husbandry using trained behaviors to increase the animal's cooperation [and comfort] during care." This includes things like a stationing, targeting, predictor cues, and consent behaviors.

If we expand the definition of cooperative care to include a more general collaboration between animals and people providing the care, then anytime we are focusing on the emotional well-being of animals and adapting our interactions based on behavioral signals from the animal, we are performing cooperative care. It becomes a dialogue between animals and people rather than a one-sided conversation controlled by people. Cooperative care *training* is the gold standard for empowering the animal and increasing their comfort level with care. In the ideal world, all pets would have cooperative care *training*. What a wonderful life skill for animals to have!

- Cooperative care training is the gold standard for empowering the animal and increasing their comfort level with care.

Stationing and targeting behaviors

One form of cooperative care training is teaching the animal to station or target their body or body part in a particular position. This could include teaching a "Treat-Ment" station. (Information regarding the Treat-Ment station and predictor cues is a collaboration of content written by Mikkel Becker and Debbie Martin.) Aspects of needed care can be done on the animal's Treat-Ment station, including examination, handling, grooming, administering oral or topical medications, and other procedures. Unlike a settle mat, where the animal's default body position is commonly a relaxed position like a down, the default body position for the Treat-Ment station is a stand, as is commonly needed during handling and procedures. From the standing position, the animal may be prompted to move into other positions as needed, such as cued to sit, lie down, or move into a side lying position.

It is important that the animal has a positive, pleasant association with their Treat-Ment station built from the start and maintained throughout the life of the pet. The Treat-Ment station's value is built and preserved by continually associating its use with high-value reinforcers. One way to do so is by feeding special treats, meals, stuffed food puzzles, and favorite chews on this area and performing short, happy handling and mock care sessions on the station. Ensuring the animal's consent or lack thereof is respected and responded to properly is also an important way to keep the animal comfortable.

It is important for the animal to always have the choice to move onto or off their Treat-Ment station. The animal should never be coerced or forced to move onto the space, but willingly offer it by choice. Moving onto and remaining on the Treat-Ment station serves as the animal's "yes" for care to start or continue. If the animal is reluctant to move onto their Treat-Ment station, or if already on the Treat-Ment station then leans away, moves off or steps away from the area, this signals a need to pause or stop and for the human handlers to reassess the situation; including the animal, the surrounding environment, and themselves, and to adjust accordingly. The animal's lack of participation may signal fear, anxiety, and/or stress and require a different approach or more gradual exposure to the situation.

A Treat-Ment station should be mobile and provide good footing and a non-slip surface. Utilize as many of the pet's senses as part of the training. For example, use calming music to signal a training session as well as using commercially available calming pheromones or a calming scent such as dilute lavender for dogs.

Video 8.6 on the companion website demonstrates the training process of teaching a Treat-Ment station with dogs (Video 8.6).

Another example of cooperative care training is teaching a target behavior. The Treat-Ment station is a body target behavior to the mat. Other target behaviors include a chin rest on a hand or towel, a sustained nose touch to a hand or object, a shoulder or hip target to an object such as a cage door. Trained target behaviors can allow the animal to be positioned for veterinary care without the need to be physically manipulated into position. Thus, creating a more cooperative and enjoyable experience.

Video 8.7 on the companion website is an example of using a chin rest behavior for husbandry care at home. This video is courtesy of Mikkel Becker, Lead Animal Trainer for Fear Free Pets, CBCC-KA, CDBC, KPA CTP, CPDT-KA, CTC, Fear Free Cert, BA Comm, co-author of *From Fearful to Fear Free*.

Predictor cues

Predictor cues are another form of cooperative care training. They are also known as communication or informational cues. Unlike a typical cue taught to prompt a behavior in the animal, a predictor cue communicates to the animal what the person is going to do next. It provides the animal with information about what to expect. This predictability and consequently lack of uncertainty, can help create ease in the pet.

- Unlike a typical cue taught to prompt a behavior in the animal, a predictor cue communicates to the animal what the person is going to do next.

Ideally, the pet should be trained to the Treat-Ment station prior to commencing with teaching predictor cues, as the Treat-Ment station is a great place to work on handling. When working on predictor cues, first pair being touched by a person with the animal getting treats (distraction and touch then reinforce techniques). Once the pet is happily anticipating or staying relaxed with being touched, start to add in a predictor cue, such as "pet," "ear," or "foot." Immediately after saying the predictor word, then do the action (Figure 8.9). Such as saying "pet"

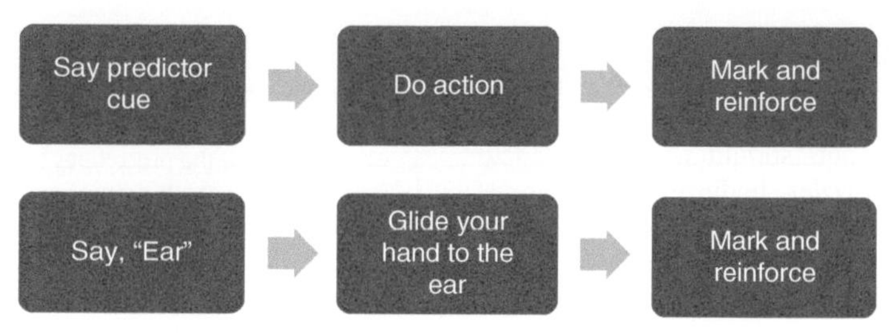

Figure 8.9 Predictor cues.

and right after touching the pet on the shoulder (the pet should show happy and expectant body language and already understand that you will touch and then give a treat). Take care in using a consistent word and not overusing the word (just once is enough prior to the handling/action). Ideally the communication cue will leave the pet with a happy anticipation upon hearing it or the pet will remain relaxed. However, if the pet acts stressed (leans away, ears go back, tail goes down, brow furrows) upon hearing the predictor cue, take it as information about how the pet is feeling in the moment about being touched in that area. It could indicate that additional training is needed to create more comfort with being touched in that area or it could be the pet is experiencing discomfort in the area. Video 8.8 on the companion website is an example of the predictor cue, "brush" resulting in the dog showing avoidance and was not associated with something the dog enjoyed at that moment (Video 8.8).

Generally, predictor cues are taught to help put the animal at ease and decrease uncertainty; however, they can also provide the pet with the option to disengage from the interaction or say no. If the cue is given and the pet displays signs of FAS and/or moves away, we can hear what the pet is saying before actually making contact as was demonstrated in Video 8.8.

Consent behaviors

Consent behaviors are trained behaviors which allow the pet to say they are ready for the next repetition. Examples of consent behaviors are stationing and target behaviors such as the Treat-Ment station and chin rest. Other examples are using eyes as a target, such as the animal staring at a bucket or treat container (a game made popular by renowned animal trainer Chirag Patel, with Domesticated Manners), providing eye contact to the handler, or targeting their nose to an object, such as the nail trimmers or brush. Through training the animal learns that when they offer the behavior, the handler will perform another repetition. This gives the animal the choice to ask for the next repetition and signal when they are ready to proceed. Of extreme importance is that if the animal is doing a duration behavior such as staring at a bucket or a chin rest, if the animal stops performing the behavior during the procedure, the handler should, if possible, pause or cease the handling immediately. Duration consent behaviors are a way for the animal to clearly communicate they need a break. Consent cues give the client and veterinary team clear communication that the patient is not comfortable with handling before an aggressive display has begun. In contrast, a short duration behavior such as targeting the nail trimmers to signal the animal is ready for the next nail to be trimmed, allows the animal to set the pace but does not have a built-in clear signal for the animal to opt out during the procedure. Both types of consent behaviors are valuable and can be useful in a variety of care situations. Video 8.9 on the companion website illustrates the beginning stages of adding in handling with a chin rest and the dog learning that lifting his head up stops the trainer's behavior (Video 8.9).

- Consent cues give the client and veterinary team clear communication that the patient is not comfortable with handling before an aggressive display has begun.

Gentle control tools

To safely provide less physical restraint, gentle control tools may be warranted in some situations. Any tool used to increase safety, should not be done at the expense of the pet's emotional well-being. The goal of using a gentle control tool is to allow for more pleasant associations and a better experience for the pet. Ideally, pets should be acclimated to things like basket muzzles, body and head wraps, toweling techniques, head collars, and Elizabethan collars at a young age (during puppy and kitten classes). To create positive experiences with care, the situation, and the gentle control tools, the pet should be introduced to these tools using treats or other high-value reinforcers.

- Any tool used to increase safety, should not be done at the expense of the pet's emotional well-being.

For more information on these tools refer to Chapter 9, Training tools. A fantastic resource on toweling techniques for cats is *Low Stress Handling and Restraint*, the book and online courses.

Gentle control summary

Cooperative care training is the gold standard for empowering the animal and increasing their comfort level with care. In the ideal world, all pets would have cooperative care training. For pets that do not have the advantage of having cooperative care training, we can still utilize effective and humane strategies for care in the moment.

We should always be asking ourselves, does the process create a behavior change for the better, worse, or no change? What works well for one learner might backfire completely for another. Previous learning is likely to affect this. For example, Debbie's clicker-trained Malinois showed more relaxed behaviors with the touch then treat techniques instead of the distraction techniques, possibly because she found it to be more predictable based on her learning history. However, this might also be because Jazmin was never taught to be touched while eating and she understood the process of X happens, then the click occurs, then she gets a treat. She had learned this game in a variety of contexts. Perhaps if we want to be able to use distraction techniques with the utmost success, we need to introduce the procedures to our learners in a variety of contexts before using it with husbandry and veterinary care.

- Perhaps if we want to be able to use distraction techniques with the utmost success, we need to introduce the procedures to our learners in a variety of contexts before using it with husbandry and veterinary care.

Debbie Martin has found that no matter how much she broke down a desensitization plan, some animals become suspicious after the first few repetitions of the touch then treat techniques. If Debbie went back to distraction to show them what she was working toward, they often relaxed immediately, and then they could switch back to the touch then treat. For some situations remaining with the distraction techniques worked better. Listen to the learner in front of you.

Have a plan before you start but be willing to change the plan if it is not working! You might ping-pong between procedures. Video 8.10 demonstrates adjusting to the dog's avoidance of the stethoscope by switching between distraction and touch then treat techniques. This technique of switching back and forth between procedures is referred to as ping-ponging (Video 8.10).

Throughout the handling watch for signs of decreased interest in the treat, shifting or moving away, a change in how the animal is taking the treats, and other body language indicators of relaxation and FAS.

Keep the session to two or three repetitions of handling then take a 30-second break to ask for other cues, play, or relax away from the handling area. Repetitive handling without little mini breaks can result in decreased enthusiasm for the "game."

Being able to read animals and modify what we are doing (i.e. having a dialogue instead of a monologue) takes practice. Every "conversation" you have with a pet will be different and just as they are learning from you, you will learn from them.

- Every "conversation" you have with a pet will be different and just as they are learning from you, you will learn from them.

The flow chart in Figure 8.10 provides a breakdown of the process of determining which techniques should be used in a given situation.

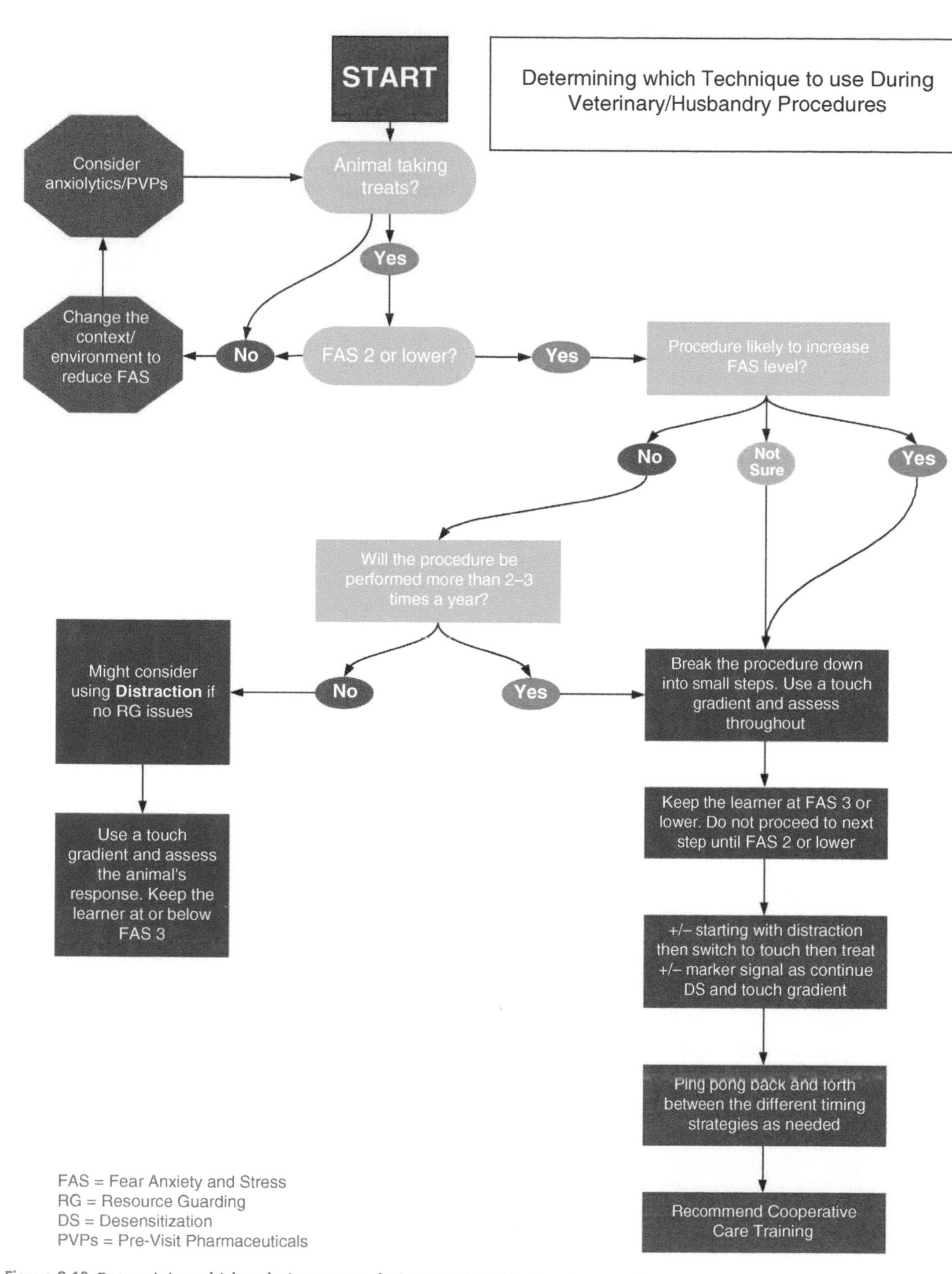

Figure 8.10 Determining which technique to use during veterinary/husbandry procedures.

Creating a plan for veterinary care

This information has been modified from a handout titled *Prior to Handling Small Animals* by Shreyer et al. 2012 and information in the original Fear Free Veterinary Certification Course Module 6.

Before starting any veterinary care procedure, take a moment to create a plan of action. This will help make the experience more efficient and successful for everyone. Box 8.3 outlines the four steps to creating a plan for veterinary care.

When creating a plan for veterinary care, first determine a reinforcement hierarchy for the patient. What does this patient enjoy that could be used as a possible distractor during a procedure or reinforcer after the procedure? Referring to the EMR can help in planning but reassess the patient's response at every visit.

Next, rank procedures as most to least important. The veterinarian will often be responsible for determining this hierarchy. When there are several procedures to be performed, prioritizing them allows for the most critical things to be completed first. Thus, if the patient requires a break due to escalating FAS levels, the patient's tolerance for procedures is not wasted on less important tasks.

After procedures have been ranked from most to least important, then rank the most important procedures as least to most aversive. Determine whether there are stopping points for breaks in the procedure and what behavioral indicators for this patient will be considered stopping points. A general guideline is three seconds/three well-tolerated tries for dogs and two seconds/two well-tolerated tries for cats. The premise is that if a dog struggles or stops accepting a distraction for three seconds, then try something else. Three well-tolerated attempts/tries (or two tries for cats) is the general limit before you should consider rescheduling or sedation (see section **Prioritizing veterinary procedures**). Depending on the EMR of the patient, these guidelines may be modified to fewer attempts or less time.

Once you have a high-level reinforcer for the patient, a plan for the order in which you will perform the procedures, and stopping or pause points, consider the three Ws.

- ***Where*** will you perform the procedure? The examination room, treatment area, or housing area? It is usually better for patients to remain where they are most comfortable. If the appointment is for a preventive care visit, can the procedure be performed in the examination room? If the pet is staying in the hospital, an examination room (if available) or the pet's housing area (if safe to do so and appropriate) can provide a quiet and less active environment than the treatment room.
- ***Who*** will be present? If possible, it is usually best for the owner or a familiar person to be present.
- ***What*** do you need to make the environment as pleasant as possible (non-slip mat, pheromones, acoustic therapy, etc.)? What items do you need for the procedure? Get everything ready before the patient is brought to the area.

Always be willing to ask for assistance from other team members as needed for re-evaluation of the plan.

BOX 8.3: CREATING A PLAN FOR VETERINARY CARE INCLUDES THE FOLLOWING

1. Assess the patient
   - Observe and note body language and behavioral indicators of FAS
   - Continuously reassess throughout the procedure
2. Assess yourself
   - Are you using Considerate Approach?
   - Ask for help if you are feeling uncomfortable
3. Assess the environment
   - Set up the environment to be patient friendly by applying Considerate Approach
   - Remove or minimize stressors in the environment
4. Create a plan for care
   - Identify reinforcers
   - Rank most to least important procedures
   - Plan least to most aversive procedures
   - Identify stopping or pause points
   - Consider the three Ws (where, who, what)

Prioritizing veterinary procedures

Procedures can be grouped into "wants" and "needs" (Koch 2015).

Wants are procedures that you would like to perform today. *Needs* are those that must be performed straightaway because they are vital to the animal's immediate health and waiting any length of time, even a few minutes, would be detrimental.

Another way to think about it: Needs are considered lifesaving treatments and wants are everything else. The table below shows some examples of wants versus needs (Table 8.5).

- Needs are considered lifesaving treatments and wants are everything else.

Table 8.5 Wants versus needs.

Situation	Want or need
A one-year-old spayed female Chihuahua is presented for an examination and vaccines. The patient was able to eat for the full examination but showed some concerning body language and stopped eating during the vaccinations. Before the patient is placed back on the ground, the owner mentions that she would like the pet's nails trimmed.	**Want:** The nail trim is not a lifesaving procedure. The veterinary team should explain the changes in the patient's body language and discuss setting up another appointment perhaps after 1–2 fun visits to proceed with the nail trim.
A five-year-old intact male DSH was presented to the veterinary hospital for elimination out of the litter box. The owner had brought this cat into their home last week and at this examination it was found that the cat was still intact. During the examination, the cat was social, interacted with the team, ate spray cheese, and even played with toys. The examination was modified as a "less is more" as the patient did begin to thrash its tail, stiffened its posture, and low growl with increased amounts of handling. The veterinarian would like to obtain a sterile urine sample via cystocentesis. This cat is a wonderful addition to their home and the owners would like to schedule the patient to be neutered as soon as possible.	**Want:** In this situation, the sterile urine collection would be a want as not obtaining the urine sample today is not life threatening. The client wants to keep the cat and is willing to have the cat neutered as soon as possible (which may also eliminate the inappropriate urination). The veterinarian should consider a trial of a PVP prior to the neuter appointment to help reduce this cat's stress and anxiety with handling. Once the cat is under general anesthesia, the team can obtain a sterile urine sample for urinalysis and culture.
A six-year-old neutered male Boxer mix is presented to the boarding facility adjacent to the veterinary hospital for boarding. The owner thought that all of the vaccines were updated but it turns out that the patient needs to have an updated Rabies vaccine to enter the boarding facility. The owner mentions that this dog is very concerned about veterinary care and is usually fully sedated by their local clinic for examinations, but the owner is on board with the veterinary team performing a physical exam and updating the vaccines. The veterinary team tries to examine the patient, but he begins to air snap with the visual presentation of a muzzle but can be restrained.	**Want:** In this situation, the vaccines are a need for boarding but not a lifesaving need. Therefore, it would be in the best interest of the veterinary team to stop and set up a kennel space for the dog in the hospital wards until they can make contact with the owner. It can be discussed that the veterinary team would be happy to move forward with the examination and vaccine after the patient has had some PVP and intramuscular sedation. After this has been completed, the patient can be moved to the boarding facility. If the client declines this plan, the patient can stay with the veterinary team in their wards at an updated charge to prevent any potential exposure of disease.
A 9-year-old neutered male DSH presents as an emergency as the owners have not seen the patient eliminate urine for over 48 h. Upon palpation, the patient begins to growl and hiss but the veterinary team palpates a large bladder.	**Need:** The cat is most likely painful and has a blocked urethra. The patient should be sedated quickly and unblocked as soon as possible.

DSH: domestic short-haired (cat); PVP: pre-visit pharmaceuticals.

If "wants" are producing FAS in the patient, it does not mean that the procedure will never be performed. Instead, other options should be considered, such as being willing to reschedule. Perhaps the patient has reached their tolerance for today. Another day may be better. In the meantime, schedule some fun visits or more structured victory visits (see Becker M 2016, http://veterinaryteam.dvm360.com/what-heck-victory-visit and the section in this chapter, **Fun visits versus formal training for veterinary experiences**, and information in Chapter 7) so that the patient can have pleasant experiences at the hospital. The veterinarian should consider dispensing PVP.

If rescheduling is not an option – the procedure is a need – the veterinarian should consider sedation to minimize a potentially emotionally damaging experience. Pets have long-lasting memories. The experiences they have in the veterinary hospital stay with them for a lifetime. Experiences that result in an adrenaline release also result in long-term memory storage. Just "getting it done" regardless of the stress level of the pet, can result in a pet who is no longer able to be attended to medically at the veterinary hospital or at home due to irreversible severe psychological damage.

- Pets have long-lasting memories. The experiences they have in the veterinary hospital stay with them for a lifetime.

CHAPTER 8

- Just "getting it done" regardless of the stress level of the pet, can result in a pet who is no longer able to be attended to medically at the veterinary hospital or at home due to irreversible severe psychological damage.

The medical treatment of FAS

An animal's behavior is a part of ALL veterinary care. Whether there is a pain-inducing problem to a pet who is just "ADR," (Ain't Doing Right) body language and overall demeanor are part of obtaining a thorough and precise physical examination. When an in-depth physical examination is unable to be performed, vital information may be missed. Unfortunately, in veterinary medicine, we cannot talk to our patients and explain to them the procedure we are about to perform. This can lead to panic, fear, stress, aggression, and anxiety that is associated with handling, restraint, the veterinary team, or veterinary setting. Consequently, causing frustration for the veterinary team and impeding the care of the patient. When we are unable to successfully provide treatment without producing detrimental emotional stress to the pet, this becomes a quality-of-life concern as the veterinary team cannot provide medical care to keep the pet healthy long term.

- When we are unable to successfully provide treatment without producing detrimental emotional stress to the pet, this becomes a quality-of-life concern as the veterinary team cannot provide medical care to keep the pet healthy long term.

Indicators for the use of anxiolytics

Anxiolytics are a class of medications used to prevent or treat anxiety symptoms. These medications are used in addition to training, behavioral, and environmental modifications to treat veterinary-related fear, anxiety, or stress. Using medication can make veterinary visits more likely to be successful while implementing the behavioral treatment plan prescribed by the veterinary team. Medications are intended to address the specific neurotransmitters that are associated with the patient's FAS within the veterinary setting. The goal of using these medications is to help the patient's veterinary visit be more enjoyable and less stressful. The goal of anti-anxiety medications is to reduce stress and anxiety so the veterinary team can work to change the way the patient feels about specific procedures such as being examined or receiving a vaccine.

- The goal of anti-anxiety medications is to reduce stress and anxiety so the veterinary team can work to change the way the patient feels about specific procedures such as being examined or receiving a vaccine.

Giving an animal a medication with the intent to sedate or slow down the animal's reaction time but then proceed with intense physical restraint is inappropriate and is not recommended. The goal should be to reduce the fear, stress, and anxiety so the pet can receive lifelong care without high levels of FAS. If these concerns are not addressed, the patient may continue to have negative associations with the veterinary team and may inhibit the amount of medical care they can receive long term. The use of anxiolytics for veterinary care should not be recommended for use alone without training, behavioral, and environmental modifications.

Just as it is a standard of care to provide appropriate pain management for our patients, the medical treatment of fear, anxiety, and stress should be a standard of care. FAS affects the physical and emotional well-being of patients.

- Just as it is a standard of care to provide appropriate pain management for our patients, the medical treatment of fear, anxiety, and stress should be a standard of care. FAS affects the physical and emotional well-being of patients.

(The following summary of short- and long-term effects of FAS on pets was modified from Landsberg and Radosta 2017, Fear Free Symposium notes.) Short-term effects of FAS can result in inaccurate diagnostics. Physiological measures and clinical pathology data are affected by stress-induced catecholamine and glucocorticoid release. These effects include an increase in blood glucose and a stress leukogram. In studies comparing a veterinary examination of cats at home versus the veterinary clinic, a significant difference was found in respiratory rate, blood pressure, and heart rate (Quimby et al. 2011; Belew et al. 1999).

A study of 30 dogs that compared veterinary examination findings in the home to those in the veterinary clinic, found stress related to travel and the veterinary environment resulted in significant increases in blood pressure, rectal temperature, heart rate, and panting (Bragg et al. 2015). In another study, urine cortisol–creatinine ratios (indicator of stress) were increased after vaccine visits, orthopedic examination, and following overnight hospitalization. The elevation in urine cortisol–creatinine ratios persisted in almost half of the dogs after 12 hours at home. Some of these results were in a range that would be consistent with a diagnosis of hyperadrenocorticism (Van Vonderen et al. 1998).

Preventive medical intervention for FAS-inducing medical procedures

Preventing FAS is no different from preemptively treating pain before a procedure. When we are able to medicate for a behavioral concern before the situation starts, our treatment will be increasingly effective. Once the pet has become afraid or anxious, medication will be less effective, and the receptor sites will be blocked.

The FAS scale provides us with a guide for how to medically address fear, anxiety, and stress based on the patient's level of FAS. However, we can also anticipate the effect a procedure will have on the patient and treat proactively.

- The FAS scale provides us with a guide for how to medically address fear, anxiety, and stress based on the patient's level of FAS. However, we can also anticipate the effect a procedure will have on the patient and treat proactively.

Many veterinary facilities have started to preemptively treat potential stress-inducing procedures such as dental cleaning, boarding, surgery, and diagnostic imaging. The use of anxiolytics is discussed as part of the procedure or the anesthetic event and is typically dispensed one week prior to the scheduled procedure. The anxiolytic(s) and dosage are prescribed by the veterinarian ahead of time so the veterinary technician team can discuss this with the client. Treating fear, anxiety, and stress preventively can also aid in reducing the amount of anesthesia that will be needed during the procedure.

The proactive use of behavior medications should be considered prior to situations that are likely to be more stressful for the pet such as being in unfamiliar surroundings, encountering unfamiliar or startling sights, sounds, smells, and tactile sensations, pain and the anticipation of pain, being away from familiar people, a change in routine, and being fasted.

Medical intervention for FAS

Using the FAS scale as a guide, we can determine whether a situation warrants the use of anxiolytics. Score baseline FAS levels (i.e. prior to handling or procedures) after the pet has had the opportunity to settle into the new environment for 5–10 minutes. This allows time for the pet to acclimate to the situation and for the veterinary team to accurately assess the pet's FAS level.

Patients with a baseline FAS score of zero or one, who will have procedures performed that are not anticipated to result in a significant escalation of FAS, require no medication.

For patients who present at a baseline of FAS 2 or higher, PVP and/or nutraceuticals for visits regardless of what procedures are scheduled should be considered. Behavioral interventions such as desensitization and counter-conditioning appointments should also be suggested.

- For patients who present at a baseline of FAS 2 or higher, PVP and/or nutraceuticals for visits regardless of what procedures are scheduled should be considered.

If the pet is already at a level 2 when no procedures are being performed, it is probable that the FAS level will escalate as soon as procedures commence. Prevent escalation of FAS with a multimodal approach of environmental and medical management.

For pets with a level 3 FAS prior to handling, there are two options. One option is to use a light level of sedation to complete the exam and/or procedures at the current visit or give the pet owner the option to return at another time with the pet treated with PVP. For more information on PVP, see Chapter 10.

Pain increases fear, anxiety, and stress

Pain, either pre-existing, anticipated, or caused by a procedure in the hospital, can create or exacerbate fear, anxiety, and stress in patients. If pain is pre-existing, like that caused by chronic osteoarthritis, for example, the pain should if possible be controlled prior to the pet's visit to the hospital. When painful procedures are planned in the hospital, keep in mind that all living beings have a similar pain pathway. This means that procedures that would be painful to humans will likely be painful to animals. Each individual animal will perceive and respond to pain differently. All patients should be evaluated for pain at every visit and throughout a stay at the veterinary hospital. Use a scoring system to identify and rate the degree of pain. These scoring systems should be an analytical assessment of patients and their behavior. Included in each pain scoring assessment should be an evaluation of the patient's body posture, facial expressions, and demeanor, a dynamic evaluation that includes actual interaction, such as petting or walking the patient, and gentle palpation of the painful area if appropriate to do so. Finally, the pain scoring system needs to include written descriptors of the pain-related markers the pet exhibited at the time of assessment. This is key to assessing changes in pain intensity between scoring times. A commonly used practical scoring system is the Colorado State University canine and feline acute and chronic pain scales.

- Pain, either pre-existing, anticipated, or caused by a procedure in the hospital, can create or exacerbate fear, anxiety, and stress in patients.

Through the proactive use of anxiolytics, sedation, and analgesia protocols, we can minimize, prevent, and alleviate fear, anxiety, stress, and pain in our patients. Analgesic drugs should be discharged with the patient for procedures expected to produce lingering pain. The psychological and physiological effects of fear, stress, anxiety, and pain are detrimental to the health and well-being of patients. With early and appropriate management of the patient's behavior and pain, the veterinary team can provide better medical care.

- Through the proactive use of anxiolytics, sedation, and analgesia protocols, we can minimize, prevent, and alleviate fear, anxiety, stress, and pain in our patients.

Fun visits versus formal training for veterinary experiences

Fun visits and formal training for veterinary experiences, also referred to as victory visits or cooperative care visits, were discussed in detail in Chapter 7. They are similar but different. Fun visits, also referred to as happy visits, are more informal and about preventing the development of FAS related to the veterinary hospital. A formal training for veterinary experiences visit is a more structured service. It could be a preventive service or an intervention for existing FAS associated with the veterinary hospital.

Fun visits are just for fun! They are appropriate and should be encouraged for all pets who do not have established FAS associated with the veterinary hospital. This is a preventive service. See Appendices 21 and 22 for fun visit forms to assist clients with conducting a visit on their own.

In contrast, a formal training for veterinary experiences visit or victory visit is a scheduled session that involves a qualified team member. The focus is not just on making the environment a good place but also acclimating the pet to gentle control, veterinary equipment, and procedures.

In situations where the pet has already had negative veterinary-related experiences, fun visits may not be appropriate. Fun visits alone will not help a pet that has had traumatic experiences with the veterinary team. A pet with a conditioned aversion or fear of the veterinary hospital likely will need PVP and a full desensitization and counter-conditioning treatment plan to recondition the patient's emotional response to the veterinary setting and gentle control. Some treatment plans may include a cooperative care training as discussed earlier in this chapter. Box 8.4 outlines an example of the steps that may be needed in formal training sessions for veterinary-related issues.

BOX 8.4: VETERINARY VISIT TREATMENT PROTOCOL OUTLINE

Step One: DS-CC to Environment:
- Car anxiety and travel
- Parking lot
- Approaching the front door of the veterinary hospital
- Veterinary lobby
- Veterinary exam room
- Veterinary treatment room (+/–)

Step Two: DS-CC to Humans in Environment:
- Veterinary reception team (at a distance)
- Veterinary technicians
- Veterinarian

Step Three: DS-CC to Equipment and Handling:
- Teach and practice these behaviors to fluency in at least one non-distracting and comfortable environment, such as at home, prior to practicing in the veterinary setting
- Reaching and touching DS-CC, including distraction and touch then reinforce
- Stationing and targeting behaviors such as a chin rest, laying in lateral recumbency or sternal recumbency, going to a Treat-Ment station
- Positive conditioning with wearing a basket muzzle, compression wraps, and sound and/or visual buffers, such as Rex Specs Ear Pro and Thundercap
- Training to various veterinary tools including, stethoscope, syringe/needle, ophthalmoscope, otoscope, nail clippers, nail grinder, brush, comb, clippers, etc.

DS: desensitization; CC: counter conditioning

Useful supplemental tools: calming pheromone diffusers/spray, species-specific calming music.

Conclusion

For decades veterinary care was focused only on treating the physical well-being of pets. That is no longer enough. The physical and emotional well-being of pets are intricately related and must be addressed concurrently. By taking a comprehensive approach, we are able to make a profound impact on the welfare and well-being of not only pets, but also the pet guardians, and veterinary professionals.

- The physical and emotional well-being of pets are intricately related and must be addressed concurrently.

Utilizing Fear Free® and Low Stress Handling® techniques during every visit and interaction with patients allows us to provide better care. Our patients learn to trust us, and we are able to provide them with better medical care. These techniques allow us to practice better medicine. Patients who are more relaxed and calmer during diagnostic tests will have more accurate results. Often, we have to disregard test results because of the stress level of our patients. Examples include hyperthermia, hyperglycemia, hypertension, tachycardia, leukophilia, and inability to evaluate orthopedic lameness because of stress-induced adrenaline and noradrenaline release. These techniques make our jobs easier. When our patients are eager to see us, and are relaxed and calm, it is easier for us to provide needed veterinary care efficiently and effectively.

Additional resources

Cooperative veterinary care: https://www.facebook.com/groups/cooperativevetcare/about

Domesticated Manners – Chirag Patel: https://www.domesticatedmanners.com

Fear Free Pets: https://fearfreepets.com

Fear Free Happy Homes: https://www.fearfreehappyhomes.com

Low Stress Handling book and course: https://cattledogpublishing.com/why-and-what-is-low-stress-handling

Video 8.1 This video demonstrates using a treat trail to encourage a dog to get on the scale on their own. Using movement and guiding the dog with your motion is also beneficial. Most dogs will naturally follow the direction your feet and shoulders are pointing. Notice how the technician turns her body sideways as the dog walks on to the scale and then stands in front of the dog once the dog is on the scale.

Video 8.2 This video shows a dog responding to known cues while waiting in the exam room. The room has a large non-slip area and the owner has brought the dog's "Treat-Ment" station from home. There is also species-specific calming music playing. Note the cue "Aboie" is French for bark.

Video 8.3 This video demonstrates the basic distraction technique. A thorough emotional medical record is available on this dog. She is a 7.5-year-old spayed female Belgian Malinois named Jazmin and she has only ever exhibited a hard look (stare) and avoidance (moving away) with handling, FAS 4. She has never attempted to bite while being restrained or handled in the 7.5 years she has been owned by the same people. She loves toys and soft, lickable food treats. Precautionary statements: If working with a new patient that you do not have a good emotional record or relationship with already, gentle control tools and safety precautions, such as acclimating to a basket muzzle, may be warranted. In the video a touch gradient is utilized throughout. If the dog stops eating, the procedure is paused. Depending on the dog, the handling may need to be decreased rather than just paused. If the dog pauses for more than three seconds, the technician, moves her hands away to allow the dog to relax further. Without the emotional record and previous learning history with the technician, the stares from the dog would be of more concern and a safety issue. Remember if you are feeling uncomfortable with a patient, do not have a good emotional record, or established relationship, do not hesitate to acclimate him/her to a gentle control tool, such as a basket muzzle, prior to attempting gentle control techniques. Notice how when the dog stops eating, the technician stops and avoids eye contact with the dog. The dog is being given the power to tell the technician to slow down. When the dog resumes eating, the technician continues.

Video 8.4 This video demonstrates a version of the modified distraction technique. The technician cues the assistant to bring in the food by saying, "Food," and then to remove the food when she says, "Done." The dog in the video is a 9-year-old spayed female Belgian Malinois named Iliana and she has shown FAS 4, escape behavior with handling but she has not escalated to aggression. Because the dog had arthritis in her legs, she was more comfortable with less contact with the legs, thus the reason a touch gradient from the shoulder to the foot was not used.

Video 8.5 This video demonstrates the touch then reinforce technique with Jazmin the Belgian Malinois you saw have her ears cleaned using the basic distraction technique. In this example, the technician cues the helper to bring a treat to the dog by saying, "treat." Once the "treat" is spoken the technician removes her hands while the helper delivers the treat. The dog is allowed to eat the treat before the next repetition begins. Notice that this dog is more comfortable with this technique than the basic distraction technique. She still shows some signs of FAS but recovers quickly. Because this is a training situation the technician decides to start at the beginning after each repetition. This could be modified, and the technician could keep her hands on the dog as the treat is delivered and progress from the previous stop point. The second part of this video demonstrates using a clicker, rather than the word "treat," to mark the acceptance of being touched and imminent treat delivery. If using this method, the clicker should have a strong reinforcement history with the individual animal prior to using it with gentle control techniques. If this dog had been more uncomfortable with being reached over, the technician could have avoided reaching over the dog's head to access the left ear by moving to the other side of the dog.

Video 8.6 This video demonstrates the training process of teaching a Treat-Ment station with dogs.

Video 8.7 Here is a video example of using a chin rest behavior for husbandry care at home. This video is courtesy of Mikkel Becker, Lead Animal Trainer for Fear Free Pets, CBCC-KA, CDBC, KPA CTP, CPDT-KA, CTC, Fear Free Cert, BA Comm, co-author of *From Fearful to Fear Free*.

Video 8.8 This video is an example of the predictor cue, "brush," resulting in the dog showing avoidance and not being associated with something the dog enjoyed at that moment. Generally, predictor cues are taught to help put the animal at ease and decrease uncertainty; however, they can also provide the pet with the option to disengage from the interaction or say no. If the cue is given and the pet displays signs of FAS and/or moves away, we can hear what the pet is saying before actually making contact as was demonstrated in this video.

Video 8.9 This video illustrates the beginning stages of adding in handling with a chin rest and the dog learning that lifting his head up stops the trainer's behavior. Video courtesy of Debbie Martin, LVT, VTS (Behavior), KPA CTP, CPDT-KA.

Video 8.10 This video demonstrates adjusting to the dog's avoidance of the stethoscope by switching between distraction and touch then treat techniques. This technique of switching back and forth between procedures is referred to as ping-ponging. Source: Fear Free, LLC.

References

Becker, M. (2016). What the heck is a Victory Visit?! https://www.dvm360.com/view/what-heck-victory-visit (accessed May 2022).

Belew, A.M., Barlett, T., and Brown, S.A. (1999). Evaluation of the white-coat effect in cats. *Journal of Veterinary Internal Medicine* 13: 134–142.

Bragg, R.F., Bennett, J.S., Cummings, A. et al. (2015). Evaluations of the effects of hospital stress on physiologic variables in dogs. *Journal of the American Veterinary Medical Association* 246: 212–215.

Howell, A. and Feyrecilde, M. (2018). *Cooperative Veterinary Care*. Wiley Blackwell.

Koch, C.S. (2015). A low-stress handling algorithm: key to happier visits and healthier pets. DVM360. https://www.dvm360.com/view/low-stress-handling-algorithm-key-happier-visits-and-healthier-pets (accessed May 2022).

Landsberg, G. and Radosta, L. (2018). Presentation notes for the 2017 Fear Free symposium series. https://fearfreepets.com/wp-content/uploads/delightful-downloads/2018/06/Symposium-Lisa-Radosta-Proceedings.pdf (accessed November 2022).

Mariti, C., Raspanti, E., Zilocchi, M. et al. (2015). The assessment of dog welfare in the waiting room of a veterinary clinic. *Animal Welfare* 24: 299–305.

Mariti, C., Pierantoni, L., Sighieri, C., and Gazzano, A. (2016). Guardians' perceptions of Dogs' welfare and behaviors related to visiting the veterinary clinic. *Journal of Applied Animal Welfare Science* 20: 1–10. https://doi.org/10.1080/10888705.2016.1216432.

Quimby, J.M., Smith, M.L., and Lunn, K.F. (2011). Evaluation of the effects of hospital visit stress on physiologic parameters in the cat. *Journal of Feline Medicine and Surgery* 13: 733–737.

Schneider, S.M. (2012). *The Science of Consequences: How they Affect Genes, Change the Brain, and Impact our World*. Amherst, N.Y: Prometheus Books.

Shreyer, T, Croney, C., and Herron, M. (2012). Prior to Handling Small Animals. Handout.

Van Vonderen, I.K., Kooistra, H.S., and Rijnberk, A. (1998). Influence of veterinary care on the urine corticoid: creatine ration in dogs. *Journal of Veterinary Internal Medicine* 12: 431–435.

Yin, S.A. (2009). *Low Stress Handling, Restraint and Behavior Modification of Dogs–Cats: Techniques for Developing Patients Who Love Their Visits*. Cattle Dog Pub.

The PowerPoint of figures, appendices, MCQ's, cited videos are available at www.wiley.com/go/martin/behavior

9 Specific behavior modification techniques and practical applications for behavior disorders

Debbie Martin[1,2]

[1]*TEAM Education in Animal Behavior, LLC, Spicewood, TX, USA*

[2]*Veterinary Behavior Consultations, LLC, Spicewood, TX, USA*

CHAPTER MENU

Canine and Feline Behavior for Veterinary Technicians and Nurses, Second Edition. Edited by Debbie Martin and Julie K. Shaw.

Companion website: www.wiley.com/go/martin/behavior

The focus of this chapter is to standardize, through terminology and description, commonly prescribed treatments, including management, training styles, specific training exercises, training tools, and commonly prescribed behavior modification techniques. Although we are attempting to standardize behavioral treatment, each patient, client, and case are unique and adaptations are warranted based on the medical and behavioral history and response to treatment.

As described in detail in Chapter 1, it is the veterinarian's responsibility to diagnose behavior disorders and prescribe the treatment plan. The veterinary technician is the "case manager" triaging and coordinating the communication cycle between the pet owner, veterinarian, and qualified trainer. The technician also teaches the pet owner why aspects of the treatment plan were chosen, how each aspect of the treatment plan will improve the problem, and how to apply them.

The veterinary technician must be a fluent communicator, teacher, and trainer to successfully instruct the pet owner on understanding and applying the prescribed treatment plan. A canine behavior plan of care form has been included in the appendix to expedite treatment plans from the veterinarian to the technician/trainer (see Appendix 8). This text will follow the plan of care form in its organization.

As the case manager, the veterinary technician will advocate for both the client and patient, making sure the treatment plan is functional and productive, while also teaching and being the support system for the pet owner. The veterinary technician must fully understand the science behind the techniques, translate the techniques into language the client can relate to, and instruct the pet owner on how to place treatment techniques into their daily routine. A complete and confident understanding of the techniques will give the technician the ability to modify techniques to best fit the individual client's lifestyle.

- The veterinary technician must fully understand the science behind the techniques, translate the techniques into language the client can relate to, and instruct the pet owner on how to place treatment techniques into their daily routine.

Common veterinary behavior disorder diagnosis and descriptions

A "diagnosis" refers to the categorization of clinical signs into diagnostic categories that provide the veterinarian with information. The clinical information suggests an underlying cause and specific treatments for the disorder. The diagnosis is not meant to label the animal but to describe a set of clinical signs and to expedite communication between professionals. For example, a dog that has been diagnosed with fear aggression toward unfamiliar people indicates the animal has displayed a set of behaviors demonstrating fear-motivated distance-increasing behaviors toward unfamiliar people. This is comparable to diagnosing an animal that cannot process sugars appropriately due to insulin production insufficiency of the pancreas as having diabetes mellitus. Just as with any medical disorder, behavior disorder diagnoses are used to describe a set of past or present conditions that may need to be treated or managed to prevent relapses.

As with any medical diagnosis, the veterinary technician must understand the general meaning of each behavioral disorder diagnosis, the specific aspects of treatment, and the effects on the human–animal bond. The following are common behavioral diagnoses with their descriptions (reference Table 9.1).

Aggression

Aggression is the most common reason dogs are presented to referral behavior practices. In general,

Table 9.1 Common behavioral diagnoses.

Behavior	Description or motivation	Species	Target
Aggression	Conflict induced	C,F	FP, UFP[a]
	Possessive	C	FP, UFP
	Petting induced	F	FP, UFP
	Disease or pain induced	C,F	A
	Fear/defensive induced	C,F	A
	Idiopathic	C,F	A
	Inter-dog (IDA) + motivation	C	UFA
	Inter-cat (ICA) + motivation	F	UFA, FA
	Inter-dog – Household (IDA–H) + motivation	C	FA
	Alliance induced	C	FA
	Status induced	C	FA
	Learned	C,F	A
	Maternal/hormonal induced	C	A
	Play induced	C,F	FP, UFP
	Redirected	C,F	A
	Territorial	C,F	UFP, UFA
Ingestive	Coprophagia	C	
	Pica	C,F	
	Predatory behavior	C,F	
Elimination	House soiling	C,F	
	Urine marking	C,F	
	Excitement urination	C	
	Extreme fear/appeasement urination	C	
Fear/Anxiety disorders	Generalized anxiety	C, F	
	Global fear	C, F	
	Separation anxiety	C, F	
	Sound/thunderstorm phobia	C, F	
	Specific fear or phobia	C, F	
	Acute conflict behaviors/stereotypy	C, F	
	Compulsive disorder	C, F	
Other	Cognitive dysfunction	C, F	
	Hyperexcitability	C, F	
	Conditioned–unwanted behavior	C, F	

[a] Conflict-induced aggression is most commonly associated with aggression toward family members and more rarely toward unfamiliar people.

C: canine; F: feline; FP: familiar people; UFP: unfamiliar people; FA: familiar animal; UFA: unfamiliar animal; A: all.

aggression refers to threatening or harmful behavior directed toward another individual or group. Often an animal is presented with multiple types of aggression with multiple causations.

Aggression is a normal communication tool and is not necessarily a pathological or abnormal behavior. Normal aggression is demonstrated in situations that warrant aggression. The intensity of the aggression by the animal is modified, depending on the situation and the relative level of the threat. For example, a normal aggressive display would be if a stranger broke into the home unannounced and was bitten. Abnormal aggression occurs when the animal perceives threat where it does not exist and has difficulty modulating its aggressive response as the perceived threat changes. However, it is important to note that the animal perceives a threat and to them it is real, regardless of our interpretation of the situation.

- Aggression is a normal communication tool and is not necessarily a pathological or abnormal behavior.

The context of the situation will determine whether the aggression is normal or abnormal and may be influenced by a combination of genetics and experience.

Often high arousal or frustration is a complicating factor to aggression. High arousal tends to cause the animal to react rather than respond to a situation, making it difficult for it to respond consciously.

Many types of aggression can be thwarted or prevented if the veterinary technician is able to detect early warning signs in puppy and kitten classes (see Chapter 7).

There remains some controversy with regard to aggressive behavior classification among veterinary behaviorists. In this chapter, diagnosis will be defined according to motivation or trigger, behavior, and target.

Conflict-induced aggression

Conflict-induced aggression is a conflict-resolution strategy, resulting from an approach–withdrawal conflict or the inability to predict the environment. Conflict-induced aggression is usually directed toward family members. It differs from fear-based aggression in that the dog or cat does not usually attempt to leave the situation, unless the motivation to withdrawal becomes greater than to remain in the situation. Many dogs that have conflict-induced aggression also show fear-based aggression in other contexts. Conflict-induced aggression is also not limited to owner-initiated interactions. The pet may be social and solicit owner interaction and attention and then display aggression toward the owner.

Fear aggression typically occurs when a person approaches the pet and tries to interact; the pet shows appeasement or displacement behaviors (curves body, sniffs ground) and aggresses if unable to avoid the interaction.

- Fear aggression typically occurs when a person approaches the pet and tries to interact; the pet shows appeasement or displacement behaviors (curves body, sniffs ground) and aggresses if unable to avoid the interaction.

Conflict-induced aggression typically occurs when the pet seeks out the pet owner, perhaps even solicits attention, then shows conflict behaviors (freezes, shifts eyes) and aggresses. The pet could leave the situation but chooses not to because of conflicting motivations (desire to be with the pet owner and uncertainty of what will happen next).

- Conflict-induced aggression typically occurs when the pet seeks out the pet owner, perhaps even solicits attention, then shows conflict behaviors (freezes, shifts eyes) and aggresses. The pet could leave the situation but chooses not to because of conflicting motivations (desire to be with the pet owner and uncertainty of what will happen next).

The pet is in a motivational approach–withdrawal conflict. The pet wants to interact with the person, but at some point becomes uncomfortable with the social interaction because of unpredictability or uncertainty. The pet anticipates that something unpleasant or undesirable (from the pet's point of view) is about to happen. The conflict is likely similar to the feeling a human gets when a person remains in your personal space too long, or a person hugs you and holds you a little longer than you would like. A hallmark with conflict-induced aggression is the display of conflict behaviors before the aggression. Unfortunately, most pet owners are unaware of what the pet is communicating, and it escalates to growling, snapping, or biting.

Conflict-induced (and other forms of) aggression is often rewarded through removal of the threat (stimulus backs off negatively reinforcing the aggression) and the conflict/fear is resolved; the animal consequently will be more likely to continue to use aggression in these contexts and may become more offensive in its behavior as the outcome becomes more predictable. Over time, the animal may stop showing fear and/or conflict behaviors or the conflict behaviors are minimized. Therefore, when working with an animal with a long history of aggression, the technician should proceed with caution and be fully aware of past bite history, as warning signs may not be displayed. We are not suggesting ignoring the warning signs a pet is giving. Backing off, although potentially negatively reinforcing the behavior, is advised to keep the pet owner safe and allow the pet to be heard. If the signals are ignored, the pet might have to escalate the level of threat. Treatment involves identifying potential triggers and chemical imbalances and applying appropriate intervention techniques.

Conflict-induced aggression is most frequently owner directed and often includes a comorbid diagnosis of possessive aggression or the guarding of resources.

- Conflict-induced aggression is most frequently owner directed.

Conflict-induced aggression is seen in dogs and cats but is diagnosed less frequently in cats. Most cases of aggression in cats are fear-induced, with the exception of petting intolerance where the cat may be in a motivational conflict of "I want to sit on your lap, but I do not want to be petted or touched."

Conflict-induced aggression may first be seen in puppyhood as inappropriate play, fear-based aggression, and guarding of the food bowl or other resources (Guy et al. 2001). It frequently begins when a puppy is sociable (mouthing, play biting, jumping on familiar people, or displaying some form of attention-getting behavior) and the behavior is then punished by the owner. The puppy still wants to interact with the owner but is afraid and in a motivation conflict. The motivational conflict occurs because the pet owner's behavior is inconsistent and unpredictable from the puppy's point of view. Some puppies may get more aroused and interact with rougher play biting rather than leaving or avoiding the pet owner. Eventually the motivation changes from play to fear, to frustration, and conflict, resulting in the development of conflict-induced aggression (Figure 9.1).

- Conflict-induced aggression may first be seen in puppyhood as inappropriate play, fear-based aggression, and guarding of the food bowl or other resources.

Treatment includes addressing how the dog is managed, addressing basic temperament issues (fearfulness or anxiety) and the cause of the conflict (owner's inconsistency). One of the most important components of treatment is structuring consistent, predictable, and positive human–pet interactions in order to reduce fear and conflict. Social interactions, in the form of cue→response→reward, add predictability and facilitate classical counter conditioning (CC) resulting in a positive emotional state.

Consistent rules provide the dog with the possibility to predict events in the environment and thus increase confidence.

Possessive aggression

Possessive aggression is described as guarding of an item from people. Aggression over a possession, food, or handling may be subcategories of conflict-induced aggression.

- Aggression over a possession, food, or handling may be subcategories of conflict-induced aggression.

Possessive aggression often begins with a puppy possessing a "valued" or stolen item, is then chased by the pet owner (which may initially be "fun") followed by the unknowing pet owner attempting to take the object away, sometimes in an antagonistic fashion. The puppy may become fearfully aggressive

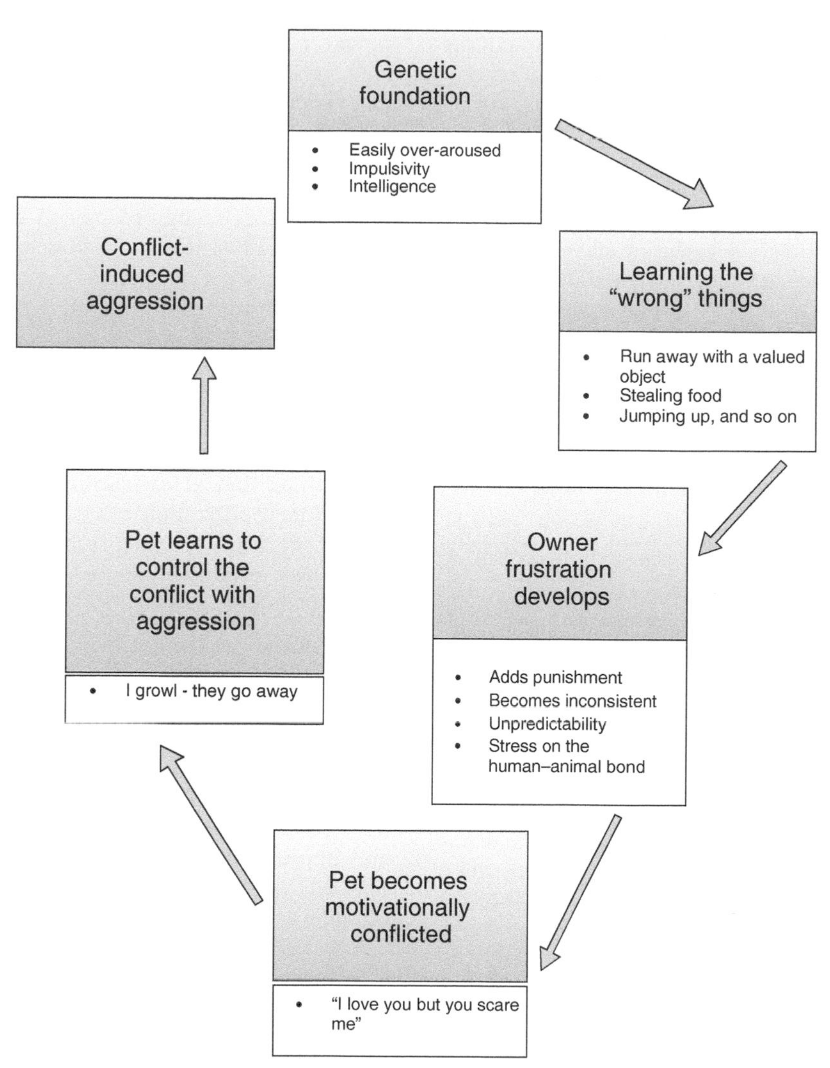

Figure 9.1 The development of conflict-induced aggression.

and when the pet owner backs off, the aggressive behavior becomes negatively reinforced, creating a strong learning component.

In the case of aggression over the food bowl, guarding food is a somewhat normal behavior of dogs, especially when directed toward other animals in the home. When excessive and directed toward animals or humans near the food bowl, it may be a subcategory of possessive aggression.

Petting-induced aggression

Petting-induced aggression in the cat can be either offensive or defensive. It is believed to be a subtype of conflict-induced aggression. The cat seems to enjoy the petting and then suddenly attacks the person petting her, jumps down, runs a short distance, sits, and grooms herself. Often the cat's pupils are dilated. In all likelihood, the cat was placed in a motivational conflict, wanting to remain on the lap but no longer desiring to be touched.

Disease-induced or pain-induced aggression

Disease-induced or pain-induced aggression occurs either primarily or secondarily from a gross medical condition. The aggression may occur primarily because the animal is more irritable because of the disease process or in the attempt to avoid or remove pain.

Aggression may occur secondarily long after the disease or pain is resolved because the animal has learned through classical conditioning (i.e. being restrained = pain, the veterinary hospital = fear.)

Decreasing pain and fear during all veterinary visits and teaching handling exercises during puppy and kitten classes may help prevent pain-induced aggression and a later veterinary hospital aversion or phobia from developing. It is critical that pets are preemptively treated for pain or sedated for procedures expected to induce pain to prevent the development of a negative conditioned emotional response to the veterinary setting and care.

- It is critical that pets are preemptively treated for pain or sedated for procedures expected to induce pain to prevent the development of a negative conditioned emotional response to the veterinary setting and care.

Fear/defensive aggression

Fear aggression is sometimes referred to as *defensive aggression* and occurs when the animal perceives a situation as threatening. Initial descriptions of the aggression may include a dog demonstrating defensive postures including head down, approach withdrawal, ears back, tail down, looking away, and lip licking. In general, cats and dogs attempt to use physical contact as a last resort in a fear-inducing situation and prefer active avoidance or withdrawal.

Aggressive responses may be followed by withdrawal and distance-increasing responses. Fear aggression occurs when the animal chooses "fight" over freezing or flight. This "choice" may occur because of not being able to leave the situation or by being in a motivational conflict about leaving the situation (i.e. "I want the stranger to leave my safe area and I do not want to leave my safe area"). Animals frequently learn to control the fear-provoking stimulus using aggression and may later become more offensive in their aggressive displays as they learn that aggression results in removal of the threat. The predictability of the consequence from previous learning experiences can result in more offensive rather than defensive aggression. However, even though there may be fewer outward signs of fear in the animal's body language, the motivation for the aggression is still fear.

"Control" in this context refers to an animal's ability to predict its own outcomes. Research conducted over decades suggests that control is an unconditional (primary) reinforcer and is especially reinforcing to animals that suffer from anxiety.

- "Control" in this context refers to an animal's ability to predict its own outcomes.

It is critical that all fear-eliciting stimuli are identified before modification can occur. The pet's emotion to the fear-provoking stimuli is modified and then a new response is taught.

Idiopathic aggression

Idiopathic aggression refers to an unexplained and intense aggression and is reserved for animals that have had a complete medical and behavioral investigation in which no identifiable aggression-provoking stimuli can be determined. The aggression has been described as explosive, out of context in its severity, and unpredictable. Idiopathic aggression is usually only diagnosed by a veterinary behaviorist who has acquired an in-depth medical and behavioral history.

Inter-dog aggression

Inter-dog aggression (IDA) is described as aggression between dogs unknown to each other. IDA does not define the motivation behind the behavior and therefore usually includes a motivation description (i.e. territorial, fear, and conflict). Common motivations may include fear/defensive, status (usually between intact males), territoriality, conflict or poor canine communication skills (undersocialized or communication skills were not learned in early puppyhood).

Underlying fear or anxiety often contributes to IDA along with learning. Some dogs that have been attacked in the past assume an offensively defensive position – "I'll attack you before you can attack me."

Inter-cat aggression

Inter-cat aggression (ICA) refers to interactions between known and unknown cats and usually includes elements of growling, hissing, spitting, attacking, chasing, and biting. ICA may also include elements of territorial aggression, redirected aggression, or fear aggression.

Status-induced aggression

Status-related aggression in cats has not been well studied or accepted in behavioral medicine but has most often been associated with densely housed cats. Cats in more natural settings tend to maintain their relationships through scent marking rather than aggression.

Inter-dog aggression – household

Inter-dog aggression – household (IDA–H) (sometimes called *sibling rivalry*) is aggression between dogs living in the same household or social group. IDA–H is not a diagnosis but a description. Several different types of aggression (some occurring simultaneously) can be exhibited between dogs in the same household, including fear, possessiveness, redirected or idiopathic aggression (see descriptions). Other types of aggression that may cause IDA–H include the following.

Alliance-induced aggression

Alliance-induced aggression refers to aggression between dogs in the same household that fight only in the proximity of the pet owner. Usually the more fearful and most owner-dependent dog becomes anxious when the other dog approaches the owner and consequently the less confident dog aggresses. If the owner leaves before it progresses to a full fight, the aggression usually subsides. This type of aggression is often inadvertently conditioned by the owner's attention.

Status-induced aggression

Status-induced aggression refers to aggression between dogs in the same household in which the relationship between the dogs is unclear. Fighting often occurs when the social relationship has changed between the dogs. The owner frequently intercedes in aggressive situations supporting the dog that would without interference likely lose the resource or conflict. The aggression is often reinforced in the less confident dog by the owner coddling or petting while often punishing the more confident dog, causing confusion and conflict in the dogs' relationship.

Learned aggression

All types of aggression have some degree of learning involved. The larger the learning component, the better the prognosis because alternate "coping mechanisms" can be taught to the animal. Aggression is conditioned through positive reinforcement (i.e. owner picks up the pet), negative reinforcement (i.e. fear or conflict-provoking stimulus retreats) and classical conditioning (veterinary clinic = pain).

Learned aggression and lack of bite inhibition is often taught to dogs in protection training or protection sports. If taught properly, it is actually a "game of tug" the dog plays with excellent cue stimulus control. In this context the motivation is not fear but instead play and high arousal.

Maternal/hormonal-induced aggression

Maternal aggression occurs when a bitch defends her puppies from people or other animals. It is considered to be normal behavior to a degree and usually is not treated as much as managed (removing the bitch before the puppies are handled).

Play-induced aggression

Canine mouthing and play biting are considered normal forms of interactions and communication for dogs but can become problematic when directed toward humans. Although not technically considered true aggression, overexuberant play can be damaging to the human–animal bond. Often the human response reinforces the behavior (i.e. attention is given) or the play escalates to the point when the owner attempts to punish the behavior, placing the dog in (from the dog's perspective) a conflicting situation of uncertainty and high arousal. Inappropriate play can then become a precursor to a more serious type of aggression, that is, conflict-induced aggression.

Feline play-induced aggression involves unsolicited attacks by a young cat targeting people or other animals within the home. It is considered a type of redirected predatory behavior, which may include hiding, chasing, stalking, and pouncing behaviors. Cats that display play-induced aggression are usually young and energetic, taken from their litter early (or orphaned) and living in single-cat households (when directed toward owners).

Redirected aggression

Redirected aggression is incidental to another form of aggression or emotional arousal. It occurs when a dog or cat cannot reach the target of its aggression and out of frustration changes its focus of aggression to an object, person, or other animal that is not the stimulus for the aggressive arousal.

Redirected aggression is very serious because the target of the aggression usually cannot modify their behavior to prevent the aggression. They are "collateral" damage in the aggressive episode.

Stimuli that may elicit redirected aggression in cats can be other cats, other animals, odors, noises, unfamiliar people, unfamiliar places, or pain. It frequently begins when a cat sees a cat outside the window or smells another cat. The aggression is then redirected toward another cat or person in the household. ICA can begin between two cats that live together as a result of redirected aggression and likely will not resolve without treatment.

Common triggers in dogs may include barking at fence lines, ringing of the doorbell, or being restrained on a leash. Redirected aggression can start IDA–H (sibling rivalry) when the "victim" dog (dog toward which aggression is being redirected) begins to anticipate the attack and fights back.

Territorial aggression

Dogs are genetically programmed to be territorial. Territorial aggression refers to aggression directed toward people or animals that are not part of the dog's immediate social group or are unfamiliar to them, when they enter the dog's perceived territory. The classic definition of territorial aggression refers to the territory being a fixed location (i.e. house, room, yard, and bed). In some literature, a mobile territory around the dog (i.e. leash, proximity to owner) is also referred to as a territory. However, a mobile territory is probably best described as just fear-based aggression in that specific context. Territorial aggression is influenced by breed, age, sex, and socialization experience. Excitement and arousal increase the aggressive behavior. Fear is an underlying component with territorial aggression and can be observed when a dog approaches and withdraws but as the person turns to leave (and becomes less threatening through the dog's eyes), the dog's territorial aggression outweighs the fear and a bite may occur to the person's backside. Fear can also be seen when dogs seem offensively aggressive through a door or window but become fearful or defensively aggressive once the door is opened.

There is also a strong learning component to territorial aggression. When the behavior is practiced it is almost always negatively reinforced by the threat (approaching person or animal) going away. This can result in less fear-related behaviors being observed as the dog learns how to keep himself safe.

Territorial aggression in cats is most often directed toward other cats, known or unknown, rather than humans. It occurs most commonly between male cats and in high-density cat areas. It can also occur when a new cat is introduced to the household or when a resident cat returns home from the veterinary hospital because it is not recognized by the other cats. Body language includes staring at the other cat, attack, chase, and paw blows. Signs of fear in the victim may trigger an attack.

Ingestive disorders

Coprophagia

Coprophagia is the ingestion of feces. It is seen most often in dogs either eating their own feces or the feces of other animals. Engaging in coprophagia is normal in most dogs although contributing factors include normal maternal behavior, puppy exploratory behavior, dietary preference, hunger, or attention-seeking behavior. Coprophagia can be a coping mechanism for high-anxiety dogs and has been identified as an oral manifestation of compulsive disorder.

Pica

Pica is generally described as the ingestion of inanimate objects. Although young animals may destroy objects in their explorations, most do not ingest objects, unlike animals that suffer from pica. Forms of pica include wool sucking in cats (sucking on fabric), rock chewing and swallowing, soil eating, or other oral fixation. Some forms of pica may be considered compulsive disorders (see section **Compulsive disorders**).

Predatory behavior

Predatory behaviors refer to a sequence of behaviors that is associated with the process of catching and killing of another animal for consumption. The canine sequence may include orient, eye-stalk, chase, grab-bite, kill-bite, dissect, consume (Coppinger and Coppinger 2001). It is linked to normal survival behavior and therefore "hardwired" in the brain. It is a highly genetically controlled behavior that is coordinated by the appetite and satiety centers of the brain; therefore, bites are usually not inhibited during a predatory attack. Through learning, predatory aggression can be redirected toward conspecifics as with dog fighting circumstances. In dogs, excitement and social facilitation can exacerbate predatory aggression; therefore, groups of dogs are more dangerous.

- Bites are usually not inhibited during a predatory attack.

As discussed in Chapter 3, manipulating, killing, and ingesting prey is a learned behavior in cats. The chase and catching of prey are an innate behavior. Cats with access to small animals (rabbits, mice, and birds) may stalk and injure or ingest them.

Elimination

House soiling

House soiling refers to elimination (either urine or stool) in locations the pet owner finds unacceptable or inappropriate. Inappropriate elimination is the most common behavioral reason pets are relinquished to shelters (Salman et al. 2000). Elimination problems can occur for multiple reasons, including medical reasons, ineffective house training or litter-box training, urine marking (see later text), separation anxiety (distress), social or environmental stressors, cognitive dysfunction, fear, extreme appeasement, or psychogenic polydipsia.

House soiling by cats usually occurs because of two primary reasons: litter-box aversion or a substrate preference.

Urine marking

Marking is a normal communicative method to call attention to objects, individuals, or an area and is frequently a sign of anxiety in both dogs and cats. Marking in the dog can take the form of visual marks created by a dog pawing at the ground or disposition of chemical cues processed through the olfactory system. Urine marking is the most common cause pet owners seek assistance for marking behaviors. Territorial urine marking is most prevalent in intact males or females.

Urine marking in cats is sometimes called "spraying" because the cat backs up to a vertical surface (less commonly on horizontal surfaces) with its tail straight up and a twitching tip. Some cats mark by urinating, emptying the bladder, or by defecating (middening). It was previously believed the volume of urine when marking was smaller than the volume of urine during house soiling, but a small pilot study done by Jacqueline Neilson, DVM, DACVB found the volume of urine amounts when spraying was similar to the amounts found when eliminating (i.e. large amounts of sprayed urine).

Urine marking in both dogs and cats frequently reflects environmental stress or anxiety.

- Urine marking in both dogs and cats frequently reflects environmental stress or anxiety.

Excitement urination

Excitement urination occurs in dogs that are overly aroused and can also be seen when a dog is in a motivational conflict, that is, the dog is excited to greet people at the door but also uncertain. Excitement urination is different from extreme appeasement urination in that appeasement behaviors are usually not shown at the same time.

Extreme fear/appeasement urination

Extreme appeasement urination is not truly an elimination problem as much as a fear issue. Appeasement urination occurs when the dog attempts to avoid a conflict by defusing the situation with the normal canine appeasement behavior of urinating small amounts. The dog is uncertain and attempting to communicate he is not a threat.

Fear/Anxiety disorders

Anxiety – Anxiety is a diffuse generalized feeling of fear, apprehension, unease or nervousness regarding an imminent event, uncertain outcome, or danger (threat). While fear is an emotional response to a real and present or perceived threat or danger, anxiety is the emotional response that occurs with anticipation of the presentation of the stimulus that induces fear. Anxiety occurs with the anticipation of an undesirable imminent event or worry about an uncertain outcome through previous learning experiences and higher order conditioning. Anxieties may build up gradually over an extended period of time and last for an extended duration (K.M. Martin, DVM, DACVB 2022, personal correspondence regarding terminology).

- Anxiety is a diffuse generalized feeling of fear, apprehension, unease or nervousness regarding an imminent event, uncertain outcome, or danger (threat).
- Anxiety occurs with the anticipation of an undesirable imminent event or worry about an uncertain outcome through previous learning experiences and higher order conditioning.

Fear – Fear can be defined as an aversive emotional state consisting of physiological, psychological, and behavioral responses to a real and present or perceived threat or danger. Fear can be adaptive and motivate the dog to avoid situations or interactions that might be dangerous. While fear can be a normal emotion, the behavior can become extreme for the given circumstance or level of threat experienced by the individual. Often with fear responses, the trigger or antecedent for the behavior can be identified and is stimulus specific (K.M. Martin 2022, personal correspondence). Abnormal fear occurs when little or no real danger threatens.

- Fear can be defined as an aversive emotional state consisting of physiological, psychological, and behavioral responses to a real and present or perceived threat or danger. Abnormal fear occurs when little or no real danger threatens.

Panic – Panic can be defined as a sudden, excessive, and profound feeling of intense fear and/or anxiety for a perceived threat or for no real danger or apparent cause. A panic attack is an abrupt and more intense feeling than anxiety and occurs for a shorter duration. Like anxieties, the trigger or antecedent may be unidentifiable or identifiable. It is important to realize sensory perception in animals is different from humans. Therefore, just because the veterinarian or pet owner cannot identify the stimulus that induces panic does not mean the animal is not reacting to a specific stimulus (K.M. Martin 2022, personal correspondence).

- Panic can be defined as a sudden, excessive, and profound feeling of intense fear and/or anxiety for a perceived threat or for no real danger or apparent cause.

Phobia – A phobia is a sudden, excessive, extreme, or profound fear response out of proportion to the situation, circumstance, or level of threat. Typically, the behavioral response is abnormal and maladaptive for the given circumstance such that it is difficult for the animal to habituate to the situation with repeated exposure. With phobias, like fears, the trigger or antecedent is often identifiable and stimulus specific. Animals with phobia may display extreme flight or escape behavior during the event. Recovery periods or the return to normal after the event is often prolonged (K.M. Martin 2022, personal correspondence).

- A phobia is a sudden, excessive, extreme, or profound fear response out of proportion to the situation, circumstance, or level of threat.
- Recovery periods or the return to normal after the event is often prolonged.

Generalized anxiety

Generalized anxiety may be defined as anxiety occurring for an extended duration of time in a multitude of different environments. It can manifest as pacing, restlessness, hypervigilance, fear/worry/nervousness, hyperexcitability, and difficulty settling. The behavior often occurs with multiple identifiable and unavoidable antecedents or for unidentifiable reasons. The behavior may occur in familiar environments and around familiar people such that it is not context specific or situational. The behavior may be worse in unfamiliar environments (K.M. Martin 2022, personal correspondence). Pets that suffer from generalized anxiety are often hypervigilant, have difficulty learning, are overreactive to stimuli and unable to adapt to new situations.

Global fear

Global fear may be defined as fear (often extreme, aka phobia) of multiple specific stimuli (often unavoidable in the animal's environment) including at least three out of five types of stimulus-specific fear – people, animals, objects, environments, or sounds.

Global fear is common in dogs or cats raised with limited social contact or early environmental experience, but the condition may also be genetic.

Animals with global fear often display fear of novelty (neophobia) and fail to habituate to people or environments over extended periods of time. Animals with global fear are often afraid of familiar people and items in the home environment (K.M. Martin 2022, personal correspondence).

Separation anxiety/distress

Dogs and cats are social animals and when they are separated from their attachment figure some degree of anxiety may occur. Signs of separation anxiety may include (only when the owner is absent) destruction at doors, general destruction in the home, rearranging of objects, house soiling, excessive salivation, distress vocalization, or self-trauma. Pet owners are placed in a deep emotional paradox. Pet owners report a high emotional value to their pet, often stating their pet is "perfect 95% of the time." Pet owners must then deal with the emotional and monetary cost of the pet's disorder.

Sound/thunderstorm phobia

Sound and thunderstorm phobias often occur in conjunction with each other or develop later. There is a genetic predisposition but phobias can also occur because of a traumatic experience and learning. Sound and thunderstorm phobias are often comorbid diagnoses with separation anxiety. The dog or cat may have a fear of thunderstorms and then experiences a storm when the owners are away. The pet then begins to associate being left alone with the potential for fear-inducing events (thunderstorms). There is evidence that the occurrence of separation anxiety or sound/thunderstorm phobias increases the likelihood that the other disorder will occur (Overall et al. 2001). Sound/thunderstorm phobia likely also occurs in cats although symptoms may be less profound and go unnoticed by pet owners.

There has also been a correlation between musculoskeletal pain and noise sensitivities in dogs (Lopes Fagundes et al. 2018). The non-pain and pain groups in the study showed similar behavioral response to loud noises. However, in the pain group the onset of noise sensitivity was later; on average four years later than the non-pain group. Dogs with pain were more likely to generalize and show avoidance of associated environments and other dogs. All dogs (pain or non-pain groups) responded well to treatment but in the pain group only once pain was treated.

Acute conflict behaviors, stereotypical behaviors, and compulsive disorders

Acute conflict behaviors

Acute conflict behaviors are an indication of conflict and stress in the environment and can be a foreshadowing of a stereotypy or compulsive disorder. They are performed in response to a specific trigger. For example, the doorbell rings and the dog runs to the door and spins in circles at the door until the person comes inside.

Stereotypical behaviors

An acute conflict behavior could develop into a stereotypical behavior. A stereotypical behavior is similar to an acute conflict behavior but tends to develop because of a more chronic stressor. For example, a lion may pace a path in an enclosure due to the restrictive nature of the environment. A stereotypic behavior is being displayed. If the lion is taken out of the context the behavior does not occur.

A stereotypical behavior is characterized by a repetitive and invariant locomotor pattern that is not a goal-oriented behavior.

Compulsive disorder

Compulsive disorders include behaviors that are usually repetitive, exaggerated, or sustained and are brought on by conflict and stress, but are then shown outside of the original context. A compulsive disorder is characterized by being a goal-oriented behavior that may be more variable in form. Compulsive disorders may be diagnosed when the presenting behaviors are pronounced and interfere with the pet's functioning behaviors. A genetic predisposition is likely present in any case of compulsive disorder but owner attention may reinforce existing compulsive behaviors. There are many medical factors that should be ruled out prior to a diagnosis of compulsive disorder. Treatment includes improving consistency in the animal's environment, behavior modification, and usually pharmacological intervention.

Compulsive behaviors are categorized into five groups.

Locomotion – tail chasing, spinning, circling, freezing, pouncing, skin rippling.

Oral – self-licking or chewing, air or nose flicking, pica, coprophagia, flank sucking, psychogenic alopecia, wool or fabric sucking, licking objects, polydipsia or polyphagia.

Vocalization – repetitive barking, meowing, whining, howling, and so on.
Hallucinatory – fly snapping, shadow and light chasing, air licking.
Aggressive – self-directed aggression or aggression toward an inanimate object.

Other

Cognitive dysfunction syndrome

Cognitive dysfunction is a progressive organic brain disorder that affects behavior. A decline in neurons, decrease in cerebral vascular blood flow, or increase of neurotoxin deposits alters awareness, decreases responsiveness to stimuli, and decreases the ability to learn and remember. Typical clinical signs include the following (DISHAAL):

Disorientation.
Interactions with humans and other animals may be altered.
Sleep/wake cycles are altered.
House training may lapse.
Activity is altered.
Anxiety.
Learning and memory are impaired.

Early diagnosis and intervention have been proven to slow the progression of the disease and sometimes alleviate early signs, thus providing improved quality of life for the pet and owner.

Hyperexcitability or hyperactive

Hyperexcitable dogs and cats are in a chronic state of excitement and tend to overrespond to even mild stimuli and show extreme lack of impulse control. Pet owners frequently also note inappropriate play and excessive attention-seeking behaviors. Hyperexcitability exacerbates all other behavior problems and disorders. If a dog is hyperexcitable and has other behavior problems or disorders, the hyperexcitability must be addressed first. Hyperexcitability was found to be a risk factor for a dog to develop conflict-induced aggression (Guy et al. 2001).

Conditioned unwanted behavior

Conditioned unwanted behaviors are not a behavior disorder but are frequently a concern to pet owners and complicate behavior disorders. Every behavior disorder described in this text has some level of conditioning involved. The veterinary technician should be fluent at functionally assessing a behavior's antecedents and consequences to direct the pet owner in teaching only the desired behaviors and explaining the extinction process. (See following general references for the above section on diagnosis terminology: Horwitz and Neilson 2007; Horwitz et al. 2009; Luescher and Martin 2010; Landsberg et al. 2013; K.M. Martin 2022, personal correspondence.)

Common veterinarian-prescribed behavioral treatments

This section is meant to describe specific aspects of the treatment plan the veterinarian may prescribe. We have intentionally not included individual treatment plans for specific disorders. It is the veterinarian's responsibility to determine what aspects of treatment will be included in the treatment plan, although the technician's insights and feedback will be integral in the development of the plan.

The technician must understand all aspects of the treatment, including the scientific basis for each recommendation, the goal or reason for each recommendation, the proper application of each recommendation and have the ability to teach the pet owner how to apply the prescribed techniques. Describing and demonstrating the techniques (when possible) with the pet owner can alert the technician to potential concerns or challenges the pet owner may have after leaving the veterinary hospital. Techniques may need to be individualized to integrate more successfully into the pet owner's lifestyle.

Treatment plans are multifaceted and usually start with management, then address the animal's temperament (fear, hyperexcitability, etc.) followed by addressing the specific problem behaviors. Below is an example of a treatment plan that might be presented to the veterinary technician to assist the pet owner in understanding and applying.

Diagnosis: Fear-based aggression toward men and generalized anxiety.
Management: Prevent access to men.
Temperament: Cease punishment; interact in a cue→response→reward format, decrease anxiety with medication.
Behavior modification and training: counter conditioning (CC) to men, begin clicker training, teach "go to a mat," teach targeting to hand, demonstrate

response substitution (RS) on walks, condition to a head collar and basket muzzle.

The veterinary technician then instructs the pet owner how each aspect of the treatment plan fits into the treatment process (i.e. utilizing a hand target can help redirect Fluffy and put her at ease in the presence of men), the function of each aspect of the treatment process, how it is to be applied, and how to make it fit into their lifestyle. Appropriate goals and expectations should be considered and discussed.

Most treatment plans will include management techniques, the specific training style to be used, training of specific behaviors, behavior modification, and specific recommended training tools. If pharmacological treatment is included (see Chapter 10), the veterinary technician should discuss potential side effects and proper administration of the medication.

Management

Management is a method of manipulating the environment (antecedent arrangement) so the animal is less likely to perform the unwanted behavior or the unwanted behavior is lessened in intensity while behavior modification is being instituted or the new behavior is being trained. Examples would be using white noise and window film to muffle stimuli of people approaching the residence. For a dog who barks at people passing by the home, these management techniques will help decrease the practice of the behavior.

In some cases, especially in cases of aggression, management can be a key point in keeping the client safe and preventing further damage to the human–animal bond while implementing the behavior modification and training components of the treatment plan.

Avoiding triggers

It is important to attempt to avoid eliciting situations or known triggers of the behavior while behavior modification and treatment are being instituted. Avoiding triggers will decrease the chances of the unwanted behavior from continuing to be practiced while training and behavior modification are being integrated into the treatment plan. It is also important to avoid triggers (especially in aggression cases) to keep the target of the aggression safe and to prevent further damage to the human–animal bond.

Specific triggers (when known) should be determined during the assessment and history-taking processes. Once specific stimuli are identified, the veterinary technician can assist the pet owner in specific methods for avoiding those stimuli. For example, if aggression is likely to occur when the pet is groomed, they are asked to avoid all grooming while the treatment plan is being instituted. If the patient becomes aggressive when disturbed while on the couch, the owner is instructed to limit the patient's access to the couch area to avoid the conflict. Another example would be walking a dog early in the morning to avoid meeting strangers on walks or avoiding walking in high-density dog areas. The veterinary technician should problem-solve with the pet owner to make sure the avoidance of triggers is manageable for the pet owner.

Goals:
- Keeps the pet and pet owner safe.
- Decreases stress for both the pet and pet owner.
- Avoids confrontations (prevent further damage to the human–animal bond).
- Keeps the patient from continuing to practice the unwanted behavior. By avoiding stimuli, the patient is no longer conditioned by the undesirable behavior producing some degree of relief from the eliciting stimulus.

Ignore attention-seeking behaviors

A treatment plan may indicate the need for the owner to avoid reinforcing certain attention-seeking behaviors. The owner should be coached on the importance of catching their dog ignoring them and being calm and subsequently reinforce those calm behaviors with an offer of attention from the owner. Having a structured routine that meets the pet's social, exploratory, and physical needs, will ensure the pet receives adequate attention and the owners are meeting the pet's daily needs.

When asked to ignore, it means not looking at, talking to, or touching the pet in response to particular behaviors and is often one of the difficult aspects of treatment for pet owners. Most pet owners do not realize they are rewarding attention-seeking or unwanted behaviors with their attention and it should not be assumed that asking a pet owner to ignore unwanted behaviors is self-explanatory. They often do not notice until it is pointed out to them that they are touching, talking, or even looking at their pet when it seeks attention. Pet owners might be asked to temporarily ignore their pet during the behavior consultation so the dependence and intensity of attention-seeking behaviors of the patient can be determined during the consultation. It is also an accurate method for determining how difficult it may be for the pet owner to ignore their pet at home. During a consultation, the pet owner may look at the pet and say "I can't pet you, I am ignoring you" without realizing he/she has just reinforced the pet's behavior. The veterinary technician can give the client specific instructions such as, "Cross your arms and pretend he is invisible" or "Stand up and look straight ahead if he jumps into your lap." Some pet owners may be taught to read a magazine instead of looking at their pet. If the pet owner has difficulty following instructions a TAG Point (see Chapter 5) maybe used. Example: When he barks at you, the Tag Point is "Look at me." The technician should shape the pet owner's behavior and reinforce any initial attempt at ignoring. If multiple family members are present, they can be taught to reinforce each other for ignoring the pet.

Owners should be advised that the behavior will likely worsen (extinction burst or frustration effect) before improving and that is a predictable part of the learning process. If providing adequate attention at set times throughout the day, this should minimize the level of frustration a pet experiences. They should also be advised that the ignoring of attention-seeking behaviors does not mean ignoring the needs of the pet. If the dog is asking to be let outside to relieve himself, he should not be ignored. This is normal communication of basic needs.

Ignoring their pet is often an extremely difficult and an emotion-laden request for clients. It is imperative that the pet owner understands how this aspect will affect the treatment process and that it is only a temporary part of treatment. Explaining that their pet may have an unhealthy dependency on them and that ignoring the excessive attention-seeking behavior will help to improve the pet's confidence is often helpful. Instruct the client with empathy, compassion, and understanding. Have the owners focus on interacting with the pet when the pet is ignoring them and is calm.

Goals:

- Decrease hyperexcitability.
- Decrease attention-seeking behaviors.
- Increase pet owner consistency and predictability.
- Increase the pet's independence.
- Reinforce calm behavior.

Ignore at specific times

The treatment plan may require the pet owner to ignore the pet only at specific times, such as prior to leaving or when returning, when treating separation anxiety. The veterinary technician should assist the pet owner in determining how to change their behaviors during the required times. For example, instead of reassuring the pet before leaving, give the pet an interactive toy. The pet owner may be asked to ignore specific pets when other pets are near, when treating IDA–H.

Goals:

- Decrease dependency on the pet owner.
- Decrease overarousal of the pet during specific times.
- Remove inadvertent reinforcing of unwanted behaviors.
- Decreasing an alliance with the pet owner when treating IDA–H.

Cue→response→reward interactions

Pet owners frequently interact with their pet casually and randomly throughout the day, speaking to them in sentences and touching them. These casual interactions are usually inconsistent (from the animal's perspective) and often inadvertently condition unwanted attention-seeking behaviors. Pets that do not exhibit anxiety or problematic behaviors can adjust to these inconsistent interactions but pets with anxiety and/or aggression issues frequently demonstrate increased anxiety, hyperactivity, and over-dependence on the owner. In those cases, the veterinarian may include in the treatment plan more consistent interactions such as a cue→response→reward (CRR) interaction.

CRR interaction suggests the owners give the animal a cue for a previously trained foundation behavior (i.e. "sit," "down," "come," "go to your bed," "watch me") when the dog is not initiating attention on its own. The owner is to give the cue, wait for the desired response, and then reward the behavior. The reward may be attention, food, or another desired reinforcer. Frequently, the veterinary technician must first teach cued foundation behaviors (see later in this chapter) before CRR interactions can occur because the pet owner may not have a reliable behavior on cue (Table 9.2). It is important to emphasize that a cue is a request not a demand. The animal should not be forced to respond to the cue. It is the animal's choice. If the dog is resting quietly on his bed, the owner asks the dog if he

Table 9.2 Cue→response→reward possible responses.

Response to cue	Pet owner's response	How to proceed
Behavior offered	Reinforce behavior	Continue with interaction
No response	Ignore or wait and cue the behavior again	Depending on the circumstances (dog resting on his bed), the dog might not be interested in interacting with the owner now, and that might be ok. If still no response, ask for another cued behavior and proceed – discuss with veterinary technician to determine if the behavior is under stimulus control
Cued behavior offered before cue given	Ask for another cued behavior	Reinforce the behavior
Animal becomes aggressive when cue is given	Avoid reacting in any way. Remain calm and end the interaction with as little conflict as possible	Call to discuss with veterinary technician

would like to come over to him by giving a known touch cue (nose touch to hand), and the dog does not respond. The dog is communicating he is not interested in interacting at the moment and that is ok.

It should be noted that CRR interactions are quite different from other historically recommended interactions commonly called *Nothing-in-Life-is-Free* (NILIF) and *deference protocols*. The aforementioned techniques are meant to change the animal's behavior by clarifying the "social status" between owner and pet. A CRR interaction places focus on changing the owner's behavior to increase consistency and predictability in the relationship. This is an important differentiation because any type of social dominance or "pack mentality" will only complicate and likely be of detriment to the treatment plan (Table 9.3).

Table 9.3 A comparison between NILIF and cue→response→reward interactions.

NILIF	Cue→Response→Reward
Based on changing the dog's attitude	Based on changing the owner's behavior
Goal is to clarify social status	Goal is to increase predictability of owner
No scientific basis	Based on laws of learning
Focus on gaining control over the dog	Giving control to the dog
Strives to create deference	Strives to create meaningful consequences
Accepts person as "leader"	Learns to trust people
About "obeying"	About choosing

Goals:

- Increase owner predictability.
- Decrease the chance of reinforcing attention-seeking behaviors.
- Pet owner focuses on desired behavior.
- Decrease over-dependence on pet owner.
- Decrease hyperexcitability and anxiety.

Change primary caregiver

Changing who takes primary care of the pet may be recommended when it is determined there is an over-dependence on one member of the household. It may also be recommended when a positive association toward an "unfavored" household member is being developed.

Goals:

- Decrease over-dependence on a family member.
- Increase a positive association with a family member.

Environmental modifications

Physical changes to the environment to decrease the chance of the unwanted behavior occurring are usually the first consideration in all treatment plans. Environmental modifications (antecedent arrangement) may include placement of barriers including outside fences, changing feeding areas, changing locations of litter boxes, covering windows with film, moving furniture to prevent access to areas, utilizing gates at doorways, acoustic therapy, pheromones, aromatherapy, and so on. The veterinary technician along with the veterinarian and pet owner should determine appropriate, functional, and acceptable environmental modifications that will fit into the pet owner's lifestyle.

Goals:
- Prevent unwanted behavior from occurring.
- Decrease stimuli.

Crate confinement or other confinement

Crate or other confinement (exercise pens, rooms, etc.) is used as a management technique to prevent unwanted behavior or to prevent the patient from access to a trigger (i.e. avoiding guests). Confinement should not be used as a punishment or associated with an aversive (yelling, physical punishment, etc.).

Conditioning to confinement is discussed in detail in Chapter 7.

The fundamental to training an animal to confinement is to classically associate the confinement area with something pleasant. Suggestions could include doing positive-based training sessions in the confinement area, feeding in the area, giving attention to the pet only when it is in the area (including play time), or allowing the pet to play with their favorite enrichment toy only while in the area.

If the crate or other confinement area has previously been associated with a negative emotional response, the following technique may be helpful.

Crate (or other confinement) reconditioning

If the animal has not generalized the negative emotional response to all confinement areas, the lack of generalization can be utilized when reconditioning to confinement.

Step 1: The "bad crate" is the crate that has been associated in the past with a negative emotional response. Create a "good crate" by making it look and seem as different as possible from the previously negatively associated crate. For example, if a plastic crate was used in the past, use a wire crate as the "good crate." Move the crate to a different room or area of the house. If at any time the pet must be crated while the "good crate" is being conditioned, use the "bad" crate, which already has a negative association.

Step 2: Shape the behavior "go in" at a non-stressful starting point. If the dog shows any anxiety about interacting with the "good crate," begin with teaching "go in" by covering a chair or table and shaping going into the covered area and place the behavior on cue.

Step 3: Once the cue of "go in" has been associated with a positive emotional response (clicker training and treats) it can then be given when shaping to go into the "good crate." Once the pet has been shaped to readily "go in" to the "good crate," continue to condition the crate as you would with a new puppy (see Chapter 7).

Step 4: Do not use the "good crate" at any time anxiety might occur (thunderstorms, fireworks, owner gone too long) until treatment has progressed (i.e. medications have taken effect).

Goals:
- Safety.
- Avoiding triggers.
- Preventing destruction.
- House training.

Tethering

Tethering is another type of confinement that allows the pet to be supervised while in the environment with the family. Tethering is frequently recommended when counter conditioning dogs within the same household to each other by tethering and training both dogs in the same room. Treats are tossed to the dog that is training and to the other dog for not reacting or for relaxation. Tethering is also frequently used for re-house training and is always recommended as a safety measure when the pet owner is teaching relinquishment exercises to a dog that has shown possessive aggression.

The animal also may be tethered to the pet owner with a waist leash or may drag a line (see section **Training tools**), allowing the pet owner to pick up the drag line to redirect the animal and do RS if the animal becomes reactive or aggressive.

Interactive toys can be tethered in confinement areas to encourage the pet to interact with the toy away from the pet owner, increasing independence from the owner.

Goals:
- Active supervision.
- Safety.
- Independence training (tethered toy).
- Assists with RS (dragline).

Dietary changes

Behavior is directly affected by diet, therefore dietary changes and/or the inclusion of supplements may be recommended by the veterinarian for various behavioral reasons including aggression, difficulty in training, coprophagia, and cognitive dysfunction (Landsberg et al. 2013).

The veterinary technician should counsel the pet owner on how to properly change diets and administer any supplements.

Goal:

- Organic benefits to brain chemistry and body health.

Regular schedule

Predictable and consistent timing of meals, play time, training, and walks helps to decrease anxiety and hyperexcitability.

Regular schedules have been found to be beneficial in general and as a preventive measure, as noted in Chapter 7.

Goals:

- Increase predictability and consistency.
- Decrease anxiety and hyperexcitability.

Meal feed dogs twice daily

A case load analysis done by Dr. Andrew Luescher at the Ontario Veterinary College reflected that dogs that were on ad lib feeding, and switched to twice daily meal feeding had a better prognosis (Unpublished data, personal communication with Dr. Andrew Luescher). Meal feeding also makes defecation more predictable and allows training to occur before meals.

Goals:

- Increases general predictability.
- Decreases anxiety and hyperexcitability.
- Increases desire for food rewards in training.
- Makes defecation more predictable.

Mental stimulation

Human studies have shown learning and brain exercises delay the onset of dementia. Canine research has found similar results and noted that mental stimulation is essential for a high quality of life and can include training and sniff walks, puzzle toys, interactive food toys (see section **Training tools**), and so on (Landsberg et al. 2013).

Mental stimulation is often recommended to prevent destructive behaviors due to lack of stimulation, improve focus and concentration, and increase trainability.

Goals:

- Improve quality of life.
- Slow cognitive dysfunction.
- Decrease destruction due to lack of stimulation.
- Increase concentration, focus, and trainability.

Walking off property

Walks off the property reduce anxiety levels and dogs that were walked regularly were shown to have less of a problem with aggression (Unpublished data, personal communication with Dr. Andrew Luescher). Owners should be encouraged to walk their dog off the property once or twice daily for 10–20 minutes (longer or shorter depending on the dog's physical needs/limitations, weather, and owner's schedule). Walking dogs off the property is believed to decrease hyperexcitability, territorial aggression, and general reactivity. Unfortunately, many owners do not walk their dog off the property because they feel the dog gets enough exercise in the backyard. This thought process overlooks the second and possibly most important benefit to walking the dog off the property, which is the mental stimulation the dog receives from visual, olfactory, and auditory stimulation (see section **SEEKING system**). Owners should therefore be informed that even if their dog has a large yard, walking off their property is very important for the mental stimulation it provides the dog. Plus, it is a great social activity that benefits both the owner and the dog.

Some patients may require fitting with a front clip harness or head halter to decrease pulling or if RS on walks is required. The veterinary technician can also teach cues for loose leash walking beside the pet owner and another cue "to go play" or sniff. Predictability is increased by giving the dog a cue for when it is acceptable to sniff and another cue for walking politely. Cues are given just before the behavior, "Go play" – dogs sniffs, followed by "Let's go" and the dog is reinforced for coming back to the side of the pet owner with a treat or by being allowed to go sniff again. Teaching the dog to "ask permission" to go sniff is another great communication tool to allow the dog to have some control over their environment. For example, if the dog lifts and turns his head in a direction to smell something, he can then be taught to look back to the owner to "ask for permission." The owner can then either cue, "Go sniff," "Let's go," or simply give a treat for the dog's offered attention depending on the circumstances.

Goals and benefits:

- Decrease anxiety.
- Decrease hyperexcitability.
- Decrease reactivity.
- Increases mental stimulation and provides an outlet for exploratory behavior.
- Provides social interaction with the handler.

Aerobic exercise

The goal of aerobic exercise is different from the goal of walking the dog off property. Aerobic exercise is exercise such as brisk walking that increases oxygen consumption. Increased aerobic exercise has been shown to improve mood, decrease depression, reduce stress, and increase the ability to cope with stress in humans (Psychology 2007–2012). Aerobic exercise is associated with the production of endorphins. Some researchers have suggested that neurochemicals such as epinephrine, serotonin, and dopamine also contribute to elevated mood. Aerobic exercise has also been found to have antidepressant-type actions (Hunsberger et al. 2007). It should be noted that some dogs may become more energetic and overstimulated by aerobic activity. Providing these dogs with additional mental stimulation via structured positive training and relaxation exercises may help counteract this stimulatory effect.

Aerobic activity in cats can be implemented by playing with the cat with interactive toys such as a feather teaser.

Goals:

- Increase endorphins.
- Decrease anxiety.
- Decrease hyperactivity and excitability.
- Decrease reactivity.

Clicker training

Clicker training is an excellent tool for increasing mental stimulation and likely activates what Dr. Jaak Panksepp calls the SEEKING system.

SEEKING system

Panksepp believed that neurochemistries lead companion animals to energetically investigate and explore their world in an attempt to seek available resources and to make sense of environmental contingencies. Others have called the system "foraging/expectancy system," "behavioral activation system" (Gray 1990), and the "behavioral facilitation system" (Depue and Iacono 1989). Panksepp believed that the SEEKING system contributes to the feelings of engagement and excitement when resources are sought (Ahn and Picard 2006) and that the basic impulse to investigate and make sense of the environment emerges from circuits in the lateral hypothalamic corridor of the brain (Panksepp 1998). This system drives human complexities such as persistent feelings of interest, anticipation, and curiosity. The SEEKING system is what is driving you to read this text.

Panksepp was convinced that clicker training (and other mentally stimulating activities) are evidence of the SEEKING system in action (Pryor 2009). This is not only in relationship to the "trainee" but also to the person training the animal. For example, the SEEKING system is activated when working closely with an animal to solve a training issue or when trying to determine the next successive approximation to reinforce. It is a puzzle that needs to be understood, creating excitement and enthusiasm. Panksepp's explanation makes it clear that a trainer using a clicker and trainee are frequently "in tune" during a training session; both are in the midst of the SEEKING system.

Punishment switches the learner away from the hypothalamus and SEEKING system to the amygdala's path of avoidance and fear (Pryor 2009).

Clicker training and the practical applications will be discussed in detail in the section **Training techniques**.

Goals and benefits:

- Increase pet owner predictability.
- Improve communication between pet and pet owner.
- Increase or repair the human–animal bond.
- Decrease hyperexcitability.
- Increase concentration and retention.
- Teach foundation and complex behaviors that can be used during CC/RS/systematic desensitization exercises.
- Keep the pet owner safe during training (hands off).

Training techniques

The American Veterinary Society of Animal Behavior states that training methods are most effective when they focus on teaching the animal what to do, rather than punishing them for unwanted behaviors (AVSAB 2021).

In addition:

1. An animal's behavior is often a "coping" mechanism for an adverse emotional state. If the motivating emotion is addressed, often the undesirable behavior is diminished or eradicated. Utilizing training techniques that positively affect the

emotional state of the animal should be used when applying behavior modification techniques.
2. The training techniques should promote and protect the human–animal bond and foster a *healthy* relationship between the pet and pet owner (see Table 4.1). Often the relationship between the pet owner and the pet has been strained or damaged by behavior concerns when they approach a veterinary professional. Training techniques that build trust and predictability will begin to heal a damaged relationship.
3. The technique should increase confidence in both the animal and the pet owner. A symbiotic relationship of mutualism between learner and trainer should be fostered. Training is a team activity that should always focus on success. If success is not occurring, the training should be modified to increase success. Learner and trainer should not focus on unwanted behavior or failure. The *information* the animal is giving should be taken into consideration and the training should be modified based on this information. For example, if the dog is unable to respond to a known cue, recognize that the situation may be too distracting, and it has not been trained to fluency. Take that information and adapt the environment to help the animal be successful. Then make a training plan to build in distractions more gradually.
4. The training technique should have a low potential for adverse side effects. Learning should be fun, enjoyable, and not something that causes anxiety or fear. Fear of punishment or failure makes learning difficult or impossible.
5. The training techniques should be based on sound principles of learning and scientific data rather than anecdotal experiences. By understanding the scientific basis for techniques, the trainer has the ability to problem solve a training challenge and resolve it in a positive manner. Utilizing techniques on the grounds that they have proved successful in the past without understanding the scientific principles guiding the techniques is neither professional nor recommended (Box 9.1).

- An animal's behavior is often a "coping" mechanism for an adverse emotional state.

BOX 9.1: GUIDELINES FOR CHOOSING A TRAINING TECHNIQUE

The training technique should
positively affect the emotional state of the animal, focus on desired behavior and success, promote, protect, and foster a healthy relationship between pet and owner, increase confidence for both the pet and the owner, have a low potential for adverse side effects, be based on scientific principles of learning and scientific data.

Why punishment is not recommended in training or the application of behavior modification

Punishment is a complex and advanced tool. It is generally misunderstood, applied improperly, and much overused. When punishment is applied incorrectly or inappropriately it becomes abusive.

- When punishment is applied incorrectly or inappropriately it becomes abusive.

Punishment, specifically corporal punishment, is defined as the use of physical force with the intention of causing pain but not injury, with the purpose of changing behavior (Mulvaney and Mebert 2007) and usually includes the use of training tools such as choke, shock, and prong collars.

Punishment-focused training is never included as part of a treatment plan and rarely recommended in behavior modification for the following reasons.

Poor learning and cognition

Research has found the unintended consequences of corporal punishment in children to include increased aggression, depression, lower self-esteem, and poorer psychological and cognitive functioning (Strassberg et al. 1994; Gershoff 2002). Another study showed children who were spanked had a significantly lower IQ than those who were not spanked (Straus and Paschall 2009). Dr. Murray

Straus reports "children who were spanked the most fell behind the average IQ development curve, and those who were never spanked advanced ahead of the average. The more the spanking, the slower the development of the child's mental ability. But even small amounts of spanking made a difference." Dr. Straus suggested that the correlation between corporal punishment and lower IQ may be attributed to the stress and fear that punishment causes.

Criteria for effective punishment are difficult to meet

As stated earlier, punishment is a complex and advanced tool. ALL of the following criteria must be met for punishment to be effective and must be successfully met by the pet owner.

The animal's motivation strength is not too high

The stronger the motivation to perform the behavior, the less likely punishment will work. Strong innate behaviors such as aggression (a defense mechanism), chasing, and hunting maybe more difficult to modify.

All animals, including humans, use a limited number of strategies to deal with dangerous situations, including escaping or avoiding, freezing, defensive aggression ("fighting back"), or appeasement. Underlying physiological changes during stressful situations are similar across species. Soldiers injured in battle fail to notice the injuries while in a traumatic experience. A rat exposed to a cat will not notice painful heat applied to its tail. The cat poses a more immediate and significant danger. In both humans and animals, stress-induced analgesia occurs as a consequence of the activation of the brain's natural opiate system (LeDoux 1996). The activation of opiates may be the reason some dogs do not respond to extreme physical punishment when motivation or emotional response is high.

Examples:

- A dog runs through the invisible fence to chase a rabbit because of a strong innate motivation.
- A dog urinates when punished – it will not decrease if punished for urinating and the punishment will likely make the urination worse.

Always contingent on behavior and only associated with the behavior

The punishment must occur every time the behavior occurs and should be associated with the behavior and not other people or animals. This is why remote punishment may be recommended in some treatment plans. See the section **Remote punishment**.

Proper intensity

The intensity of the punishment must be high enough to interrupt the behavior immediately after application of the punishment but should not be so intense as to create intense fear. Motivation strength or high emotional state (higher motivation requires a higher level of punishment) must be seriously considered. If the motivation or emotional state is high, the intensity level of the punishment may reach inhumane and cruel levels to become effective, if effective at all. At such levels, learning maybe inhibited.

If the intensity of the punishment is too low, the animal will get habituated to the punishment. Eventually harsh or cruel punishment will be required to stop the undesired behavior.

Timing

For punishment to be effective, it must be delivered within 0.5 seconds of the start of undesired behavior. The ideal time to apply punishment is just as the behavior begins. Any delay will cause punishment to be ineffective. When delivered late, it is no longer associated with the undesirable behavior and likely becomes associated with something else in the environment. For example, a dog eliminates on the floor when left alone. The pet owner returns home and punishes the dog. The dog then shows appeasement behaviors (often described by pet owners as "looking guilty") when the pet owner returns home because the dog has associated urine on the floor as the cue the pet owner will punish him. The behavior of eliminating on the floor was not punished, it was reinforced by the feeling of relief when the pet eliminated.

Alternative behavior choice

Behavior is usually performed to reach a goal or reward. Therefore, an alternative behavior should be taught and rewarded in the place of the undesirable behavior that is to be punished. The alternative behavior should be taught and placed on cue and fluent before being used as an alternative choice. Example: If a dog is punished for jumping up by the stranger turning away, it should alternatively be taught to sit to greet strangers.

Punishment (including negative punishment, see Chapter 6) should significantly decrease the behavior within three to four applications. If the behavior is not significantly diminished within that time, the punishment should immediately be ceased, and the criteria reviewed.

Punishment is counterproductive to treatment

Fear is a defense system that produces responses that maximize survival. Those responses "represent the operation of brain systems that have been programmed by evolution to deal with danger in routine ways. Although we can become conscious of the operation of the defense system, especially when it leads to behavioral expressions, the system operates independently of consciousness" (LeDoux 1996). In other words, punishing an animal's method for coping with a highly emotional situation (fear provoking) without addressing the underlying emotional state is neither appropriate nor humane and will likely not be successful in reaching the desired goal behavior.

Example 1: A dog growls when being touched on its head because a past otitis has created a negative emotional response to having his ears touched. The growling is a "coping" mechanism to make the fear-provoking stimulus retreat. Punishing the growling may decrease the behavior (growling) but does not address the underlying anxiety of being touched on the head and will likely increase overall anxiety.

Example 2: A child seeks out a parent and says he/she is afraid there is a "monster in the closet." If the parent were to spank the child, it may decrease the coping mechanism of going to the parent for consoling but do nothing to decrease the fear of the "monster."

The AVSAB Position Statement states, "Aversive training methods have a damaging effect on both animal welfare and the human–animal bond. There is no evidence that aversive methods are more effective than reward-based methods in any context." AVSAB therefore advises that aversive methods should not be used in animal training or for the treatment of behavior disorders (AVSAB 2021).

- Punishing an animal's method for coping with a highly emotional situation (fear provoking) without addressing the underlying emotional state is neither appropriate nor humane and will likely not be successful in reaching the desired goal behavior.

Punishment is not generally recommended for training or in the application of behavior modification for the following reasons:

- Slows learning and cognition.
- Increases fear and fear-based aggression.
- Is very difficult to apply consistently and therefore becomes unpredictable.
- Inadvertent or unintended negative associations are made, including toward the pet owner, other animals, other people and the environment. In this regard, punishment is more like a bomb going off than a solution that pinpoints the exact issues.
- Confrontational – Owner-applied punishment is almost always confrontational and is directly correlated to the development of conflict-induced aggression. Confrontation often leads to aggression, putting the pet and the pet owner in danger and further damaging the human–animal bond.

When treating behavioral disorders, it is imperative to decrease fear, unpredictability, and confrontations.

- When treating behavioral disorders, it is imperative to decrease fear, unpredictability, and confrontations.

Generally positive punishment is not effective for problem behaviors because all criteria for punishment cannot be met.

- Generally positive punishment is not effective for problem behaviors because all criteria for punishment cannot be met.

Why the prevalence of punishment-based training and domination techniques persist

Punishment is a complex technique, and it is often misunderstand and frequently overused (Luescher and Shaw 2007). With the knowledge of potential side effects, why does punishment remain so prevalent in the animal training world? The answers may lie in two historical experiments.

In 1961, Yale University psychologist Stanley Milgram created an experiment to test how much pain an ordinary citizen ("teacher") would inflict on another person ("learner") because he was ordered to by an authority figure ("experimenter")

(Milgram 1963). The experiment consisted of the "experimenter" instructing the "teacher" to administer electric shocks to the "learner" for incorrect answers. Unbeknown to the "teacher," the "learner" was not really receiving shocks but was acting as if he had. The "teacher" was told to move one level higher on the shock generator each time the learner flashed a wrong answer. The shock generator indicated available voltage from 15 to 450 V. Additional verbal designations included slight shock, moderate shock, extreme intensity shock, danger: severe shock, and lastly two switches labeled "xxx." At 300 "fake" voltage level, the acting "learner" was to pound on the wall to make sure the "teacher" was aware of the discomfort being caused. At 325 V, the "learner" stopped answering questions and the "teacher" was told to treat each non-answer as a wrong answer, increasing the voltage. Sometimes the "teacher" asked the "experimenter" if the "learner was liable to suffer permanent physical injury" and the experimenter said, "Although the shocks may be painful, there is no permanent tissue damage, so please go on."

The results were astounding and not predicted. Of the 40 "teachers," 14 refused to continue the experiment past 300 V, the point the "student" banged on the wall. The 26 remaining "teachers" followed the "experimenter's" direction until they reached the most potent shock available, two steps beyond the designation: danger: severe shock. Some expressed reluctance to administer shocks over the 300 V level yet complied with the authority of the "experimenter." Milgram believed two findings were surprising. The first was in regard to the strength of obedient tendencies even in the fundamental breach of moral conduct to hurt another. To disobey the "experimenter" would have not resulted in a punishment to the "teacher" yet 26 subjects abandoned their own personal values to follow the direction of the authority figure. The second was the amount of stress the experimenter caused to the "teacher." Many showed severe tension and emotional strain, yet continued as directed (Ksenych and Liu 1992).

The second experiment was the 1971 Stanford Prison Experiment conducted by psychology professor Philip Zimbardo, which tested the psychological effects of becoming a prisoner or prison guard. Dramatic, albeit controversial, results were found in both the behavior of the "prisoners" and "guards."

A mock prison was created in the Stanford psychology building. Twenty-four male undergraduates were chosen for their lack of psychological issues, crime history, and medical disabilities. A flip of a coin determined which 12 would become "guards" and which 12 would become "prisoners."

The guards were given little instruction but were told to do whatever they thought was necessary to maintain law and order and to gain the respect of the prisoners. The guards created punishment techniques which included verbal harassment, humiliation, isolation, spray from a fire extinguisher, forcing prisoners to do repetitive menial work such as cleaning toilet bowls with their bare hands, placing bags over prisoners' heads, and requiring prisoners to do jumping jacks and push-ups while weight was put on the their back. Punishment was imposed for infractions including disrespect or disobedience from the prisoners. As the experiment progressed, the guards began to see the prisoners as "troublemakers" who were out to get them and consequently steadily increased their coercive aggressive tactics. Prisoners became distressed and fatigued. Acute emotional disturbances, disorganized thinking, uncontrollable crying, and rage appeared in the prisoners.

Three types of guards were identified. Some of the guards were "tough but fair," others were "good guys" who rarely punished the prisoners. One-third of the guards were hostile, arbitrary, and inventive in the different forms of punishment administered. Initially some prisoners rebelled and fought the guards. Others developed psychosomatic illness or broke down emotionally. Some tried to cope by attempting to do whatever the guards asked, to please them. In the end, the guards won total control and commanded blind and unquestioning obedience from each prisoner.

On the sixth day of the proposed 14-day experiment, the study was ended as the prisoners were withdrawing and behaving pathologically and some guards were behaving sadistically. The "good guy" guards were beginning to feel helpless although no guards quit the study, called in sick, requested to leave early, or requested pay for overtime work.

What implications could the Milgram's behavioral study of obedience and the Stanford Prison Experiment have on teaching people to train dogs?

Pet dog owners seek veterinary professionals and dog trainers to give them advice on how to teach their pet. Many of these novice dog owners are advised to use punishment techniques, techniques they may feel quite uncomfortable administering, but they often continue with the recommended techniques. Could the veterinary professional or dog trainer take on the role of "experimenter," the pet owner the role of "teacher," and dog the role of "learner" as in the Milgram experiment? Most clients seen at the Animal Behavior Clinic at Purdue University and Veterinary Behavior Consultations in Spicewood, Texas were relieved when they were told they should no longer use the choke collar, pinch collar, or domination techniques that they had been advised to use by others.

The Stanford Prison Experiment demonstrated that when given the ability to punish, dominate, and control another, it was reinforcing to some of the guards. Control is a primary reinforcer. Punishment-based and dominance-type training is reinforcing to the person administering the punishment.

Some owners may use punishment techniques because they do not have the knowledge or understanding of alternative methods. Some may go to a professional who advocates punishment-based techniques and because that professional is an authoritative figure, they comply even though they may not feel comfortable with the techniques. Some professionals may recommend a complete authoritarian relationship between pet and pet owners, including complete obedience at all times. Such a recommendation does not build a symbiotic relationship and sets up both pet and owner for failure.

Veterinary technicians must be aware of different training styles and recommend pet owners to qualified trainers who use the most up-to-date, relationship-building, and humane training styles available.

Lure reward training

Lure reward training is a style of training that consists of giving a cue for a behavior ("sit"), luring or prompting (in a nonconfrontational manner) the behavior (treat held over the animal's head) and rewarding the behavior (sit).

For the cue to become the discriminative stimulus for the behavior, it is important that the cue be given before the lure, otherwise the cue may be overshadowed by the hand movement of the lure. This can be tested by asking the dog to "sit" with no hand movement; if the "sit" does not occur, imitate the hand signal moving over the head as if using a lure without saying the word "sit." If the dog sits without the verbal "sit," it indicates the cue is the hand movement/lure rather than the verbal "sit" cue.

The advantage of lure reward training is that if done properly and without confrontation it is a technique that can be used by almost all pet owners including children.

The challenge is teaching owners how to successfully fade the lure from the behavior either by placing the behavior on a verbal cue or fading the movement of the lure into a hand signal as a cue for the behavior. Otherwise, the behavior may only occur when the pet owner uses a treat as the lure, as the treat in the hand becomes part of the cue for the animal.

Lure reward training may be recommended as the training style of choice if the pet owner has difficulty using a marker or if minimal and less precise training is required. Although when dealing with animals with significant fear and anxiety issues, you are likely to encounter some that are not trusting of being reached for or even handed a treat. Lure reward training may be perceived as threatening to the animal.

Event marker (clicker) training

The following text will use "event marker," "marker" and "clicker," and "conditioned reinforcer" interchangeably.

This section will only discuss positive reinforcement markers and not punishment markers.

Marker training is a cross-species communication technology that allows us to communicate clearly and precisely with animals. It is a system of using positive reinforcement in conjunction with a consistent event marker (usually a clicker). The sound of a clicker is both a conditioned reinforcer (see Chapter 6) and a signal marking a desired behavior (event marker).

The fundamentals of marker training can be broken down into three steps: observe the behavior, mark the behavior, and reinforce the desired behavior. More advanced and necessary steps including cueing and fluency are discussed later in this chapter.

Benefits of clicker training, both in training and in the application of behavior modification techniques

Accelerated learning

A small research project done in 2006 tested the difference between a verbal- and clicker-type marker with regard to a comparison of training time and the number of required reinforcements. They found that training with a clicker as the event marker not only reduced the required amount of training time, but also fewer reinforcements were needed to successfully teach the behavior. The results of this study suggest that the clicker provides more accurate information than the verbal bridging stimulus, thereby increasing the rate of reinforcement and decreasing the amount of required training time (Wood 2008).

Improved retention time

The phenomenon of long retention has been abundantly proven with conditioned punishers. Conditioned reinforcers (a clicker for this discussion) are known to take parallel pathways in the brain and behave like conditioned punishers, while triggering different brain chemicals and emotions than punishers.

In practice, if the click is indeed a conditioned reinforcer and is being used correctly as a marker, the association will be retained permanently unless the training is extinguished (Pryor 2009).

Hands-off and non-threatening

Many patients suffering from behavior disorders require a non-threatening and hands-off approach to training, especially when there is a history of aversive training in the animal's past. It also allows the pet owner to train from a distance, which is often helpful when working with animals displaying fear or aggression. One family member can mark a behavior while another reinforces it. This allows the elderly or very young children to assist in the training process (Figure 9.2).

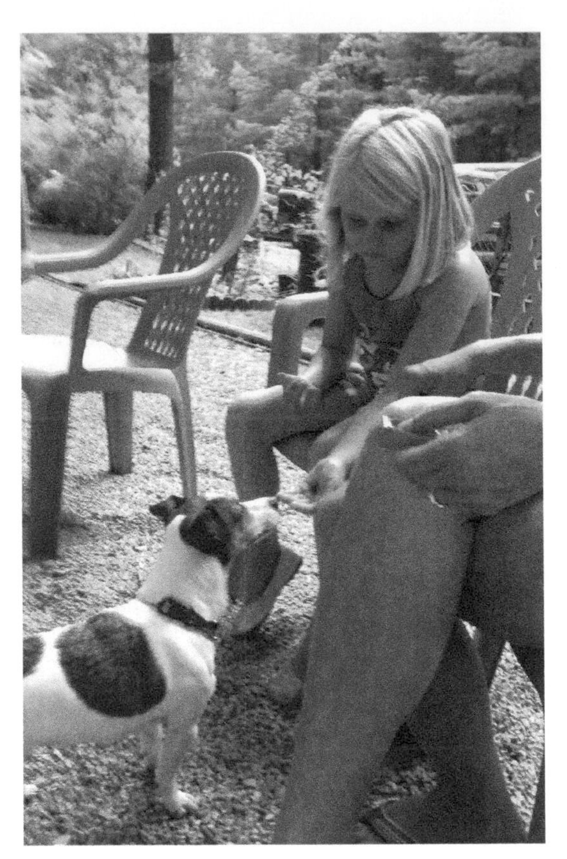

Figure 9.2 Adult marking desired behavior while a child delivers the reinforcement.

Marker training as a tool in behavior modification

A marker can be used in behavior modification to change the emotional response to a stimulus, teach an alternate response, and clearly mark subtle steps in a desensitization program.

See details about using a marker in behavior modification later in this chapter.

Strengthens the human–animal bond

As mentioned earlier in this chapter, punishment-based techniques are usually administered inconsistently and unpredictably, creating a relationship based on stress. Clicker training is very consistent and predictable. Nothing "bad" happens and a bond built on a foundation of trust and teamwork flourishes. The animal's responsibility is to offer behavior and the trainer's responsibility is to choose the behavior to be marked and reinforced while setting their pet up for success. It is a team approach. One member of the team is not more important than the other. Owners quickly realize their pet is offering behaviors to get them to click. Frequently owners realize they have drastically underestimated the intelligence of the animal and a new relationship founded upon mutual respect, trust, and understanding is created.

Assists in repairing the human–animal bond

Often the human–animal bond has been damaged in cases of aggression directed toward the owner. The target of the aggression may no longer trust the pet and the pet may not trust the person because of past communication inconsistencies (specifically if punishment was previously used). Because clicker training is hands-off, consistent, and focuses on desired behavior, it can be the first step in rebuilding a damaged relationship.

Builds confidence and creativity

Clicker training does not initially require a relationship of trust but rather builds that relationship. Animals become curious, enthusiastic, and more outgoing. The animal learns the click is reinforcing because it is assured a reinforcer will follow. The click is also reinforcing because it gives the animal information. Knowing "what will happen next" and trusting that it will be a pleasant experience creates a confidence and tolerance for even slightly stressful experiences. The animal gains some degree of environmental predictability, which is beneficial to all animals but especially to animals with fear or anxiety issues.

Challenges:

- Some pet owners, either due to physical or psychological restraints, may have difficulty accurately using a clicker. In such cases, another person can mark the behavior and the challenged pet owner can toss the reinforcement. Another solution would be to teach the pet owner to use a word as the marker. Although less accurate than a clicker, it is still a practical choice for some pet owners.
- Deaf animals or geriatric patients who are losing their hearing may require a more creative marker such as a light or hand signal.
- Some sound-sensitive animals may require desensitization to the clicker by using a modified clicker initially (see Figure 9.15) or using a verbal marker.

Other training

The following are not training styles or techniques but rather sports or activities that may be recommended in a prescribed treatment plan.

Agility training

Agility training is a dog sport that combines physical and mental skills as the handler directs the dog through a sequence of obstacles such as tunnels, hoops, weave poles, and seesaws with voice and hand cues and without touching the dog or the equipment (Figure 9.3).

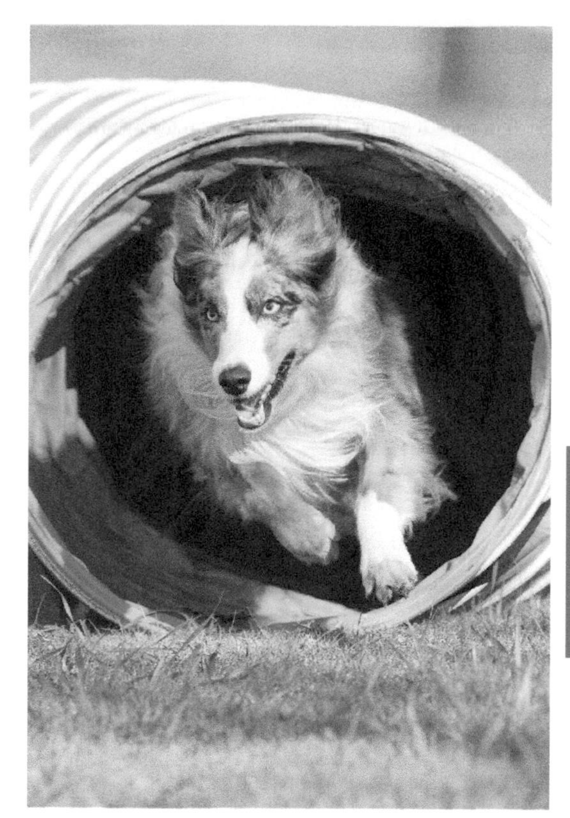

Figure 9.3 Agility training is beneficial for both aerobic exercise and mental stimulation. *Source*: Photo courtesy of Tia Guest, KPA–CTP. Photo credit to www.fastclicksphoto.com.

When agility training is combined with clicker training, dogs with low confidence learn to interact with novel objects, increasing their confidence in a variety of settings and that confidence begins to permeate other areas of their life. They become more likely to approach and investigate novel objects, including people and other dogs in other situations once a strong reinforcement history for investigating unfamiliar items and situations has been developed. Novel items that were previously a cause for concern begin to represent an opportunity to earn rewards.

Additionally, agility training strengthens the bond between dog and human as the handler and pet learn to read one another on a unique and deeply satisfying level, communicating well beyond basic cues such as "sit," "stay," and "down."

Disadvantage:

- Some patients may not be able to compete or train, unless in a controlled environment specific to their needs.

Concept training

Concept training is an advanced training model that infers a general or abstract idea from specific occurrences and teaches the ability to see connections and patterns in a situation.

Examples of concept training include

Discrimination – Discrimination training uses cues (discriminative stimulus) to teach an animal to discriminate between objects (Figure 9.4). This technique is used often in service dog training to teach the name of specific objects such as "shoe," "purse," and so on.

Modifiers – Modifier cues limit or qualify another cue. Examples of modifier cues are left/right, up/down, in/out, and large/small, and are combined with another cue. Example: Ball – big – get it.

Match to sample – Match to sample has been used in bomb and narcotic dog training and is now being used in some service dog programs. The animal is shown an object and then must locate a matching object.

Although concept training is in its beginning in the companion animal training area, this type of training may become a staple for slowing cognitive dysfunction and when working with animals that require a more challenging form of mental stimulation. Concept training is also stimulating to the trainer because it breaks up the monotony of typical foundation training.

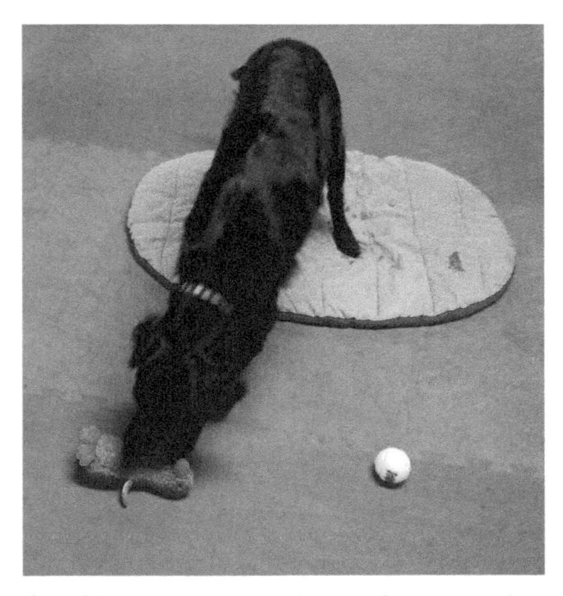

Figure 9.4 "Luna" discriminating between objects. *Source*: Photo courtesy of Susan Kennedy, KPA–CTP.

Scent/odor detection training

There are a variety of venues offering scent/odor detection training and sports for pet dogs. K9 Nose Work®, an activity and sport inspired by working scent-detection dogs, teaches dogs to find a specific odor (e.g. birch, anise, and/or clove) and locate its source (Figure 9.5).

Developed by Ron Gaunt, Amy Herot, and Jill Marie O'Brien, Nose Work was designed to help most dogs have fun and succeed in an activity that allows them to use their most acute sense – olfaction.

The activity was designed to be inclusive to dogs with issues that might normally preclude them from participating in other group activities. Dogs work one at a time, and while one dog is out of his crate, the other dogs are covered in their crates or confined in another area. Dogs are unable to see each other and no aversives or punishments are allowed in class. Because emphasis is placed on controlling the environment and not the dog (e.g. using a leash or blocking off an area where you do not want the dog to search), each class or lesson becomes a safe zone where the dogs do not have to worry about either intentional or inadvertent corrections.

Many patients have had their lives shrink because they are not successful in the world at large. A controlled scent-detection class or competition run by certified and knowledgeable positive-reinforcement trainers can provide the opportunity for some patients to gain confidence and socialize within a

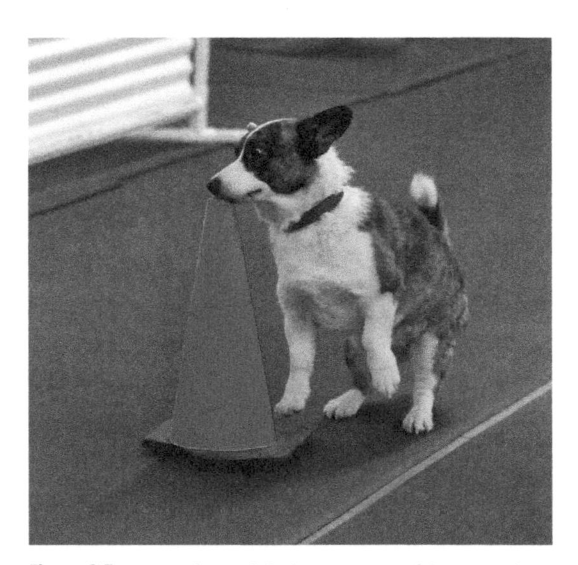

Figure 9.5 "Siren" alerts while doing Nose Work®. *Source*: Photo courtesy of Becky Hart.

BOX 9.2: BENEFITS OF SCENT DETECTION TRAINING TO THE BEHAVIOR PATIENT

Increases confidence and sociability
Increases mental stimulation
The dog learns an activity that may be more comforting than scanning in times of stress
Raises the arousal threshold (it takes longer to become frustrated or aroused)
Improves the ability to focus on a task
Strengthens the owner–pet bond (often damaged by repeated "failures" in other activities)
Provides passive CC to other dogs, people, and the environment

safe environment where they also have a chance to fulfill a natural drive and solve puzzles. It also allows geriatric patients to remain mentally active. The benefits of scent/odor detection training are also often advantageous for problem prevention and intervention treatment plans (Box 9.2).

Training tools

Training tools are used to temporarily or permanently assist in changing behavior. There are a myriad of behavior tools and equipment that veterinary technicians can call upon to help owners work with their pets. No single piece of equipment is suitable for every situation. Therefore, one should carefully consider the animal, the owner, and the problem before reaching into their toolbox.

Animals exhibit individual reactions that are based upon a combination of genetics and learning. Although you cannot change the genetic component, with the aid of appropriate equipment, skill, and knowledge in using them, it is possible to manage and then teach the animal an alternative, more acceptable response.

Successful resolution of a problem behavior entails evaluating and recognizing why the animal performs the behavior (see section **Functional behavior analysis**) and then applying the principles of management and training to encourage an appropriate response.

Owners must become knowledgeable about the safe and effective application and use of equipment before beginning any behavior modification that will include the use of that equipment. Training equipment is comparable to a surgical instrument – it can be used effectively and without adverse effects if applied properly. It is often helpful to train the pet first and acclimate it to the training tool, then turn attention to teaching the pet owner. Initially, it may be beneficial to demonstrate with a stuffed animal, and then introduce the pet. If multiple pet owners are present, one pet owner can then demonstrate teaching the technique to the others, with the technician's input and guidance. This technique often builds a pet owner's confidence level by watching it, doing it, and then teaching it.

Introducing a training tool to pet owners without teaching them the proper use will likely cause the tool to be reported by them as ineffective or cause the problem to worsen.

It is equally important for owners to understand the importance for all interactions with training tools to include positive, relationship-building methods that avoid causing confrontation or fear-induced behaviors, which would be detrimental to the treatment plan.

The appropriate use and application of any training tool is frequently crucial in regard to the outcome of some cases. For example, in the case of redirected aggression to the owner when on leash, a head halter and basket muzzle may be imperative to avoid further overt aggression toward the owner and prevent further deterioration of the human–animal bond while the treatment plan is introduced.

In such a situation, training tools such as a head halter and basket muzzle would allow the pet owner to provide exposure on walks but be able to intervene safely, prompt another behavior (i.e. Let's go), and then increase distance from the provoking stimulus. Without such training tools, it could be nearly impossible to redirect some animals without increasing their fear or risking the pet owner's safety.

Example: A dog diagnosed with owner-directed, conflict-induced aggression may guard space or objects. In this situation, the pet owner may need to intervene in an emergency situation to remove an item and a dragline may be required to prompt the behavior of leaving the object, which can then be reinforced.

In any situation, a training tool should be used only to manage a behavior, prompt an appropriate response that can be reinforced, or intervene in an emergency situation (i.e. stimulus suddenly appears and an aggressive reaction is occurring).

In cases where episodes of intervention are occurring frequently, management and other aspects of the treatment plan should be reassessed.

Example: An unplanned visitor rings the doorbell, the dog charges to the door barking, the pet owner cues "come" and prompts the dog to turn toward him/her with a dragline. The behavior of moving with the pet owner can then be reinforced with a treat. The doorbell should be disconnected and access to the front door should be managed with barriers.

As treatment progresses (i.e. medications reach therapeutic levels, management and behavior modification techniques have been successfully implemented, and the pet owner begins to gain confidence) the dependence on some tools, such as draglines, should lessen quickly. While in severe cases or in situations in which the pet owner would prefer to rely on the training tool, they may always be required to some degree.

Listed below is a small sampling of the equipment that may be part of a prescribed treatment plan and tools that behavior technicians commonly rely upon when working to manage and change behavior while at the same time maintaining safety. Please note, this list is not all-inclusive.

All tools should be introduced to the animal using desensitization and treats or another high-value reinforcers. The tool should have a positive conditioned emotional response, evidenced by the pet eagerly approaching the tool and showing happy expectation. If the harness or head halter is pulled out and the dog runs away, this is not an appropriate tool to use with this patient. Proper conditioning must occur prior to use with behavior modification. If a pet is unaccepting and uncomfortable with a particular tool, even with an appropriate introduction process, the tool should not be used.

Head halters

There are several different types of head halters currently available, each with its own pros and cons. This section will not discuss specific brands but will instead focus on the general concept of head halters.

Most head halters (also referred to as head collars) have a loop that encompasses the muzzle and a strap that fastens around the neck. When head collars were originally marketed in 1987, it was thought there was a "pack instinct" relationship to the head collar. It is now known that is entirely incorrect. Rather, head halters work by applying pressure behind the neck and around the muzzle so that the dog can be encouraged to display the chosen response by prompting a head turn. The principle is similar to that of a horse halter; where the nose goes, the body follows.

Practical applications and uses

Head halters are suitable for most dogs that pull on-leash, bark at people or other animals, grab hands, clothing, or the leash, jump up on people, or perform other behaviors that require better control.

Head halters employ negative reinforcement (release of tension), as do all collars and harnesses, and should be paired with positive reinforcement (offering a treat) to prompt the dog for desired behavior that can be reinforced. For instance, a dog who has a history of lunging and barking at other dogs while on a walk, the head halter would limit the dog's forward movement and allow the owner to redirect the dog more easily with a "Let's go" cue and a change in direction to move away from the stimulus. A treat is given to the dog as a reward for following the owner.

Shaping loose leash walking, reinforcing for offered attention (unprompted attention to the owner), and slack in the leash should be taught separately (i.e. without the stimulus present) in a non-distracting environment and then the learned behavior applied in behavior modification.

Many treatment plans include walks off the pet owner's property to increase the pet's mental stimulation and frequently a head halter is required for the pet owner to walk safely.

When using a head halter, the leash should always be slack unless the dog is pulling or needs guidance and redirection. Leash corrections should never be applied.

- When using a head halter, the leash should always be slack unless the dog is pulling or needs guidance and redirection.

Dogs that pull while using a head collar have not been taught properly. The handler has likely continued to walk forward while the leash was taut, therefore reinforcing a taut leash. The leash may also be tight because the stimulus has increased too rapidly or is too close.

If the patient pulls ONLY due to a lack of training, the dog is not stronger than the handler, and the dog is not motivated by an adverse emotional state, a front clip harness may be more applicable and usually requires less acclimation by the pet. The goals for each patient's treatment plan should be considered along with the pet owner's abilities when determining which harness is more appropriate for that patient's specific situation.

As mentioned previously, a head halter is often a necessity for practicing some response substitution, at least initially.

In moments of intervention, it may be necessary to use the head halter to prompt turning away from the stimulus by giving gentle pressure on the collar, as if touching someone on the shoulder to gain their attention, and then reinforcing the dog for walking away. Often the best reinforcement for a frightened animal is to increase distance from the fear-provoking stimulus.

Benefits

The use of a head halter can be a quick method (almost instantaneous) for pet owners to walk their dog without pulling, therefore making it more likely that the pet owner will walk the dog more frequently. Some head halters can be used for young puppies. This can be useful as a problem prevention tool when the size of the puppy will become out of proportion with the pet owner's abilities to walk the dog (e.g. Great Dane puppy owned by geriatric pet owners).

A head halter allows the handler to turn the dog's eyes, head, and body away from a stimulus without physically harming the dog and provides added safety for dogs displaying reactivity or aggression on walks while working to modify their behavior. Head halters are frequently a key to initially and successfully applying RS.

Properly fitted head halters can be worn for long periods of time, which may be necessary in extreme aggression cases, but they should never be left on an unsupervised pet at any time.

Disadvantages and cautionary comments

An introduction and acclimation period are necessary and may require CC and DS before a head halter can be used properly. If not acclimated properly, if a previous negative association has occurred (some dogs generalize muzzles to the nose strap of the head halter), or if not fitted properly, some animals can find a head halter aversive.

Some dogs seem to have more difficulty acclimating to a head halter than others. Brachycephalic breeds may not be physically able to wear a head halter. Having multiple brands of head halters available will allow testing for the best fit. A head halter can be uncomfortable for a dog suffering from allergies because the nose strap could be irritating. In such cases, a different brand of head halter can be tried to improve comfort or a head halter may need to be removed from the treatment plan entirely until the allergy issues are at least somewhat resolved.

Some social stigma to head halters remains (i.e. mistaken for a muzzle). Explaining to pet owners that the head halter is only a temporary tool and that their pet can eat, drink, bark, and even bite (even when fitted properly) while wearing the head halter can sometimes decrease the stigma. Emphasize that their pet may require the head halter only initially, to enable their pet to progress through the treatment plan. One analogy I often use to convince pet owners who are even slightly uncomfortable with their pet wearing the head halter is that of a person walking with a cast as their leg heals. Like a head halter, the cast will hopefully not be needed after the leg heals, although some injuries require an aid for the rest of the person's life. Using the head halter may be a useful tool for the patient's life, and that is neither inappropriate nor unacceptable.

Caution should be taken when working with a pet owner who has done extensive punishment-based training with a choke or pinch collar. Jerking (applying leash corrections) on the leash could be a "muscle memory" behavior and care should be taken to teach the pet owner to never jerk on the leash reflexively. A retractable leash should never be used in conjunction with a head halter. If the dog were to suddenly run to the end of a long leash (more than 4–6 feet) a neck injury could occur.

Some patients with handling issues may be extremely difficult to safely and properly fit with a head halter, and may require extensive CC and DS before the head halter can be utilized by the pet owner. In extreme cases, the head halter fitting may either be done as the veterinary technician observes the pet owner and instructs him/her step by step on the fitting and use of the head halter (TAG Points would be helpful in this case, see Chapter 5). In severe cases, the head collar first needs to be CC and DS at home before other aspects of the treatment plan are in place (i.e. walking the pet off property). On these occasions, the head halter can be sent home with the pet owner to first CC the head halter and then revisit the situation at a follow-up appointment.

Head halters should never be used as punishment but rather as a prompt to induce a reinforceable desired behavior (like turn away from a stimulus). Often a head halter provides a safe way for the owner to manage the pet on leash while applying behavior modification.

- Head halters should never be used as punishment but rather as a prompt to induce a reinforceable desired behavior (like turn away from a stimulus).

Basket muzzles/other muzzles

It may be assumed that many dogs will require wearing a muzzle at some point in their lives. The ability to comfortably wear a muzzle can be critical when treating some behavior disorders and some communities have laws requiring specific breeds of dogs to wear a muzzle whenever out in public.

Muzzles may be used to help keep a dog from biting or causing injury during the treatment process. They can also be used for dogs with coprophagia and pica to prevent the dog from picking up inappropriate items while outside.

The two types of muzzles that will be discussed in this section include nylon and basket muzzles.

Nylon muzzles

Veterinarians and groomers often use nylon muzzles for short procedures. They surround the dogs muzzle and are held in place by two straps that fasten at the back of the neck. Nylon muzzles are easy to size, easy to apply, and equally easy to remove.

One significant disadvantage of nylon muzzles is that the patient's mouth is closed or almost completely closed, thus preventing panting and could result in overheating if used for long periods of time, especially during hot weather, or if used on a struggling dog. Another consideration, depending upon how the muzzle is made, is that the person restraining the dog may accidentally slip a finger through the front opening and a bite can still occur. It is also difficult to use classical CC with a nylon muzzle because often the patient is unable to readily take a treat. Consequently, even for short procedures, basket muzzles are preferred over nylon muzzles.

Basket muzzles

The basket muzzle is aptly named. It has a wire or hard plastic basket-type cage that fits over the dog's muzzle and buckles at the back. They come in sizes suitable for any breed of dog. Some basket muzzles have a strap that runs up and over the top of the dog's head and fastens to the strap on the muzzle. This holds the muzzle in place, a feature very useful for dogs with short faces.

Dogs wearing this type of muzzle are able to open and close their mouth to pant and drink water. Basket muzzles often have openings wide enough so the dog can receive treats through the muzzle (Figure 9.6).

Basket muzzles can be worn for longer periods of time than a nylon muzzle. They can be useful when performing behavior modification by giving an added "safety zone" in case a mistake is made during training and the animal becomes aggressive. This gives the veterinary technician and owner a "buffer" and helps them to focus on the procedure being desensitized. The basket muzzle may also help pet owners to relax as they implement behavior modification exercises.

Basket muzzles can also be used as a management tool while treatment is being implemented for dogs that compulsively eat unacceptable objects or compulsively self-mutilate.

Example: A dog with a history of pica has had surgery several times due to ingesting rocks from the yard. It has become a contest as the dog attempts to eat the rocks before his owner can intercede. Although the owner must still supervise the dog, it is possible to allow the dog outside for a longer period of time with minimal worry about ingesting inappropriate objects.

Cautions

Muzzling a dog is not a guarantee of safety, and caution should still be exercised when working with a dog displaying aggression.

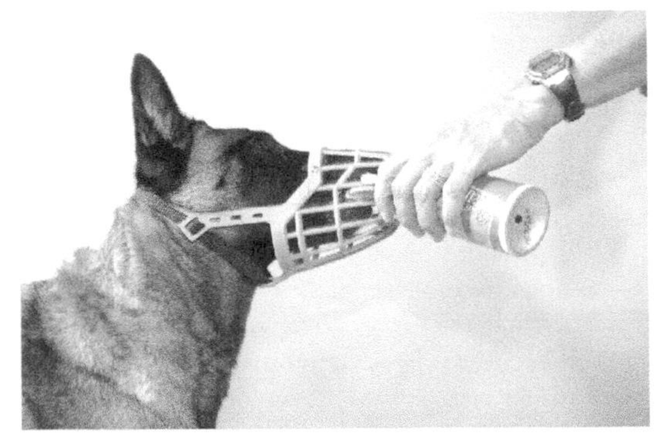

Figure 9.6 Dog receiving canned cheese through the basket muzzle.

Dogs wearing hard basket muzzles can still cause injury by performing a "muzzle punch," an act where the dog forcefully jabs his mouth at a person or other animal. Additionally, the openings in the basket are often wide enough for a finger to slip inside and a bite to occur.

Muzzles should never be considered a replacement for training or safe confinement for dogs displaying aggression. Instead, they are used to safely implement training and while assessing progress. They are not in themselves the treatment. Simply putting a muzzle on a dog that is aggressive toward strangers and then allowing the dog around strangers (without implementing DS and CC) is inappropriate and is not treating or improving the underlying problem. Similarly, when using a basket muzzle to allow for less restraint during veterinary or husbandry care, the dog's emotional state should continue to be assessed and responded to appropriately. See Chapter 8 for in-depth information regarding handling in the veterinary hospital.

Body harnesses

Harnesses come in several different styles, depending on the purpose and unique use of the harness. Harnesses described in this section will include front clip harnesses and standard harnesses. Each has its own unique use.

Front clip harnesses

Front clip harnesses attach the leash to a clip that is in the middle of the harness across the front of the dog in the thoracic inlet area. They stop pulling by steering the dog to the side and directing their attention back to the owner. To explain the physics of how it works, you might compare it to a line on the bow of a boat. No matter which direction the water flows, the boat pivots around to face front.

The front clip harness is a good choice for dogs that pull hard but are able to be redirected easily by their owners and are not at risk of pulling the owner over. A front clip style harness may be beneficial to dogs with medical problems impacting their neck area. Usually, only a short acclimation period is needed to condition the dog to the harness being placed on it and attached.

Considerations

Front clip harnesses can be difficult to fit properly. If the harness is not fitted properly, or if the dog is taken for a run while wearing a front clip harness, the harness may rub and cause sores to develop under the dog's front legs. Some dogs learn to pull through the harness. The biggest drawback to a front clip harness is that it provides no or little benefit for overly reactive dogs and dogs that jump or mouth because the dog is difficult to redirect without controlling its head. Front clip harnesses are not a good choice for dogs that like to grab the leash simply because the leash is easy for them to reach. Wiggly dogs or dogs with short legs can sometimes slip out of a harness.

Standard harnesses

Standard harnesses provide no control against pulling and clip at the back.

Standard harnesses can be used for small dogs with neck, spine, or trachea problems. Many cat owners relish the idea of allowing their cats to enjoy the great outdoors, but are unsure about how to accomplish it safely.

Young kittens can easily be taught to walk on a leash. There are harnesses specifically created that allow cats to safely enjoy outside time with their owners.

Standard harnesses function similarly to those used for training sled dogs. They use the dog's opposition reflex to encourage pulling and some animals are able to slip out of a standard harness.

CHAPTER 9

Treats

The importance of treats and the way they are used cannot be stressed enough. Owners often select a treat "they" consider desirable only to discover that the animal does not share their opinion (see section **Determining a reinforcement hierarchy**). The value of a treat is determined by the animal.

Practical applications and uses

Treats can be used as a distraction, a reinforcer, or to develop positive associations during a procedure. Some popular and easy-to-keep options for dogs include peanut butter, cream cheese, string cheese, canned dog food, canned cat food, canned baby food (no onions), canned chicken, freeze-dried chicken or beef, and hot dogs. Cats often enjoy dry/soft cat treats, canned cat food, baby food, tuna, sardines, and chopped chicken. Technicians can use pretzel rods, food-dispensing mats or toys, and empty syringe cases as treat-dispensing tools in addition to hand-feeding treats (Figure 9.7).

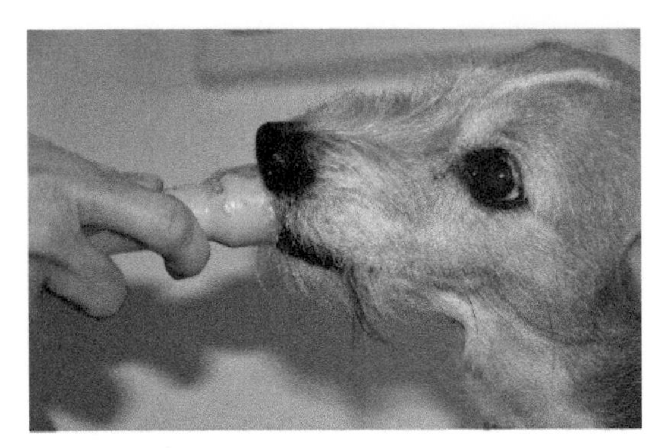

Figure 9.7 An empty 12-cc syringe case can be recycled as a treat dispenser.

Example 1: If a pet is sensitive to having its feet handled, begin by briefly touching the shoulder while feeding a high-value treat. Repeat this process several times. The next step is to touch the pet's shoulder and provide a treat just after the touch. Continue starting at the shoulder than begin to slide the hand down the leg, then treat. Working up to sliding the hand to the foot and then treating. By using this sliding motion, referred to as a Touch Gradient (see Chapter 8), the animal can be assessed throughout the increasing intensity of touch and responded to appropriately. Once the animal is looking forward to having his foot touched so he can get a treat, begin to maintain contact a little longer before treating. Slowly work up to holding the paw, then giving gentle squeezes, and eventually touching between his toes. How much time this takes depends upon the animal and past learning history.

Example 2: When vaccinating a cat, it may be helpful to allow it to lick a treat off a tongue depressor or off the exam table, thus providing a distraction.

Considerations

There are several challenges with using treats. Large quantities of treats can result in weight gain. This can be offset in several ways. Special high-value treats can be given when teaching difficult behavior, while a portion of the pet's regular diet can be fed as a reward for behaviors it already knows. Additionally, once a pet is able to reliably perform a behavior, it is possible to substitute something else that the animal likes for food, including play, walks, or petting.

If owners are not careful while training, pets can learn that the cue to performing a behavior is only when the pet owner has treats. This can easily be remedied by instructing the pet owner to train throughout the day without treats in plain sight (i.e. in a container on a shelf).

Treat bags

Treat bags can be a fancy bag that hooks to your belt or something as simple as a carpenter's apron with large pockets. Treats can also be stationed in areas where behavior modification is likely to occur, such as at the front door for quick access (Figure 9.8). Easy access to treats helps with keeping a high rate of reinforcement, and reminds the pet owner to reinforce behavior. If the apron or bag has multiple pockets, it is easy to separate high-value treats from low-value treats.

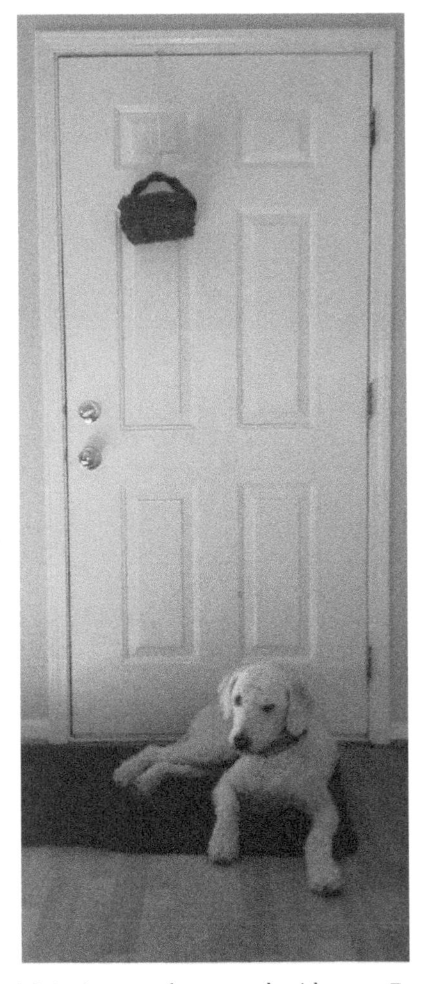

Figure 9.8 Station treats for easy and quick access. Treats in a bag at the front door.

Target sticks

A target stick can be commercially made or homemade, using a small dowel rod with a wooden ball securely fastened to the end.

Targeting is a universal skill that has many different functions and is useful in all animals. Zoos often use targeting with large animals for drawing blood or other husbandry duties that would otherwise require force or use of sedation.

The first step is to teach the pet to touch the stick and immediately reward. The target should be held close to the animal to encourage success but avoid moving the target toward the pet. Instead have the animal move forward to touch the target.

For animals that are fearful or reluctant to touch the target stick, the pet owner can use hands or fingers and then change over to a target stick. It may be necessary to shape the behavior by reinforcing any movement toward the target and increasing the difficulty in incremental amounts.

One of the benefits of targeting is that the patient can transfer touch from someone familiar to a new person or object. Targeting can be used as a way to redirect a patient when faced with a distraction. Recalls and loose leash walking can easily be taught with targeting (Figures 9.9 and 9.10).

Calming cap

Behaviors can be affected by a dog's emotional reaction to people, places, and objects encountered in the environment. Triggers, such as the sight of a person walking by, another dog close to their home, or riding in a car, may result in a sudden and intense fearful or stress-related reaction. Dogs in such a highly aroused state are difficult to work with because they lose the ability to focus on other behaviors that can be rewarded.

Calming caps are lightweight fabric masks with a sheer panel that filters a dog's vision (Figure 9.11). The calming cap addresses sensory overload and may be helpful in creating a non-stressful starting

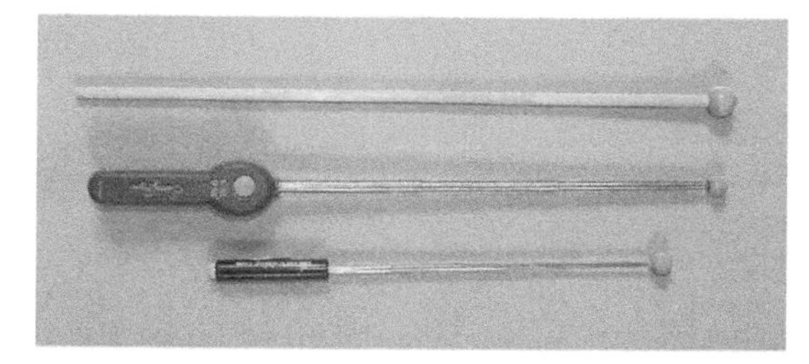

Figure 9.9 Various target sticks.

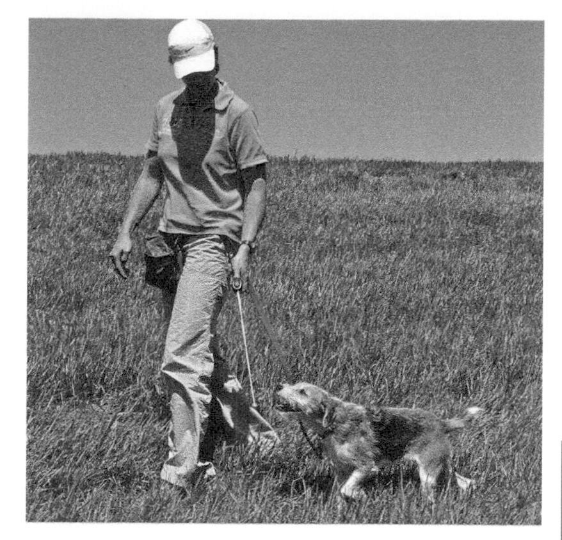

Figure 9.10 Teaching "Iris" to walk by the person's side using a target stick.

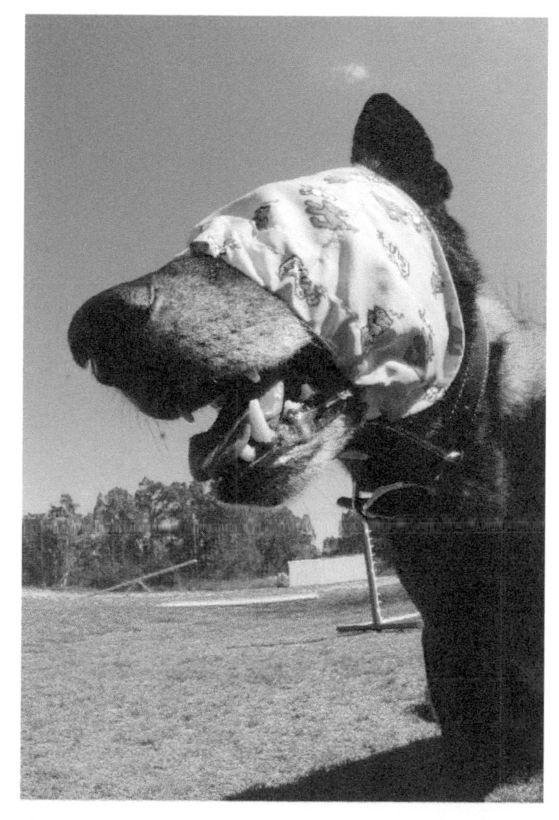

Figure 9.11 A calming cap could be used as a "visual filter" during behavior modification.

point for DS to occur. For example, if a dog is triggered by another dog even when it is a block away, a calming cap can be used to decrease the visual aspect of the stimulus, possibly creating a point for DS to occur. This in turn may help lower the dog's arousal response. It is not a blindfold but rather a visual filter – some sight still occurs. Dogs are still able to perform normal behaviors that rely upon vision, such as maneuvering around his environment while on walks.

The calming cap does not "cure" the dog but helps manage the situation while the technician works to modify the underlying cause. It can be used along with a body wrap for dogs with thunderstorm phobia, especially if the problem involves sensitivity to lightning.

Calming caps are lightweight and available in various sizes and most dogs can easily be conditioned to wear the calming cap for long periods. This helps the dog to better tolerate longer trips in the car or lengthy periods of stormy weather.

Considerations

Some animals with global fear or that have severe anxiety disorders may not do well with a calming cap. Either their anxiety worsens or the animal goes into learned helplessness, which is not beneficial to the application of behavior modification. The calming cap should not be used to place an animal into learned helplessness to expedite a medical treatment. As with all tools, it should be properly acclimated prior to use.

Anxiety clothing

"Anxiety clothing" relies upon pressure to help calm dogs and cats. One of the most commonly used brands is the "Thundershirt." A 2011 study conducted by CanCog Technologies and overseen by veterinary behaviorist, Gary Landsberg, DVM, revealed significant improvements during a thunderstorm test for dogs wearing a Thundershirt.

Some experts believe the success of anxiety clothing is directly related to the calming effect of pressure on the nervous system. It is thought that this pressure is responsible for the release of calming hormones. This concept has been observed in humans for many years.

Examples: Wrapping an infant snuggly in a blanket is frequently used by parents and in hospital nurseries to encourage calmness in fussy infants. Dr. Temple Grandin discovered how applying gentle pressure to the body relieves the anxiety commonly experienced by people with autism.

Anxiety clothing may bring immediate relief to some animals, require several repetitions for other animals, or have no effect. It is often used as an adjunct to behavior modification and can be worn for extended periods of time when necessary.

Considerations

Some anxiety clothing uses velcro as a way to close and connect sections together. Dogs with extreme noise sensitivity may startle at the sound of the velcro being pulled apart and CC and DS to the sound may be required prior to using it on the pet.

Waist leashes, tethers, draglines, long lines

Waist leashes

Waist leashes are multipurpose tools. They can be specially designed leashes that buckle around the waist with a leash that attaches directly to the belt. Waist leashes can simply be a leash that is tied around the owner's waist or clipped using a strong carabiner.

The waist leash is recommended for puppies or adult dogs that require constant supervision to prevent house soiling or inappropriate chewing. They can also help encourage attention to the owner as the pet learns to watch and anticipate movements. Runners often use them to keep their hands free while jogging with their dogs. Loose leash walking is often taught using a waist leash.

Owners who employ the waist leash for supervision are not forced to hold the leash and thus can go about their normal routine. When used for training, owners learn how to maintain attention without pulling on the leash. When training a dog that has shown reactivity or aggression in public, the waist leash maybe used as a second leash and as a safety back-up.

Considerations

Waist leashes offer many benefits, but also have some drawbacks. Some owners forget they have a dog attached to the end of the leash and may trip over their pet and fall, or step on the pet, causing injury. Very strong dogs may have the ability to pull their owners over when excited.

Tethers

Toy tethers are usually made of plastic-coated wire cables with snaps on one or both ends. They are offered in different lengths. Using a wire cable prevents the dog from chewing through the tether. The plastic coating provides protection for nearby objects.

Wall tethers are often used during training and behavior consultation to practice hands-free behaviors, but are also a safety tool during behavior consultations (see section **Staying safe**).

The tether provides an opportunity to safely observe the dog's behavior. It also takes the leash out of the owner's hands, allowing him/her to answer questions and provide information without worrying about the pet.

Short tethers, approximately 3 ft in length, are generally used to prevent dogs from becoming tangled. Anchoring the tether to an eyebolt secured to the wall or floor provides stability when faced with large strong dogs in practice behavior modification sessions (see Figure 1.9).

Considerations

Tethered dogs must always be supervised. Avoid long tethers as it is possible for dogs to become tangled. Check tethers and anchors frequently to detect any weakness. Do not allow dogs to chew on the tether as it can cause harm to teeth.

Draglines

Draglines are often considered interchangeable with long lines. However, there are some differences. Drag lines are used for close work inside the house and tend to be made of a lighter material and are narrower than a regular leash, with a length of no more than 10 ft. Although similar to a regular leash, it has no handle and is much less likely to become snagged on objects.

As the name indicates, the dog drags the leash around with it. It offers an easy way indoors to interrupt undesirable behaviors and gain control of a dog that darts out of open doors, jumps on furniture, or jumps on guests. The owner is quickly able to pick up the leash and guide the dog away from what it is doing without being confrontational.

A benefit of a dragline is that owners never need to physically touch the dog, making it much less likely that any negative association will be made with hands and provides increased safety for the pet owner.

Considerations

Even though these make useful training tools, dogs should never be left unattended when wearing a dragline. It is also important never to grab and yank on the line; they are meant to gently redirect the dog's attention if the dog is unable to respond to a cue. A dragline may be necessary in the early stages of training. Once the dog is able to respond reliably to the owner even when distracted, a dragline would no longer be necessary for response substitution.

Long lines

Long lines are most frequently used outside. They are usually made of nylon, cotton, or leather and may extend anywhere from 20 to 100 ft.

One of the most common uses for a long line is teaching the recall outside, around distractions.

A benefit of long lines is that they provide more room for exploration, while keeping the dog safe and ensuring it will not run away.

Considerations

Long lines should never be used with head halters but should instead be fastened to the dog's regular collar or harness.

Owners should never allow the dog to run and "hit" the end of the line. This can cause severe injury to the dog. There is risk a dog could become tangled in a long line and panic.

Additionally, owners should be careful when holding a long line. If the dog begins to run and the owner allows the line to slip through his/her hands, a rope burn can easily occur. This possibility can be greatly decreased by tying knots in the line at several different spots to provide a better grip.

Using a long line when working with a dog that lunges or chases stimuli can be dangerous and the pet owner must always be aware of the environment and changes in the environment before the dog is, otherwise it may charge to the end of the leash, injuring itself and the pet owner.

Interactive toys or puzzles

The use of interactive toys or puzzles for preventing behavior problems and disorders has been discussed at length in Chapter 7. Interactive toys and puzzles are frequently recommended in treatment plans as a way of increasing mental stimulation and enrichment. They offer an opportunity to practice a variety of problem-solving techniques and are often recommended in the treatment of separation anxiety and teaching independence from the pet owner.

Pheromones

Pheromones are chemicals released by one animal that send messages to other animals of the same species. Pheromone-based products for pets were introduced in the United States in 2001. They mimic naturally occurring dog and cat calming and appeasing pheromones and may relieve stress in pets. Pheromone-based products are available as sprays, plug-in diffusers, and gel diffusers. There are also pheromone collars for dogs.

Feline pheromone products have been recommended to help with marking, spraying, and aggression problems but they are also used to help alleviate stress while traveling, when a cat is being boarded, or during veterinary visits. One of the most recognized feline pheromone products currently on the market is Feliway®. It imitates the F3 facial pheromones cats deposit when cheek rubbing to mark something in the environment as safe and not to be feared.

Canine pheromones are used in adult dogs for stress, separation anxiety, and noise sensitivity to thunderstorms or fireworks. They can be used to help puppies deal with the stress of entering new homes. Dog appeasing pheromones are released by nursing dogs to calm their puppies.

As pheromones are species-specific, they should have no impact on other animals exposed to them. Although pheromones may not work in every animal, there are no reports of negative reactions to the products. Therefore, they are considered safe to use in almost any situation where animals could potentially experience stress.

Considerations

Pheromones used alone are often not sufficient to ameliorate stress-related behavior. Instead, they should be employed as part of a comprehensive modification plan. It is equally important for animals to first be examined by a veterinarian to rule out medical problems before assuming a situation is behavior related.

Aromatherapy

Different from pheromones, aromatherapy uses specific scents in the environment to affect behavior and mood. Aromatherapy is the therapeutic exposure to aromatic essential oils or natural plant extracts to enhance physical and emotional well-being. The scent might be something that is thought to elicit calm behavior, but a specific scent can also be used to help provide environmental stimuli associated with safety or training which can then be generalized to other locations. For example, when working on a Treat-Ment station (Chapter 8), utilizing a dilute lavender scent on the station associates the positive learning experiences with the station and the smell. Thus, when generalizing the station to other locations, the familiarity of lavender can assist with prompting feelings and memories of safety.

Aromatic essential oils are detected by animals through olfactory means. Some aromatic essential oils that may alter canine behavior include lavender, chamomile, rosemary, and peppermint. Some aromatic essential oils that may alter feline behavior include lavender, catnip, silver vine, valerian, and Tatarian honeysuckle.

In dogs, topical application of lavender oil affects vagal activity and may produce relaxation (Komiya et al. 2009). Diffused lavender odor may calm dogs with travel-induced excitement (Well 2006). Dogs spent significantly more time resting and sitting and less time moving and vocalizing when exposed to lavender (Well 2006).

Diffused oil of lavender or chamomile may promote relaxation in dogs housed in a shelter environment. Dogs spent more time resting, less time moving, and vocalized less upon exposure to lavender or chamomile than any of the other olfactory stimuli (Graham et al. 2005). In that same study, diffusion of rosemary or peppermint into the dogs' environment encouraged significantly more standing, moving, and vocalizing (Graham et al. 2005). Therefore, diffused rosemary or peppermint may promote behaviors associated with arousal in dogs housed in a shelter environment.

In cats, aromatherapy with lavender can significantly reduce behaviors associated with stress and anxiety (Goodwin and Reynolds 2018). Catnip produces estrus-like behavior, encourages play-like behavior, and is also associated with behaviors indicative of reduced activity. About one-third of domestic cats do not respond to nepetalactone, the chemical compound found in catnip (Bol et al. 2017). Silver vine, Tatarian honeysuckle, and valerian have similar behavioral effects (increasing play) and are alternatives to catnip for felines (Bol et al. 2017). Silver vine encourages sitting and playing in cats (Myatt 2014). Cats are more sensitive than dogs to potentially toxic effects of some aromatic essential oils. Others not listed above, but considered safe to use around cats are copaiba, helichrysum, and frankincense.

Considerations

Improper use of oil can be toxic, produce adverse central nervous system effects, and lead to respiratory problems. Because dogs and cats have an exceptional sense of smell, odors should be dilute to prevent irritation to airways. Aromatic essential oils may be diffused (as simple as a drop of oil on a cotton ball placed in a glass jar with a lid with holes in it) into the environment in a variety of ways but caution and close observation of pets and people in the environment should always be maintained.

Acoustic/sound therapy

Acoustic therapy may be used with dogs and cats. Sounds can be used to lessen or reduce the impact of auditory stimuli associated with fear, anxiety, stress, or reactivity. Sounds can be used to promote positive emotional responses, physiological responses, and desirable behavioral responses. Sounds can be cues to perform desired behavior in specific contexts (doorbell is a cue to find the owner, thunder is the cue to go to a safe place). The pet's association with the sound will be dependent on classical conditioning, operant conditioning, and patient familiarity. The sound may be paired with treats or a relaxed behavior to help promote desirable responses and reduce fear, anxiety, and stress (FAS).

Humans and animals respond differently to various auditory stimuli with different sounds producing different behavioral responses. In humans, slow tempo music (50–60 beats per minute) decreases heart rate and blood pressure, whereas fast tempo music (120–130 beats per minute) increases heart rate and blood pressure (Edworthy and Waring 2006). In human newborn infants, both white noise and heartbeat sounds have been demonstrated to produce calming effects (Kawakami et al. 1996). In dogs, short rapidly repeated notes increase motor activity whereas long, continuous notes have been shown to decrease motor activity (McConnell 1990). In a study of dogs exposed to heartbeat sounds and classical music, there were tendencies to decreased average heart rate (Fukuzawa and Kajino 2018). Kenneled dogs exposed to music, regardless of genre (Soft Rock, Motown, Pop, Reggae, and Classical), spent significantly more time lying and significantly less time standing. Dogs were significantly more likely to bark following cessation of auditory enrichment. Heart rate variability, indicative of decreased stress, was significantly higher, when dogs were exposed to Soft Rock and Reggae, with a lesser effect observed with Motown, Pop, and Classical genres. A variety of auditory enrichment can be beneficial and prevent habituation (Bowman et al. 2017).

Another small study found that kenneled dogs exposed to audiobooks compared to other auditory conditions, including classical music, spent more time resting, and less time vocalizing, sitting, or standing (Brayley and Montrose 2016). The authors speculated that the sound of a person talking provided an illusion of human companionship.

Classical music can be used to calm cats. Classical music in the operating room may contribute to a reduced anesthetic dose in cats anesthetized for elective ovariohysterectomy. Most cats in the study exhibited lower values for respiratory rate and pupil diameter when exposed to classical music, intermediate values to pop music, and higher values to heavy metal music (Mira et al. 2016a). All cats experienced lower values in arterial blood pressure, systolic blood pressure, and heart rate when exposed to classical music, intermediate values when exposed to pop music, and higher values when exposed to heavy metal music (Mira et al. 2016b). Species-specific modified music has been shown to reduce stress in cats in the veterinary clinic setting. Stress scores and handling scores were lower during examination when cats were exposed to species-specific music (Hampton et al. 2020). Cats may find species-specific music to be more appealing than music made for humans; in one study cats preferred music with a higher pitch and a tempo based on purring and the suckling sound made during nursing (Snowdon et al. 2015).

Considerations

Acoustic therapy should be tested in the individual pet to assess the individual's response. Likely, there are individual preferences and aversions based on past learning experiences or a lack of experience.

Reward markers

Reward markers are often used without owners even realizing it. There can be multiple reward markers, but the three basic types are the clicker, a verbal marker, and a visual marker. They all communicate to the pet that whatever behavior the animal is doing at that time is correct and a reinforcer is coming. In order for a marker to work, it must be used as the behavior occurs and before the dog has performed a different behavior.

Example: A dog is being taught to sit. As the dog's rear end makes contact with the ground, mark the behavior and then bring the reward. The dog has been reinforced for sitting. An easy mistake is for the dog to sit and then immediately stand up before the owner uses the reward marker. If the owner gives the reward marker at that time, the dog is rewarded for standing.

Clickers are devices that make a short, distinct "click" sound. They are often preferred by trainers because they are so precise that it is easy for any animal to hear and understand the behavior that is being rewarded. See section **Event marker (clicker) training**.

Verbal markers are probably one of the most widely used tools. Owners often tell their pets "Good dog" or "Good!" when a desired behavior has been performed. When owners use a verbal marker, it is important to select short and distinct words and always follow the word with a reinforcement. To prevent confusing an animal, avoid phrases frequently used in everyday conversations (i.e. yes, okay) and instead select seldom-used words.

Deaf dogs cannot hear audible markers. However, there are several ways to compensate for this situation. Owners may use a pen light or small flashlight, there are vibration collars owners can activate, or even a hand signal such as thumbs up, to signal a well-done behavior.

Visual and sensory markers help owners to easily communicate with a pet that otherwise might be difficult to train. They can be tailored to meet the needs of the situation and the animal.

Remote reward

A remote reward system allows owners to quickly and efficiently reinforce desirable behaviors from a distance, without being directly associated with the process. They are lightweight and portable, so they can easily be used in many different locations. The most recognized of these systems, Treat and Train®, was developed by veterinarian Dr. Sophia Yin. In a 2008 issue of *Applied Animal Behavior Science*, Dr. Yin published results of research that appeared to confirm the efficacy of a behavior modification protocol for dogs with a history of excessive barking and jumping that used a remote control food reward dispenser.

The systems employ operant conditioning and shaping to train new desired behaviors. Many provide a strong tone prior to dispensing the treat, so the pet learns that the tone predicts a treat.

The remote reward system is appropriate for use in puppies, adult dogs, kittens, and adult cats. It is an effective part of a modification protocol for behaviors like jumping, barking, and door-charging, as well as serving as an aid for working with separation anxiety. Owners of competition and agility dogs have reported improvement in performance using remote reward systems. Remote rewards can help cats and kittens to learn to love their crates and use appropriate areas for scratching.

Most remote reward systems are lightweight and portable. Those with a tone mark the appropriate behavior and indicate a treat will follow. With some models it is possible to program automatic ongoing rewards between three seconds and one hour apart.

Considerations

Most systems require batteries that can go dead in the middle of a training session. Occasionally, there can be a defect in the remote control. Some models may not handle all types of dog food and will become jammed. In multiple-pet households, remote reward devices might result in conflict or guarding behaviors between the pets.

Double leashing

Double leashing is used to provide an extra degree of safety to prevent escape and possible injury to the dog.

The double-leash technique is a great tool, especially when working outside. The main leash is attached to the head collar or harness and held by the owner. A second handsfree waist leash is then attached to the dog's harness or buckle collar. In case the dog becomes startled and lunges away, or some type of equipment malfunction happens, there is a backup system to provide security (Figure 9.12).

Decoys

Decoys are life-size stuffed animals that can be used when assessing a dog's level of aggression toward

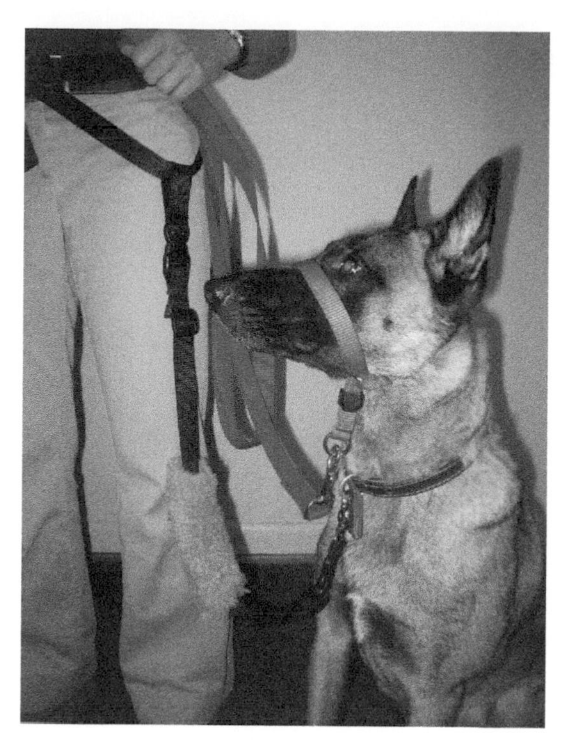

Figure 9.12 A second handsfree waist leash attached to the dog's harness or buckle collar for increased safety.

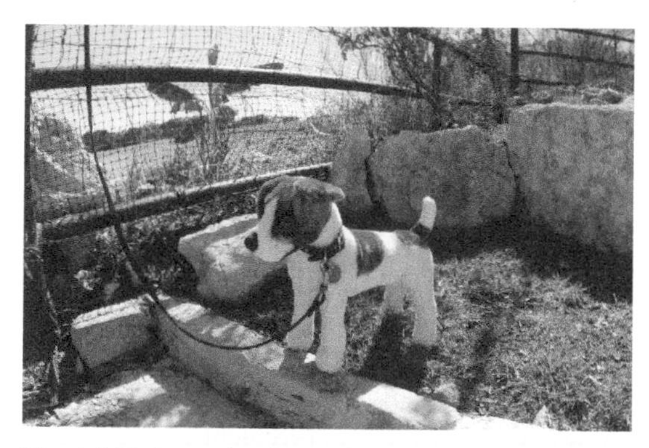

Figure 9.13 Decoys can be used for assessing behavior and during desensitization.

other dogs and are often useful as a non-stressful starting point when practicing DS to other dogs (Figure 9.13).

This chapter has provided information on a few of the most commonly used tools available for technicians working to manage and modify behavior. Technicians can use these items to begin establishing their own individualized tool kit for training.

Marker training techniques and skills

Markers can be used as either a conditioned reinforcer or as a conditioned punisher. This text will focus on the use of a marker as a conditioned reinforcer to teach desired behavior. See Table 9.4 for general guidelines on marker training.

Table 9.4 General guidelines for marker training.

Mark, then reinforce.	Reinforcement before or at the same time as the click will make the click meaningless.
Keep the treat hand still until after the click.	Movements before the click will overshadow the marker.
If you click you must reinforce.	Not reinforcing after a click will deteriorate the classical association of the marker and reinforcement.
Keep sessions short (2–5 min).	Training sessions are intensely mentally stimulating. A 5-min training session can be as mentally stimulating as a 20 min walk.
End session early rather than later.	End session while a high rate of reinforcement is maintained.
Smoothly lower and raise criteria to keep a high rate of reinforcement.	Don't always increase criteria, at times slip back to a lower criterion for reinforcement.
Work on only one new (not on cue) behavior per training session.	This will help to decrease confusion for both the learner and the trainer.
Initially train with low distractions.	Once the behavior is learned and on cue, begin adding distractions incrementally.
Start to reinforce within ½ second.	Late reinforcement can cause frustration and miscommunication.
Initially reinforce every desired behavior, once the behavior is on cue, under stimulus control and fluent reinforce with variable reinforcements and/or intermittently and with reinforcement variety.	Variable reinforcement and reinforcement variety will maintain the behavior.

(Continued)

Table 9.4 (*Continued*)

Do not apply aversives (something the animal will work to avoid) to teach a behavior.	If the expected response does not occur, do not reinforce. The opposite of reinforcement is NO REINFORCEMENT.
Test cued behaviors for stimulus control.	See Table 9.9
Generalize	Once the behavior is on cue, generalize to different people giving the cue and in different locations. Begin in most familiar location with low distractions, then add various locations followed by adding low-level distractions.

Functional behavior analysis

Dr. Susan Friedman describes applied behavior analysis (ABA) as the technology of behavior change based on the experimentally derived principles of learning and behavior. The primary focus of ABA is to (i) determine the functional relationship between observable behavior and environmental events: What does the animal DO? (ii) explain the function of the behavior by its consequences: Why does the animal do that? (iii) intervene by redesigning the environment to provide an alternate way for the animal to achieve the same purpose served by the problem behavior: What can the animal be taught to do instead? (iv) teach new skills to make the problem behavior less likely to occur.

Functional behavior analysis is a technique of assessing the antecedent, behavior, and consequence and then functionally assessing whether the hypothesis about the antecedent and consequence is accurate. Behavior analysis is an essential tool for creating behavior change, whether in teaching a foundation behavior or in addressing problem behaviors (Friedman 2009a, b).

A veterinary technician (trainer) can influence operant conditioning by influencing the antecedents (what happens prior to the behavior) and the consequences (what occurs immediately following the behavior). The behavior (what the animal DOES) is not manipulated but rather changed by the trainer's influence on antecedents and consequences.

Functional assessment

Dr. Susan Friedman describes the steps in a functional assessment as the following:

1. Observe and operationally define the target behavior.
   (a) What does the animal do that can be observed and measured?
2. Identify the distant and immediate physical and environmental antecedents that predict the behavior.
   (a) What general conditions or events affect whether the problem behavior occurs; medical or physical problems, sleep cycles, eating routines and diet, daily schedule, etc.?
   (b) What are the immediate antecedents (predictors or triggers) for the problem behavior? When, where, and with whom is the behavior problem most likely to occur?
3. Identify the consequences that maintain the problem behavior, that is, the immediate purpose the behavior serves.
   (a) What does the animal gain by behaving in this way, such as attention, an item or activity, or sensory feedback?
   (b) What does the animal avoid by behaving in this way, such as particular people, a demand or requests, items or activities, or sensory stimulation?
   (c) To what extent does the animal's natural environment support the behavior (i.e. what function might it serve)?

Once the above assessment is complete, intervention can proceed (Friedman 2009a, b). Refer to the behavior solutions model outlined in Chapter 7.

Foundation trainer skills

Ability to observe behavior

The skills needed to use a marker successfully are the same qualities required of a good behavior technician: excellent observation of behavior, precision and consistency in training and communication skills, and the ability to be generous with and knowledgeable about reinforcements.

The ability to accurately and objectively observe behavior during training enables the trainer to determine what actions occur naturally by the animal and are therefore more likely to occur in specific situations. The trainer can then capture these naturally occurring behaviors by marking them or by shaping a more complex behavior by incrementally marking more extreme behavior through successive approximations.

Astute observers can note the subtle precursors of the desired behavior (e.g. cat dips its head just before picking up its foot to groom). Lifting of the foot can then be better predicted and consequently improve the marker timing.

Species differences

Before training an animal, as much as possible should be learned about the animal's natural history, social structure, feeding habits, and other naturally occurring behaviors (Ramirez et al. 1999).

The laws of learning and marker training techniques discussed in this chapter are the same, regardless of the species being trained but there are differences between species (and between individuals within that species) in regard to their physical abilities and patterns of behavior, reinforcement hierarchy and how reinforcement is delivered (Table 9.5).

Physical abilities and patterns of behavior include the following: What does the animal do naturally? When is its most active time of day? Which behaviors occur most frequently? Do certain behaviors always lead to other behaviors? (i.e. stretching before yawning, spinning before lying down.) How does the animal respond to different sights, sounds, and environments?

What reinforcement to use and how to deliver the reinforcement also varies between species. For instance, cats tend to take a long time to consume their reinforcement, stopping to groom in between reinforcements. For that reason, a helpful training tool to deliver reinforcement to a cat is a clicker taped to the handle of a spoon, which allows the cat to quickly lick a reinforcement (canned food, tuna, ice cream, etc.) and then the spoon can quickly be removed to set up for another opportunity to perform behavior (Figure 9.14).

Table 9.5 Species considerations.

Observation	Use in training
What behaviors does the animal do naturally?	Identifying naturally occurring behaviors for the species will help identify appropriate behaviors to capture and shape.
Which behaviors occur most frequently?	Choosing a frequently occurring behavior will improve the rate of reinforcement.
Do certain behaviors always lead to other behaviors?	Identify precursor behaviors to better predict and time the marker
How does the animal respond to different sights, sounds?	Species differences in response to sights, sounds, etc. will determine an appropriate event marker and assist the trainer in avoiding fear-provoking stimuli in the environment.
What does the animal find reinforcing?	Will help to determine the reinforcement hierarchy for that specific species and individual.
How can that reinforcement be given quickly and efficiently?	The method and delivery of reinforcement will affect the rate of reinforcement.

Choosing an appropriate event marker

Conditioned reinforcement markers are used to systematically "explain" or give information about a behavior. During learning of a behavior, the information the marker delivers becomes as important as the reinforcement itself. Once the behavior is under a stimulus-controlled cue and is fluent, the marker is no longer required.

The marker chosen should be able to precisely pinpoint a behavioral moment as it is used to inform the animal that the current criterion of behavior has been met.

The event marker should be brief so only a specific increment of the behavior is marked, for example, a muscle relaxing in the shoulder. The marker should not be something the animal must discriminate from similar stimuli in the environment (Table 9.6). For example, a verbal marker of "yes" must be discriminated from other words the animal hears throughout the day. Although the voice can be used as an event marker when a clicker is not available or

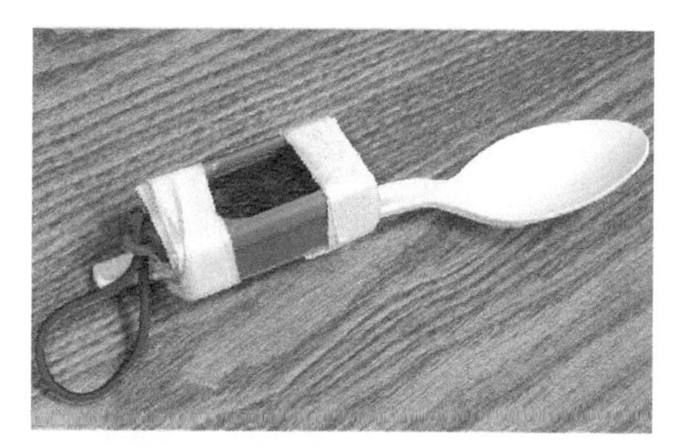

Figure 9.14 A clicker taped to the handle of a spoon for quick reinforcement for cats and other animals.

Table 9.6 Qualities of an appropriate event marker.

Brief	A specific behavior is pinpointed
Distinct	Easily noticeable
Different	Not easily confused with other environmental stimuli; unique
Neutral	Has no previous associations (when first introduced)
Easy to deliver	Improves speed and accuracy of the event being marked

CHAPTER 9

suitable, it might not be as efficient. Research has suggested that using the voice as an event marker slowed learning and required more reinforcements than a mechanical marker (Wood 2008).

The marker should not have a previous association. For example, a whistle that is a cue for "come" should not also be used as a marker. This can occur if a pet owner has improperly used the clicker to "call the dog." Some animals, specifically sound-sensitive animals, may generalize the marker sound to previously negatively associated events. In that case, the technician must determine a different type of event marker (a flash of light) or desensitize the animal to the marker (Figure 9.15).

The marker must be easy to deliver quickly and efficiently so the desired event or behavior is marked accurately and precisely.

Conditioning the event marker and teaching contingency

The event marker is a conditioned secondary reinforcer that is classically conditioned to an unconditioned reinforcer (UR) (something that is intrinsically reinforcing to the animal) and is therefore under the same requirements for classical conditioning to be effective.

- The presenting order must be correct (i.e. mark then treat). The click must always occur before the UR.
- The CR and the UR must occur at a 1:1 ratio (i.e. if you click, you must reward). Because the event marker does not have an intrinsic value to the animal, the 1:1 ratio maintains its reinforcement value.
- Secondary environmental stimuli, such as the trainer's body movements, distractions, and other sounds in the environment should be minimal, decreasing the possibility that the animal will make an association with outside environmental stimuli rather than the sound of the marker. Animals that are astute at noticing the subtle movements of the handler often associate a movement just before a click as the marker; therefore, handler movements should remain at a minimum until after the marker, including facial expressions and eye movements.

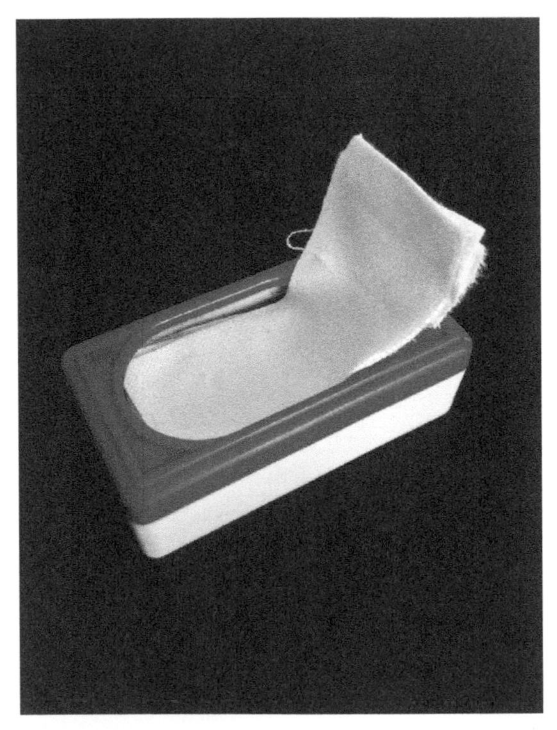

Figure 9.15 Placing tabbed tape pieces on the dimple of the clicker and systematically removing pieces can aid in desensitizing the sound of a clicker for sound-sensitive animals.

The animal needs to learn two things before the event marker can be used to teach new behaviors. First, the animal needs to pair the event marker with something it really likes. Second, the animal must learn that his behavior makes the human mark and then reinforce him.

The conditioning of the marker must occur for it to have intrinsic value to the animal but can often occur within one to two repetitions. It was once believed that conditioning of the marker should be a separate and specific procedure from teaching the animal that the click/marker was contingent on his behavior. It is now understood that many animals may learn very quickly that the marker means reinforcement and that teaching them that the click is contingent on their behavior can and should occur almost simultaneously with conditioning of the clicker (see Video 7.17).

When initially conditioning the marker and teaching the animal that the marker is contingent on its behavior, it is best to use a variety of very special, flavorful, soft, food treats. Food is most often the chosen UR because it is commonly near the top of most animals' reinforcement hierarchy.

Small (the size of a pea, one lick, etc.), soft food treats can be eaten quickly, so many repetitions of reinforcement can be completed in a short training session. The value of the food reinforcer is not necessarily in its size but in the experience itself. For example, people often play penny slot machines for hours. Small food reinforcements also prevent the animal from becoming satiated quickly. Increasing the variety of the food reward improves learning because it maintains interest in the training session. Creating "trail mix" so that the treat hierarchy can be varied smoothly and fluently throughout the training session is helpful.

To teach contingency of the marker to the animal's behavior and classically condition the clicker, follow this process:

- Only introduce the event marker to an animal if they are relaxed and taking treats. Introducing an event marker when the animal is in a heightened state of fear or anxiety, can result in the animal finding the marker unpleasant.
- If the animal is relaxed (FAS 2 or lower – see Chapter 8), mark and treat one to two times for "nothing," just to assess the animal's response to the event marker. If a startle or fear response is noted, modify the marker and test again.
- Immediately begin to capture (clicking/marking) some behavior the animal does (i.e. glancing toward the trainer) and follow each click with a treat (Video 7.17).

It is important that the animal learns early on that it makes the click happen by doing something. Spending too much time classically conditioning the animal to the clicker (i.e. clicking and treating for no specific behavior) can make teaching that the click is contingent on the animal's behavior more difficult.

Targeting is very useful in teaching the animal to offer a behavior and also aids the trainer in practicing accurate timing of the click. The goal behavior is for the animal to touch the end of a target stick (or other target such as a hand) with their nose, paw, or other body part. Targeting once taught can be used as a prompting technique (detailed below). Most animals will quickly investigate an object held in front of them. A target could also be a specific object lying on the floor (i.e. a head collar) or a spot on the wall or floor. With a relaxed patient, you might multitask by using a training tool (as long as the animal is relaxed with the object), such as head halter or basket muzzle placed on the floor or held in the trainer's hand, as a target when teaching behavior contingency. This process will also help create a positive emotional response to the training tool. At the moment the animal's nose touches the target, the trainer should mark and reinforce the behavior. Eventually the animal will begin following the target because it understands touching the target will be reinforced. The animal then understands that the click/marker is a promise of a reinforcer and he can "earn" the reinforcer by offering a behavior.

- Only introduce the event marker to an animal if they are relaxed and taking treats. Introducing an event marker when the animal is in a heightened state of fear or anxiety, can result in the animal finding the marker unpleasant.

The click has become a conditioned event marker when, after the click, the animal turns toward the trainer for reinforcement, and after eating the treat repeats the behavior (Table 9.7).

- The click has become a conditioned event marker when, after the click, the animal turns toward the trainer for reinforcement, and after eating the treat repeats the behavior (Table 9.7).

Determining a reinforcement hierarchy

An individual reinforcement hierarchy should be determined for each learner and for specific situations. The hierarchy will vary depending on species of animal, current environmental factors, and the learner's current emotional state. For example, an animal that is highly motivated to chase prey will probably not be reinforced by food in that situation. An animal displaying signs of fear may not find food reinforcing at the moment it is placed on the examination table but may find the food treat reinforcing when the fearful stimulus is decreased (i.e. when the animal is placed back on the floor). In such a situation, try a higher-value reinforcement while it

Table 9.7 Functions of the event marker.

Function	Message to learner
Precise acoustic event marker	"That's it! What you were doing at that exact moment was what I wanted."
Bridges the event and reinforcement	"Reinforcement is coming."
Click ends the behavior	"Criteria for that repetition have been reached."

is still on the table; if unsuccessful, remove the animal to the floor and try the reinforcement again. If the animal readily takes the higher-level food reinforcement from the table but does so more roughly than previously, do not increase what you are doing but wait until it is taking the treat more gently. If the animal takes the treats without "snatching" them, the procedure may continue. Dogs experiencing fear and anxiety often first grab treats roughly just before they stop taking treats entirely, which is an indication that the stress level is too high. If the animal will still not take the high-value reinforcement, the stress in the environment must be decreased before training can commence.

Difficult to perform behaviors or an animal in mild emotional distress must be reinforced with a higher-value reinforcement.

- Difficult to perform behaviors or an animal in mild emotional distress must be reinforced with a higher-value reinforcement.

Manipulating motivations

Just as with humans, reinforcement value will be affected by competing motivations. For example, I may want to go for a walk and it is raining outside, therefore I find the smell of fresh baked cookies more reinforcing than walking and I stay in the house and eat the cookies. If it had been sunny outside, I may have found the walk more reinforcing than staying in the house to eat the cookies.

Animals are faced with competing motivations that are driven by senses that we humans cannot completely understand. It is critical that the animal's reinforcement hierarchy in various situations be determined and then applied for more effective and faster training.

Astute trainers are able to subtly manipulate motivations.

Example 1: "Todd" is a two-year-old neutered male mixed-breed dog that finds playing with the other dogs at class more reinforcing than food treats. Todd pulls at the leash in an attempt to make contact with another dog while his owner pushes a treat into Todd's face. The trainer manipulates the reinforcement by asking the pet owner not to feed Todd before class, to bring steak in the treat pouch, and come to class 20 minutes early to play with another dog. The motivation to play is decreased while the motivation for the food reward is increased.

Example 2: With a dog that is charging forward toward another dog, the reinforcement type and rate will likely need to be at a higher level, depending on the underlying motivation (excitement, frustration, fear, or a combination thereof). The trainer must be perceptive and increase the value of the reinforcement (i.e. freeze-dried chicken) while also decreasing the motivation (i.e. the target dog moves further away). In some cases, until the negative emotional response of a situation is altered, the only reinforcement the animal desires may be increasing distance from the fear-provoking stimulus.

Once it is determined what reinforcements the subject desires, a reinforcement hierarchy can be developed. For example, the tennis ball may be preferred over kibble, but freeze-dried chicken may be preferred when a cat is present, and a tennis ball may be more reinforcing than steak when training in the back yard. The top of the hierarchy can be used to train the most difficult task and above-average responses, while lower-ranking reinforcers can be used for easier tasks or only average responses.

Animals that are the easiest to train are animals that have a vast reinforcement hierarchy and are easily reinforced. For example, the stereotypical Labrador retriever; the reinforcement possibilities for these dogs are endless because there is so much that they want. This is one reason cats can be more difficult to train. Their reinforcement hierarchy is usually smaller and more difficult to determine and manipulate. This in part might be due to early learning history and expectations (see Chapter 3).

Reinforcement schedules

The schedule of reinforcement refers to the pattern of reinforcement that is chosen (see Chapter 6). Continuous reinforcement is best used during the initial stages of training to expedite and solidify learning. A continuous or 1:1 ratio should be maintained during the early stages of teaching the behavior, although the type of reinforcement can and should be varied. For example, a dog may receive a food treat for coming to the owner and other times a toss of a toy may be the reinforcement.

Not all behaviors must be continuously reinforced once they have been well learned (placed on cue, fluent and generalized to multiple situations). Once a behavior is well learned, one usually moves on to an *intermittent reinforcement schedule*, whereby not every correct response is rewarded. The effect of intermittent reinforcement is that the behavior will become resistant to extinction.

Difficult or problem-solving behaviors (tasks that require ingenuity and creativity such as some service animal tasks) or highly desired or valued behaviors should continue to be reinforced continuously.

Most pet owners generally and routinely *under* reinforce desired behaviors and therefore the technician's focus should be more on how the pet owner can continuously reinforce behaviors they like. Using a variety of reinforcements (petting, talking to the animal, clapping hands, etc.), intermittent reinforcement will occur naturally.

Reinforcement delivery

Delivery of the reinforcer should occur, as a general rule, within one second of the marked behavior and before another behavior occurs. Delays will slow the training process considerably.

"Clean" and efficient treat delivery is imperative to making sure the strong association to the marker is maintained. Any unintentional movements by the trainer before the event marker will cause the marker to lose value. Keep the actual delivery of the reinforcement separate from delivery of the event marker. If treat delivery occurs at the same time as the marker, overshadowing will occur, causing the marker to be ineffective because the marker has no predictive value.

- Keep the actual delivery of the reinforcement separate from delivery of the event marker.

The placement of the treat after the click is also a tool to assist with the next repetition of the behavior. This is different from luring because it comes after the marker and does not prompt the behavior and therefore does not need to be faded (see section **Luring – handler prompts**). The strategic placement of the food reward can set the animal up to easily perform another repetition, thus avoiding the performance of other unnecessary behaviors between repetitions.

Example: When teaching a dog to go to a mat or bed, click the dog for looking at the mat on the floor and toss the treat beyond the mat. The dog goes out past the mat to eat the treat. After the dog has completed eating the treat and turns back toward the mat (because the handler is in that direction), click again as it moves toward the mat but before it moves past the mat. Tossing the treat beyond the mat sets the dog up to turn again toward the mat after eating the treat, increasing the likelihood the behavior of approaching the mat can be captured.

Treat delivery from the hand

When delivering food reinforcement from the hand, the animal's head or eyes will often orient toward the treat. Drifting toward the treat can be advantageous when rewarding the animal in a stationary position or when the movements required are in close proximity to the trainer.

For example, a dog is clicked while walking close to the handler on the left side. The treat is delivered by the hand closest to the dog's head (left hand) to encourage staying in that position for the next cue or repetition (Figure 9.16).

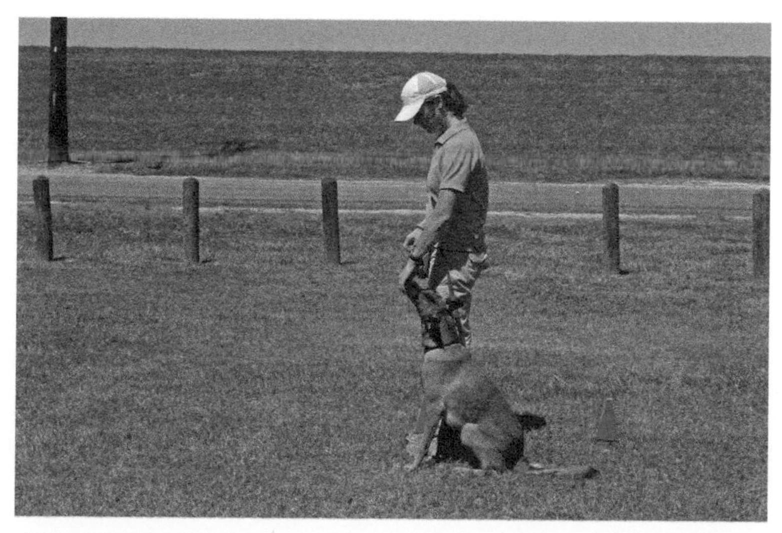

Figure 9.16 A treat delivered by the hand closest to the dog's head to encourage staying in that position for the next cue or repetition.

Hand delivery of treats can also help to gauge the animal's frustration, excitement, or anxiety level. Animals that have previously taken treats gently but begin to "snatch" or grab roughly at the treat are likely demonstrating an increase in anxiety. Take note and only raise criteria once the animal is again taking the treats gently. Criteria may need to be raised slowly or a break may be necessary.

Precautions:

- Learn the animal's food-guarding history. Some dogs with serious guarding issues may become aggressive when treated from the hand. In such cases, tossing the treat is better until trust by the animal has been gained.
- Some animals may "suddenly" realize they are in close proximity to the technician and find themselves in a motivational conflict (wanting the treat but not wanting to be too close to the veterinary technician) and consequently, feel the need to aggress.

Tossing the treat

As mentioned previously, conscious and accurate placement of the treat allows the trainer to "set up" for the next repetition. When it is advantageous for the dog to work at a distance from the handler or the trainer is working to shape the dog's path, tossing the treat along that path will generate anticipation and increase the likelihood of the behavior. Tossing of the treat may also allow for the additional reinforcement of chasing and "catching" the treat for dogs that enjoy that activity.

For example, teaching a dog to walk onto a scale by tossing the treat onto the scale after clicking the dog for approaching the scale will set up the likelihood of the next criterion, stepping one foot onto the scale.

Tossing treats is a skill that should be practiced and developed. Inaccurate or random tossing can result in lost treats and consequently create frustration in the learner.

Precaution:

Pet owners should be cautious while tossing treats in a household with multiple pets. When teaching something new or if tossing treats during a training session, it is best to place other pets in another area.

Timing

Accurately predicting the behavior and clicking at the precise moment that the behavior occurs is a fundamental and critical skill. Habitually late clicks will communicate inaccurate information to the pet about what is being marked and reinforced. Before timing can be accurate, the trainer must have a clear picture of what the desired behavior is and have a plan for when they will click. Being unsure or indecisive of the criteria can often cause the click to be delayed.

Once a behavior is on cue, the click can be incrementally delayed to shape the fluency of duration of the behavior.

Capturing behaviors

Any behavior that can be detected by the human senses can be marked and reinforced.

> • Any behavior that can be detected by the human senses can be marked and reinforced.

Capturing is the technique of waiting for a behavior to occur and marking the behavior as it happens naturally. For example, "sit" or "down" may be taught by simply marking the behavior when it occurs. Tossing a treat away from the animal will cause the animal to get up from the "sit" or "down," which will create another opportunity for the animal to offer another "sit" or "down." Behaviors like yawning or deep breaths can be captured to encourage relaxation. This is an excellent technique when training animals who display fear and/or aggression and that cannot tolerate close interactions.

> • Behaviors like yawning or deep breaths can be captured to encourage relaxation.

Behaviors such as play bows, sneezing, or scratching are easily captured and can become cute tricks. The challenge of capturing behavior is that many behaviors are not offered frequently and therefore are more difficult to mark and reinforce.

Shaping

Shaping is the process of "building" a behavior by successively reinforcing bits or "criteria" of the behavior that are approximations of the final behavior. The animal's behavior is molded into an end response by the trainer's differential reinforcements of the behavior. The process of differentially reinforcing some behaviors and not others is called *successive approximation*.

Gradually the trainer "expects more" (raises criteria) until the desired behavior is reached. For example, to teach a dog to walk backward you would click shifting of the weight backward, any movement of a back or front foot, greater movement of the feet, and so on, until the dog moves backward. An excellent training technique used to teach trainers how to watch for small increments of behavior is to have the trainer sit in a chair with his/her back against the chair at all times; the dog is directly in front of the chair and the trainer must teach the dog to walk backward without allowing his/her own back to leave the chair. Good observational skills and excellent timing are critical in shaping the behavior.

The first approximation of the behavior is initially captured and marked and rewarded several times. Then the criterion for the next approximation is set. In a "perfect" training session, approximations should look as shown in Figure 9.17.

In reality, shaping is not usually a steady upward staircase but more comparable to a "dance," with criteria being raised and lowered to keep a steady stream of information flowing to the animal (Figure 9.18). If a criterion is raised too quickly, the response rate of the animal becomes *slower* and the situation becomes increasingly *stressful* for the animal. If pushed to the extreme, an animal may quite simply quit working altogether and show signs of distress and will have to be retrained using more frequent reinforcements. Before this occurs, drop the current criterion to the last successful approximation and continue raising criteria but within smaller increments of the approximations. See general shaping guidelines in Table 9.8.

Creating a shaping plan

A shaping plan is a framework for developing a behavior. The trainer considers potential increments of behavior to reach a criterion and creates successive approximations of the behavior into their plan

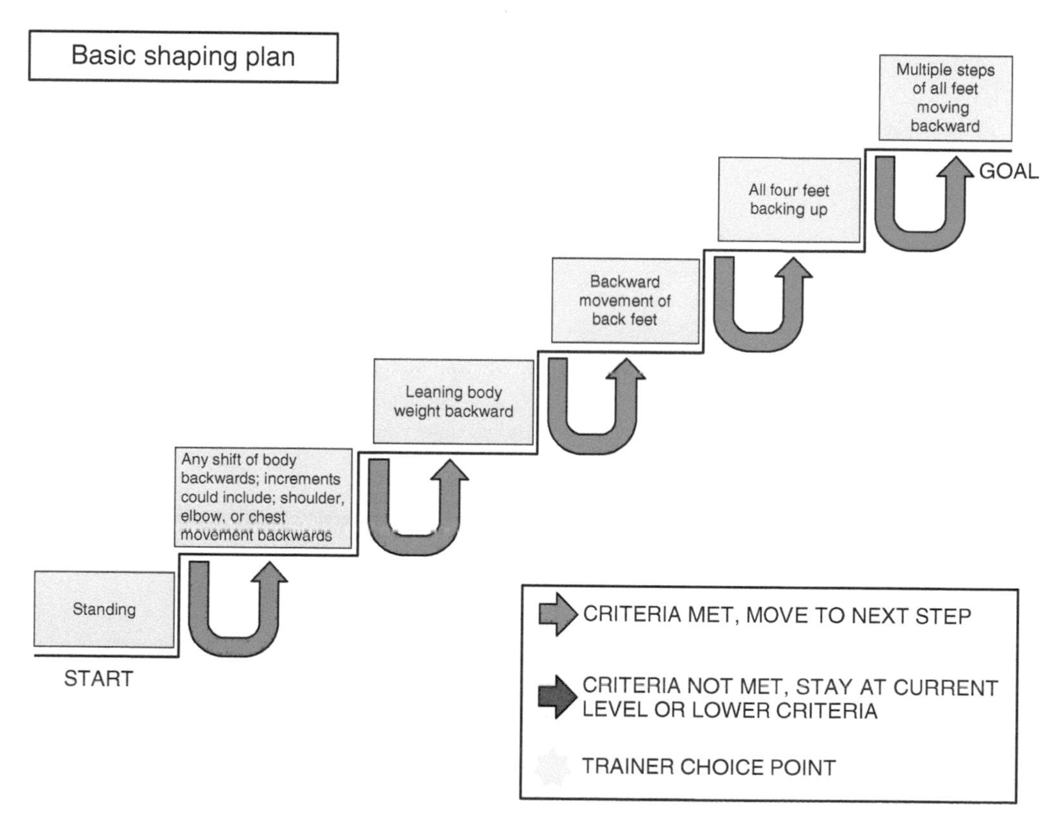

Figure 9.17 Basic shaping plan example for "back up"; in a "perfect" training session approximations occur at each step in a steady incline. *Source*: Photo courtesy of Melissa Spooner, LVT, VTS (Behavior), BS, KPA–CTP.

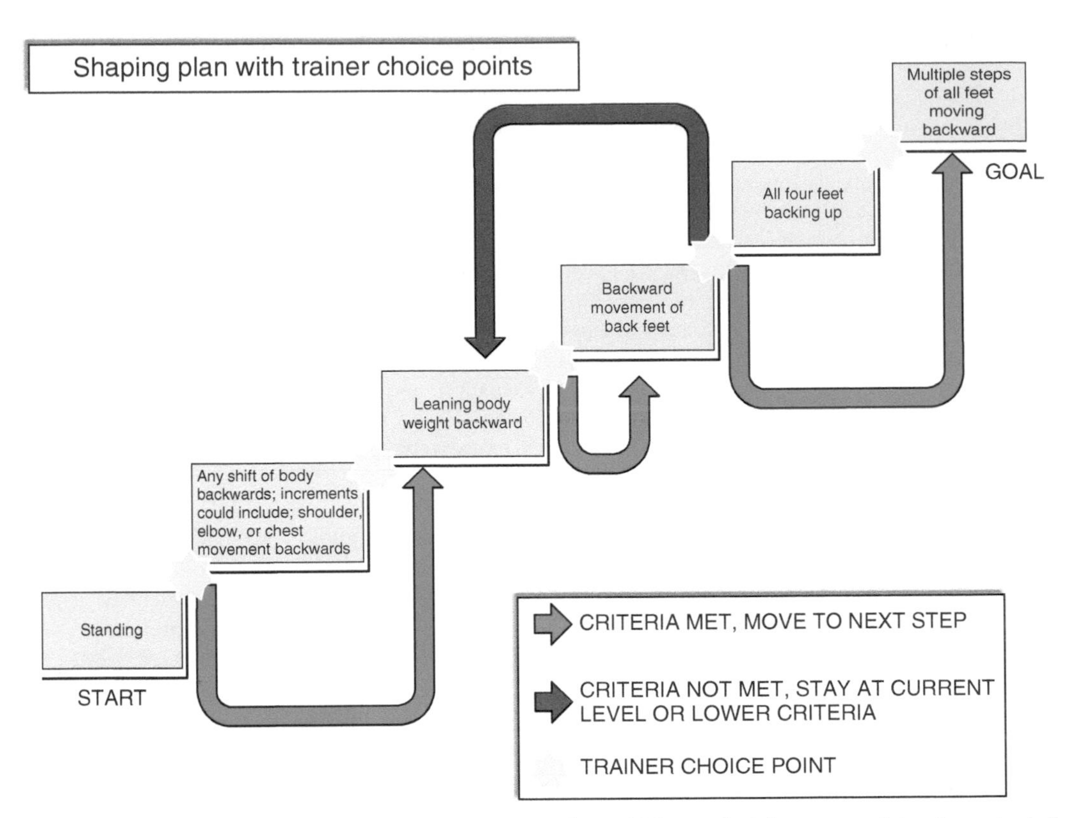

Figure 9.18 In reality, shaping is a raising and lowering of criteria to keep a high rate of reinforcement and therefore a steady flow of information to the animal. *Source*: Photo courtesy Melissa Spooner, LVT, VTS (Behavior), BS, KPA–CTP.

Table 9.8 Shaping guidelines.

Be prepared before you start.	Set up an appropriate environment and have all your supplies easily accessible. Be ready to mark and treat immediately as the training session begins.
Ensure success at each step.	Create a shaping plan and include the specific criteria for each step. Break the behavior down into small enough increments that the learner has a realistic chance to be successful.
Train one criterion at a time.	Don't try to shape for two criteria of a behavior simultaneously. For example, when working on speed of the behavior, do not require the criterion of precision.
Relax criteria when something changes.	When introducing a new criterion, temporarily relax the old ones. For example, if working on precision, lower the criteria for speed.
If one door closes, find another.	There are many ways to "get behavior"; if one plan is not working "think outside the box" and create another plan.
Keep training sessions continuous.	The animal should be continuously engaged throughout the session. This includes keeping a high rate of reinforcement.
Go back to kindergarten, if necessary.	If a behavior deteriorates, go back to an easier step in the shaping process. Behaviors are likely to regress if marker timing is late or if the criteria are not appropriate. Review and revise your shaping plan.
Keep your attention on your learner.	Disengaging from the training session and learner, can result in the learner losing interest or feeling punished. If you need a break, give the animal a "goodbye present" or redirect him to another fun activity.
Stay ahead of your learner.	Be prepared to "skip ahead" in your shaping plan if your learner makes a sudden leap.
Quit while you're ahead.	End each session with something the learner finds reinforcing. Ideally, end a session on a strong behavioral response and with the learner eager to continue training.

Source: Adapted from Pryor 2014.

CHAPTER 9

with the final desired behavior at the top of the staircase. A shaping plan is used to guide the training process and should be reevaluated, assessed, and modified frequently during the shaping process.

As noted previously, shaping of behavior is really a combination of science and art. The trainer must be knowledgeable and subtly raise and lower criteria while keeping a high rate of reinforcement (see subsequent text).

Rate of reinforcement per minute

A high rate of reinforcement (reinforcements per minute) provides the learner with a continuous stream of information over a small period of time, keeping the learner engaged. It can also be used as a guide to the trainer as to when to place a behavior on cue. The rate of reinforcement is highly variable between subjects due to the differences between the speed at which the animal can perform the behavior and the time it takes to reinforce behavior. For example, when training a dog to lie down, a Great Dane will likely receive fewer reinforcements per minute because it takes longer to assume the down position than it does for a Jack Russell terrier. Therefore, the highest reinforcement rate (rr/minute) that can be successfully achieved for that behavior with that specific animal should be the guide to when to add a cue. Each animal and each behavior should have its own ideal rate of reinforcement per minute and be determined by keeping accurate training records. A very general guide is to aim for an rr/minute of around 8–20.

A "jackpot" is a term used to describe giving a high-value reward or several high-value treats in a row to emphasize to the learner the significance of the behavior just performed. It is to be used when a learner masters a particularly difficult behavior or is making an effort to get back into the training game. The problem with a "jackpot" is that if the training session is continued, the subsequent reinforcements for repetitions of the same behavior will be less.

When an animal makes a breakthrough in training, it is a good time to end the training session. End on a good note while the learner is still engaged. However, abrupt discontinuance of a training session can be upsetting to the learner. So, to end a session, dole out several treats one after another, scatter several treats on the floor, or play a game of tug or fetch. An "end of training" session routine, although not a "jackpot," may look like one in action. So if tempted to give your learner a "jackpot," consider this an appropriate time to give a special reward and take a short break from the training session.

Prompting

Prompting can be a (humane) way of inducing a behavior and is sometimes incorporated into the shaping process to cause a specific behavior or criterion of the desired behavior to occur. The most common types of prompts are physical or environmental prompts, luring, and targeting.

The behavior is prompted, marked, and reinforced. The eliciting behavior (prompt) becomes the cue to do the behavior. Later training sessions gradually reduce the intensity of the prompt, eventually fading it entirely and transferring to a different cue or incorporating it into the new cue. For example, movement of a hand over a puppy's head makes the behavior of bending the rear legs more likely to occur and therefore can be reinforced. The hand movement over the head will continue to be the prompt (cue) until it is transferred to another cue, such as the word "sit."

Physical and environmental prompts

Physical and environmental prompts include such things as touching a puppy's rear to prompt a "sit" (physical prompt) or teaching a dog to heel by walking with the dog next to a wall (environmental prompt). Physical prompts are not commonly recommended because they can cause fear or resistance in some animals, especially animals suffering from fear and anxiety disorders. Environmental prompts can be used to increase the likelihood of a behavior being offered and promote precise muscle memory with early learning and repetitions.

Luring – handler prompts

Luring is an advanced skill and is the process of holding a food treat or toy in front of the pet's nose to guide the pet into the desired position. Examples would include holding a treat over a puppy's nose to guide her into the sit position or throwing treats onto a mat to teach "go to your bed." While luring is a very useful prompting technique, it can have the drawback of the dog becoming so focused on the food treat that she does not think about what she is doing to get the reward. In such cases, a better prompting technique would be targeting.

Luring is an advanced skill because it requires consideration and thought in the training plan as to how the lure will be faded. If a lure is used to prompt the behavior, it should be faded within one or two repetitions.

- If a lure is used to prompt the behavior, it should be faded within one or two repetitions.

Luring can also be beneficial as a management tool when a dog is in a situation that he is perhaps not equipped to handle. A food lure may distract the dog and allow the handler to move the dog away from the situation.

Targeting

Targeting is the prompting technique of teaching the animal to touch or follow an object such as the trainer's hand, a stick, or other object. Targeting is very useful in teaching a dog to heel at your side by having it touch the target of your hand occasionally as you walk (see Figure 9.10). Targeting can also be used to teach body placement. For example, to get a puppy to step onto the scale to be weighed, the puppy can be taught to target and follow your hand directly onto the scale. Large zoo animals and horses have been taught to target their nose on a spot, which acts as a stationing behavior to aid in medical care.

Targeting is a technique that is very easy and quick to teach. Simply hold the target in front of the animal and click any movement toward the target. Many animals tend to investigate a novel item that appears in their environment and the trainer should be prepared to capture the first investigation of the target. If the animal grabs the target with its mouth, initially mark the behavior but then raise criteria for only nose touches. This might be accomplished by clicking as the animal approaches the target prior to putting his mouth on it. The next step would be to gradually move the target so the animal will follow it. The animal can also be taught to maintain the target position by the trainer gradually withholding the click for longer durations. Video 7.19 on the companion website provides a demonstration of teaching a nose touch to the trainer's hand. Video 9.1 demonstrates using a target stick to begin to teach a new behavior.

Fading prompts

When a prompt is used, it often becomes the cue or discriminative stimulus for the animal to perform the behavior and therefore it may be desirable to transfer to another cue quickly. Often the ultimate goal is for the behavior to be on a verbal or hand cue, without the prompt being presented. For this reason, when using prompts, a plan should be in place as to how the prompt will be faded. A prompt should only be needed for one to three of the offered behaviors and then quickly faded out. The trainer can then switch back to shaping the behavior if needed after removing the prompt. Tactile prompts are more difficult to fade than visual prompts.

Prompting a behavior is an advanced skill.

- Prompting a behavior is an advanced skill.

When using a food lure to teach a puppy to lie down, it is useful to gradually decrease the size of the treat held in your hand. Eventually the trainer holds their hand in the same luring position but without a treat. This hand movement can then be turned into a hand signal for the down position or transferred to a verbal cue. A target can be faded by gradually decreasing the size of the target.

Cues

This text has attempted to use the word "cue" instead of "command." A cue is simply information, a signal as to which behavior is to be performed at that moment and a promise of a desired result. A cue can be thought of as a request. A command, in contrast, has a level of threat involved: do this or else… (Pryor 2009).

Cues are learned antecedents and discriminative stimuli that predict the potential for positive reinforcement.

Cues give the animal information and provide a common language between trainer and learner. Cues also differentiate between behaviors and are key to building complex behavior chains.

Once the concept of cues has been learned by the animal, it will become easier and faster to associate his behavior with cues.

Cues improve the quality of an animal's life by providing information; that information is reinforcing in itself. It tells the animal, "Do THIS behavior at

THIS moment and the opportunity for reinforcement is in place." Karen Pryor compares cues to a green light at a stop light in *Reaching the Animal Mind*, 2009. "Think about that little sense of joy or relief you feel when the traffic light turns green; that's a cue, identifying a behavior that you want to do. Every cue is a green light, permission to go do the thing it names. The cue thus becomes reinforcing in itself. Any time you give a well-learned cue, you are actually reinforcing what the individual you are cuing happens to be doing at the time."

- Cues improve the quality of an animal's life by providing information.

As learning is constantly occurring, any event or situation can become a meaningful and predictive cue or antecedent for other behaviors and consequences. Dogs may show fear reactions only in certain places (where previous learning has occurred), or only respond to cues when the pet owner's treat bag is present.

For example, the garage door going up is a cue that you will be entering the house. Seeing a dog in the distance can become a cue to the dog that his choke collar will be jerked. The doorbell cues a person at the door. Often the technician and trainer must analyze behaviors to determine how to manipulate previously associated cues (like the doorbell).

Cues can be predictors of our behavior. For example, when walking with your dog say "left" just before you turn left. After only a few repetitions the dog will associate the verbal "left" with the behavior that is about to occur: the trainer turns. The trainer can then say "left" before turning, pause, and reinforce any left turning movement the dog does. Another example is to say "up" just before picking a dog off the floor. The dog will quickly associate the cue "up" with what you are about to do. If the dog enjoys being picked up, this informational cue will provide the dog with increased predictability and decreased anxiety with the situation, which is very important for animals.

Cues can also be used to build other behaviors. For example, the known behavior of "down" can be used when shaping "go to a mat" and later faded out so "got to a mat" means go to your mat and lie down without requiring the "down" cue.

Types of cues

Cues should be easy to give consistently, distinct, and easily perceived by the animal and easy to transfer to another cue if needed. Cues can be anything the animal perceives; for example, words, sounds, scents, sight of an object, movement, or an environmental situation can become a cue. Motion cues are usually more salient to the dog and easier to perceive then verbal cues.

How and when to add the cue

A cue can be added when the behavior can be reliably predicted (or prompted) and begins to occur regularly with more intensity and intention. What "regularly" is will be determined by the animal's learning history. A long learning history of clear and properly applied cues will likely make it possible for the animal to generalize the use of cues more quickly. The rate of reinforcement per minute (rr/minute) for these animals may be lower than for a novice. A very basic rule of thumb is to add the cue when the rr/minute has reached 8–15 clicks.

The cue is given just before the behavior occurs. The behavior is then rewarded only after the discriminatory stimulus (cue) has been given and not reinforced when the behavior is offered without the cue. Through discrimination, the animal learns the behavior will only be reinforced when the cue precedes the performance of the behavior.

It was once believed that a cue should not be added until the behavior was "perfect." As marker-based training has progressed in understanding techniques and as animals have progressed because of better training, it is clear that cues are valuable information for the animal and should not be withheld until fluency has been achieved, but added early. Cues can be readily transferred and changed. Thus, a trainer who wants a high degree of precision in a behavior may elect to first use a nonformal cue for a less precise behavior and then transfer to a for mal cue for the precise polished behavior.

Example of properly adding a cue:

- Dog offers rear end on the ground, click then treat (C/T).
- Trainer gives the cue "sit" as the dog sits, C/T.
- Trainer gives the cue "sit," just before the dog sits, C/T.
- Trainer gives the cue "sit," before the dog offers the sit, C/T.
- The trainer pauses, if the dog offers the "sit" there is no reinforcement or response from the trainer.

The dog gets up from the sit and considers what was different; at that moment the trainer gives the cue "sit" and the dog learns the cue is the key to reinforcement. It is the trainer's responsibility to teach the dog to discriminate when the behavior will be rewarded (cue is given) and when it will not be rewarded (cue not given). The trainer can set the animal up for success by providing the cue frequently: 10–20 repetitions where the cue is given prior to the dog offering the behavior. The trainer pauses slightly and if the dog orients to the trainer, the trainer can mark and reinforce the offered attention. If the dog offers the "sit" behavior it is not marked or treated. But then the trainer gives the cue for the behavior, helping the animal discriminate. The dog should be successful more often than not and the waiting for a cue (i.e. looking to the trainer) should be reinforced often. As the cue is added, the animal's behavior will likely slightly decrease in quality as the animal perceives the addition of the cue and then recognizes its meaning.

Waiting for the cue demonstrates a degree of impulse control, a very valuable and useful skill for companion animals. Once the animal makes the connection and association between the behavior and the cue the animal can be shaped to wait for the cue rather than randomly offering the behavior. The animal learns only behaviors that occur immediately after the cue will be reinforced and other offered behavior will not.

The cue can be strengthened by alternating between different cues (i.e. "sit," "down," "touch"), minimizing cues so they are subtle, removing any prompts, and generalizing the cue to different situations and environments.

Video 9.2 on the companion website illustrates teaching a puppy to sit and the process of adding a cue.

Generalization

Generalization is the concept of learning that the cue means the same thing in a multitude of environmental contexts. For example, do the cued behavior regardless of changing variables like location, person giving the cue, and so on. The more generalization is practiced, the faster behaviors are generalized.

Lack of generalization history in regard to problem behaviors and behaviors associated with fear is beneficial when applying behavior modification. A location or situation that looks and feels different from previously associated events is often the first place to apply behavior modification (i.e. a nonstressful starting point).

Transferring cues

Frequently, cues for a specific behavior will need to be changed. For example, the cue may currently be a hand signal over the dog's head (likely from being prompted with a treat over the head and not faded) and the pet owner would prefer the cue to be verbal.

When transferring cues, it is important to give the cues in the correct order. It is very important that the two cues, the new cue and the old cue, do not occur simultaneously as the unlearned, new cue may be blocked.

- It is very important the two cues, the new cue and the old cue, do not occur simultaneously as the unlearned, new cue may be blocked.

Example of transferring a hand signal for sit to a verbal cue, "sit"

- New cue "sit" followed by known cue (hand signal), dog sits, C/T. Repeat several times.
- Verbal "sit" pause … old cue (hand signal), behavior, C/T. Repeat several times.
- Verbal "sit," pause, pause, old cue (hand signal), but given more subtly to fade it out, behavior, C/T.
- Verbal "sit," pause, pause, pause, very slight hand signal given, behavior, C/T.
- Verbal "sit," pause, pause, pause, dog offers sit without the old cue, C/T.

"Poisoned" cues

Frequently a cue develops a negative emotional association or is "poisoned."

A cue that has been associated with an aversive (whether intentionally or unintentionally) becomes a cue that is no longer "safe" and predictable of a positive outcome. "The cue becomes a conditioned negative reinforcer, signaling the opportunity for avoiding punishment. The shift becomes visible in the learner's attitude, which switches from attentive eagerness to reluctance, often with visible manifestations of stress" (Pryor 2002).

"Poisoning" of a cue is commonly seen when treating companion animal behavior problems and disorders. In many situations, the pet owner applies many different training styles, including punishment-based training and is inconsistent with cues and reinforcements. An analogy would be if a person were told, "Go sit in the chair" and every time he/she sat in the chair something "bad" occurred. Soon, when the person heard "Go sit in the chair" he/she would have a negative emotional response to the cue. An example of a pet owner inadvertently "poisoning" a cue would be when the pet owner cued "come" and the dog ran to the pet owner and was then punished (i.e. inappropriately punished for running away). In such situations, the behavior should be retaught through shaping, capturing, or targeting and a new cue should then be attached to the behavior. As the new positive relationship builds between the pet owner and pet, the new cue can be utilized without association to the previous negative emotional response.

Stimulus control

When a response is under the influence of a cue and meets the following conditions in a training situation, it is considered to be under "stimulus control" and may then be taught to fluency. A behavior cannot become fluent until it is under stimulus control. The cue can now be generalized to new environments and conditions and stimulus control should be retested.

The four conditions for a behavior to be under stimulus control are given in Table 9.9.

Fluency

Fluency refers to the animal's ability to perform a cued behavior with speed and accuracy. Each criterion for fluency should be trained separately. When one criterion of fluency is being shaped, it is necessary to lower criteria for the other aspects of fluency. For instance, when shaping for speed or latency the precision of the behavior may deteriorate (Figure 9.19).

Precision – Precision is how a finished behavior should look. The trainer must first have an image of the precise behavior and then gradually shape the behavior toward those qualifications. For instance, a straight sit with the dog's shoulders by the handler's left knee, head looking straight ahead, and muzzle parallel to the ground.

Low latency – Low latency refers to the lag time between a cue being perceived and the time the animal begins the behavior. Low latency is a sign that the cue is clearly understood, and the animal is attentive to the trainer. The animal often generalizes latency and later new cued behaviors will decrease in latency from the beginning. Low latency can be shaped by determining the current average length of latency and then shaping lower latency by C/T only shorter latency.

Speed – Speed of the behavior refers to how quickly the animal performs the behavior. The goal is to have the behavior performed as quickly as possible, with consideration for the animal's physical abilities. Determining the current average speed

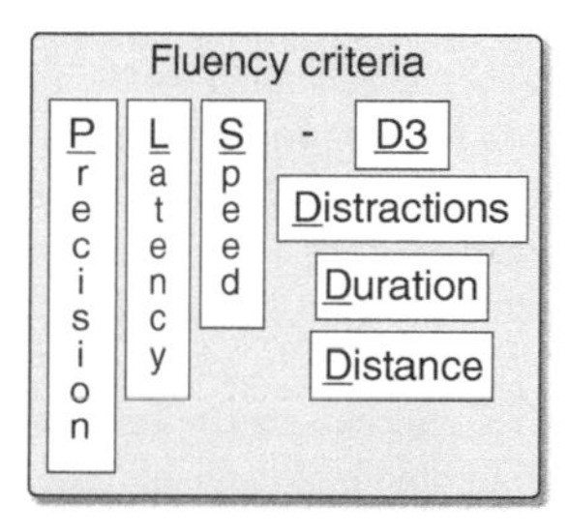

Figure 9.19 Fluency criterion: precision, latency, speed, distractions, duration, distance. Each criterion of fluency should be shaped separately.

Table 9.9 Four conditions to test for stimulus control of a trained behavior.

Condition	Description	Example
C = B	Cue given and the desired behavior occurs	Verbal cue, "sit" = Dog sits.
No C = no B	No cue results in the behavior not being offered	During a training session the sit behavior is not offered without the cue, "sit."
AC ≠ B	A different cue is given and it does not result in performance of the behavior being tested	Handler cues "down." The dog does not sit.
C ≠ AB	Cue given does not result in a different behavior	Handler cues "sit." The dog does not lie down.

C: cue; B: behavior; AC: different cue; AB: another behavior; ≠: does not equal.

of the behavior and reinforcing for faster completions of the behavior will shape faster speed of the overall behavior.

Distraction – Distractions, such as the smell of other animals, are a constant occurrence in the environment and may not even be distinguishable to a human. The trainer should identify specific distractions and then introduce them in a controlled manner (sometimes requiring desensitization). The animal is taught to associate the presence of a distraction as an opportunity for reinforcement.

Duration – Duration is the length of time a behavior can be sustained. Duration is gradually shaped by systematically delaying the C/T for longer periods of time. It is important to vary the duration. For example, when working on an average duration of 10 seconds, some repetitions may take 3 seconds, others 12 seconds. When the criteria are varied, the learner is less likely to anticipate the end of a repetition.

Distance – This criterion of fluency usually applies to stationary behaviors such as sit–stay or response to a cue from a distance, such as a recall. Another circumstance would be when the trainer gives the cue while at a distance from the animal and the animal responds without approaching the handler. For example, the trainer asks the dog to sit and the trainer walks 20 ft away from the dog, and then cues the dog to lie down. This can be the most difficult aspect of fluency for dogs that have only been trained near their handlers or who are overly attached to the handler and have separation issues. Often when cued from a distance, these animals will run to the handler before performing the behavior. It may be that proximity to the handler has become part of the cue.

Behavior chains

Behaviors chains are behaviors linked together by a sequence of cues. Each behavior has been previously trained, is under stimulus control and trained to the desired level of fluency before it is placed into the chain. Cues for the sequence may be environmental or delivered by the handler. Learned cues are reinforcing and are used to reinforce the previous behavior, therefore creating a behavior chain. Each behavior in the chain is reinforced by the next cue until the last behavior in the chain is marked and reinforced. Each cue in the sequence is both a marker for the current behavior and a cue to perform the next behavior.

Complex chains are commonly required for a sequence of behaviors to be performed. For example, "explosive" dogs must search, locate the bomb, sit, and bark. Service animals must target an item, retrieve the item, and deliver the item to a person's hand (Figure 9.20). Chains of behavior also occur naturally. The dog focuses attention on a stimulus, the pet owner tightens the leash, the dog aggresses, and the stimulus leaves.

Behavior chains are often assembled by backchaining the behaviors. Each skill in the chain is first taught individually and the last behavior of the sequence is conditioned first. The situation in which the last behavior is performed becomes the discriminatory stimulus for the next behavior. The second to the last behavior is then conditioned, followed by the third to the last behavior, and so on.

Backchaining utilizes the concept that familiar is reinforcing. By adding the last behavior in the chain first, the second to the last behavior in the chain is reinforced by the familiarity of the next behavior. "Knowing what to do next" is very reinforcing to animals.

When the dog has learned the entire chain, the primary reinforcement would only be given at the end of the sequence. To prevent breakdown of a chain, it is important to continue to practice components of the chain individually.

Behavior modification

It is the veterinarian's responsibility to diagnose a behavior disorder and prescribe the treatment plan, although input from the entire treatment team (veterinarian, veterinary technician, trainer, and pet owner) is critical for creating a practical and successful plan.

We will first discuss general theoretical concepts and general applications of each behavior modification technique, followed by specific exercise examples. Commonly prescribed exercises that a veterinary technician may be asked to teach a pet owner are included along with practical applications for the general hospital setting.

Using a marker in the application of behavior modification

A positive event marker (clicker) is an invaluable tool in behavior modification. It can be used in behavior modification to simultaneously change the emotional response of a stimulus or event, teach an

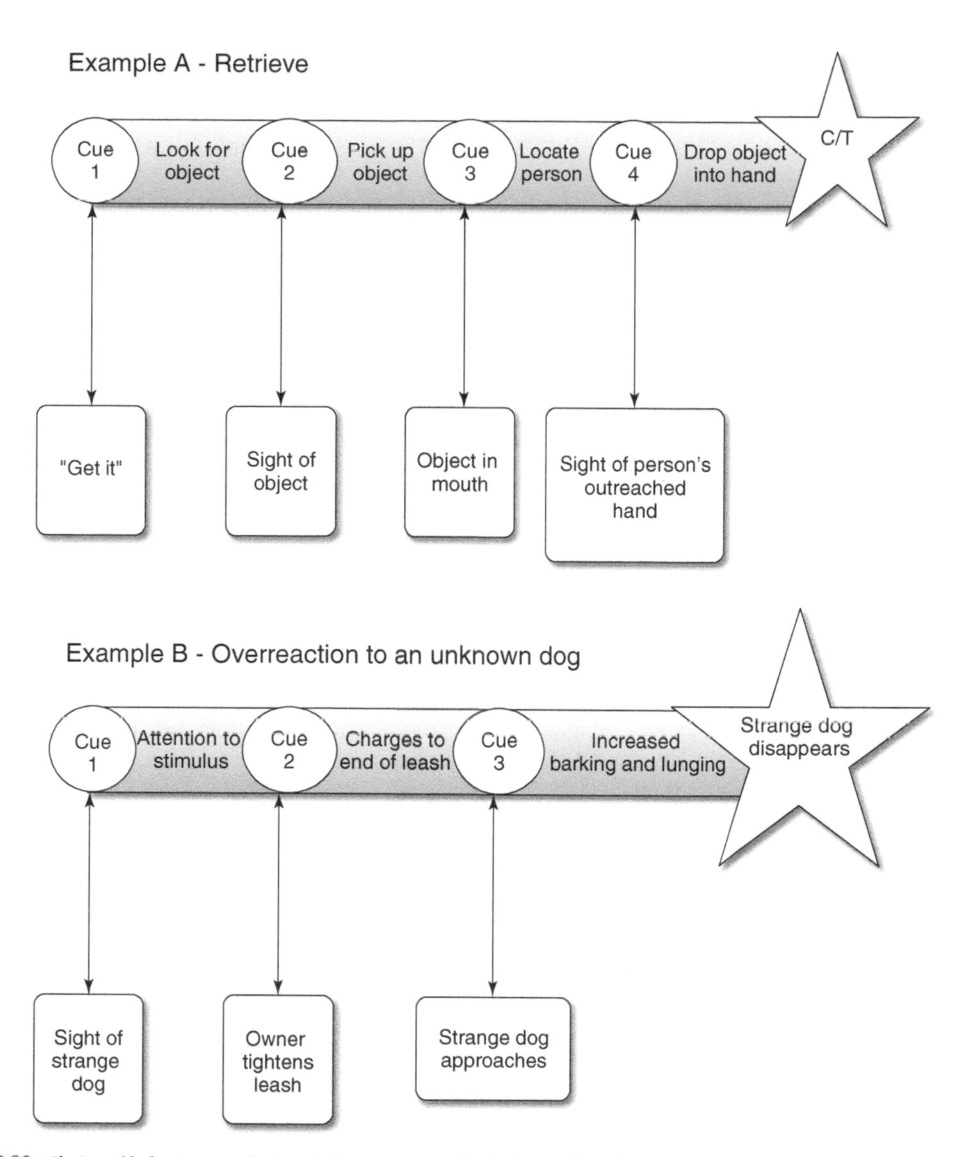

Figure 9.20 Chains of behaviors can be taught to create complex behaviors but also occur naturally.

alternate response, and clearly mark subtle steps in a desensitization program.

It must be emphasized that before using the clicker for behavior modification, the animal should have a long and positive history with the clicker and associate a positive emotional response to the clicker (Figure 9.21a, b).

Without this strong association, the clicker may inadvertently become associated with or predictive of a negative stimulus and become aversive and will no longer be a positive way to communicate with the animal.

A clicker must have a sufficiently positive association before being used in the application of behavior modification.

• A clicker must have a sufficiently positive association before being used in the application of behavior modification.

A clicker will likely be ineffective if the animal is too stressed (not taking treats) or if the animal is too

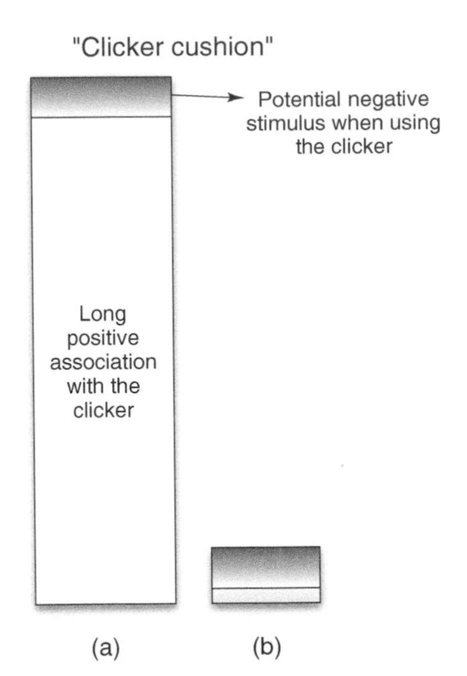

Figure 9.21 (a) A long positive learning history with the clicker (or other positive event marker) should be in place before using it in behavior modification. (b) Without this strong association the event marker may inadvertently become associated with or predictive of a negative stimulus and become aversive.

stimulated to acknowledge the clicker. In both cases the stimulus should be decreased to a level at which the animal is less emotional and can focus on training.

The clicker is a valuable tool to expedite behavior modification and should therefore be used appropriately and accurately to keep its value and positive association.

Throughout this text we will use C/T (Click/Treat), CC (Classical Counter Conditioning), RS (Response Substitution), and DS (Desensitization).

Generalization and behavior modification

As described in the section **Marker training techniques and skills**, generalization means to generalize a behavior to different situations. With regard to behavior modification, lack of generalization can be used to benefit the behavior modification process. When applying any of the behavior modification techniques described, the technician should attempt to create a situation that is different from the past learning history. It is comparable to trying to write on a blackboard that is already filled with writing (previous learning history) versus starting with a clean, unmarked blackboard. The goal should be to create a fresh "clean" learning history whenever possible. For instance, if the animal has had a bad experience in an examination room, training should begin at home and then be transferred to different locations and eventually the veterinary hospital. If a negative emotional experience was created with one style of nail clippers, a different style of nail clipper should be used in behavior modification.

Classical counter conditioning

Whenever we interact with animals in training or otherwise, classical conditioning is taking place. The animal will associate the situation and circumstances with a positive (pleasant), negative (unpleasant), or neutral (not pleasant or unpleasant) experience. These associations occur all of the time, whether we are conscious of them or not.

Classical counter conditioning in veterinary behavior modification is a technique used to change a specific, previously created negative emotional response to a stimulus to a positive emotional response. In other words, a current situation that is frightening or upsetting to the animal, for example, fear of large dogs, is to be changed from the negative emotional response of fear to tolerance or pleasantness; it is then taught an alternate operant response (RS: see subsequent text).

When the animal's emotional state (i.e. fear) is modified, the behaviors that often drive that emotion (distance-increasing behaviors, overreactivity) are also decreased. This will make the application of RS and DS easier.

The positive emotional response should then quickly prompt subtle changes in the operant response of the animal. For example, if currently the sight of a large dog causes fear followed by the operant response of charging to the end of the leash to occur, when the driving emotion of fear is decreased, a change in the operant response of charging to the end of the leash also begins to be seen. Once the emotional state of the animal changes to a less reactive state, cognitive options and choices become more obvious to the animal. Charging at the end of the leash becomes slightly less intense, and/or the dog (the patient) is able to pause before reacting, which is the moment to incorporate RS by giving a cue for an alternate foundation behavior (let's go, target, etc.).

For example, operant behaviors like a slight pause before reacting or turning attention away from the stimulus will begin to occur. Those subtle changes can be reinforced with a clicker and therefore produce a change in the emotional response to the stimulus (if a strong positive association with the clicker is in place). You might have noticed we are combining a focus on CC and marking specific behaviors that the pet is doing (i.e. operant behaviors). Because classical and operant conditioning are happening simultaneously, there will always be some behavior the animal is doing when he receives the counter-conditioner.

The previously fear-provoking stimulus becomes the cue for an alternate response and the animal begins to anticipate the introduction of the fear-provoking stimulus as an opportunity for reinforcement. The pet can then be cued by the presence of a stimulus to look at the pet owner (attention) or to target the pet owner's hand (note: hand targeting of the animal's nose to the pet owner's hand should not be recommended for animals that are highly aroused and could redirect to the presented hand).

CC is also the easiest for owners to understand and apply. A pet owner can be told, "First, we will change how 'Spot' feels about the situation (e.g. other dogs, veterinary clinic) so he will be less afraid. Once he is less afraid of and even begins to LIKE_, we will teach him other coping skills (rather than barking and lunging) that he can use in those situations."

As the improved emotional state should be seen relatively quickly if CC is applied properly, the pet owner is also reinforced therefore increasing pet owner's compliance and confidence.

Some mild issues may require only a focus on CC to change the behavior. For example: A rescued four-year-old Sheltie, "Tag," nips at the pet owner's ankles (sometimes leaving marks) when the dishwasher makes a chiming sound. "Tag" is placed on leash (so the behavior cannot occur), a chiming sound is produced (it is helpful to find an easily producible and controllable chiming sound, other than the dishwasher, that triggers the response), immediately followed by a treat. Beginning this process in a room or environment where the previous behavior of nipping ankles has NOT occurred (no past or little past learning history) will expedite the CC process.

Classical counter-conditioning benefits:

- Is usually the easiest technique for pet owners to apply.
- Often a relatively quick emotional change is seen.
- Positive emotional response makes it easier for the pet to learn other coping skills (see section **Response substitution**).
- Makes the application of RS and DS easier or possibly not needed in mild cases.

Practical application of counter conditioning

To make a strong classical counter-conditioned emotional response the following should occur:

- The current stimulus that causes the negative emotional response must be at a low enough level that the patient does not react or reacts only very mildly.

  When applying CC, DS is usually also occurring because the stimulus (e.g. sight of large dog) is first introduced at a tolerable level. The stimulus should be noticed by the animal and acknowledged but not at a level at which the animal reacts strongly.

  Example: If the trigger is the presence of a large dog, the large dog must be far enough away so there is very little or no response from the patient.

  Example: If the stimulus is touching of the feet, touching a foot must occur at a level that does not elicit a significant response. Touch the foot = reinforcement. If touching of the foot is too high a stimulus, then touching the shoulder may need to occur first (DS). This may mean touching of the shoulder is first treated.
- The presenting order must be correct.

  Example: large dog in sight, food is presented. Dog leaves, food stops.

  Example: Touch the foot, give a treat, release the foot and the treat disappears.

  It is helpful to cue YOUR behavior first, for example, say "foot," technician touches foot, C/T. The cue "foot" begins to predict the foot touch (predictability can decrease anxiety), food reinforcement, C/T.
- Outside environmental stimuli should be decreased; otherwise the animal may make an association with something in the environment.

  Example: Presentation of a basket muzzle containing food. Once the dog is enjoying eating out of the muzzle, put the muzzle away and ignore the dog for five minutes. NOTHING good happens to the dog until the muzzle reappears. The goal is for it to become very clear to the dog what is making the fun/food appear again (the muzzle).
- Once reactivity to the stimulus has decreased (large dog can be closer before there is any

response from the patient or the intensity of the response is decreased) response substitution can be added.

Example: Large dog in the distance, dog turns to pet owner anticipating a treat. Other responses, like targeting and/or loose leash walking away from stimulus, can now be incorporated into the treatment plan.

- Fear and aggression cannot be reinforced or increased with food (Garcia and Koelling 1966; Luescher and Martin 2010; Martin and Martin 2011).

More examples of CC:

- Counter conditioning in a situation where a dog is displaying signs of fear at the veterinary office
  Dog enters the veterinary clinic and receives treats.
- Counter conditioning in a situation where a dog is showing signs of fear with thunderstorms
  Thunderclap = peanut butter in mouth or other desired reinforcement.
- Counter conditioning in a situation where a dog is showing signs of fear and/or aggression to a new baby
  When the baby is in the room, dog gets a stuffed food toy and attention. The toy is removed and the dog is ignored when the baby is not present.
- Counter conditioning in a situation where a dog is showing signs of fear of a head halter
  Head halter is presented, and the dog receives attention and treats. Head halter disappears and attention and treats cease until the head halter is produced again.

Response substitution

Response substitution is operant counter conditioning. CC, as described earlier, is a classically associated response and focus while RS is an operant-associated response and focus.

The aim of RS is to replace undesirable behavior with desirable behavior in a given situation, the situation being the cue (discriminative stimulus) for the current undesirable behavior (Figure 9.22). Response substitution uses the situation in which undesirable behavior usually occurs (e.g. person at the door) as a discriminatory stimulus for the substituted desired behavior (i.e. go to a place – see section **Foundation behaviors**). The new, desired behavior should be incompatible with the undesirable behavior (i.e. go to crate or other place when person comes to the door is incompatible with charging the front door).

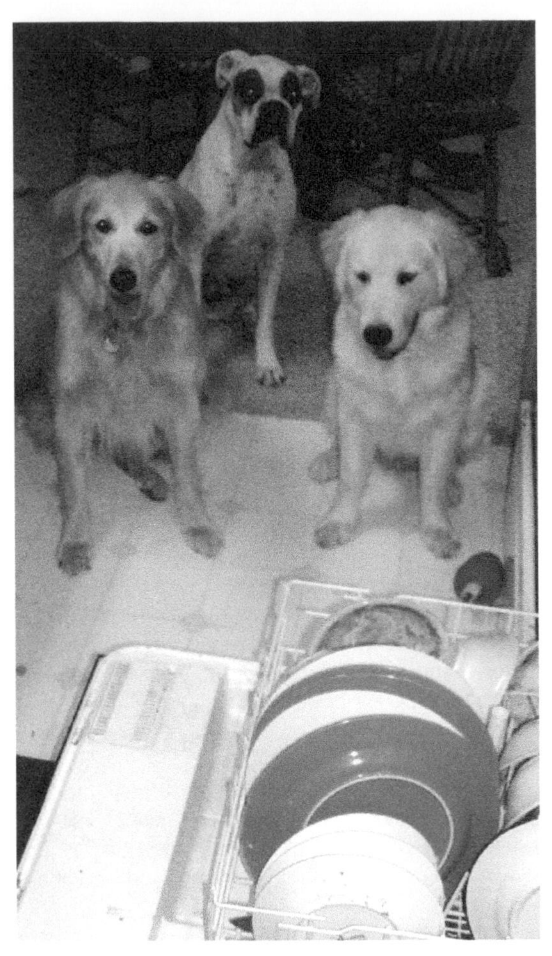

Figure 9.22 These dogs are cued to "sit" while the dishwasher is being loaded and then reinforced by getting to investigate the dishwasher.

Response substitution is often used in conjunction with desensitization and positive reinforcement. For example, training relaxation or another foundation behavior, while gradually exposing a dog to increasingly intensive stimuli and reinforcing with treats.

Response substitution can be explained to the pet owner as "teaching the pet a new, more appropriate coping skill" and explained further as, "Spot's current 'coping' skill when he is afraid is to charge the leash and try to make the scary thing go away, and it usually works, or so it seems to him. We are going to teach him a new coping skill and we will substitute that response for the current one. Over time, he will know that you will tell him what to do before he becomes upset and therefore the unpredictability of the situation will lessen and he will become calm. It will also help you because you will also know what to do and also become calm. It is response substitution for you too!"

If the dog's current "coping skill" is charging at the front door to "greet people" the dog is taught an alternate coping skill of going to a bed or "place" for a reward when the doorbell rings. Both CC (stranger = food) and RS (go to a bed) occur simultaneously.

When the animal performs an unwanted behavior he should be distracted before cuing the alternate behavior to prevent chaining or linking of the unwanted behavior to the substituted behavior. For example, a dog barks at the window, the owner gently claps his hands or makes a kissy-kissy sound to interrupt the behavior (not to frighten or scare the dog); dog turns attention toward pet owner, cue "go to your bed" is given; dog is rewarded for going to his bed. Interrupting the behavior with a soft hand clap prevents the behavior chain of the dog barking at window and then going to its bed for a reward. It might be necessary to do several behaviors in an unpredictable manner to prevent a chain from forming. Ideally, the pet owner is proactive and redirects and rewards the dog before the barking occurs (see the Behavior Solutions Model in Chapter 7).

RS is usually easier and more smoothly applied after some classical CC has already occurred because a more positive emotional response has already been developed with the stimulus.

- RS is usually easier and more smoothly applied after some classical CC has already occurred because a more positive emotional response has already been developed with the stimulus.

It is important for owners to understand that the preferred behavior must be trained before attempting to use it in the desired situation. For example, it is not appropriate and much more difficult to begin initial training to sit to greet people the moment the dog is jumping on a visitor. Create calm training situations; then generalize the situations before attempting to apply the newly trained behavior in a specifically needed situation (visitor at the door).

RS benefits:

- Gives the animal an "alternate coping skill" when unsure in a situation.
- The pet owner begins to focus on desired behavior rather than the undesired behavior.
- Response substitution also gives the pet owner an "alternate coping skill." For example, instead of tightening the leash in anticipation of barking and lunging, asking the dog to target away from the stimulus utilizing a fast-paced loose leash walking with turns and sits to increase distance from the stimulus.

Practical application of response substitution

- Choose an alternate and appropriate behavior to train that will not allow the unwanted behavior to occur but will still meet the needs of the animal. What is the function of the undesirable behavior? The new behavior should meet that function for the animal.
- Shape or capture the behavior. Place it on a cue and train to fluency.
- Begin applying the new on cue and fluent behavior in a quiet environment. Training should be done in a situation unrelated to one in which the unwanted behavior occurs. Possibly begin "go to your bed" in a room away from the front door. Once the behavior has been learned in that situation, move "the bed" closer to the goal area (e.g. across the room from the front door).
- Once the dog is consistently responding fluently to the cue in a quiet environment, presentation of the stimulus that causes the unwanted behavior at a low intensity can be introduced (DS). For example, if the dog barks every time someone comes to the door, have a known person walk up to the front door, and stand quietly without knocking. Before the dog reacts to the person, cue the dog to go to his bed. When he goes to his bed, immediately reward him. Often a remote reinforcement tool is beneficial.
- Gradually increase the intensity of the eliciting stimulus (DS) – have people approach the door, ring the bell, and enter. If the dog fails to perform the behavior at any stage, return to the previous level and concentrate on training at the level of stimulus intensity until the dog is responding correctly, every time, before progressing to the next stage.
- Once training and behavior modification have begun, it is important to manage situations to prevent the dog from continuing to practice the undesirable behavior. Training will progress much more quickly if the dog's opportunity to perform the unwanted behavior is eliminated. When someone comes to your door unexpectedly, prevent the dog from barking at the door by confining the dog in a room or crate when the guest

CHAPTER 9

first arrives. Bring the dog back out into the living area once everyone is settled.

More examples of RS:

Ask the pet owners what behavior they want the pet to do: Instead of ________ I would like him to __________.

- Instead of jumping on people I would like him to sit for greetings.
- Instead of begging at the table I would like him to go to his bed when we eat.
- Instead of jumping at the front door when the doorbell rings I would like him to go to his crate when he hears the doorbell.

Systematic desensitization

This is a technique used to reduce or eliminate a response (e.g. fear or aggression) to a stimulus (e.g. loud noise, strangers) through gradual and systematic exposure. The animal is trained to quiescence and relaxation before beginning the DS process. The stimulus is then introduced at a low intensity (i.e. recording of a noise at low intensity, stranger from a distance) and the animal is rewarded (CC) for relaxed behavior or performing an alternate behavior (RS). Once the animal has habituated to the stimulus at a low intensity, the intensity is systematically and gradually increased, and the procedure repeated.

Specific aspects of the stimulus are systematically added without causing a full or intense reaction in the animal.

This aspect of DS is often the most difficult because identifying the specific aspects of the stimulus and then placing them into a systematic hierarchy must be determined and extrapolated from watching the animal's body language and getting the pet owner's observations and input from past experiences.

Once the characteristics of the stimulus can be determined and are placed into a DS hierarchy, variables are added one at a time, decreasing one variable as another is added.

DS can be explained to pet owners by instructing them: "We are going to figure out, to the best of our ability, what characteristics of strangers bother 'Spot' the most. Then we are going to create a plan to introduce those aspects gradually and one at a time."

Requirements for the systematic desensitization program

To utilize DS properly the following must occur:

- Identify the cause of the fear.
- Reproduce the cause of the fear.
- Identify a starting point where the animal is not afraid (relaxed and still taking treats).
- Control the intensity of the fear-provoking stimulus.
- Control exposure to the fear-provoking stimulus (it does not occur spontaneously or randomly).

If the above criteria cannot be met, DS cannot be effectively applied and behavior modification should focus around CC and RS with combined pharmacological intervention. As other aspects of the treatment plan are successfully put into place, DS can be reconsidered (if still needed).

Creation of a systematic desensitization plan

The goal of DS is to increase tolerance to a stimulus. This is comparable to building a muscle; the patient may be slightly uncomfortable at times but learns that it can tolerate the stimulus at that specific level, even if slightly uncomfortable. At the next application of DS, the patient learns to tolerate a bit more as its tolerance "muscle" grows in size.

1. Identify characteristics and variables of the stimulus that influence the animal's stress level and response. This can increase your insight into the causes of the distress and make it easier to create an accurate hierarchy.

   Examples of possible variables:

   - Distance away from the stimulus.
   - Sound/loudness of the stimulus.
   - Speed/movement of the stimulus.
   - Specific characteristic of the stimulus.

   Example: "Spot" was diagnosed with fear-induced aggression toward unfamiliar men.

   Discuss with the pet owner the possible characteristics of unfamiliar men and ask the pet owner to rank the characteristics on a scale of 1–10, with 10 being a strong reaction.

2. Prioritize the characteristics into a graded (on a scale of 1–10, for example) stress hierarchy, and then break down those characteristics into manageable components. Place the characteristics that bother the animal the most at the end of the list.

   The stress hierarchy is a graded list of the situations related to the fear-provoking stimulus.

   Constructing an accurate hierarchy is very important as it provides the framework for approaching the problem. To create an accurate hierarchy, thought and discussion with the pet owner are critical as well as continual reevaluation based on the animal's response during DS.

First analyze the problem with the pet owner into situational components. Ask the pet owner, "What situation is the most difficult for Spot?" Constructing the stress hierarchy has its own therapeutic value by helping the pet owner analyze the pet's specific fears into an objective format, thereby increasing understanding of the problem and the specific triggers of that fear.

(a) Ask the pet owner to describe a situation in which Spot is least likely to respond aggressively to the stimulus (i.e. the least scary), and to describe the worst-case scenario the behavior would occur in (the most scary).

For example, Spot would not react to a familiar, dark-skinned, non-bearded man in shorts and a shirt at a distance of 100 ft while out on a walk in the neighborhood. Spot would be most upset by a bearded, light-skinned man, wearing a dark coat, sunglasses, and carrying an umbrella, at the front door in the evening.

Grade the characteristics on a scale of 1–10 (10 being the most difficult or upsetting) and place the items in order from the least upsetting to the most upsetting by asking the pet owner to think about each situation and rate the difficulty of that situation for the pet.

Begin with items so mild that they are practically nonfrightening. The smaller the steps, the faster the DS process goes. Raising a characteristic too quickly or adding multiple characteristics at once without decreasing other characteristics might cause the problem to worsen (actually sensitizing rather than desensitizing).

This ranked list of fear-evoking items constitutes the hierarchy that you will use in your treatment. Modifications, additions, combining of items, and further breaking down of items on the hierarchy may be made at any time during the desensitization therapy (Table 9.10).

3. Determine a non-stressful starting point.

Determine what contexts or interactions the animal can tolerate without a stress reaction. A good barometer that a characteristic has been increased too quickly is that the dog suddenly stops taking treats or starts roughly grabbing at the treat. Subtle body language signals, such as conflict and displacement behaviors (see Chapters 2 and 3), may also indicate the animal is starting to reach his threshold of tolerance for the situation. The animal might also begin to show a decrease in fluency (lack of precision, higher latency, slower speed) in response to a usually fluent cue. If a non-stressful starting point cannot be determined, DS cannot be properly applied and a non-stressful starting point may need to be created using drug desensitization first.

4. Create "practice" situations.

(a) Each characteristic should be increased individually, not simultaneously.

(b) As one characteristic is intensified, another characteristic may need to be temporarily lessened. For example, the patient may have learned to tolerate a stationary man in close proximity but when introducing a moving man, the distance from the patient should be increased.

(c) The intensity of each characteristic should be increased gradually – always striving to stay below the threshold for reactivity (see Figure 9.29) for the individual and preventing distress in the animal.

(d) Progression to the next level of intensity should be accomplished without eliciting undesirable behavior (i.e. noticing and looking at the stimulus is necessary, but a hard, tense stare is an indication that the level has been increased too quickly).

(e) Clicker training can be a very valuable tool in the desensitization process to influence the emotional response of the animal and mark desired behavioral responses.

A marker or clicker is extremely valuable in the desensitization process because it is possible to pinpoint the exact reinforceable moment, for example, the relaxation of a shoulder during desensitization of restraint. Probably the most important use of the clicker in behavior modification is in changing the animal's emotional state before it becomes distressed. It is possible to influence the animal's

Table 9.10 "Spot's" anxiety hierarchy for fear of men.

Characteristic of stimulus	Anxiety rating
Women	2
Carrying an object (book)	2
Dark clothing	6
Volume of voice	7
Light skin tone	8
Men with facial hair	9
Close proximity (3 ft)	10

In this DS plan for Spot's fear aggression toward men, the first stimulus to be incorporated would be a woman at a distance. Other variables are added according to the anxiety hierarchy without adding multiple variables at the same time.

reaction to the stimulus by clicking before it reaches his reactivity threshold or by clicking just as it begins to reach the threshold. In other words, click before the aggressive response occurs – the moment before it makes the decision to react can swing the animal away from previously learned behaviors (charging at the end of the leash, aggressing during restraint). At that point, the stimulus should not be increased but instead it might be decreased or maintained at that level.

Helpful hints:

- The smaller the steps, the faster the progress made.
- DS always "works" when applied properly. If progress is not being made, likely multiple variables are being added simultaneously, variables are being raised too quickly, the characteristics of the stimulus were not prioritized properly, or a non-stressful starting point was not determined.
- Think about what you are about to do and decrease it by 50%.
- Implementing systematic desensitization inconsistently or too rapidly can cause the problem to worsen.

Behavior modification conclusion

A combination of the behavior modification techniques is almost always occurring simultaneously, but it is important for the veterinary technician to be able to tease aspects of those techniques out of the treatment plan to properly understand and then be able to explain them to the pet owner.

For instance, a dog that has had an adverse emotional response to a nail trim in the past can quickly be taught to target its paw to a hand while being clicked and treated (operant and classical counter conditioning), therefore changing the emotional response of the event (having the feet touched). The paw is gradually held for longer lengths of time in the hand. When pressure on the paw is added, the length of time the paw is held is decreased (DS).

Drug desensitization

The goal of drug desensitization is to address the suspected pathologic dysfunction of the neurotransmitter system leading to or worsening the problem behavior or behavior disorder.

Antianxiety medications (not sedatives) are administered to the animal at a high enough level to prevent the fear reaction to the stimuli. The intensity of the stimuli may stay the same, but there is a gradual reduction of the drug over time so that the animal becomes gradually more aware of the frightening stimuli.

Drug desensitization is used when the intensity of the stimulus cannot be controlled, a non-stressful starting point cannot be identified, or when there are too many frightening stimuli to use systematic desensitization.

Additionally, it can help to make behavior modification easier to apply, giving the owner a starting point for desensitization, and improving compliance and treatment success (see Chapter 10).

Systematic desensitization and drug desensitization can be used simultaneously.

Other

Interruption of behavior

Interrupting behavior is *not* meant to teach a specific behavior or to punish a behavior but is used to temporarily stop a behavior so that an alternative cue can be given. If a behavior is not disrupted before giving another cue, the behaviors may be inadvertently chained together (i.e. stimulus outside becomes cue to bark and the barking becomes the cue to go to the mat). If behavior is interrupted, it is less likely that behaviors will be chained.

Interruptions could include softly clapping hands, patting your leg, making a kissy-kissy sound, or picking up a dragline to get the dog's attention. The interruption should not elicit fear or panic in the animal. It should be performed in a nonconfrontational manner and be just enough to get the pet's attention and interrupt the thought process so that another cue for an alternative behavior can be given.

Cease punishment

Pet owners should also stop all scolding or physical punishment. Punishment is likely to increase or cause fear. Fear produces unpredictable side effects and rarely the desired effects. Punishment is comparable to a bomb going off; unpredictable and unfocused damage is caused with collateral damage occurring in the process. Especially pet owner-applied punishment (i.e. scolding, physical punishment, dominance techniques) is detrimental and counterproductive to any treatment plan.

As it is nearly impossible for pet owners to apply punishment correctly, such punishment becomes unpredictable, increasing stress. Instead of using punishment, pet owners should be taught to set the pet up through environmental management (antecedent arrangement) to make it less likely for the undesired behaviors to occur and when necessary, gently interrupt behavior and use response substitution to cue another behavior.

Remote punishment

Remote punishment involves the application of an aversive stimulus without the pet owner being present.

As discussed previously, punishment should not be associated with the pet owner (or another person or stimulus) and must occur when the behavior occurs and must occur every time the behavior occurs. The remote punishment should not be operated by the pet owner but instead only be activated by the pet's behavior (i.e. cans falling off counter when the pet investigates the counter).

Side effects for remote punishment remain the same as with other punishment. Inadvertent associations can be made, including fear of sounds or fear of entering the space where the punishment occurred.

The primary advantage of remote punishment is that it is less likely that the pet owner will be associated with the punishment. Therefore, the pet should learn to cease the behavior even when the pet owner is absent (Landsberg et al. 2013). Rarely, if ever, should a remote punishment technique be necessary if appropriate environmental management has been implemented.

Euthanasia or rehoming

Euthanasia may be a responsible and appropriate decision when the quality of life for the pet, the pet owner, or other pets in the home is poor, or when animals and people are at risk for serious emotional and physical harm, and treatment is not a viable option. It is a complex decision that the veterinarian will make along with the pet owner after obtaining an extensive history and possible referral to a veterinary behavior specialist.

The veterinarian may recommend rehoming as an option if the pet's behavior problem or disorder is not likely to persist or worsen in a new home or if the environment in the new home can be controlled in such a way that triggers are no longer an issue (i.e. a home without other pets or a home with no children).

If the pet owner is not at peace with the decision, then the owner should be given the option of a behavior consultation with a veterinary behaviorist. Additional support from an appropriate mental health professional within the community should also be offered to the client.

Grief counseling of client

Chapter 5 detailed grief counseling for pet owners. Grief will occur whether the pet owner is euthanizing, rehoming the pet, or when accepting the pet they have. Grief is a process that the veterinary technician may be able to assist the pet owner through, being aware of grief that is not progressing, and being able to refer the pet owner to an appropriate mental health professional when needed.

The practical applications of behavior modification

Foundation behaviors

Foundation behaviors are trained behaviors that are likely to be required to successfully apply the prescribed behavior modification techniques. These behaviors and skills are useful to teach any animal (with species modifications) and should be included in all preventive behavior plans (i.e. puppy and kitten classes).

Targeting

Targeting is a very useful behavior tool and can be used in many applications of behavior modification. How to shape targeting has been discussed earlier in this chapter.

Target to hand

Targeting to the handler's hand can be cued when a potential problem stimulus (i.e. unknown animal or person) is seen by the handler and used as a prompt to turn the pet away from the stimulus before it can react (emergency U-turn) (Video 7.19). Once turned, fast-paced loose leash walking with numerous sits and turns can be added to increase the distance from the stimulus. A hand target should not be used when the patient is overly aroused or has a history of redirecting bites.

- A hand target should not be used when the patient is overly aroused or has a history of redirecting bites.

Targeting to a hand is also useful for teaching loose leash walking. The hand can be presented as a prompt to help show the dog the desired position of walking beside a person.

Hand target recall

Very frequently the pet owner's recall cue has been "poisoned" and associated with a negative emotional event. This can happen inadvertently. For example, a dog that shows signs of separation anxiety may begin to associate being called in from outside with the owner's departure. The owner lets the dog outside to eliminate just before leaving the home. The dog is called inside and then the owner leaves.

In instances where the recall cue has been "poisoned," the behavior must be retaught using a new cue. If targeting has a strong positive emotional response, it can be used to prompt the recall behavior. Later, should the handler so desire, the cue for the recall can be changed to a different cue, such as a whistle or novel verbal cue.

Attention

Attention is really another targeting skill, targeting of the eyes to the handler. Eye contact can be captured and shaped (Video 7.17). The behavior of making eye contact may need first to be desensitized if in the past eye contact was discouraged or if the animal is not comfortable with looking directly at the owner. Initially, any eye contact is C/T. Once it is predictable it can be placed on cue. Distractions and duration can be added systematically to the behavior.

Offered eye contact (without a cue from the pet owner) to the owner on walks and during training is a behavior that should be highly reinforced throughout the life of the dog. When working with a dog that displays reactivity to stimuli, the owner should be coached to mark and reinforce offered eye contact in a variety of contexts even without distractions present. The dog quickly learns *offering* calm attention to his owner results in good things. A verbal cue, such as "Eyes" or "Watch," should also be taught because this can be beneficial when playing a game of opposites; "Look" and "Watch" (see subsequent text).

- Offered eye contact (without a cue from the pet owner) to the owner on walks and during training is a behavior that should be highly reinforced throughout the life of the dog.

Game of opposites: "look" and "watch"

Just as people notice changes in the environment, so do dogs. It is natural for all animals to notice a sudden change in the environment. This awareness is a natural survival mechanism and it keeps us safe. We notice it, assess the threat, and then usually recognize the stimulus as nothing to worry about. For example, you are sitting in a coffee shop and you see a person walk in the front door, you assess the situation and as long as the person appears to be of no threat, you return to your conversation. Some dogs are anxious and unsure about certain stimuli in the environment and assess what we would consider non-threatening stimuli as a threat. Initially expecting a dog to just ignore and look away from such stimuli is impractical and perhaps impossible for the dog.

Teaching a game of opposites, "look" and "watch," can help change the dog's emotional response to stimuli. These cues will initially be taught in a non-distracting environment using capturing and shaping and should not be associated with the presence of triggers during the early stages of training. They are a pair of opposite behaviors. "Look" will be used to mean look at something away from the handler and "watch" will mean look at the handler. A directional cue (finger point) may be useful with "look" in order to indicate what direction the dog is to look. *Control Unleashed* by Leslie McDevitt is a great resource for teaching the skills and adding in distractions systematically.

Initially the handler will use the cues "look" and "watch" in a variety of contexts within the house and yard and with inanimate objects such as a toy or chair. Once the dog has learned the cues and CC to the fear-provoking stimulus has already occurred on walks, the owner can ping-pong back and forth between "look" and "watch" (and other known cues) in the context of previous triggers.

Default looking at stimuli and offered eye contact (without a cue or prompt from the handler) should still be rewarded as well but eventually they will be placed on a variable ratio of reinforcement. Stimulus control with the cues is not realistic or expected. The dog will still look at the handler at times and will notice things in his environment whether cued to do so or not.

Ultimately, if the owner is consistent with marking and reinforcing for the sight of triggers, two things will start to happen. First, the dog will begin to anticipate earning a C/T for the presence or sound of a stimulus/distraction and will begin to anticipate the stimuli/distraction as an opportunity for reinforcement. This moment often occurs when the click is delayed slightly. The dog looks at the stimulus and then turns toward the pet owner, curious as to why it was not clicked for seeing the stimulus. This turning away from the stimulus should be highly rewarded. The second side effect is that the dog will start to look for triggers not because he is worried or concerned, but because it has become a game; the motivation of the behavior has changed. This change in the emotional response will also be evident in the body language of the dog. Review Videos 7.18, 9.8, and 9.10 on the companion website.

Basic cued behaviors – sit, down, come, loose leash walking

Cued behaviors are critical for applying and building on any behavior modification plan. When a patient has no available handler-given on-cue behaviors such as sit or down, the behavior technician must begin by teaching cued behaviors that can be used in later aspects of the treatment plan (i.e. RS and DS).

The ability to successfully cue a behavior that produces a reliable response will be necessary any time the pet owner needs to assist the pet when it is unsure what to do or before it reacts to a stimulus. Without handler-given cued behaviors it is difficult to communicate to the animal an alternative method for getting out of a situation.

For example, a frightening stimulus is approaching in the distance, the pet owner can cue other behaviors like "look" or "touch" and then cue fast-paced walking, while increasing distance from the stimulus with quick turns and sits (or a combination of behaviors). Initially the steady flow of information is a distraction from the frightening stimulus. Later, as the dog's anxiety decreases, the learning history becomes, "I can do this and get reinforced AND the scary things weren't so scary after all."

Practice tip: These cues and fast-paced walking should be practiced often without any triggers present. Otherwise, the owners change in pace and quick cues will become a predictor of stimuli in the environment.

• Practice tip: These cues and fast-paced walking should be practiced often without any triggers present. Otherwise, the owners change in pace and quick cues will become a predictor of stimuli in the environment.

The veterinary technician often teaches the pet owner how to train the basic cued behaviors of targeting, watch, look, come, sit, down, and loose leash walking. Techniques for capturing and shaping, adding a cue and basic fluency should be covered and written materials should be provided for the owner to refer to. Cued behaviors will be used during CRR (cue→response→reward) interactions, RS, DS, and to guide pet owners in focusing on what behavior they want the pet to DO rather than undesirable behavior.

Only the behaviors that are required to apply the treatment plan should be taught at the initial consultation to keep from overwhelming the pet owner. Later, the veterinarian and veterinary technician should refer the pet owner to the veterinary hospital's qualified trainer for further training.

Before training foundation behaviors, the veterinary technician should determine by discussion with the pet owner and by assessing the animal's body language if a previous cue for any of these behaviors has been "poisoned" (see cueing). If so, a different type of cue should be used to reteach the behavior.

Place – go to a specific location

Teaching a dog or cat to go to a specific location is useful as a preventive tool as discussed in Chapter 7 but stationing will also be utilized during many behavior modification exercises. It should be noted that teaching an animal to go to a "place" is not the same as teaching relaxation, a Treat-Ment station, or safe place, although "place" is frequently used in the shaping of some of these behaviors. These other stationing behaviors are used for specific contexts, such as promoting relaxation, working on cooperative care training, or safe place training for noise aversions. Specifically, go to a place might be used in a desensitization program with an animal that has separation anxiety, fear, and aggression toward other animals in the home, or for situations when the dog needs to be managed away from the owner.

Shaping "place" example:

- Place a nonslip mat on the floor as a target.
- Mark the animal for looking or turning its head toward the mat; toss the treat toward the mat.
- Mark the animal for any movement toward the mat; toss the treat past the mat.
- Mark as the animal turns from picking up the treat and turns toward the mat; toss the treat onto the mat.
- Mark for 2 ft on the mat, toss the treat off the mat.

- Mark for 3 or 4 ft on the mat, toss the treat off the mat.
- Once the animal is readily going to the mat cue a "down" (taught in a previous session), mark and toss the treat off the mat.
- Fade out the verbal cue "down" by waiting for the dog to offer the behavior before the C/T.
- Once the dog is readily offering the behavior of going to the mat and lying down, the cue "place" can be added.
- Fluency of the "down" on the mat can be gradually shaped by working on distractions, duration, and distance.

Video 9.3 on the companion website demonstrates teaching a place cue utilizing a remote treat dispenser. In this example, once the behavior can be prompted with the chime from the dispenser, the verbal cue is added.

Relaxation

Foundation skills needed: "Down," "Go to your Mat"

Training tools needed:

- A portable mat, different from a favorite bed or a place previously used to teach "place." The new mat will initially be the cue for relaxation. Later the cue will be transferred to the verbal cue "relax" (or whatever cue is chosen).
- Leash.

Teaching relaxation can be added to "place" but is different in that the focus is on shaping relaxation rather than going to a specific location. "Relax" can then be generalized to multiple environments, even when the mat or "place" is not available; for example, on a walk or during thunderstorms.

Because the clicker can cause a strong emotional response of excitement, the clicker may not be effective in shaping relaxation with all dogs.

Teaching to relax on cue is a behavior that can be included in many aspects of behavior modification and should be considered a foundation skill. Relaxation can become a default offered behavior when the dog is unsure of what to do and should become a problem prevention tool taught early in the dog's life. The following protocol was modified from *Chill Out Fido* by Nan Arthur.

1. Ask the pet owner what the dog looks like when it is most relaxed. That will be the behavior that is shaped. The position described by the pet owner can also be captured by C/T when the dog assumes the position but the following shaping should occur to teach deep relaxation in many situations and environments.
2. With the dog out of the room, scatter 5–10 treats on the mat, ensuring a positive response to the mat.
3. Bring the dog into the room on leash and passively allow him to investigate the treats on the mat. Begin every relaxation training session in the same manner. The leash may be held or dropped and stepped on. The leash restriction is used to associate relaxation with the leash and also keeps the dog from wandering during the training session.
4. As the dog eats the treats off the mat, drop a few more treats onto the mat; as the dog begins to eat those treats, drop one treat at a time between the dog's front paws, also on the mat. Quietly dropping the treats rather than treating from the hand should occur because being given a treat from the hand overly excites some dogs. Dropping the treat also prompts the dog to lower its head.
5. It was noted previously that a clicker is not usually recommended when training relaxation because excitement is often an emotional response to the clicker. Instead, use a quietly spoken word as the marker, a quiet verbally spoken "good" could be the marker, for example. Begin by first assuming a relaxed position yourself. Do not interact with the dog; become completely disengaged from the dog. Pretend the dog is invisible.
6. Once the dog begins interacting with the mat do not reinforce the dog for staring at you. Reward instead when he diverts his attention away from you. Begin reinforcing for sniffing the mat or otherwise disengaging from you.
7. Once the dog begins to understand that less activity is being reinforced, begin shaping for less intense behavior such as less intense sniffing, sitting, lying down, or lowering head, and marking the behavior with the verbal "good" and treat. It should also be noted that a treat lower on the reinforcement hierarchy may be the best treat of choice, creating less excitement. Excitement is counterproductive to shaping relaxation.
8. Next begin shaping for more obvious signs of relaxation. A yawn or deep breath can be captured. Reinforce as close and quietly to the dog's front feet as possible, reinforcing lowering of the head.
9. Practice with the leash on the dog with you standing, which teaches the dog to relax on leash while you are standing. Place the behavior on a cue ("chill," "relax," etc.).

10. Transfer the cue of the sight of the mat to the verbal cue. Practice the exercise with the dog on leash but without the mat present. Give the new verbal cue, pause, present the mat, and continue transferring the cue as previously described.
11. Generalize and train to fluency.

Applications of behavior modification

The following exercises are examples of behavior modification exercises that may be included in a prescribed treatment plan. The discussed techniques are only examples of how the behavior modification exercises might be applied. The veterinary technician may need to modify the exercises for each patient and situation and communicate any significant modifications to the veterinarian. Significant changes may indicate a change in the treatment plan is required.

As the patient and pet owner progress through treatment, the techniques may be modified at follow-up appointments. All aspects of CC/RS/DS should be reviewed before applying these techniques.

Behavior and environmental modification for unfamiliar people in the home

Foundation skills needed: Comfortable in a confinement area out of sight of the door and on leash in the house, at least three behaviors on cue, basket muzzle conditioning, learning history of being marked and reinforced for offering attention to the owner and also noticing stimuli, settle on a mat.

Possible training tools needed: A remote reward system is very helpful for reinforcing at a distance. Leash and collar, basket muzzle, mat, special treats. A head halter may be required for some dogs for extra safety.

When addressing behavior modification with unfamiliar people in the home, it can be broken down into three specific exercises. Success with level 1 must be accomplished prior to beginning the level 2 exercise. Once success has continued with levels 1 and 2, the final level 3 exercise might be considered.

Level 1 exercise for addressing unfamiliar people in the home avoids the front door or the dog seeing people come into the home. There is often a rich learning history associated with visitors entering the home and overcoming that learning will take time. Thus, instead of starting with that aspect, the dog is managed out of sight of the door when guests arrive. The level 1 exercise should be routinely practiced (daily if possible) without any visitors to the home. The dog and pet owner must be comfortable with the exercise. If the setup is only performed when there is a visitor, the dog will learn the setup predicts unfamiliar people. Make the training session mundane by practicing it often without any visitors.

Environmental modifications include avoiding visualization outside the home (consider window film to prevent the practicing of territorial barking). Use white noise and/or acoustic therapy to minimize outside noises that might prompt a response from the dog. Avoid negative associations with visitors in the home during the treatment period. If the pet owner cannot focus on the training, the dog should be safely managed out of sight.

Do these exercises with the dog on leash and collar for safety and keep the dog under the handler's control. Use a basket muzzle to minimize the risk of injury prior to close contact with unfamiliar people.

Level 1 exercise for behavior modification for unfamiliar people in the home – Gradual introductions

1. The dog should be comfortable being confined briefly in a room or crate out of sight of the owner. Daily the owner should practice cuing the dog to go to the confinement area and give the dog a few treats or a puzzle feeder. Utilize calming music and a white noise machine to dampen sounds outside of the room.
2. Next, while the dog is in his confinement area, the owner pretends to invite a guest into the home by opening the door and verbally acknowledging and inviting an imaginary guest into the home. Instruct the owner to place a box or novel object in a chair or seat where a guest might sit.
3. Once the "guest" has come in, the owner returns to the dog. If the dog is barking, ideally the pet owner should wait for the dog to settle slightly before returning to the dog. The owner should place the dog's collar and leash (and muzzle if indicated and properly conditioned) and do a warm-up marker training session in the confinement area. The owner is assessing the dog's stress level based on body language, response to cues, and treat consumption.
4. The owner then takes the dog on leash throughout the house while training. The three markable (C/T) moments are: responding to a known cue, offering unprompted attention to

the handler/owner, and noticing stimuli (the box or novel object) on the chair.

5. After a few weeks of completing this exercise without a visitor, then a familiar person the dog is comfortable with would be added into the training. For example, if the spouse of the pet owner is out of the house, she would call when she is five minutes away. The pet owner would place the dog in his confinement area. The spouse would use the entrance a guest would use and sit in a chair and ignore the dog while the pet owner trains the dog around the person who just returned.
6. Maintain the fluency of this exercise with doing "mock" (i.e. no person arriving) visits at least two times a week.
7. Work up to less familiar guests. Guests should ignore and avoid threatening body language (approaching, staring, leaning over, or reaching for the dog). Guests should not pet the dog.
8. The majority of treats should come from residents of the home and not guests. Expose the dog on leash and at a distance from guests such that he is not reactive. Use treats for classical counter conditioning (changing of a negative emotion to a positive emotion). Keep the dog busy with various cues. Mark and treat the dog for looking at the guest and offering autofocus on the handler. Reward nonreactivity. Foster positive rather than neutral associations.
9. Gradually reduce the distance from guests without reactivity over several training sessions. Use the distance away from guests and visual barriers (furniture, hallway, kitchen island) to lessen reactivity (fear, anxiety, or aggression). The dog should get more and more comfortable visualizing people from a distance while on leash. End the session on a good note and after a short positive exposure session, place the dog away to prevent a negative experience.
10. Gradually, the duration out in the environment (under control of a leash) may be increased with specific visitors to the home. The dog might be able to settle on his mat near the owner for short periods of time or in an exercise pen, on a secure tether, or behind a secure baby gate. Guests should be instructed not to approach the dog. If there is any concern for aggression, the dog should wear a basket muzzle prior to close contact with unfamiliar people in the home.

Video 9.4 on the companion website demonstrates this Level 1 introduction process.

Once the owner and dog are successful with the Level 1 exercises, they may opt to work on teaching an alternate behavior for the arrival signal. Depending on the living situation, the arrival signal might be a doorbell, knock, phone call or ding, the creak of a gate opening, or intercom. Many dogs pair the arrival signal with guests' arrival after just a few pairings. Common behaviors triggered by the arrival signal, which owners often find problematic, include the dog running to the door, barking, and jumping at the door. The stress and excitement level on hearing the arrival signal can rise quickly making it difficult for the owner to successfully redirect the dog or for the dog to be present cognitively. Level 2 teaches the dog to perform a new behavior when they hear the arrival signal. Conditioning the dog to do an alternate behavior in response to the signal can make everyday management easier for the pet owner and dog.

Level 2 exercise for behavior modification for unfamiliar people in the home – Transfer the arrival signal to an alternate behavior

1. The first step is to determine the alternate behavior for the dog to perform. Traditionally, teaching the dog to go to a place has been used as an alternate behavior. This can be the most challenging and should only be used once success with earlier phases of training has been accomplished. Remaining stationary on a location can be destressing for a dog if they are encountering a fear-evoking stimulus. Other options can be to grab a toy and run to the owner or go to a room, crate in another room, or a backdoor to be released into a secured backyard.
2. Teach the alternate behavior and put it on cue and generalize the behavior.
3. Then transfer the cue (see section **Transferring cues** in this chapter) to the arrival signal by recording the arrival signal and introducing it in a novel location (i.e. not in the house). Play the new cue/arrival signal. Follow it immediately with the known cue for the alternate behavior. Reinforce the dog for performing the behavior. Repeat 10 times.
4. Start to pause for one or two seconds after giving the arrival signal and see if the dog starts to perform the behavior. If not, give the known cue. Continue working on transferring the cue over several sessions until the dog can respond to the arrival signal with starting to perform the desired behavior.

During the learning process, dismantling the arrival signal is necessary to prevent continued practicing of the undesired behavior and to assist with the transfer of the cue. If possible, it is best to install a new arrival signal. Wireless doorbell systems are inexpensive and easy to install and often offer a variety of sounds to choose from, thus making it a novel sound. If using the existing arrival signal expect the training process to take longer as there is a learning history associated with it. Video 9.5 on the companion website illustrates the process of teaching an alternative behavior for the arrival signal and transferring the cue.

The final behavior modification exercise (Level 3) to consider for addressing unfamiliar visitors in the home is the door exercise. This will be the most challenging exercise for the dog. Generally, owners should have made progress with Level 1 and 2 before doing the door exercise. The following exercise should be controlled with the dog on leash and collar for safety. A basket muzzle can minimize the risk of injury prior to close contact with unfamiliar people. The premise of this exercise is to teach the dog to be relaxed at the door and have a positive association with the space and people appearing on the other side.

Level 3 exercise for behavior modification for unfamiliar people in the home – Training at the door:

1. Teach the dog to do a stationary behavior (sit or down) at the door for a food treat without any visitors at the door. If a place or settle mat has been trained it can be used for this exercise. It may also be beneficial to do practice sessions at an interior door or a back door where there has been less learning history, especially if the front door of the house is too exciting initially.
2. Several times during the day, go to the door, ask the dog to perform a stationary behavior, and offer a food reward for a correct response.
3. Next, with the dog in a stationary position at the door, jiggle the doorknob or crack the door, and reinforce the dog for remaining in position. The dog should be on leash prior to opening the door or a barrier should be in place to avoid accidental escapes from the property. If the dog gets up during a repetition, do not respond or reprimand him. With the next repetition, decrease the stimulus; touch or reach for the door handle rather than jiggling it.
4. Eventually, work up to being able to open and close the door without visitors there and reward the dog for remaining in position.
5. Repeat the above but add a light knock before you open and close the door.
6. Gradually, you can increase the intensity of the knock with the dog remaining stationary.
7. Next, start with someone familiar to the dog at a distance (20 ft) from the door. Repeat steps 1–6 but acknowledge the person's presence. Say "Hello," the other person should respond accordingly. If the dog remains stationary, mark and treat and close the door.
8. Gradually the person's distance from the door may be reduced each time the door is closed. Start with the person about 20 ft away, and gradually reduce the distance to 19 ft, 18 ft, etc. while repeating the above exercise.
9. Eventually, the person should be able to stop 6 ft away from the door. The handler should reinforce the dog for remaining in position.
10. Once the dog is comfortable and successful with several familiar people, repeat the above exercise with less familiar people.

It is advised to do only one to four repetitions before giving the dog a mini break and walking away from the door.

Video 9.6 on the companion website exemplifies the door exercise training process.

Introducing a muzzle or head halter

Training a dog to wear a basket muzzle or head halter utilizes the same techniques and will be used interchangeably in the following text.

A pet owner may be instructed to acclimate their dog to wearing a muzzle or head halter if the dog has a well-established bite history, or if the owner is in doubt of their ability to manipulate the environment so that the dog can remain below his threshold consistently.

A basket muzzle can be used to reduce the risk of injury. A head halter can be used to redirect a dog that is reactive to a stimulus. The basket muzzle and head halter are not a treatment for aggressive behavior because they do not change the underlying motivation. They are used as a management and safety tool while implementing behavior modification. They serve to minimize injury if an incident should occur and can be used as a step in many DS processes. For example, when the dog has been DS to a stimulus while behind a gate but the next step of the behavior modification plan involves the dog being on leash and moving more freely in the home, having a basket muzzle on the dog allows for increased safety. It is comparable to the dog wearing a "moving" gate. Steps to classical (counter) condition and desensitize the dog to a basket muzzle or head halter:

1. Short training sessions that last five minutes or less are best.
2. Take the basket muzzle out and put cheese or peanut butter inside the basket so the dog is prompted to stick his nose in to lick the treat out. This is to assist with creating a positive conditioned emotional response to the muzzle.
3. Lower the muzzle down to your side and allow the dog to approach and stick his nose in on his own. Keep your hand still and allow the dog to approach. NEVER reach forward with the muzzle (or head halter nose loop); instead let the dog push his nose into the muzzle. Reaching forward toward the dog is likely to make the dog back away.
4. If the dog is wary and will not approach the muzzle, place a leash on the muzzle, so the dog cannot pick it up and run away with it, and place the muzzle on the floor. Begin marking and reinforcing for targeting the muzzle on the floor. C/T for any interaction. Once interacting with the muzzle has become an opportunity for reinforcement, begin again at step 3.
5. The muzzle or head halter should disappear along with all attention and treats. Ignore the dog for 15–30 seconds. Bring the muzzle/head halter out and resume attention and treats again; the dog should become excited when he sees the basket muzzle or head halter, indicating CC has occurred.
6. After the dog is showing excitement when you get the muzzle out and readily pushing his nose into the muzzle to eat the treats, you may start placing the strap around the back of his head.
7. An alternate step is to mark and reward the dog for putting his nose in the muzzle or head halter nose loop as an offered behavior (without food to prompt him). This step can be incorporated once the classical conditioning component has occurred.
8. After attaching the neck strap, it is important to give the dog treats through the muzzle. Canned cheese is ideal for this.
9. The muzzle and head halter should be incorporated into a variety of activities to prevent them from becoming a predictor of potential stressful situations. If the muzzle or head halter are only used when visitors come to the home or the dog goes to the veterinarian, the positive association may be diminished.

Video 9.7 on the companion website introduces methods to condition a dog to a muzzle.

Behavior modification for exposure to a person, animal, or other stimulus on a walk

The requirements to apply behavior modification are the same regardless of the stimulus. This approach uses a systematic approach to addressing the dog's reactivity to stimuli and breaks the components into four possible stages of training. We use the acronym ACES (Figure 9.23) to illustrate the four stages.

Foundation skills: marker training, watch, look, target/touch, sit or down, fast-paced heeling, and emergency U-turns (Let's go and leash pressure cue).

Possible training tools needed: Clicker and treats, a well-fitted collar or harness, and a 4 to 6 ft leash, possibly a head halter and/or basket muzzle or double leash system for extra safety.

The first step is working on *associations*. The goal is that stimuli become associated with earning really good stuff. The focus is on classical counter conditioning (i.e. changing the conditioned emotional response) but it also includes the marking of operant behavior. A marker or clicker is used to help pinpoint the exact moment the dog earns the reinforcer.

On these association walks the owner is instructed to focus on clicking and treating two things.

1. The first is offered "check ins" with the owner. Whenever the dog looks at the handler, the dog is marked and treated.
2. The second context that is a "markable" moment is when the dog notices stimuli in the environment. The key is to click or mark the alert or noticing of stimuli in the environment. This should occur before the dog escalates his reaction. Non-reactivity earns reinforcement. Handlers or owners should maintain a substantial distance

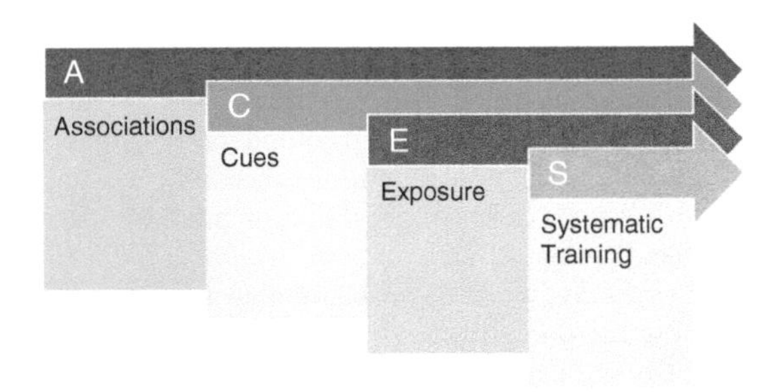

Figure 9.23 ACES: the components of behavior modification for reactivity to stimuli on walks.

between the dog and stimuli. The goal at this point is not to get close to the stimuli but instead have brief exposure to stimuli from a distance that does not elicit reactivity from the dog. The focus is on new positive associations to occur on walks.

For example, a dog has a history of barking and pulling on leash with the sight of unfamiliar people and/or dogs on walks when the stimulus is a half block away. The handler would start with marking/clicking the first instance the dog notices a stimulus. The owner is walking the dog and notices the dog's ears perk forward and fixation of the gaze in the direction of a person getting out of a car about a block away. The handler/owner should mark/click the instant the dog notices the stimulus and then give the dog a high-value treat. Treats may be given every one to two seconds or continuously as the dog navigates past the stimuli. Alternately, the handler/owner may elect to change direction to avoid further arousal or escalation of the undesirable behavior (this will depend on the individual dog). Since the dog will already be conditioned to the clicker, it should be expected that upon hearing the click, the dog will orient towards the handler/owner for the reinforcer. If the dog is unable to reorient after hearing the click, that is information to the owner that the dog is too distracted by the stimulus. The owner will need to redirect the dog and get further away from the stimulus. If a non-stressful starting point cannot be identified, medication will likely need to be considered.

- If the dog is unable to reorient after hearing the click, that is information to the owner that the dog is too distracted by the stimulus. The owner will need to redirect the dog and get further away from the stimulus.

Ultimately, if the handler/owner is consistent with marking and reinforcing for the sight of stimuli, two things will start to happen; one the dog will begin to anticipate earning a click and treat for the presence or sound of a stimulus. The owner will often report that when they are late on clicking the presence of a stimulus, the dog will turn and look at them like, hey where is my click? The second side effect is that the dog will start to look for triggers not because he needs to be vigilant, but because it has become a game; the motivation of the behavior has changed. This will also be evident in the body language of the dog when it notices stimuli. Distractions and stimuli have become an opportunity to receive a reward from the owner. Video 9.8 on the companion website illustrates capturing offered attention to the handler and noticing stimuli.

While owners are working on associations, they can also work on teaching the *Cues*: "Look," "Eyes/Watch," "Touch," "Let's go" and a tactile cue of leash pressure. These cues should be taught in a non-distracting environment initially and should not be associated with the presence of triggers during the initial training phase. They are a pair of opposite behaviors ("Look" and "Eyes/Watch"), a target behavior ("Touch"), and a tactile cue (leash pressure), and/or a verbal cue, "Let's go." "Look" will be used to mean look at something away from the owner. A directional cue (finger point) might also be added with "Look" to indicate which direction the dog is to look. "Eyes" or "Watch" will mean look at the handler for reinforcement. "Touch" cues the dog to touch its nose to the handler's hand/palm. The touch cue is not recommended to be used with a dog that has displayed redirected aggression towards the handler. "Let's go" will mean go with the handler on leash. Leash pressure or tension on the leash will first be classically conditioned with treats and then operantly conditioned to be a cue to go in the direction of the pressure. Visit the companion website to watch Videos 7.18 (Look, Eyes, Touch), 7.19 (Touch), 9.9 (leash pressure cue).

These behaviors can all be taught with clicker training using capturing and/or shaping. Once on cue, the owner will use the cues in a variety of contexts within the house and yard, with inanimate objects such as a toy or chair, and when possible, with neutral or positive stimuli (i.e. a person or animal with whom the dog lives and has a good relationship with).

Once the dog has learned these cues and the dog has started to associate stimuli with earning a click/treat (associations exercise), the owner may now start to incorporate some of these cues during *exposure* walks. They will ping-pong back and forth between, look, eyes, let's go, and touch (and other known cues) throughout the walk and also in the presence of previous stimuli for undesirable behavior. The touch cue can be given as the owner pivots to change direction or to redirect the dog while walking past a stimulus. Owners should practice these cues throughout the walk without stimuli present that would induce reactivity. Default (offered or uncued) looks and eye contact in the presence of a distraction should still be reinforced. Video 9.10 on the companion website illustrates putting this into action.

There are *systematic training* exercises utilizing desensitization and counter conditioning (operant and classical) with a controlled stimulus which can be very valuable as part of a treatment plan for addressing reactivity to stimuli on walks. These training exercises are more important when the dog needs to be introduced to another dog or person. Controlled setups are required to implement these exercises because the stimulus needs to be able to be controlled. Common exercises include: Stimulus stationary – desensitization and classical and operant counter conditioning to a stationary stimulus (patient moving and stimulus stationary); Moving together – desensitization and classical and operant counter conditioning to a moving stimulus (patient and stimulus moving); Stimulus approach – desensitization and classical and operant counter conditioning to the approach of a stimulus while the dog patient is stationary.

With the stimulus present but stationary, utilize desensitization, classical counter conditioning, and response substitution. This step may be explained to the owner with the analogy – "If you were afraid of spiders would it be easier for you to approach the spider or have the spider approach you?" It is usually less stressful to approach the stimulus then to have the stimulus approach you. Gradually decrease the dog's distance from the stimulus while performing fast-paced walking, turns, look, watch, and sit. Simultaneously reward the dog with high-value reinforcements (classical counter conditioning) frequently after each behavior (Figure 9.24). Utilize inanimate objects, familiar people/dogs, and working in a familiar environment before working with a real trigger for the dog. For the owner and the dog to be successful in a distracting or slightly stressful situation, they need to be fluent with the exercise through routine practice with neutral or pleasant stimuli. For a video example of this exercise, visit the companion website and watch Video 9.11.

Note: Each step will involve several repetitions. With the reset for another repetition, start again at the same starting point. With successive repetitions the ending point will be gradually closer to the goal behavior. Varying the difficulty level is beneficial to incorporate some very easy repetitions. Thus, the exercise does not seem to always be getting more and more difficult.

Once the dog is comfortable working around the stationary stimulus from a distance of 8–10 ft, increase the distance from the stimulus and now incorporate some slow movement by the stimulus. The stimulus still stays in place but shifts their weight or walks in place, while the dog works closer to them. After success at this step with the dog remaining calm, nonreactive, and able to easily respond to known cues at a distance of 8–10 ft, progress to the next behavior modification exercise, Moving together.

The Moving together exercise incorporates the stimulus and the dog/handler simultaneously walking parallel with each other or in concentric circles and at a distance that the dog is relaxed. Gradually the distance from each other can be reduced but it should be done at a pace that allows the dog to remain calm. Each time the handler cues the dog to perform a stationary behavior, the distraction person should also slow down or stop moving. Variations of the same exercises, adding in other stimuli, may be repeated as needed, before progressing to the final step. Watch Video 9.12 on the companion website for an example of the Moving together exercise.

The final behavior modification exercise is Stimulus approach; the patient remains stationary with the handler and the stimulus gradually approaches. This usually is much more difficult for the dog. Begin with the patient in a sit or down position by the pet owner and directly facing the stimulus. Sit is usually easier at this point but if the down position is associated with previously taught relaxation it may be the behavior of choice. Ideally, relaxation has been previously taught and can then be used during this step. The distraction person or stimulus is at a non-stressful starting point. The handler cues "sit" which cues the distraction person to begin slowly walking in a zigzag (parallel to the dog and gradually decrease the distance) pattern toward the patient. At any point if the dog glances toward the stimulus, C/T. C/T any attention toward the handler and for responding to the look and watch cues or any other cued behaviors. A high rate of reinforcement is ideal. While the dog is still relaxed but may be showing subtle indicators of increased distraction, for example, he is slower to respond to cues or is having difficulty looking away from the stimulus, the handler will cue the dog to sit again (even if he is still sitting) and reward him. This is also the cue for the distraction person to stop walking, pause briefly, and then walk away and return to the original starting point. This reset acts

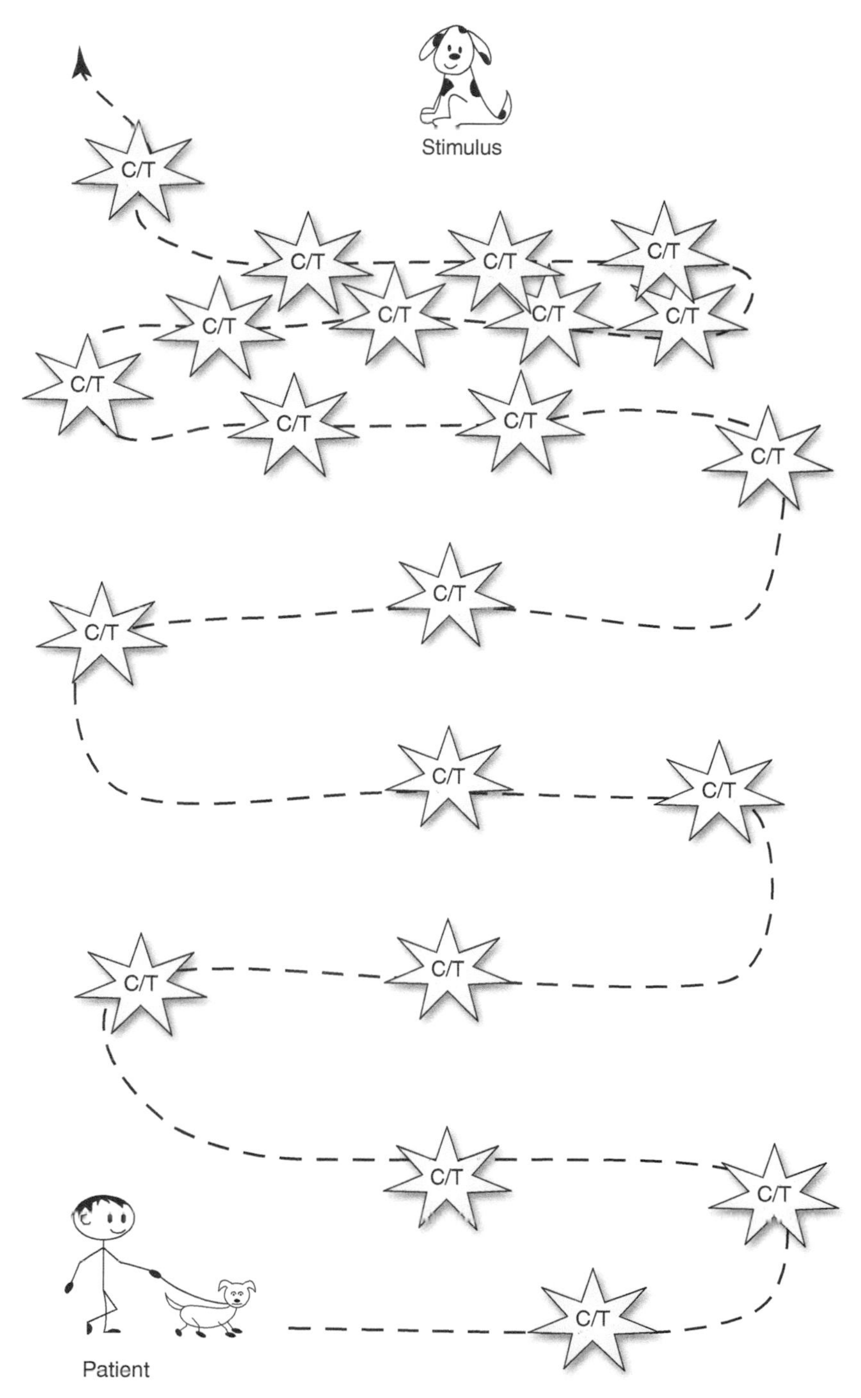

Figure 9.24 Stimulus stationary: With the stimulus present but stationary, utilize DS, CC, and RS to the stimulus. Gradually decrease the patient's distance from the stimulus while performing fast-paced walking, turns, look, watch, and sit and C/Ting at each response. A higher rate of reinforcement may be required as the distance to the stimulus is decreased.

as a functional reward for the dog and is a form of negative reinforcement; the intensity of the stimulus is decreased (social pressure is removed). Ideally this reset should happen before the dog begins to show conflict or displacement behaviors, such as prolonged staring, taking treats roughly, or trying to avoid the stimulus. It is beneficial to increase and then decrease the criteria (distance the stimulus approaches) with repetitions on this exercise rather than making each repetition more difficult. Incorporate the stimulus walking in a curved path toward the patient, then walking at an angle, and finally straight toward the patient. Add other variables but always decrease one characteristic before adding another characteristic (see section **Systematic desensitization**) (Figure 9.25).

This example is using the sit cue as the signal to the stimulus to stop their approach but another cue such as touch, as demonstrated in Video 9.13 on the companion website, could be used as well. Visit the companion website to view Video 9.13 for an example of the Stimulus approach exercise.

Implementation tip: Take frequent breaks and alternate between these exercises during the training session. Going back to easier versions or taking a short play break help to rejuvenate the DS process and allow for faster progress.

Behavior modification for thunderstorm/noise aversions

Foundation skills: relaxation and other foundation behaviors

Possible training tools needed: treats, mat, food puzzle, controllable sound source

Goals: This exercise has two goals. The first is to promote relaxation and CC to the sounds that have previously induced fear or anxiety. The second is to teach the animal a "safe" place to go when it hears these sounds. For thunderstorm anxiety, it is beneficial for the safe place to be located in an interior room, such as a walk-in closet that is void of windows (decreasing lightening) where the sound of thunder is muffled (Figure 9.26).

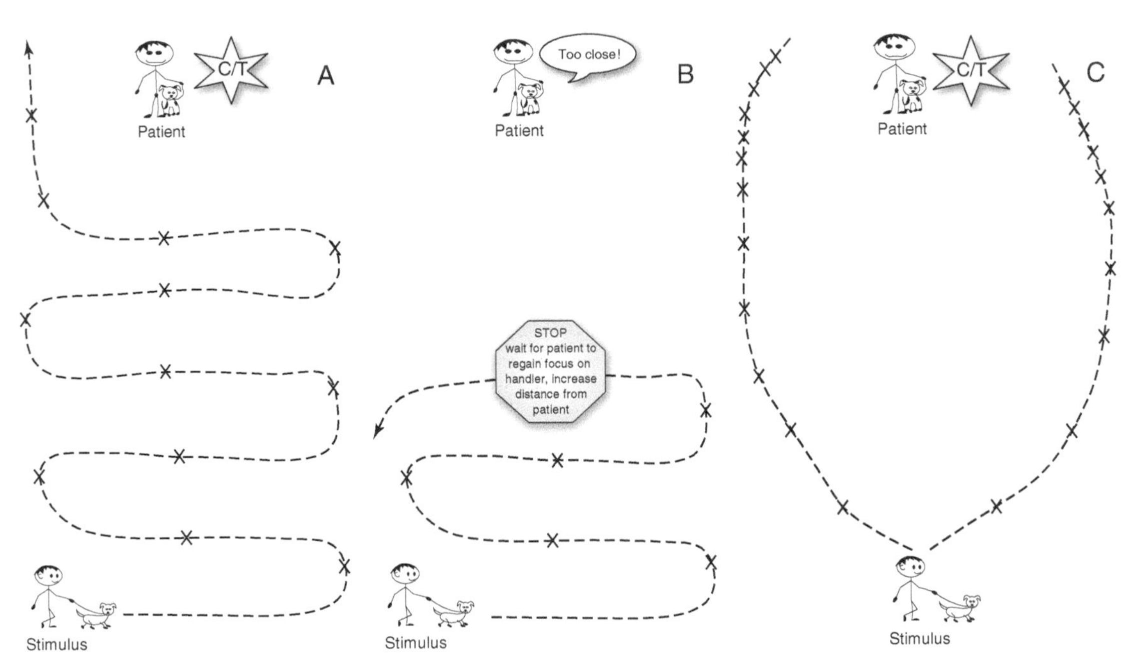

Figure 9.25 Walking patterns for Stimulus approach. (a) Stimulus approaches in a zigzag pattern while the patient is reinforced for an alternative behavior. "X" notes potential reinforcement opportunities for the patient, just as the stimulus turns toward or passes in front of the patient. (b) While the dog is still relaxed but may be showing subtle indicators of increased distraction, for example, he is slower to respond to cues or is having difficulty looking away from the stimulus, a cue should be given to the patient which also indicates to the person approaching to stop, when the patient calms and can again focus on the handler the stimulus increases distance from the patient and approaches at a more gradual pace. (c) Incorporate the stimulus walking in a curved path toward the patient. (d) Incorporate the stimulus walking at an angle toward the patient. (e) Incorporate the stimulus walking straight toward the patient.

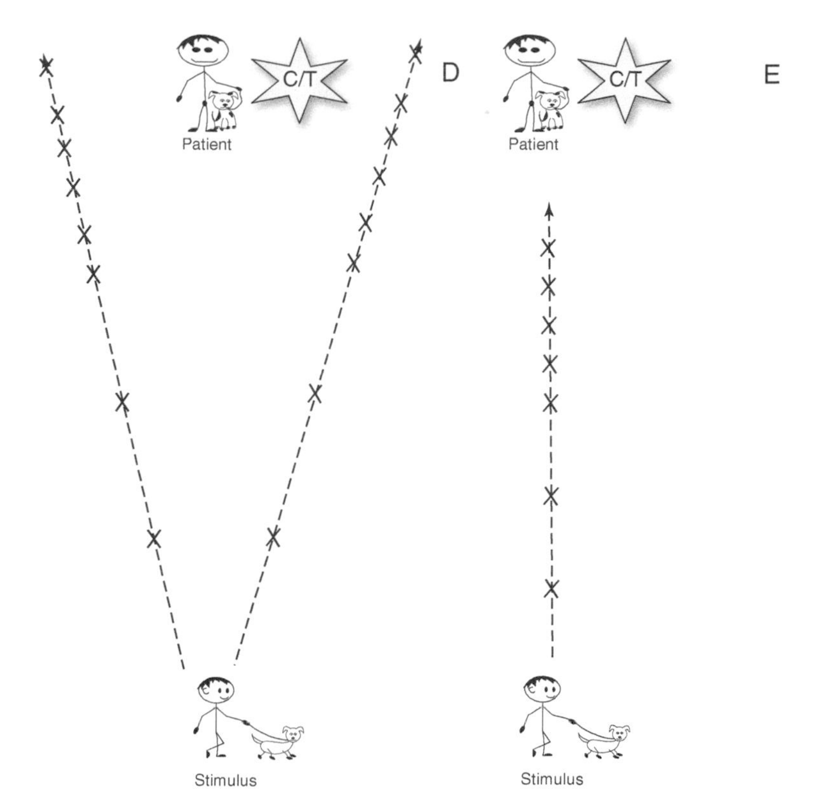

Figure 9.25 (*Continued*)

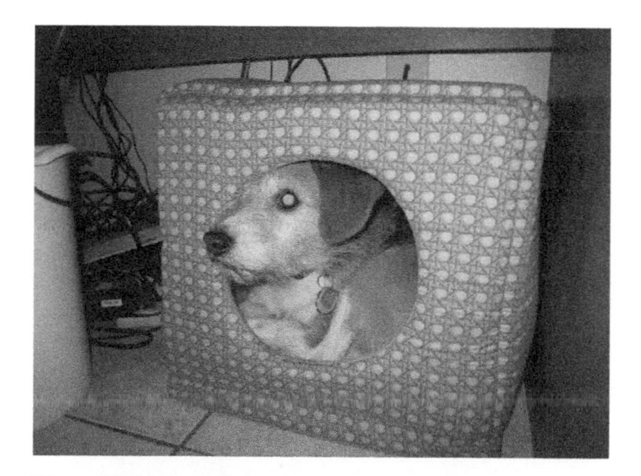

Figure 9.26 "Iris" in her safe place during a storm.

There are four main steps to safe place training for noise aversions. One, teach the dog that the safe place is AWESOME! Two, add a verbal cue to the behavior so you can prompt it. Three, incorporate desensitization and counter conditioning to sounds with the safe place training. Finally, transfer the cue to go to the safe place to the noises.

1. The Safe Place is Awesome!

   The first step is creating a strong positive emotional response to the safe place. Engage as many of the dog's senses as possible by using calming pheromones or aromatherapy and species-specific calming music. In the initial stages of training the safe place station will only be out during training sessions. Choose something that is mobile such as a bathmat or towel. If the dog already has a trained relaxation or place behavior, you can start by adding it to that behavior.

   Training should be started in a location where the dog is calm and relaxed and when the frightening sounds are not likely to occur – for thunderstorms that would mean only on good weather days. To create a positive association with the station, you can train known behaviors on the station but since the goal of this behavior is eventually to be an independent self-soothing behavior that does not rely on a person being there, the majority of the time in the safe place should involve independent activities such as eating a meal out of a snuffle mat or special treats out of a food puzzle.

2. Add a Verbal Cue

   Once the behavior is predictable, add a cue, such as "Go hide." In a training session, just before the dog goes to the safe place, say the cue. Reinforce the dog for performing the behavior. Toss a treat to reset him off the safe place and allow for another repetition. Generalize the station to a variety of places in the house and even outside.

3. Desensitization and Counter Conditioning to Sounds

   Once the dog is excited about his safe place, the behavior is on cue, and you have generalized it to several locations – this usually takes a minimum of three days but could take a few weeks, you will now be ready to start adding in the desensitization to sounds.

   Before playing the sounds with the safe place training, FIRST test the dog's reaction to the recording without the safe place setup. We want to make sure we have a non-stressful starting point. Play the recording on a low volume with the dog relaxing nearby. As long as the dog does not appear to become nervous about the sound, you are now ready to start using the safe place training with the sound recording. Start in a location where you have previously worked on safe place training but it should not be the final safe place location. Just in case the dog becomes frightened with the sound, it will not be associated with the desired safe place location.

   Always start each new session with the sound on a low volume, bring out the station and let the dog relax and eat treats on it while the volume of the recording is slowly increased. Pay careful attention to the dog's responses. The goal is for the dog not to show any anxiety with the sound. If the dog shows early signs of anxiety (ears back, tail down, looking around, furrowed brow, slow to take treats), the volume should immediately be decreased. If the dog starts to slow down or stop eating, you know the stimulus is too much. Decrease the volume or take a break altogether if needed.

   Generalize this training to multiple locations in the home as well. Eventually working up to the final safe place location. The dog may have already chosen a place he prefers such as a bathroom or closet. Once you are able to play the recording at a high volume and the dog is relaxed and eating, the station can remain out in the environment at all times.

4. Transfer the Cue

   The final step is teaching the dog that the sound is the cue to go to his safe place. Have the dog resting nearby you. Warm up by cueing the dog to go to his safe place and reinforce him. Then with him resting nearby, play the sound recording, cue him "Go hide" and reinforce when he does it. After a few repetitions, pause after the sound happens and see if he chooses to go to his safe place. Now the sound has become the cue to go to his safe place giving him a coping strategy to help him handle his fear of the sound.

Video 9.14 on the companion website illustrates the safe place training process.

Relinquishment exercises

Foundation skills needed: Sit

Possible training tools needed: The dog should initially be tethered to a stable point for this exercise and should be comfortable with being tethered.

Food bowl exercises

A common situation in which dogs show aggression is over their food. Management by feeding the dog in a location away from people and animals will need to be implemented. Some owners may decide that management rather than treatment is their preferred option. In treating severe food bowl aggression, the following protocol is recommended:

1. Feed the dog in a new place and use a different food bowl (preferably an old saucepan with a long handle) so that the dog does not associate feeding with past learning experiences (Figure 9.27).

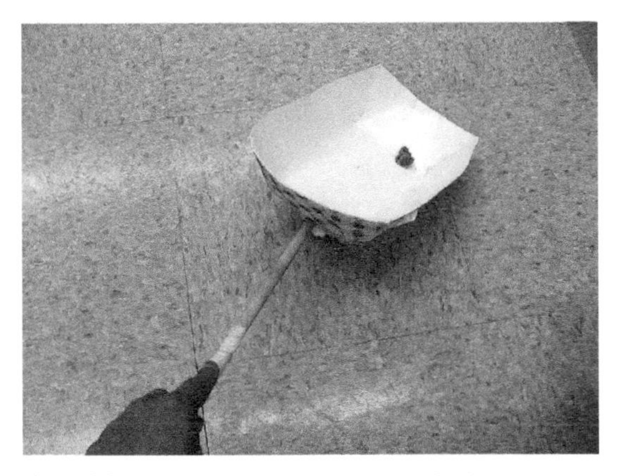

Figure 9.27 An adapted food bowl to begin the desensitization process for food bowl guarding.

2. Tether the dog securely with a leash and a buckle collar.
3. Measure out the amount of food to be fed in a different container that is out of reach of the dog. Cue the dog to "sit," place three kibbles in the saucepan, lower the pan to the dog so that he can eat the food out of the pan. The owner should continue to hold the saucepan and be turned sideways and avoid direct eye contact while the dog is eating. Many dogs will stand up to eat the food. It is acceptable for the dog to stand up while eating the food.
4. Prior to pulling the empty pan away, cue the dog to sit again (even if the dog is still sitting). This adds predictability. When the dog sits, move the pan away and add a few more kibbles into the pan.
5. Continue in this manner until all the food is fed.
6. If the dog shows any aggression at any time, (which would be unusual due to the gradual nature of the exercise), leave the area for a few minutes until the dog is no longer aroused. Return and continue as before but with less kibble or kibble of lower value. The exercise may need to be discontinued if aggression reoccurs.
7. Once the dog is comfortable with being fed in this manner, gradually start adding more food into the bowl with each repetition.
8. The next step involves gradually lowering the bowl to the floor. Go back to only three kibbles at a time in the bowl. With each repetition the bowl will be closer and closer to the ground until it is resting on the ground.
9. At this point, let go of the saucepan handle for a short period of time, and gradually increase the time. The dog will be cued to sit prior to removing the empty pan to add more food to it.
10. Gradually increase the amount of food being added to the pan each time.
11. Once you place one-third of the ration into the saucepan at once, using a ladle, start adding the remaining food into the saucepan as the dog eats.
12. Finally, all the food is placed into the saucepan at once and while the dog is eating, add or toss special treats such as cheese and hotdogs from a distance that does not elicit aggression.
13. Do not pet the dog while he/she is eating.
14. Progress should be gradual; do not be tempted to move forward too quickly or you could destroy any progress that has been made.
15. In the future, when walking past the food bowl, say the dog's name in an upbeat tone and toss a high-value treat into the bowl.

Video 9.15 on the companion website provides a quick demonstration of the food bowl exercise.

Exchange desensitization exercise

Dogs are natural resource guarders. Edible objects such as bones or rawhides, as well as non-food objects such as socks, Kleenex, or plastic wrappers may be guarded. These objects become much more valuable as the owner tries to get the stolen item away from the dog. Often the dog has been conditioned to run with the item as the pet owner chases. A behavior chain is created; obtaining a valuable object cues the pet owner to give chase (conflict situation created), which prompts the dog to defensively guard the object. During treatment, the goal is to change the dog's emotional response from one of fear to one of anticipation of reinforcement for relinquishment. The initial circumstance of having a valuable object must be changed to a positive emotional response of anticipating an opportunity for reinforcement and a "drop it" cue taught. This can be accomplished by teaching a release cue, such as "drop it," using positive reinforcement. While teaching "drop it," further conflict should be avoided. This may require using management by picking up or making unavailable any items which may be guarded by the dog.

1. The pet owner should be encouraged to capture "drop it" anytime the dog drops an object (toy) throughout the day by C/T at the moment the object is dropped. The dog should begin to associate dropping objects with the C/T and begin to offer the behavior. The cue "drop it" can be added.
2. Create a DS hierarchy listing the dog's least valued items to the most valued items. Start with low valued items. For safety tether the dog to a stable point with a leash attached to its buckle collar.
3. Start by showing the dog an object that has no value, such as a large rock at the end of the dog's reach on the tether.
4. Place the object about 3 ft away from the dog and cue "drop it." As you pick up the object C/T, tossing the treat to the dog. Next place the object 2.5 ft away. Give the "drop it" cue, pick up the object, C/T. As the exercise progresses and the dog begins anticipating a reward, chain "sit" and "drop it" together. Cue "sit"→dog sits→cue "drop

it"→pick up the object, C/T. Repeat the exercise while continuing to place the object closer and closer to the dog. Note: even though the dog is not releasing the object in response to the "drop it" cue, the cue is providing information about what the owner is about to do (pick up the object then give the dog a treat).

5. If at any time the dog tries to grab the object, cue "sit." And continue as long as the dog is not anxious or aggressive.
6. Set up exchanges in the same manner with slightly more coveted objects.
7. Gradually move up the previously prepared DS hierarchy, moving to more valuable objects.
8. Do exchanges with objects the dog has spontaneously taken possession of. Use special food rewards for releasing the object. When safe to do so, return the object to the dog or offer an alternative appropriate chew toy. The counting game as detailed in Chapter 7 (Video 7.11) could also be used.
9. Do exchanges with "hot" objects the dog has spontaneously taken possession of. Use special food rewards for releasing the object. When safe to do so, return the object to the dog or offer an alternative appropriate chew toy.
10. Generalize the above exercises in different environments with different people.

Video 9.16 on the companion website demonstrates a quick progression of what the relinquishment exercise might look like.

Independence training

Foundation skills needed: Sit, down, place, relaxation

Possible training tools needed: Video camera

Independence training is often used when it has been determined that the pet has an unhealthy over-attachment to the owner or as a preventive exercise. Any behaviors that can be performed without being in direct or visual contact can be used to shape independence.

For example, going to a place or mat can be trained initially next to the pet owner. Gradually the distance between the mat and the owner is increased. Later, sending the dog to a mat out of the pet owner's vision can be included. A tethered interactive food storage toy can be used when he is resting on the mat away from the pet owner. Tethering the food storage toy makes it impossible for the dog to carry the toy while following the owner (Video 9.19).

Sit–stay and down–stay should be trained to fluency as described below:

The three Ds of fluency are focused upon when teaching duration behaviors such as sit–stay or down–stay and should be added separately and in sequence.

i. **D**uration
ii. **D**istance
iii. **D**istractions

1. Initially, cue "sit" and then pause before giving a C/T. The dog in essence has to hold the position longer before receiving the reward.
2. Some people choose to make the "sit" or "down" cue the only cue used and duration is gradually taught with the single stationary cue. Others prefer to have a separate cue to signal to the dog to continue doing what they are doing, such as a verbal cue, "stay," or a hand signal (hand out in front as if motioning to stop). While teaching duration avoid repeating the cue or continue to hold your hand out.
3. Train duration first without moving away. Be aware that staring at the dog to hold him in place could quickly become part of the cue. Then when the handler looks away from the dog, the dog gets up. Vary the time. Do not always make it longer. End on a good note and set the dog up to succeed. If you see the dog getting ready to break the stay, it is best to avoid clicking and treating. Otherwise, you are likely to reinforce the early movement of breaking the stay and inadvertently teach the dog to break the stay. Instead, reset the dog and make the next repetition easier, so that the dog is successful.
4. Once you have worked up to a 30-second stay without moving away from the dog, start adding the next variable – distance. You will need to make the duration shorter when adding the new variable.
5. Cue the dog (sit, stay). Take a half step or one step away from the dog, click, return immediately, and treat.
6. Continue in this fashion. When you start to add distractions, decrease the other variables. Distractions could be the handler doing something (jumping jacks, turning around, singing, etc.), other people, dogs, or toys. Always set the criteria at a level at which the dog has a realistic chance at being successful. If you are not progressing, most likely it is because multiple criteria are being raised at once. Reassess.

CHAPTER 9

7. It is important to time the click when the pet owner is away from the pet and has not begun to return to the pet. This will encourage a positive emotional response to the pet owner leaving. Dog thinks, "Move away from me so I can get clicked!"

Videos 9.17–9.19 on the companion website demonstrate teaching independence with three different methods.

Desentization to departure cues and planned departures

Pet owners often have a predeparture pattern that predicts to the pet that the owner is preparing to leave. The pet suffering from separation anxiety often gets more anxious as it recognizes that the owner is preparing to depart. The goal with DS to departure cues is for these cues to lose their predictive value as a signal the owner is going to leave the pet and thus minimize the pet's anxiety associated with predeparture routines.

The owner should make a list of things they do prior to a routine departure. An example of a predeparture list might include turn off the TV, turn on the radio, take phone off the charger, let the dog outside, put on shoes, brush teeth, confine the dog to the bedroom, pick up keys, open the garage, set the alarm and exit the garage door.

Several times throughout the day when the owner is not leaving, some of these behaviors should be performed. For example, the owner may put on her shoes, brush her teeth, then sit down and watch a movie. The owner should not attempt to agitate the dog or get the dog's attention. In fact, the owner should just ignore the dog during this time and be nonchalant. Ideally the owner should attempt to avoid the dog seeing these departure cues when she does actually have to leave the dog. The owner might exit out a different doorway or put things in the car at night. Another option is to create a positive association with some of the departure cues by pairing them with a treat. Video 9.20 on the companion website demonstrates using a remote treat dispenser to counter condition the jingle of keys.

Once DS to departure cues has been accomplished, the next step may be to desensitize the dog to planned departures. The early stage of this is combining a relaxed down stay with the departure cues as a distraction (Video 9.21). A remote treat dispenser can be helpful in this process to disassociate the treat from the owner. Another alternative is to give the dog a long-lasting food storage toy tethered by his bed.

Safety cues (music and bed) signify to the dog that this is training. Until the owner has progressed in training to being able to leave the dog for gradually longer periods of time, the safety cues would not be used with an actual departure. The owner cues the dog to settle on his bed and performs departure cues randomly without leaving the dog or going out of sight. The dog is rewarded for calm behavior with either the food storage toy or remote treat dispenser, or the owner clicks and tosses a treat to the dog. Eventually the goal is for the owner to progress through the departure routine and then leave for short periods of time. Gradually the time the owner is gone is increased but should be variable (some short and some longer). At this point it would be important to be utilizing a long-lasting food storage toy. Upon return of the owner, the dog should initially be ignored to avoid overexcitement with return.

This process can be very time consuming and difficult to perform without sensitizing the dog. Many owners are eager to work on the departures as they are feeling trapped in their home because leaving the dog is anxiety-inducing for the dog and for them. However, if the dog becomes anxious during the process, the frequent departures and leaving of the dog may create more anxiety with departure. If working on planned departures, it is recommended to only do one out-of-sight session a day. Video can be helpful to allow the owner to assess the dog's behavior while the owner is out of sight. While working on DS to planned departures, it is important to avoid leaving the dog or have a different routine that signals an actual departure versus the training session (i.e. the dog is confined to a specific room for actual departures and is loose in the house during training). DS to departure cues and planned departures should be used in conjunction with a complete treatment plan for separation anxiety, which may include medication options.

Behavior modification for fear with veterinary or husbandry care

Unfortunately, patients often develop a negative emotional response to the veterinary hospital. Chapter 8 has provided detailed information regarding the prevention and treatment of FAS associated with veterinary and husbandry care. Please refer to Chapter 8 for details about restraint and handling alternatives.

It is imperative to create a detailed DS plan for addressing all criteria associated with the situation.

Most patients not only have a fear of the location (the veterinary hospital) but also with the physical manipulation or handling involved with the care. When developing the DS plan it is best to work on changing the emotional response to these two aspects (handling and environment) separately before working on them together. A typical behavior modification protocol would involve working on distraction techniques and cooperative care training (Chapter 8) in a location where the pet feels relaxed and comfortable and has no learning history of veterinary or husbandry care taking place. This is often a room in the pet's home. The training should also be performed with a person the animal trusts and has an established relationship with and ideally, no negative learning history with care. Once training has advanced in the comfortable environment, then take the training on the road and generalize it to a variety of contexts the pet enjoys. This might be different rooms in the house, the car, a familiar park, pet store, and so on. When adding in new criteria such as other people or veterinary or grooming equipment, return to the most familiar and safe environment. This safe location is where all changes in criteria with handling should start.

If car travel is an issue for the pet, that must also be addressed separately if vehicular travel is required for a visit to the veterinary hospital. See Table 8.1 for a DS-CC plan for car travel.

While working on the handling aspect, the pet owner can begin to counter condition the pet to the veterinary environment. A non-stressful starting point must be found to begin this training. Where will the pet take a highly valued reinforcer? Initially it may be in the car in the parking lot. CC should occur first, taking the pet to the hospital and only give treats and then leave. The next step may be taking treats in the parking lot and doing training – then leaving. If the sight of other people and dogs is a trigger, it would be necessary to do this training at times when the hospital is closed or not busy. Work up to entering the lobby, then an exam room. When entering an examination room, it should not be a room in which the dog has had a previous bad experience. The dog is anticipating being restrained and instead should be given treats and then leave the examination room. Once the dog is eagerly (no hesitation) visiting various areas of the hospital, taking treats and responding to known cues, then the generalized handling exercises discussed earlier can be added into the veterinary environment.

Because previous negative and traumatic experiences with veterinary and husbandry care will be a memory the pet carries with them for life, behavior modification will take time. Anxiolytic medications are often warranted in these cases to help facilitate the learning process, assist with developing a non-stressful starting point, and for the welfare of the pet.

Staying safe

When a pet is being seen for a behavioral disorder, it is likely that the pet is experiencing fear and anxiety and may or may not have exhibited aggression. Before interacting with the pet, the veterinary technician minimally should have obtained the following information:

1. Age of the animal. The age will give insight into the length of learning history of the animal, in other words, how much time the animal has had to practice the coping skill it has utilized to control the environment in the past. The "coping" behavior may be actively avoiding the situation (leaving), aggressing to make the stimulus increase distance, or some other behavior like a stereotypic stress-relieving behavior. A dog that has had a lengthy history of conflict-induced aggression may no longer demonstrate conflict behaviors before a bite.
2. Past bite history. Past behavior will be the best predictor of future behavior. How many times has the animal bitten? Does it give warning signals (i.e. conflict behaviors)? How easily is the behavior triggered? Has the pet inhibited his bite in the past and does the animal bite multiple times or leave after the first bite?
3. Known and identifiable triggers. Usually the pet owner can identify triggers of aggression when the veterinary technician asks, "What would you tell me not to do with 'Fluffy' because it might upset her and trigger the response?" If the owners cannot identify triggers, the veterinary technician should continue to listen to the history being obtained by the veterinarian before moving forward. The triggers will likely be identified as a more detailed history of prior episodes is obtained. Use extreme caution when working with an older patient who has displayed aggression, does not inhibit his bite or bites multiple times, and triggers are unknown. Such cases should be referred to a veterinary behaviorist.

4. Have punishment-based techniques been used in the past to attempt to correct aggressive behavior? If so, the animal may give little or no warning signs before aggressing.

Safety techniques for the behavior consultation room

When working with an animal with a history of fear and/or aggressive behaviors, the following suggestions can help decrease the chances of an aggressive episode during a behavior consultation:

- Keep interruptions to a minimum – Any change of environment, including knocks on the door or people entering and leaving the consultation room can incrementally push the patient toward the threshold for reactivity (Figure 9.29). Keep all interruptions, noises, or other "surprises" to a minimum during the consultation.
- Keep movement and variables low during the consultation. Although having all members of the family present is important for obtaining the behavioral history and it is important to have all members present to discuss the prescribed treatment plan implementation, it is also important to keep distractions and uncontrolled stimuli to a minimum. Very young children may not be appropriate for the consultation.
- Tethers: A wall or floor tether can be used if the bite threshold and bite history are unclear. Identify triggers as quickly as possible so they can be avoided or applied systematically and not accidentally (see Figure 9.28).
- Mobile chair: A rolling desk-type chair can be used by the technician to move out of the tethered space if needed. The chair can also be used to turn away from the dog if conflict behaviors are seen or if an aggressive situation occurs. Use a chair that can turn and be pushed away if needed.
- Although a valid veterinarian–client–patient relationship must be established based on local regulations, for patients with high levels of FAS, the bulk of a behavior consultation might be better received by the pet owner and the pet via tele-medicine. Video consultations provide for the least amount of stress for the pet and the client. This mode of consultation should be an option for patients whose welfare will be compromised by being in a novel environment or around unfamiliar people.

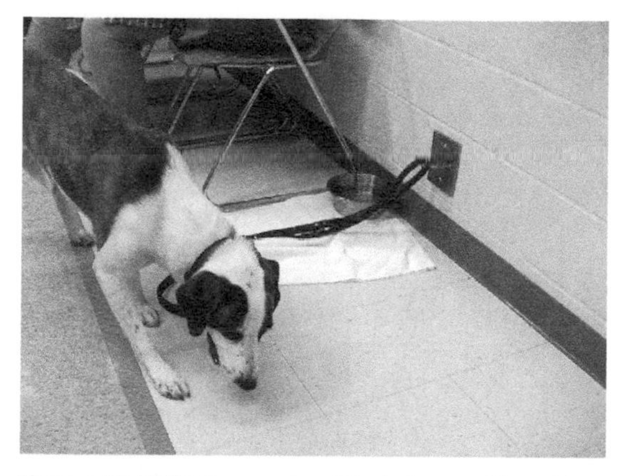

Figure 9.28 Wall tethers can be utilized when working with an animal with a bite history or unknown bite history.

Understand the animal's threshold for reactivity

All dogs have a level at which they will bite. They also have thresholds for other levels of threat, such as growling, snarling, and snapping. The first step is to determine potential risk factors. Typical risk factors include categories of people to whom the dog was not socialized, certain ways of being touched, pain, presence of food, and other dogs. Presentation of any one of these risk factors by itself may elicit reactivity or biting, depending on the dog's particular threshold level.

A combination of more than one risk factor at the same time usually evokes a higher level of threat. In many situations, a dog that has bitten "for no reason" may have been exposed to a novel combination of risk factors at once, pushing him over his "threshold for reactivity" (Figure 9.29).

For example, Stanley, an eight-year-old poodle, was not socialized to children, is uncomfortable around loud noises and is arthritic. Stanley has never bitten anyone before. One day the neighbor's three-year-old child comes over blowing a whistle and falls on Stanley. Stanley bites the child. The pet owners say the bite was unprovoked. Stanley was pushed over his threshold. Helping pet owners understand their dog's threshold for reactivity will help them to realize the bite was not unprovoked and they can then learn to recognize when they are reaching the dog's threshold and change the environment before a bite can occur.

Greeting a patient displaying signs of fear

If the patient has been known to display fear behaviors in the examination room in the past, the

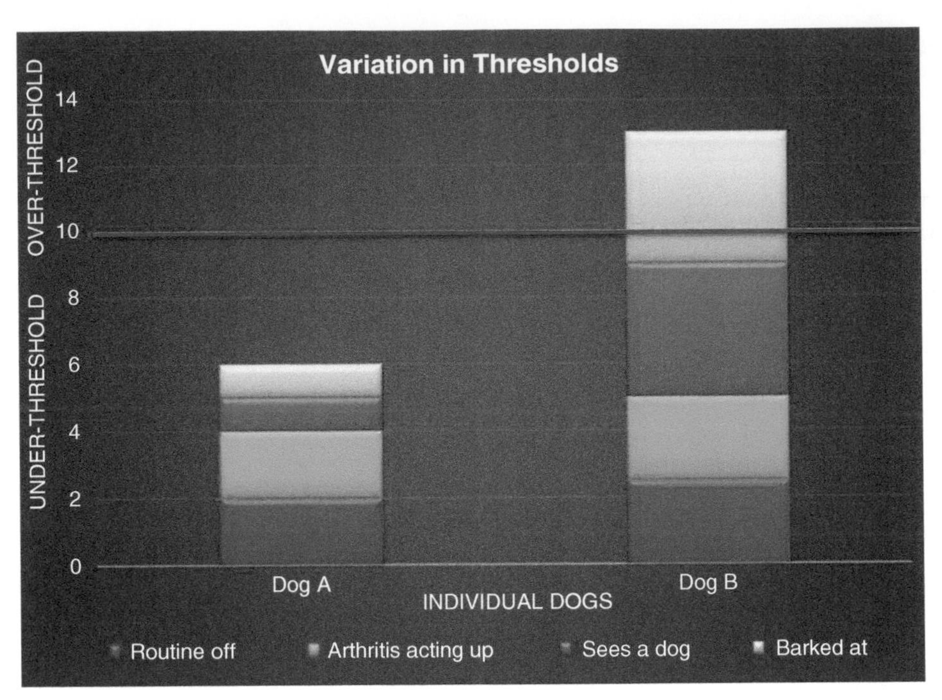

Figure 9.29 Threshold for reactivity: Dog A has a high threshold. Dog B more easily reaches his threshold for reactivity when triggers are stacked.

following suggestions should be incorporated for his next visit but can also be incorporated with all patients regardless of their previous learning history. Using a considerate approach with all patients will put them at ease (see Chapter 8 Approach and Behavior of Veterinary Team Members) and create a more pleasant experience.

Control as many antecedents as possible

Make sure the pet does not have to wait in the reception area but can enter the examination room immediately. Have the pet owner keep the animal in the car until the examination room is ready. This will keep arousal and anxiety related to anticipation from rising. Be in the exam room before the patient enters. Many dogs will almost immediately begin guarding the space in the examination room unless the technician is in the room first. As said previously, the best predictor of behavior is past behavior. If the dog has had issues in the past, ask the owners not to feed him on the day of his appointment, if medically and behaviorally appropriate. Have a range of food reinforcements available but also ask the pet owner to bring the pet's favorite treats. Ignore the patient when they enter the room and explain to the owner that you are trying to be non-threatening toward the pet.

Counter conditioning and desensitizing to your presence

As the medical history is obtained, ignore the dog but toss the very best treats possible (i.e. chicken) (see Figure 9.30). Every veterinary examination room should have a can of cheese, canned dog food, hot dogs, or cooked chicken chunks in the freezer.

If the patient will not take the treats you have tossed, ask the owner to offer the treats to the dog. Frequently, it only takes an offered "safe" treat from the owner for the dog to sample what you have tossed.

If the pet remains hidden behind the owner, ask the owner to walk across the room away from the pet (Figure 9.31). At this point the patient will decide whether it is "safer" to hide alone or to follow the owner. By getting the dog to walk across the room you are creating an opportunity for him to gain confidence when nothing "bad" occurs when he walks across the room. An area of safety has

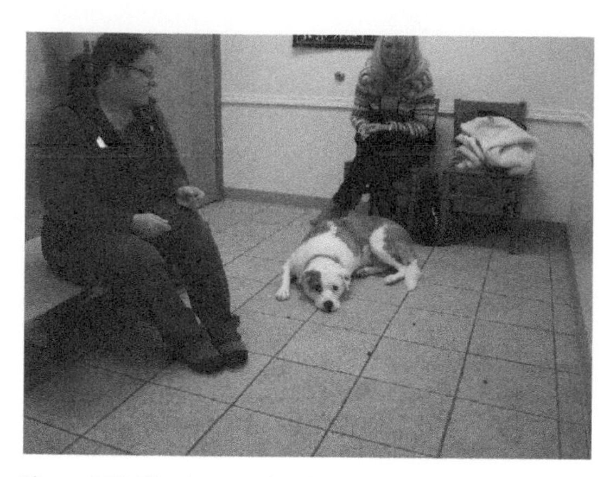

Figure 9.30 Veterinary technician tossing treats to a patient. *Source*: Alicea Howell RVT, VTS (Behavior), KPA–CTP, CPDT–KA.

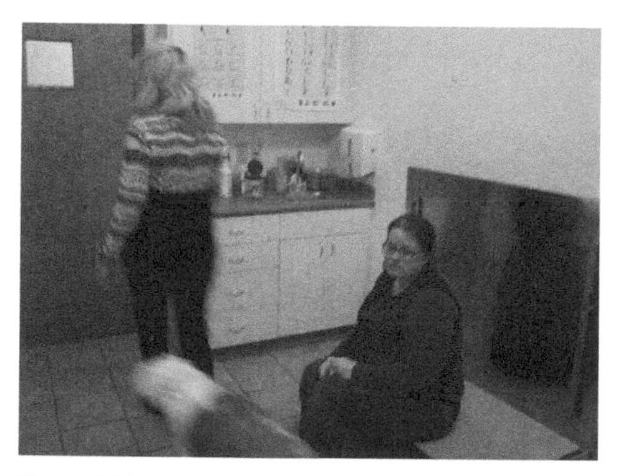

Figure 9.31 Pet owner walking to opposite side of the examination room with the patient following. *Source*: Alicea Howell RVT, VTS (Behavior), KPA–CTP, CPDT–KA.

been created. If the dog does not follow the owner, have the owner kneel and offer or toss a treat across the room to the pet.

Once the pet and owner have left the "safe" area, the technician can sit where the dog was previously hiding (Figure 9.32). The technician should turn sideways, avert his eyes from the pet and nonchalantly toss treats to the pet creating a "breadcrumb trail" leading to the technician. DO NOT TALK TO THE PET OR LOOK DIRECTLY AT IT. Continue calmly talking to the pet owner in a relaxed fashion, regardless of what the pet does. Pet owners often feel ashamed of the way their pet behaves at the veterinary clinic. It is important that you assist the client to relax by telling him/her that the pet is only afraid and it is ok, you are hoping to calm his fears.

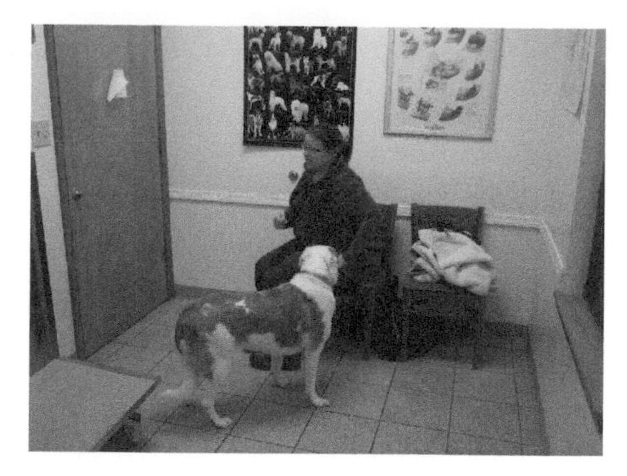

Figure 9.32 Technician sitting sideways and where the pet owner and patient were sitting previously. *Source*: Alicea Howell RVT, VTS (Behavior), KPA–CTP, CPDT–KA.

As the pet begins to take treats closer to you, offer a treat from your upturned hand. Make sure not to remove your hand until the pet has turned to walk away (Figure 9.33). The movement of your hand can cause a dog to startle and to become aggressive. If the dog is "stretching" or "snatching" the treat from your hand, be very still and do not increase any aspect of the interaction until the dog chooses to move away on its own.

Once the dog is comfortable and not showing signs of fear when taking treats out of your flat hand, hold the treat closer to your body for the dog to take it from you. Continue until eventually your hand

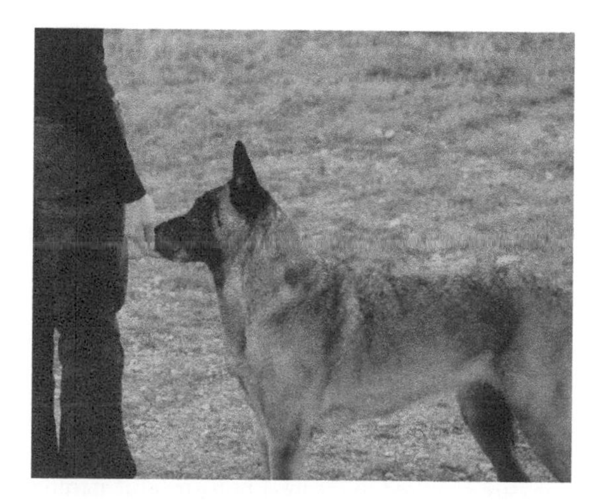

Figure 9.33 Hand offering treat with palm up and avoiding reaching into the dog's space. The hand may be moved once the patient has moved away or initiated further contact.

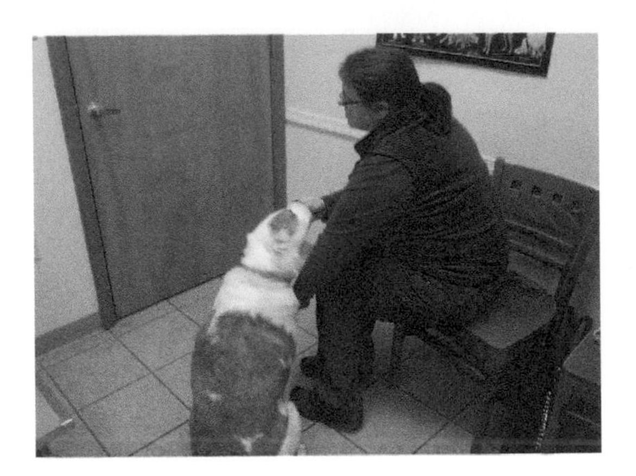

Figure 9.34 Dog beginning to relax as the technician scratches chest, still sitting sideways and avoiding eye contact. *Source:* Alicea Howell RVT, VTS (Behavior), KPA–CTP, CPDT–KA.

with the treat is next to your body. At this point the dog may not leave once it has eaten the treat. This is the point where you can offer another treat while you scratch the dog's chest (Figure 9.34). Always allow the dog to retreat whenever it feels the need, allow the dog to be in control of the interaction. Eventually the dog will begin not leaving you and may even lean against you. Even at this point, do not stand or change your posture until the pet leaves on its own. You can toss treats across the room to move the dog away from you if needed.

Next, stand and toss treats again. The pet should now trust you enough to begin seeking your attention. Quietly ask for a "sit" and then reward. It is likely at this point you have just won a permanent friend.

If the dog will not take any treat at any point during the appointment, a "non-stressful" starting point has not been found. If appropriate for the situation, a tele-medicine consult might be an alternative to offer. If the dog is truly hungry (the owner has restricted food before the appointment) and you are using a treat "that cannot be refused" then this patient is in extreme distress. The next step is to determine when the patient stopped taking treats. Would he take treats in the owner's car in the parking lot? Then that is the place to begin the process. This may also be a case in which anxiolytic medications are required to create a non-stressful starting point. See Chapter 8 for more information on providing veterinary care in an emotionally protective manner.

Conclusion

Veterinary technicians are an instrumental asset in the positive resolution of behavior problems and behavior disorders that threaten the human–animal bond. By understanding the motivations that drive behavior, potential diagnosis and treatments that may be prescribed, and with practiced applications, they can become the pet's behavior case manager, working with the veterinarian, the qualified trainer, and pet owner to successfully apply prescribed techniques.

Acknowledgement

The author acknowledges the contribution of Julie K. Shaw to the first edition chapter.

Video 9.1 Targeting with "Iris." This video demonstrates using a target stick to begin to teach a new behavior.

Video 9.2 Teaching sit. This video illustrates teaching a puppy to sit and the process of adding a cue. Initially the puppy is lured into a sit but then the technician switches to capturing the sit. A cue is added once the behavior is predictable. Source: Fear Free, LLC.

Video 9.3 Place. This video demonstrates teaching a place cue utilizing a remote treat dispenser. In this example, once the behavior can be prompted with the chime from the dispenser, the verbal cue is added.

Video 9.4 TA intros. This video provides instruction and demonstrates the Level 1 exercise for CC/RS/DS to unfamiliar people in the home – Gradual introductions.

Video 9.5 Transfer arrival signal. This video illustrates the process of teaching an alternative behavior for the arrival signal and transferring the cue.

Video 9.6 Door exercise. This video exemplifies the door exercise training process.

Video 9.7 Muzzle. This video introduces methods to condition a dog to a muzzle.

Video 9.8 Auto check in and looks. This video illustrates capturing offered attention to the handler and noticing stimuli.

Video 9.9 Leash pressure cue. Teaching the dog to move in the direction of gentle pressure on the leash (i.e. the gentle pull is the cue) is advantageous as it conditions a positive association with pressure on the leash.

Video 9.10 Putting it all together. This video illustrates putting together offered attention and noticing stimuli as well as known cues (eyes, look, touch, let's go) while working on stimuli at a park with a dog.

Video 9.11 Stimulus stationary. This video demonstrates the stimulus stationary exercise. It is usually much easier for the patient to be moving rather than stationary with the first stages of behavior modification and training for reactivity to stimuli.

Video 9.12 Moving together. This video is an example of moving together.

Video 9.13 Stimulus approach. This video depicts the Stimulus approach exercise.

Video 9.14 Safe place training. This video illustrates teaching a dog to go to her safe place when hearing the sound of thunder. Please note that at one point in the video the volume is increased to a point where the dog slows down eating. The trainer should have decreased the volume of the thunder at that point but she did not. Instead the volume was increased and the dog lifts her head and stops eating.

Video 9.15 Food bowl. This video depicts the process of using a tether, saucepan, and sit cue, while quickly progressing through the steps for demonstration purposes only. The actual desensitization process would take weeks with daily practice.

Video 9.16 Relinquish objects. Watch the following video demonstrating a quick progression of what the relinquishment exercise might look like. If this dog had had severe guarding issues, the trainer should have modified her position to avoid leaning into the dog's space when placing or picking up the object. If the dog has displayed significant aggression, a grabber tool may be used for additional safety.

Video 9.17 Clicker training a down stay on mat. In this video the distance of the owner from the dog and the duration of the stay is varied. The click is given when the owner is at a distance from the dog. The treat is tossed to reset the dog for the next repetition. Prior to adding duration and distance the dog was taught to go to the bed on cue ("Place").

Video 9.18 Remote treat dispenser to reinforce staying on the mat. A remote treat dispenser is used to reinforce the dog for remaining on the mat, while the owner walks away. The owner has a remote that controls when the machine dispenses the treat. This also disassociates the reward from the owner which can be beneficial with teaching independence.

Video 9.19 Tethered food storage toy to help teach independence. A food stuffed toy is tethered to a fixed point by the dog's bed. The owner is then able to gradually move away to help build independence. The toy is tethered to prevent the dog from picking it up and following the owner.

Video 9.20 Desensitization to departure cues. Many dogs with separation anxiety start to become anxious when they perceive the owner is preparing to leave. This is an example of using a remote treat dispenser to change the meaning of and emotional response associated with the jingle of keys.

Video 9.21 Desensitization to planned departures. This is a training session to teach the dog to become comfortable with the steps leading up to an actual departure. It is a combination of the relaxed down stay on a mat with departure cues. Safety cues (music and bed) signify to the dog that this is training. Until the owner has progressed in training to being able to leave the dog for gradually longer periods of time, the safety cues would not be used with an actual departure. The owner should progress in a gradual manner and the dog should remain relaxed at all times. Video monitoring is needed once the owner is out of sight.

References

Ahn, H. and Picard, R. (2006). Affective cognitive learning and decision making: the role of emotions. *Proceedings of the 18th European Meeting on Cybernetics and Systems Research*, Vienna, Austria (April 18–19, 2006).

American Veterinary Society of Animal Behavior (AVSAB) (2021). Position statement on Humane Dog Training. https://avsab.org/wp-content/uploads/2021/08/AVSAB-Humane-Dog-Training-Position-Statement-2021.pdf (accessed August 2022).

Association for Applied Sportpsychology (2007–2012). Psychological benefits of exercise. http://www.appliedsportpsych.org/resource-center/health-fitness-resources/psychological-benefits-of-exercise/ (accessed May 22, 2014).

Bol, S., Caspers, J., Buckingham, L. et al. (2017). Responsiveness of cats (Felidae) to silver vine (*Actinidia polygama*), Tatarian honeysuckle (*Lonicera tatarica*), valerian (*Valeriana officinalis*) and catnip (*Nepeta cataria*). *BMC Veterinary Research* 13: 70.

Bowman, A., Scottish, S.P.C.A., Dowell, F.J., and Evans, N.P. (2017). The effect of different genres of music on the stress levels of kenneled dogs. *Physiology and Behavior* 171: 207–215.

Brayley, C. and Montrose, V.T. (2016). The effects of audiobooks on the behaviour of dogs at a rehoming kennels. *Applied Animal Behaviour Science* 174: 111–115.

Coppinger, R. and Coppinger, L. (2001). *Dogs: A Startling New Understanding of Canine Origin, Behavior & Evolution*. New York City, New York, USA: Scribner.

Depue, R.A. and Iacono, W.G. (1989). Neurobehavioral aspects of affective disorders. *Annual Review of Psychology* 40: 457–492.

Edworthy, J. and Waring, H. (2006). The effects of music tempo and loudness level on treadmill exercise. *Ergonomics* 49 (15): 1597–1610.

Friedman, S.G. (2009a). Behavior fundamentals: filling the behavior-change toolbox. Paper presented at the annual North American Veterinary Conference, Orlando, FL (January 2009).

Friedman, S.G. (2009b). Functional assessment: hypothesizing the predictors and purposes of problem behavior. Paper presented at the annual

CHAPTER 9

North American Veterinary Conference, Orlando, FL (January 2009).

Fukuzawa, M. and Kajino, S. (2018). Auditory stimuli as environmental enrichment tool for family dogs. *International Journal of Biology* 10 (3): 19–26.

Garcia, J.K. and Koelling, R.A. (1966). Relation of cue to consequence in avoidance learning. *Psychonomic Science* 4: 123–124.

Gershoff, E.T. (2002). Physical punishment by parents and associated child behaviors and experiences: a meta–analytic and theoretical review. *Psychological Bulletin* 128: 539–579.

Goodwin, S. and Reynolds, H. (2018). Can aromatherapy be used to reduce anxiety in hospitalised felines. *The Veterinary Nurse* 9 (3). Published Online: 20 Apr.

Graham, L., Wells, D.L., and Hepper, P.G. (2005). The influence of olfactory stimulation on the behaviour of dogs housed in a rescue shelter. *Applied Animal Behaviour Science* 91 (1–2): 143–153.

Gray, J. (1990). Brain systems that mediate both emotion and cognition. *Cognition & Emotion* 4 (3): 269–288.

Guy, N.C., Luescher, U.A., Dohoo, S.E. et al. (2001). Risk factors for dog bites to owners in a general veterinary caseload. *Applied Animal Behaviour Science* 74 (1): 29–42.

Hampton, A., Ford, A., and Kox, R.E. (2020). Effects of music on behavior and physiological stress response of domestic cats in a veterinary clinic. *Journal of Feline Medicine and Surgery* 22 (2): 122–128.

Horwitz, D. and Neilson, J.C. (2007). *Blackwell's Five–Minute Veterinary Consult Clinical Companion: Canine and Feline Behavior*. Ames, Iowa: Blackwell Pub.

Horwitz, D., Mills, D.S., and British Small Animal Veterinary Association (2009). *BSAVA Manual of Canine and Feline Behavioural Medicine*. Quedgeley, Gloucester England: British Small Animal Veterinary Association.

Hunsberger, J.G., Newton, S.S., Bennett, A.H. et al. (2007). Antidepressant actions of the exercise–regulated gene VGF. *Nature Medicine* 13 (12): 1476–1482.

Kawakami, K., Takai-Kawakami, K., Kurihara, H. et al. (1996). The effect of sounds on newborn infants under stress. *Infant Behavior and Development* 19 (3): 375–379.

Komiya, M., Sugiyama, A., Tanabe, K. et al. (2009 Jun). Evaluation of the effect of topical application of lavender oil on autonomic nerve activity in dogs. *American Journal of Veterinary Research* 70 (6): 764–769.

Ksenych, E. and Liu, D. (1992). *Conflict, Order, and Action: Readings in Sociology*. Toronto: Canadian Scholars' Press.

Landsberg, G.M., Hunthausen, W.L., and Ackerman, L.J. (2013). *Behavior Problems of the Dog and Cat*. Edinburgh: Saunders/Elsevier.

LeDoux, J.E. (1996). *The Emotional Brain: The Mysterious Underpinnings of Emotional Life*. New York: Simon & Schuster.

Lopes Fagundes, A., Hewison, L., McPeake, K. et al. (2018). Noise sensitivities in dogs: an exploration of signs in dogs with and without musculoskeletal pain using qualitative content analysis. *Frontiers in Veterinary Science* 5: 17.

Luescher, A. and Martin, K.M. (2010). *Dogs! & Cats: Diagnosis and Treatment of Behavior Problems*. Purdue University.

Luescher, A. and Shaw, J. (2007). *DOGS! Principles and Techniques of Behavior Modification Notes*. West Lafayette, IN: Purdue University.

Martin, K.M. and Martin, D. (2011). *Puppy Start Right: Foundation Training for the Companion Dog*. Waltham, MA: Sunshine Books, Inc.

McConnell, P. (1990). Acoustic structure and receiver response in domestic dogs, *Canis familiaris*. *Animal Behaviour* 39: 897–904.

Milgram, S. (1963). Behavioral study of obedience. *Journal of Abnormal Psychology* 67: 371–378.

Mira, F., Costa, A., Mendes, E. et al. (2016a). Influence of music and its genres on respiratory rate and pupil diameter variations in cats under general anaesthesia: contribution to promoting patient safety. *Journal of Feline Medicine and Surgery* 18 (2): 150–159.

Mira, F., Costa, A., Mendes, E. et al. (2016b). A pilot study exploring the effects of musical genres on the depth of general anaesthesia assessed by haemodynamic responses. *Journal of Feline Medicine and Surgery* 18 (8): 673–678.

Mulvaney, M.K. and Mebert, C.J. (2007). Parental corporal punishment predicts behavior problems in early childhood. *Journal of Family Psychology* 21 (3): 389–397.

Myatt, A. (2014). *An olfactory enrichment study at the Ashland Cat Shelter*, 1–40. Ashland University https://etd.ohiolink.edu/apexprod/rws_etd/send_file/send?accession=auhonors1399629978&disposition=inline (accessed December 2022).

Overall, K.L., Dunham, A.E., and Frank, D. (2001). Frequency of nonspecific clinical signs in dogs with separation anxiety, thunderstorm phobia, and noise phobia, alone or in combination. *Journal of the American Veterinary Medical Association* 219 (4): 467–473.

Panksepp, J. (1998). *Affective Neuroscience: The Foundations of Human and Animal Emotions*. New York: Oxford University Press.

Pryor, K. (2002). The poisoned cue: positive and negative discriminative stimuli. Karen Pryor Clicker Training. http://www.clicker training.com/node/164 (accessed May 22, 2014).

Pryor, K. (2009). *Reaching the Animal Mind: What the Clicker Training Method Teaches us About Animals*. New York: Scribner.

Pryor, K. (2014). *The Modern Principles of Shaping*. Karen Pryor Clicker Training.

Ramirez, K., John, G., and Shedd Aquarium (1999). *Animal Training: Successful Animal Management Through Positive Reinforcement*. Chicago, IL: Shedd Aquarium.

Salman, M.D., Hutchinson, J.M., Ruch-Gallie, R. et al. (2000). Behavioral reasons for relinquishment of dogs and cats to 12 shelters. *Journal of Applied Animal Welfare Science* 3 (2): 93–106.

Snowdon, C.T., Teie, D., and Savage, M. (2015). Cats prefer species appropriate music. *Journal of Applied Animal Behaviour Science* 166: 106–110.

Strassberg, Z., Dodge, K., Pettit, G., and Bates, J. (1994). Spanking in the home and children's subsequent aggression toward kindergarten peers. *Development and Psychopathology* 6: 445–445.

Straus, M.A.M. and Paschall, M.J.M. (2009). Corporal punishment by mothers and development of children's cognitive ability: a longitudinal study of two nationally representative age cohorts. *Journal of Aggression, Maltreatment & Trauma* 18 (5): 459–483.

Well, D.L. (2006). Aromatherapy for travel-induced excitement in dogs. *Journal of the American Veterinary Medical Association* 229 (6): 964–967.

Wood, L. (2008). *Clicker Bridging Stimulus Efficacy*. New York: Hunter College.

The PowerPoint of figures, appendices, MCQ's, cited videos are available at www.wiley.com/go/martin/behavior

10 Introductory neurophysiology and psychopharmacology

Kenneth M. Martin
Veterinary Behavior Consultations & TEAM Education in Animal Behavior, Spicewood, TX, USA

CHAPTER MENU

Introduction

This chapter explores the most important cells of the nervous system – neurons. The nervous system is the information highway of the body. This multicellular system is directly responsible for the vast communication that is occurring every second of every day. The brain is the supervisory center of the nervous system and is the most complex organ in the body. The anatomy and physiology of

Canine and Feline Behavior for Veterinary Technicians and Nurses, Second Edition. Edited by Debbie Martin and Julie K. Shaw.

Companion website: www.wiley.com/go/martin/behavior

the brain are discussed; however, owing to its intricacies, information will focus on the functional anatomy pertaining to behavior. Because the brain is such a convoluted organ, it has mechanisms protecting it from the general circulation. The blood–brain barrier (BBB) is described, and the basic anatomy and physiology underlying drug effects are considered. Neurotransmitters in the brain producing behavioral effects are elaborated on, and pharmacokinetics and psychopharmacology are discussed.

- The nervous system is the information highway of the body.

Basic neurophysiology

The nerve cell is the functional unit of the nervous system. There are four main structures to every neuron; the soma, dendrites, axon, and presynaptic terminals. Each neuron has a specific purpose: to transmit messages through electrical impulses to adjacent neurons until this information reaches the brain.

The soma is also referred to as the *cell body*. It contains the nucleus and the organelles necessary for cellular life and communication (Meyer and Quenzer 2005).

Dendrites branch out from the soma and are the major receiving apparatus responsible for taking signals from other neurons and transmitting them into the soma. Dendrites branch out similarly to a tree and are covered with spines. These specialized dendritic spines vary in morphology and receive excitatory input from other neurons. It is hypothesized that the abrupt changes occurring with these structures are involved in learning and memory (Hedges and Burchfield 2006).

Axons are much longer than dendrites, often extending several feet in length in some animals. Axons act as the conduction unit of the neuron. They are covered with a fatty layer called the *myelin sheath*, which serves as an insulator. The myelin sheath wraps around the tubular axon and is interrupted at regular intervals called *nodes of Ranvier*. These interruptions accelerate the conduction down the axon. Electrical impulses are carried through the axon to presynaptic terminals (Cunningham and Klein 2007; Figure 10.1).

Presynaptic terminals branch out from the end of the axon and contain presynaptic vesicles that secrete neurotransmitters to other cells. The axon fires and these neurotransmitters are released into the synaptic cleft. Neurochemicals cross the synaptic cleft and attach to specialized receptors on adjacent nerve or muscle cells specific for that chemical (Figure 10.2). Depending on the neurotransmitter released and the receptor site bound to, excitement, inhibition, or initiation of enzymatic reactions will occur. It is here where most psychotropic medications initiate their effects (Hedges and Burchfield 2006). Impulse communication is about a third of a millisecond at which time the neurotransmitter must be deactivated. Neurotransmitters are deactivated from the receptors by diffusion into the extracellular fluid, enzymatic metabolism, or reuptake into the presynaptic terminal to be used again (Grilly 2006).

An average neuron forms thousands of synapses with other neurons. These interactions between neurons are responsible for all perceptions, memories, thoughts, and behavior. Learning is the process in which specific experiences alter our nervous system and influence our behavior. The Hebb rule states that learning involves strengthening of a synapse that is repeatedly active when the postsynaptic neuron fires (Carlson 2002).

- These interactions between neurons are responsible for all perceptions, memories, thoughts, and behavior
- Learning is the process in which specific experiences alter our nervous system and influence our behavior.

The central nervous system (CNS) consists of the brain and the spinal cord. The brain is divided into several major parts, the hindbrain, the midbrain, the forebrain, the basal ganglia, and the olfactory bulb (Meyer and Quenzer 2005; Figure 10.3).

Hindbrain

The hindbrain consists of the brainstem, connecting the brain to the spinal cord, and the cerebellum. The brainstem is made up of the medulla oblongata and the pons (Figure 10.4). These structures are primarily responsible for respiratory and cardiac function.

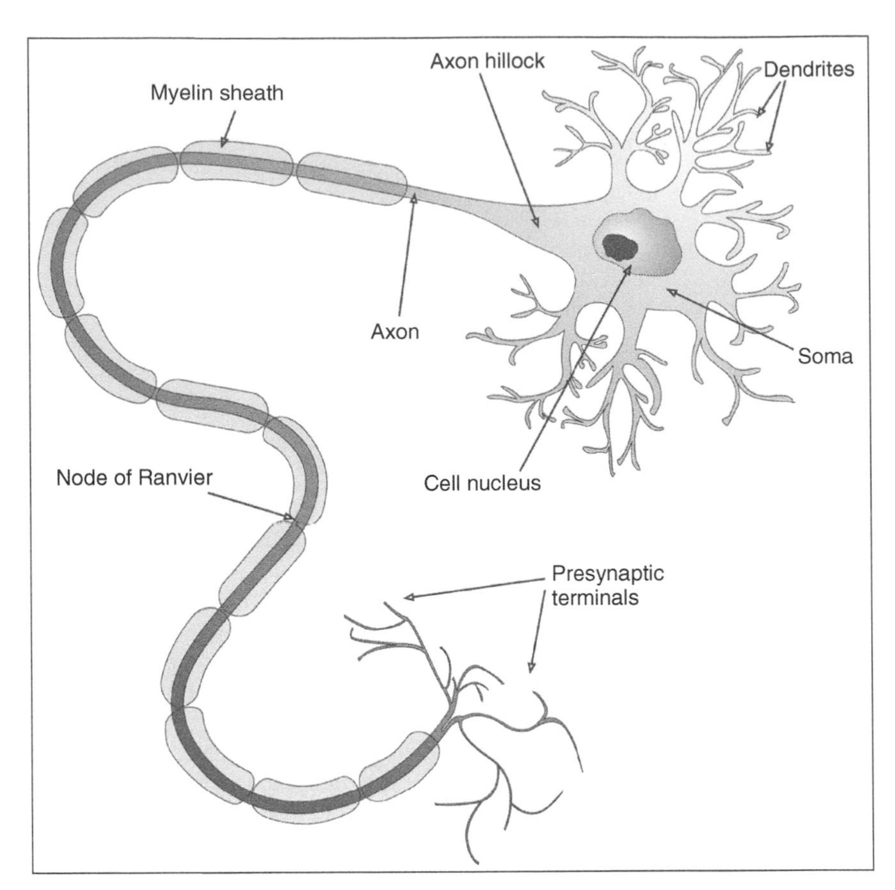

Figure 10.1 Neuron. Illustration by Carol Bain, DVM.

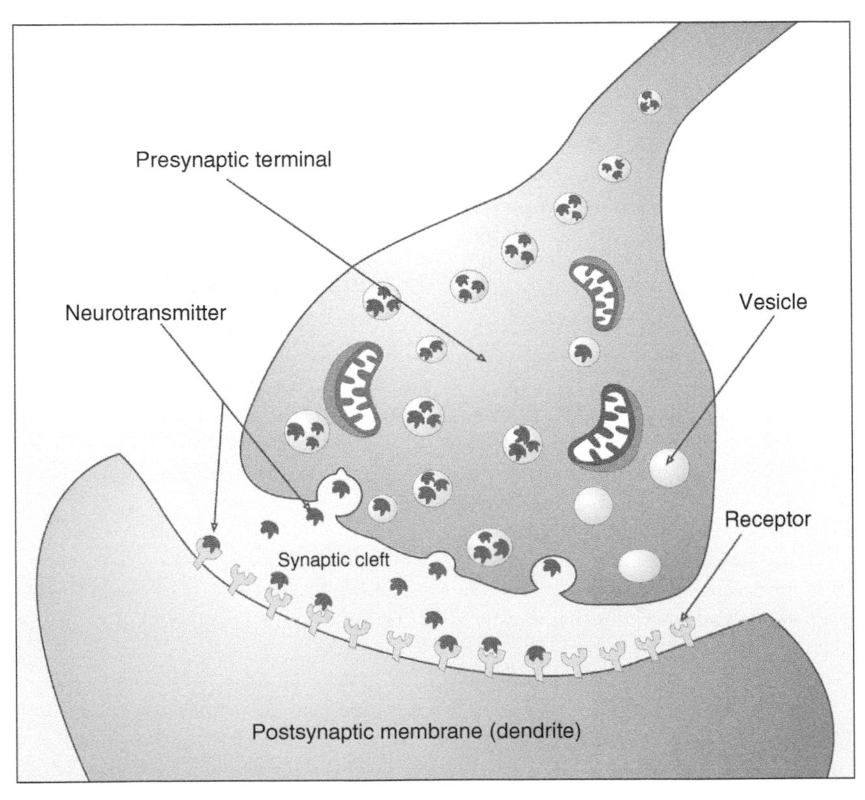

Figure 10.2 Neurotransmission. Illustration by Carol Bain, DVM.

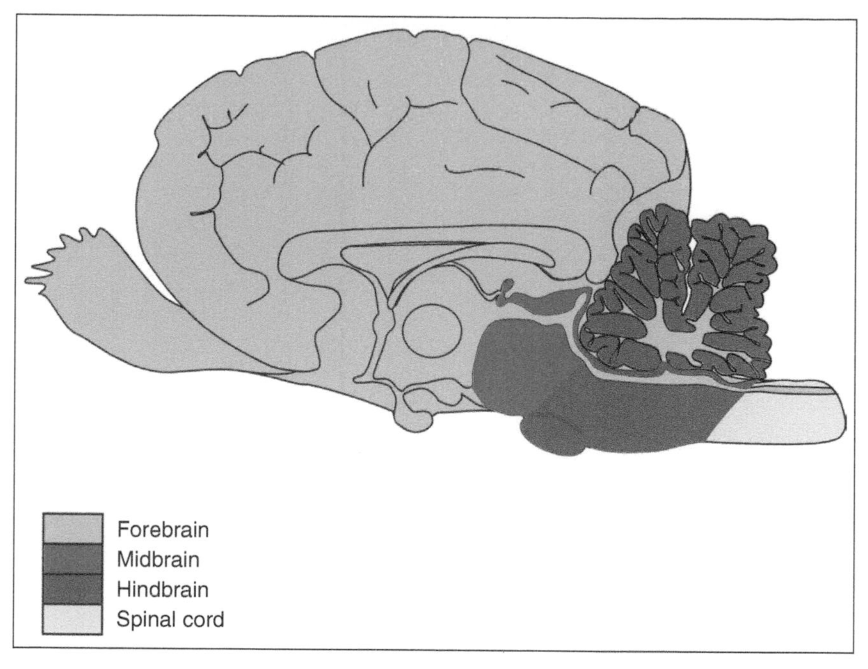

Figure 10.3 Color-coded brain structures (forebrain, midbrain, hindbrain, and spinal cord). *Source*: Illustration by Carol Bain, DVM.

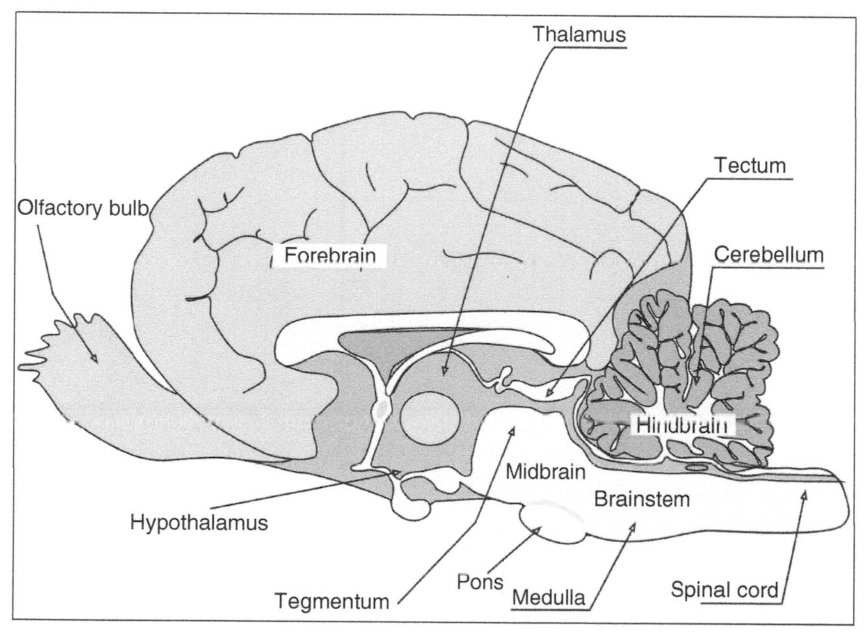

Figure 10.4 Brain anatomy (color, but not necessarily color coded). *Source*: Illustration by Carol Bain, DVM.

Cranial nerves pass through the medulla to transmit information from the head and the neck to the spinal cord. Therefore, damage to this area can result in a wide range of neurologic deficits (Hedges and Burchfield 2006). The pons incorporates a portion of the reticular formation, a collection of nuclei forming a network responsible for attention and arousal (Carlson 2002). The cerebellum is primarily involved with coordination but has also been implicated in attention and cognition (Hedges and Burchfield 2006).

Midbrain

The midbrain is located dorsal to the brainstem and envelops the tectum and tegmentum (refer to Figure 10.4). These structures play a role in visual reflexes and reactions to moving stimuli. They are also involved in arousal, attention, and behaviors modulated by rewards (Carlson 2002; Hedges and Burchfield 2006). Within the tegmentum are several other structures, some of which are important for organizing behaviors such as predation and defensive rage (Meyer and Quenzer 2005).

Forebrain

The forebrain is the largest portion of the brain and contains a wide array of structures involved with learning. The forebrain is predominantly comprised of gray matter and is covered by the cerebral cortex. The cortex is divided into two hemispheres that are connected by millions of axons. The largest of these axon pathways is called the *corpus callosum* (Meyer and Quenzer 2005). The cerebral cortex is further divided into four lobes in each hemisphere: the frontal, the parietal, the temporal, and the occipital lobes (Figure 10.5). Other structures of the forebrain that are not necessarily associated with a specific lobe include the thalamus/hypothalamus, basal ganglia, and olfactory bulb (refer to Figure 10.4). Each lobe of the cortex consists of several structures responsible for specific functions. Each lobe transmits electrochemical impulses to other areas of the brain in which the information is further analyzed and perceived. This vast and intricate communication coordinated within the brain is how memories and perceptions are formed (Meyer and Quenzer 2005).

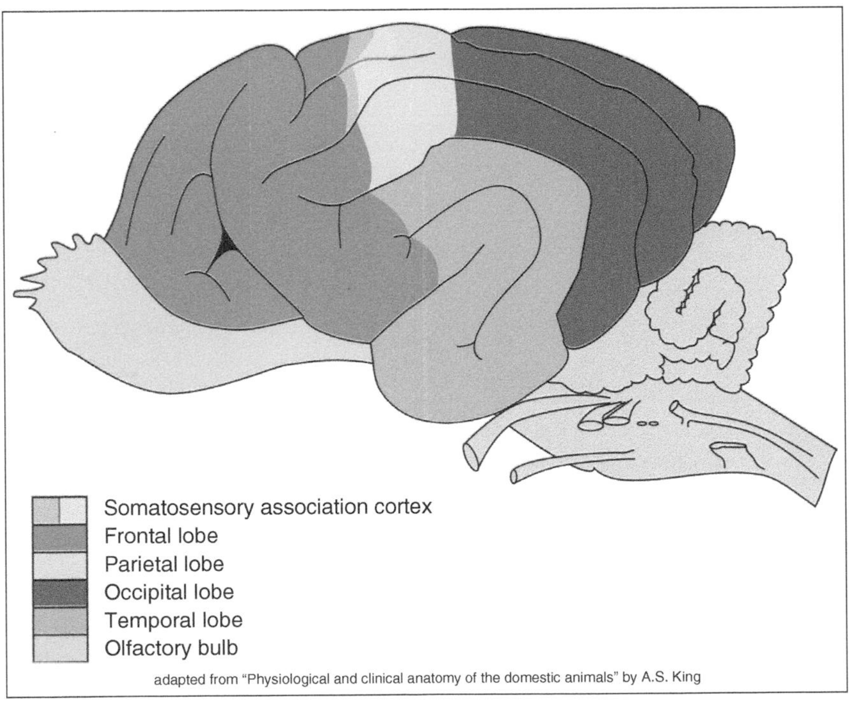

Figure 10.5 Color-coded brain lobes (somatosensory association cortex, frontal lobe, parietal lobe, occipital lobe, temporal lobe, and olfactory bulb). *Source*: Illustration by Carol Bain, DVM.

Parietal lobe

The parietal lobe lies caudal to the frontal lobe and dorsal to the temporal lobe (refer to Figure 10.5). The rostral portion of the parietal lobe consists of the somatosensory association cortex. It receives electrical impulses from the body and the head relative to pain, temperature, touch pressure, and position of the limbs and sense of joint movement. The caudal portion is responsible for cognition and selective attention.

Occipital lobe

The occipital lobe is considered the visual cortex and interprets sensory information from the eye. With regards to behavior, the occipital lobe functions in conjunction with the parietal lobe to form the cognitive association area (King 1987).

Temporal lobe

The temporal lobe is considered the interpretative association area and is concerned with learning and memory. The temporal lobe harbors the limbic system, which is comprised of the hippocampus and the amygdala (Figure 10.6). The limbic system is important in behavior because it is considered the emotional center of the brain. It is involved with fear, aggression, affection, initiative, imagination, and anxiety. All of these emotions contribute to individual personality. Specifically, the amygdala interprets facial expressions, processes stressful stimuli, and modulates fear and aggressive responses. The hippocampal formation is involved with learning and spatial memory rather than emotion, but it is also implicated with the stress response (Hedges and Burchfield 2006; King 1987).

Basal ganglia

The basal ganglia are a group of nuclei that lie deep within the brain and encompass a variety of complex structures. This area of the brain is not as well understood as other areas but is known to receive signals from the cerebral cortex and project these signals to other regions (Cunningham and Klein 2007). They are most often associated with movement regulation but appear to possess functions associated with obsessive compulsive disorder, depression, and dementia (Hedges and Burchfield 2006).

Frontal lobe

Although the frontal lobe is not as developed in dogs as it is in humans, it has many responsibilities pertaining to behavior. The frontal association area contributes to general alertness, intelligence, and temperament of each individual (King 1987; refer to Figure 10.5).

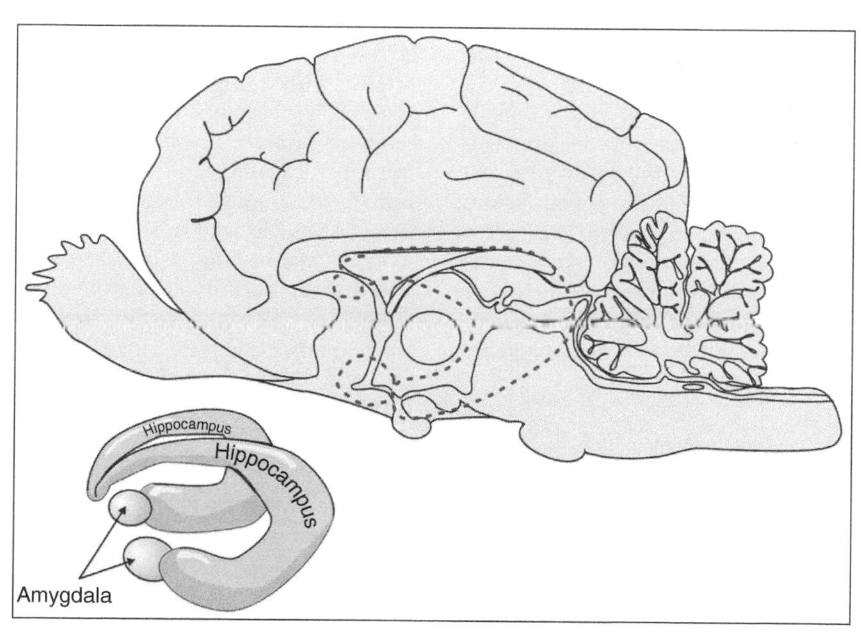

Figure 10.6 Amygdala and hippocampus. *Source*: Illustration by Carol Bain, DVM.

Hypothalamus/thalamus

The hypothalamus and the thalamus are a major division of the forebrain (refer to Figure 10.4). The hypothalamus is most commonly known for its role in homeostasis. Specific to behavior, the hypothalamus works in conjunction with the hippocampus and amygdala to control the emotions of rage and aggression. The thalamus is a distribution center taking information from one region of the brain and projecting it to the appropriate portion of the cerebral cortex (Carlson 2002; Meyer and Quenzer 2005).

Olfactory bulb

The olfactory bulb is located in the most rostral part of the brain in most animals (refer to Figures 10.4 and 10.5). Axons from the olfactory bulb project to the amygdala, limbic cortex, and the piriform lobe. All of these structures are important in reproductive behavior (Carlson 2002).

Blood–brain barrier

The brain and the spinal cord are bathed in the cerebrospinal fluid (CSF), which acts as a cushion for the brain, nourishment for cells, and a conduit for hormones. Cells in the brain form tight junctions around the capillaries, preventing extracellular fluid from entering the CNS. This semi-permeable barrier is considered the blood–brain barrier (BBB). The BBB is directly responsible for protecting the CNS from toxins and fluctuations of extracellular fluid. It also prevents neurotransmitters from leaking into general circulation. Because of this protective barrier, only specialized medications can penetrate into the CNS. Solubility, ionization, and polarity are a few of the important characteristics of every medication that directly affects the absorptive quality of the drug. Only lipid-soluble, unionized, and nonpolar medications can cross the BBB (Cunningham and Klein 2007; Bill 2006).

Neurotransmitters

Neurotransmitters are the chemicals released from presynaptic vesicles under specific stimulation and used in the brain to transmit information from one neuron to another. Hundreds of chemicals have been identified in the nervous system as being, or having the potential of being, a neurotransmitter. This section focuses on the most common neurotransmitters pertaining to behavior (Grilly 2006).

- Neurotransmitters are the chemicals released from presynaptic vesicles under specific stimulation and used in the brain to transmit information from one neuron to another.

Acetylcholine

Acetylcholine (ACh) is synthesized in nerve terminals from a vitamin, called *choline*, and acetyl-CoA (Figure 10.7). This neurotransmitter is primarily excitatory and is distributed throughout the CNS and the peripheral nervous system (PNS). The functions of ACh on the CNS are not well understood but are implicated in chemosensory associations and are responsible for triggering rapid eye movement (REM) sleep. ACh is also involved in facilitating perceptual learning and controls functions of the hippocampus, including the formation of memories (Carlson 2002; Table 10.1). In the PNS, ACh activates muscles and is the major neurotransmitter in the autonomic nervous system. ACh will bind to two receptor types referred to as *nicotinic* and *muscarinic*. Nicotinic receptors are located in both the CNS and the PNS and are considered the "fast" receptors. Evidence suggests that when they are activated, other neurotransmitters are released, resulting in a myriad of effects (Grilly 2006). Muscarinic receptors are considered the "slow" receptors and are involved with the formation of memory, learning, and movement (Hedges and Burchfield 2006). An enzyme called *acetylcholinestrase* (AChE) located in the synaptic gap degrades ACh by hydrolyzing it into acetate and choline. This degradation is different from other neurotransmitters in which postsynaptic activity is regulated via reuptake. Choline is then actively taken back into the cell and reused for more ACh synthesis (Grilly 2006).

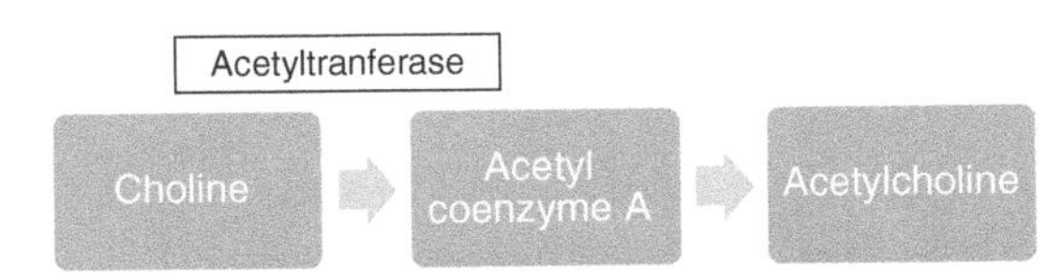

Figure 10.7 Synthesis of acetylcholine.

Table 10.1 Neurotransmitters, functions and primary locations.

Neurotransmitter	Function	Location
Acetylcholine	Perceptual learning	Throughout CNS and PNS
	Formation of memories	Hippocampus
Dopamine	Attention	CNS
	Cognition	Basal ganglia
	Sociability	Limbic system
	Motivation	
	Reward	
Norepinephrine	Arousal	Throughout CNS and PNS
	Dreaming	Pons
	Anxiety	Hypothalamus
	Fear	Frontal cortex
	Mood	Hippocampus
	Attention	
	Processing information	
Serotonin	Regulates mood	CNS and PNS
	Anxiety	Brainstem
GABA	Reduces anxiety	Throughout CNS
	Promotes sleep	
	Muscle relaxation	
Glutamate	Learning/memory	Throughout CNS
	Cognition	
	Psychosis	
	Anxiety	

CNS, central nervous system; GABA, gamma-aminobutyric acid; PNS, peripheral nervous system.

Monoamines

There are four neurotransmitters that belong to the monoamine family. These include dopamine (DA), norepinephrine (NE), epinephrine, and serotonin (5-HT). The first three are further classified as catecholamines, whereas 5-HT is considered an idolamine (Carlson 2002).

Dopamine

Dopamine (DA) is synthesized through a series of interactions of various enzymes. Two amino acids, called *phenylalanine* and *tyrosine*, are directly involved with the synthesis of L-dopa. The final product of these reactions is DA (Cunningham and Klein 2007; Figure 10.8).

This neurotransmitter is found exclusively in the CNS because L-dopa does not cross the BBB. It is found in the basal ganglia and limbic system as well as other areas of the brain. Depending on the receptor site, it can be both excitatory and inhibitory. DA is responsible for autonomic functions, posture, fine motor movements, attention, cognition, sociability, motivation, and reward (Hedges and Burchfield 2006; refer to Table 10.1).

There have been five receptor sites identified for DA, but only two of them are commonly used. DA is degraded by two different enzymes, monoamine oxidase (MAO-B) and catechol-O-methyltransferase (COMT). Both of these enzymes are found in the synaptic gap and deactivate DA. The majority of DA is reabsorbed by active transport back into the vesicles to be reused (Grilly 2006).

Norepinephrine/epinephrine

Norepinephrine (NE) and epinephrine are also called *noradrenaline* and *adrenaline*, respectively. They are synthesized in a similar manner to DA because DA is a precursor of NE and epinephrine (Cunningham and Klein 2007; Figure 10.9).

These catacholamines are produced throughout the CNS and PNS, including the pons, hypothalamus, frontal cortex, hippocampus, and adrenal gland (Hedges and Burchfield 2006). NE and epinephrine are responsible for arousal, dreaming, anxiety, fear, mood, hunger, thirst, attention, and the processing of information (Meyer and Quenzer 2005). These neurotransmitters have been implicated in attention-deficit hyperactivity disorder as well as depression (Hedges and Burchfield 2006; refer to Table 10.1).

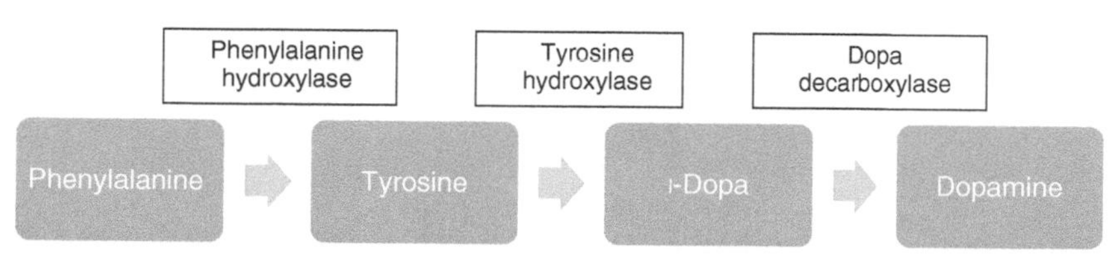

Figure 10.8 Synthesis of dopamine.

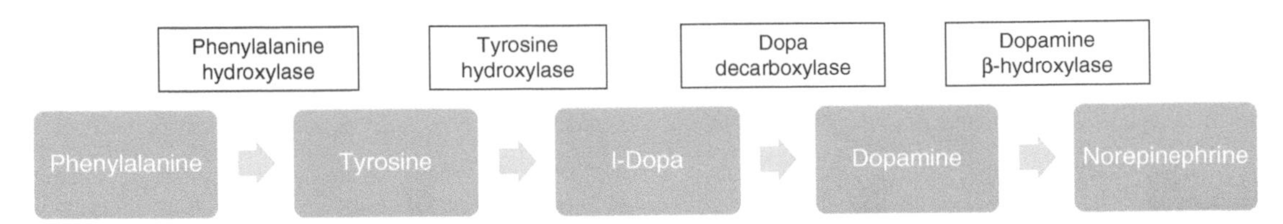

Figure 10.9 Synthesis of norepinephrine.

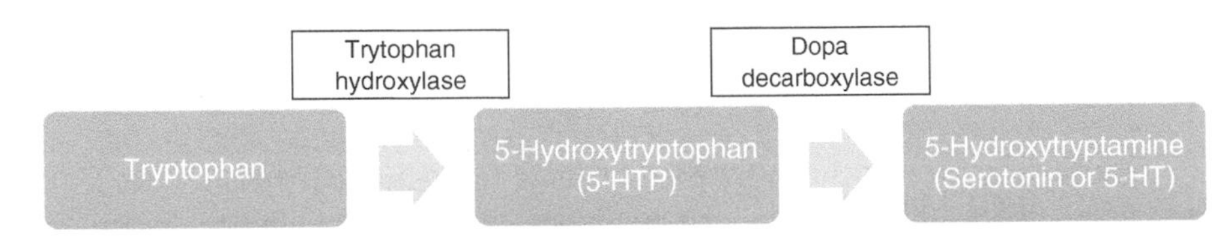

Figure 10.10 Synthesis of serotonin.

There are two catecholamine receptors that differ in shape and affinity. These receptors are referred to as *alpha* and *beta*. Each of these receptor types is responsible for specific physiological effects. Similar to DA, MAO-B and COMT can degrade NE and epinephrine, but the primary mechanism is reuptake into the vesicles (Meyer and Quenzer 2005).

Serotonin

The synthesis of 5-HT occurs in two steps and involves the essential amino acid tryptophan (Figure 10.10; Carlson 2002).

5-HT is found in both the CNS and the PNS and is involved in a wide array of physiological processes. In the CNS, 5-HT is synthesized in cell bodies found in the brainstem (Hedges and Burchfield 2006). 5-HT regulates mood, anxiety, appetite, sleep, arousal, metabolism, the regulation of pain, and, to some degree, aggression (refer to Table 10.1).

Nine receptors have been identified and mediate the effects of 5-HT. The receptors most commonly associated with behavior are the type 1A and 2A receptors. The primary mode of termination is by reuptake through active transport (Carlson 2002; Grilly 2006).

Gamma-aminobutyric acid

Gamma-aminobutyric acid (GABA) is a product of glucose and glutamic acid and is widely distributed throughout the CNS. GABA is the primary inhibitory neurotransmitter in the brain and is responsible for reducing anxiety, promoting sleep, reducing seizure activity, and producing muscle relaxation (Carlson 2002; refer to Table 10.1).

GABA receptors are complex and involve five binding sites. Each binding site has an affinity for a different drug. The first site is for GABA itself, the second is for a class of drugs commonly used in behavior modification called the *benzodiazepines*, the third is for barbiturates, the fourth for steroids, and the fifth for a poison found in an East Indian shrub (Carlson 2002; Grilly 2006).

Glutamate

Glutamate is the primary excitatory neurotransmitter and is widely distributed throughout the CNS. It is involved in sensory and motor function, learning, memory, and cognition (refer to Table 10.1). Glutamate interacts with other neurotransmitters to achieve numerous functions (Hedges and Burchfield 2006).

Glutamate has three main receptors: kainate, metabotropic, and N-methyl-D-aspartate (NMDA). The kainate receptor is involved with epilepsy, the metabotropic receptor is implicated with anxiety, and the NMDA receptor plays an important role in learning, memory, and in the development of psychosis. The NMDA receptor is complicated and is continually under investigation for its potential involvement in learning and a variety of mental disorders.

Pharmacokinetics

Pharmacokinetics is defined as the movement of drugs into, through, and out of the body and includes the processes of absorption, distribution, metabolism, and excretion (Bill 2006).

The most common methods of medication administration include intravenous injection (IV), intramuscular injection (IM), subcutaneous injection (SC), oral administration (PO), orotransmucosal (OTM), and transdermal (TD) absorption. Once drugs have been administered, they are absorbed from the site of administration into systemic circulation and distributed to the site of action (McCurnin and Bassert 2006). Drugs interact with biologic tissues and vary in their effectiveness based on the binding affinity and specificity with receptors at the site of action. In the case of psychoactive medications, these sites of action are generally receptors in the CNS. However, most medications have more than one site of action and can produce undesirable side effects. The goal of medication therapy is to administer a dose that maximizes the intended effect and minimizes side effects (Bill 2006; Grilly 2006).

- The goal of medication therapy is to administer a dose that maximizes the intended effect and minimizes side effects.

Medications may be either metabolized and excreted or excreted without being metabolized. Although enzymes in the brain destroy certain drugs, most metabolism of drugs occurs in the liver. Drugs or their metabolites are primarily excreted by the renal and hepatic systems. Other routes of elimination include skin, lungs, saliva, and through breast milk (Hedges and Burchfield 2006; McCurnin and Bassert 2006).

The half-life of a drug is the measurement of time that it takes for the maximum blood concentration to decrease to half after equilibrium. Therefore, the half-life is the amount of time for half of the drug to be eliminated from the system (Bill 2006; McCurnin and Bassert 2006).

Steady state is attained when serum concentrations from repeated administrations reach a state of equilibrium between doses administered and the amount of drug eliminated in a given time interval. The steady state can be calculated by multiplying the half-life by five (McCurnin and Bassert 2006). The therapeutic window is the ideal range of a drug concentration. Drug concentrations below the range of the therapeutic window generally do not produce therapeutic effects. Alternately, drug concentrations above the range of the therapeutic window may show signs of toxicity. The goal of medication therapy is to reach steady state within the therapeutic window (Bill 2006).

- The goal of medication therapy is to reach steady state within the therapeutic window.

Drugs act through receptors. Medications that bind to a receptor and block a natural neurotransmitter are called *antagonists* and inhibit the effects of a neurotransmitter. Medications that bind to a receptor and activate the receptor to stimulate the cell are called *agonists* and facilitate or imitate the effects of a neurotransmitter (Bill 2006). Psychoactive medications work primarily through their variable agonist or antagonist roles, resulting in a shift in the balance of neurotransmitters or other active nervous system chemicals.

- Psychoactive medications work primarily through their variable agonist or antagonist roles, resulting in a shift in the balance of neurotransmitters or other active nervous system chemicals.

Drug categories

Medications for behavior problems are used as an adjunct therapy in combination with behavior and environmental modification. With a multifaceted approach to treatment, therapy is more likely to be successful than if either drugs or behavior modification is used alone (Overall 2001; Horwitz and Mills 2002).

- With a multifaceted approach to treatment, therapy is more likely to be successful than if either drugs or behavior modification is used alone (Overall 2001; Horwitz and Mills 2002).

A goal of using behavioral medications in animals is to reduce underlying fear, anxiety, and/or stress which contribute to the behavioral condition being treated. Behavioral medications help to facilitate learning when combined with behavioral and environmental modification and improve the animal's ability to cope with exogenous and endogenous stressors.

Before adding a medication as part of a treatment plan to address a behavioral problem, certain requirements should be met. First, it is imperative that a valid veterinarian–client–patient relationship has been established before prescribing behavioral medications. The pet should undergo a thorough medical and behavioral history, as well as a physical examination and ideally a complete laboratory evaluation, including a complete blood count, chemistry profile, urinalysis, and thyroid panel. The clinician overseeing the case should have determined a working behavior diagnosis or diagnoses. In addition, he or she should be aware of side effects, drug interactions, and contraindications associated with the medications of choice (Overall 2004). It is imperative that a diagnosis is made so an appropriate medication can be chosen; this prevents just treating behavioral signs (symptoms). These medications are intended to address the specific underlying neurochemical mechanisms associated with the behavioral diagnosis and to help make implementation of the behavioral treatment plan easier to accomplish for the owner (Overall 2004).

Most behavioral medications are used off label for animals. Only a few have been approved for veterinary use by the United States Food and Drug Administration (FDA) in dogs to treat specific behavioral problems. Whenever possible, FDA-approved medications should be used before an alternative or generic medication. When an FDA-approved medication is not available for the diagnosis or for the species of intent, the owner should be counseled on the off label use of the chosen medication.

There are several different indications for the use of medications in a behavioral treatment plan. General indications include drug desensitization, failure of a treatment plan that was initially comprised of behavior modification alone, or to address a behavioral problem that has a medical component.

The goal of drug desensitization is to address the suspected pathologic dysfunction of the neurotransmitter system, leading to or worsening the behavioral disorder. In addition, it can help to make behavior modification easier to apply, giving the owner a starting point for systematic desensitization, and improving compliance and treatment success.

Specific indications include anxieties, such as separation anxiety, generalized anxiety, fears, and phobias; compulsive disorders, cognitive dysfunction syndrome (CDS), hyperkinesis, which is a rare pathologic hyperexcitability disorder, and aggression. When addressing a problem that includes aggression as a symptom, it is important to keep in mind some critical points. First, there are no FDA-approved drugs for use in aggression. Second, there is always a degree of risk of disinhibition (loss of conscious control of the aggressive response), although this risk varies with the drug class chosen. Understanding the mechanism of action as well as label indications and contraindications of all drugs is imperative before prescribing or administering them. There is also a significant liability risk when treating aggression. The use of liability release forms for aggression as well as off label drug use is encouraged.

- Understanding the mechanism of action as well as label indications and contraindications of all drugs is imperative before prescribing or administering them.

Several drug classes are discussed in this section. They include the tranquilizers/neuroleptics/antipsychotics, the anxiolytics, the antidepressants, including the tricyclic antidepressants (TCA), selective serotonin reuptake inhibitors (SSRI), and the monoamine oxidase inhibitors (MAOI), the mood stabilizers, the atypical antidepressants, CNS stimulants, and a few anticonvulsants (Table 10.2).

Tranquilizers/neuroleptics/antipsychotics

In this category, phenothiazines have historically been the most commonly used for behavioral reasons. In people, they are used for tranquilization and for the treatment of psychosis and behavioral arousal.

The mechanism of action mainly centers on the blocking of DA (D2) receptors, which leads to a decrease in spontaneous activity. In people, this is called *ataraxia* or a blunting of both normal and abnormal responses. While in this state, the ability to learn is often impaired.

Side-effect presentation and severity typically depend on whether a high-potency or low-potency phenothiazine is administered. The most common presentation seen in dogs and cats is tranquilization,

Table 10.2 Common veterinary behavior medications.

Class	Drug family	Drug	Indications	Time to effect	Side effects	Contraindications
Tranquilizers/ neuroleptics/ antipsychotics	Phenothiazine	Acepromazine PromAce	Chemical restraint, tranquilization, preanesthetic	Oral: 1–2 h Injectable: 15 min	Hypotension, decreased seizure threshold (?), tranquilization, behavioral disinhibition, decreased learning, paradoxical excitation, potential increased reactivity to noises	Not beneficial for anxiolysis, noise phobia, separation anxiety. Caution or avoid use with cases of aggression. Should not be used alone because it does not provide any anxiety or fear relief.
Anxiolytic	Azapirones-serotonin 1A receptor agonist	Buspirone, Buspar®	Anxiety, fear, mild phobias, anxiety-related urine marking in cats	Oral: 4–6 wk for maximal effect	Bitter tasting	Do not use in conjunction with MAOI
	Low affinity partial agonist for the benzodiazepine binding site of GABA A receptors	Imepitoin Pexion™* *Pexion is FDA approved for treating noise aversions in dogs	Fear, anxiety, panic	Oral: For noise events, twice a day starting 2 days prior to event	Ataxia, increased appetite, lethargy, vomiting, potential to increase aggression	Caution or avoid use with cases of aggression
	Benzodiazepine–GABA receptor potentiation	Diazepam, Valium®	Fear, anxiety, panic	Oral: 1–2 h prior to anxiety-producing stimuli	Sedation, ataxia, muscle relaxation, polyphagia, behavioral disinhibition, paradoxical excitation, acute hepatic necrosis (cats), impaired memory/learning, short acting	Caution or avoid use with cases of aggression, avoid oral use with cats
	Benzodiazepine	Alprazolam, Xanax®	Fear, anxiety, panic- strong anti-panic effects	Oral: 1–2 h prior to anxiety-producing stimuli	Same as diazepam, thought to be less sedating	Caution or avoid use with cases of aggression
	Benzodiazepine	Clonazepam, Klonopin®	Fear, anxiety, panic	Oral: 1–2 h prior to anxiety-producing stimuli	Same as diazepam; thought to produce less sedation and less polyphagia, and longer acting	Caution or avoid use with cases of aggression
	Benzodiazepine	Lorazepam, Ativan®	Fear, anxiety, panic	Oral: 1–2 h prior to anxiety-producing stimuli	Same as diazepam; possibly safer on the liver in cats	Caution or avoid use with cases of aggression
	Alpha-2 agonist	Clonidine, Catapres	Anxiety, fear, panic	Dogs, Oral: 1–2 h prior to anxiety-producing stimuli	Vomiting, diarrhea, sedation, hypotension, tachycardia or bradycardia, increased anxiety, irritability, anticholinergic effects	Do not use in conjunction with MAOI, do not use with cats, avoid in dogs with severe cardiovascular, respiratory, liver or kidney disease, or in conditions of shock, severe debilitation, or stress due to extreme heat, cold or fatigue

(Continued)

Table 10.2 (*Continued*)

Class	Drug family	Drug	Indications	Time to effect	Side effects	Contraindications
	Alpha-2 agonist	Dexmedetomidine oromucosal gel, Sileo®* *Sileo is FDA approved for treating noise aversions in dogs	Treatment of noise aversions in dogs; off-label for acute situational fear, panic	Dogs, OTM: 30 to 60 min prior to noise event	Pale mucous membranes, vomiting, sedation, gastroenteritis, periorbital edema, inappropriate urination	Do not use in conjunction with MAOI, do not use in cats, avoid in dogs with severe cardiovascular, respiratory, liver or kidney disease, or in conditions of shock, severe debilitation, or stress due to extreme heat, cold or fatigue
Antidepressant	Selective serotonin reuptake inhibitor (SSRI)	Fluoxetine, Prozac®, Reconcile®* *Reconcile is FDA approved for treating separation anxiety in dogs	Anxiety, chronic fear, compulsive disorder, aggression	Oral: 4–6 wk for maximal effect	Mild lethargy, anorexia nausea, vomiting, diarrhea, constipation, insomnia, increased agitation, tremors, increased anxiety, increased aggression	Do not use in conjunction with MAOI, TCA, other SSRI; Avoid abrupt discontinuation after 3–4 wk of use. Caution with tramadol, other serotonergic drugs
		Paroxetine, Paxil®	Same as fluoxetine	Oral: 4–6 wk for maximal effect	Same as fluoxetine plus: Urinary retention, constipation	Same as fluoxetine; caution with male cats due to potential for urinary retention
		Sertraline, Zoloft®	Same as fluoxetine	Oral: 4–6 wk for maximal effect	Same as fluoxetine	Same as fluoxetine
		Citalopram, Celexa®	Same as fluoxetine	Oral: 4–6 wk for maximal effect	Same as fluoxetine plus: Increased cardiac sensitivity in dogs	Same as fluoxetine
	Tricyclic antidepressant (TCA)	Clomipramine, Clomicalm®* *Clomicalm is FDA approved to treat separation anxiety in dogs	Anxiety, chronic fear, compulsive disorder	Oral: 3–4 wk for maximal effect	Sedation, anticholinergic effects: dry mouth, dry eye, mydriasis, urine retention, constipation. tachycardia or other arrhythmia; antihistaminic effect; aggression	Do not use in conjunction with MAOI, SSRI, other TCA; Glaucoma, keratoconjunctivitis sicca (dry eye), cardiac arrhythmias, seizures, urinary retention, or thyroid disease. Avoid abrupt discontinuation after 3–4 wk of use.
		Amitriptyline, Elavil®	Same as clomipramine	Oral: 3–4 wk for maximal effect	Same as clomipramine	Same as clomipramine
		Imipramine, Tofranil®	Same as clomipramine	Oral: 3–4 wk for maximal effect	Same as clomipramine	Same as clomipramine
		Doxepin, Sinequan®	Same as clomipramine	Oral: 3–4 wk for maximal effect	Same as clomipramine plus: Strong antihistaminic effect	Same as clomipramine
	Monoamine oxidase inhibitor (MAOI)	Selegiline, L-deprenyl, Anipryl®* *Anipryl is FDA approved for treating cognitive dysfunction syndrome in dogs	Cognitive dysfunction syndrome, anxiety, pituitary dependent hyperadrenocorticism in dogs	Oral: 4–8 wk for maximal effect	Increased motor activity, vomiting, diarrhea, agitation, restlessness, disorientation, stereotypic behavior with high doses, "cheese effect"	Do not use in conjunction with other MAOI (including amitraz), SSRI, or TCA. Tramadol, St. John's Wort, Griffonia seed extract, other opioids, alpha-2 agonists

Mood stabilizer	Anti-epileptic drug, tricyclic compound	Carbamazepine	impulsive, explosive aggression	Unknown in animals	nausea, dizziness, elevated liver values, blood dyscrasias, dermatologic lesions; aggression	Do not use in conjunction with MAOI
Atypical antidepressant	Mixed serotonin agonist/antagonist	Trazodone, Desyrel®	Anxiety, fear, phobias	Oral: 2–3 h	Vomiting, diarrhea, sedation, increased anxiety, irritability or aggression	Do not use in conjunction with MAOI
	Tetracyclic antidepressant/ serotonin and norepinephrine reuptake inhibitor	Mirtazapine, Remeron®, Mirataz™* *Mirataz is FDA approved for the management of weight loss in cats	Anxiety, chronic fear, appetite stimulation	Oral: 1 h	Polyphagia, agitation, tremors, muscle twitching, tachycardia, decrease seizure threshold, anti-nausea, anti-emetic effects	Do not use in conjunction with MAOI
CNS stimulant		Methylphenidate, Ritalin	Hyperkinesis, narcolepsy	Unknown in animals	Hyperactivity, agitation, aggression, hypertension, lower seizure threshold	Do not use in conjunction with MAOI
		Dextroamphetamine (injectable)	Hyperkinesis, narcolepsy	30 min to 2 h	Same as Methylphenidate plus: tremors, GI upset, dry mouth	Same as Methylphenidate
Anticonvulsants	Gabapentinoid	Gabapentin, Neurontin®	Fear, anxiety, phobia, panic, chronic neuropathic pain, patients with epilepsy, pre-veterinary visit medication, situational anxiety	Oral: 1 to 2 h	Dose-related ataxia/sedation, may intensify sedation from other medications	When using high dosages, sedation and ataxia may occur.
	Gabapentinoid	Pregabalin, Lyrica	Same as gabapentin; although more potent, readily absorbed, better anticonvulsant than gabapentin	Oral: 90 min	Same as gabapentin	Same as gabapentin

CNS: central nervous system; GI: gastrointestinal; MAOI: monoamine oxidase inhibitor; OTM: orotransmucosal; SSRI: selective serotonin reuptake inhibitor; TCA: tricyclic antidepressant.

hypotension, and some concern of decreased seizure threshold (Plumb 2002). However, a 2006 retrospective study did not find a correlation between acepromazine maleate (a phenothiazine) administration and increased seizure activity (Tobias et al. 2006). Additional side effects may be seen with longer term use or the use of high-potency medications. These may include neuroleptic malignant syndrome, extrapyramidal signs, and tardive dyskinesia. Neuroleptic malignant syndrome is a rare and idiosyncratic syndrome mainly seen in people. It is expressed as autonomic system instability manifested by muscle rigidity, altered levels of consciousness, hyperthermia, and tachycardia (Simpson and Simpson 1996). Extrapyramidal signs include resting tremors or stiffness or decreased movement of the facial muscles. Akathisia, identified by motor restlessness, agitation, and pacing, has been noted in some animals (Simpson and Simpson 1996). Acute dystonia, described as abrupt onset facial and neck muscle spasms, has also been noted (Simpson and Papich 2003). Tardive dyskinesia, described as facial contortions, abnormal movements of the tongue and mouth, or twisting postures that can affect the face, limbs, and trunk, is mainly seen in people after long-term administration of antipsychotics (Simpson and Simpson 1996; Simpson and Papich 2003).

Acepromazine is a low-potency phenothiazine and historically has been one of the most frequently used drugs to decrease mobility and reactivity in veterinary patients. It has a wide variety of uses, including a preanesthetic agent, an antiemetic (Plumb 2002), and for "aid in controlling intractable animals" (PromAce® Package insert, Fort Dodge 2000). A state of profound sedation with a poor anxiolytic effect is typically seen. Profound sedation along with the antiemetic effect makes it an appropriate choice for preanesthesia. Acepromazine can leave the animal more reactive to noises potentially resulting in a startle response, so caution should be taken when handling an animal under the influence of acepromazine. If used as a preanesthetic, consider utilizing commercially available ear protection for dogs or cotton balls placed in the ear canal to minimize noise perception. Unfortunately, acepromazine's effect merely slows down the pet's physical reaction, whereas the mental anxiety the pet is experiencing remains minimally affected. This makes acepromazine an inappropriate choice for use alone in animals with noise phobias or other anxieties, as it has been historically used.

- Acepromazine's effect merely slows down the pet's physical reaction, whereas the mental anxiety the pet is experiencing remains minimally affected. This makes acepromazine an inappropriate choice for use alone in animals with noise phobias or other anxieties.

Additional side effects that can be seen with the use of acepromazine include inhibition of learning, making the implementation of behavior modification challenging; and paradoxical excitation, primarily in horses and cats, but can include increased aggressive response and/or the loss of bite inhibition in any species. Therefore, extreme caution should be used, and safety measures such as basket muzzles should be implemented when acepromazine is used in animals with a history of aggression.

- Extreme caution should be used, and safety measures such as basket muzzles should be implemented when acepromazine is used in animals with a history of aggression.

Anxiolytics

Anxiolytic drugs commonly used in veterinary behavior medicine include three medication groups; benzodiazepines, azapirones, and alpha-2 agonists.

Benzodiazepines

Benzodiazepines work by potentiating the inhibitory effect of GABA. This occurs by binding to the GABA A receptor and strengthening the binding of GABA to this receptor. The effects seen include sedation, decreased anxiety, muscle relaxation, seizure control, although these effects tend to be dose dependent. Behaviorally, these medications are used to help treat events connected to fear, anxiety or panic, such as thunderstorm or other noise phobias, separation anxiety, or to decrease the fear response in "pariah" or the victim cat in cases of inter-cat aggression (Lindell et al. 1997). For the maximal anxiolytic effect to be seen with oral administration, most benzodiazepines must be administered at least one hour, sometimes as early as two hours, before initiation of anxiety-producing stimuli.

Some additional effects may also be seen with the use of benzodiazepines. Increased appetite, sometimes profound, can be noted; this may be beneficial in counteracting the anorexia seen secondary to the use of some antidepressants. Similar to acepromazine, memory deficits can be identified as well. These can be recognized by difficulty in learning new material, or the animal may seem to forget what has been previously taught. Decreasing the ability to learn may be a useful side effect if used during fearful situations, such as a visit to the veterinarian's office when a stressful procedure must be performed on the pet.

Paradoxical reactions, such as idiosyncratic excitation, agitation, and restlessness can also be seen in dogs and cats.

In addition, disinhibition of behaviors can also occur. In people, a loss of conscious inhibition of hostility, aggression, or rage has been documented. In animals, these medications should be used with extreme caution in aggression, as they can decrease bite inhibition, similar to what can be seen with acepromazine.

Acute hepatic necrosis in cats is a rare, but often fatal, potential side effect of benzodiazepines. It has been documented with oral diazepam, but the risk is present with the other benzodiazepines as well. There have been cases reported with almost every drug in this class. It is recommended to evaluate liver values before and within five days of starting medication when benzodiazepines are used in cats (Center et al. 1996).

- It is recommended to evaluate liver values before and within five days of starting medication when benzodiazepines are used in cats (Center et al. 1996).

Benzodiazepines are schedule IV controlled substances by the Controlled Substances Act and carry a risk of abuse by owners; therefore, additional monitoring and recording of prescriptions is necessary.

These medications are commonly used only as needed for event treatment, such as fireworks associated with holidays or fear, anxiety, and stress associated with veterinary visits. If they are administered chronically, as may be done with separation anxiety or generalized anxiety, they should be weaned gradually before being discontinued. The general rule is to decrease the administration by 25–30% per week or slower (Schwartz 2005). This helps prevent recurrence of behavioral signs and withdrawal, such as nervousness, tremors, or seizures.

There are several different drugs in this class that have been used for anxiety control in dogs and cats, but only one is FDA approved for use in dogs with noise aversions.

Imepitoin tablets (Pexion™) is an FDA-approved benzodiazepine-type medication for treating noise aversions in dogs. Unfortunately, the drug has had a delayed launch in the United States and has been slow to become commercially available. It is a low-affinity partial agonist for the benzodiazepine binding site of GABA A receptors and has been used as an antiepileptic and anxiolytic drug in Europe. Because the drug has been used as an antiepileptic, imepitoin may be classified by some as an anticonvulsant. For use situationally with noise events, imepitoin must be administered twice a day starting two days prior to the event. Sedation may be less than other full agonists, but also the effect may be less than other full agonist benzodiazepines. Common adverse effects include ataxia, increased appetite, lethargy, and vomiting. Pexion may disinhibit behavior in dogs and lead to signs of increased aggression, such as growling at a young child and a lack of self-control around other dogs. Therefore, caution is advised, or avoidance should be considered in cases of aggression.

Some other commonly used benzodiazepines include diazepam (Valium®), alprazolam (Xanax®), clonazepam (Klonopin®), and lorazepam (Ativan®). Each has a relatively short half-life, much shorter than is seen in people, making frequent dosing important. Variation does occur with the half-life, frequency, and intensity of side effects with each drug in the class. All benzodiazepines are metabolized in the liver and excreted through the kidneys, although intermediate metabolites and their effect on the liver vary.

Diazepam may have duration as short as four hours in dogs, leading to a frequent dosing requirement. Some patients may experience significant sedation and ataxia which may be a side effect related to muscle relaxation. Rare, but fatal acute hepatic necrosis may occur with use in cats. Clonazepam may be longer acting, less sedating, and have less of a polyphagia effect relative to some other benzodiazepines. Individual responses and variation to dose and effects do occur. Alprazolam has strong anti-panic effects and has less sedative effect compared with other benzodiazepines.

Some veterinary behaviorists believe that lorazepam may be safer for the liver, especially in cats, because it is believed not to have any intermediate metabolites that must be processed by the liver.

Azapirones

The azapirones are another drug class that can be classified as anxiolytic but they also have antidepressant effects. Buspirone (Buspar®) is the drug most commonly used in veterinary behavior medicine from this class. It is classified as a 5-HT (serotonin) 1A receptor agonist, as it has very specific affinity for the 5-HT 1A receptors. Its mechanism of action is interesting in that it initially activates autoreceptors, which actually potentiate negative feedback. Over time, however, these receptors will become progressively desensitized as with SSRI. This leads to enhanced activation of postsynaptic 5-HT 1A receptors (Blier and de Montigny 1998).

The degree of anxiety control is mild, making buspirone inappropriate for profound panic states. The late receptor reregulation effects results in a delayed anxiolytic response compared to the benzodiazepines. It may take up to four to six weeks to see the full effect of this medication. The degree of specificity for the 5-HT 1A receptor makes side effects associated with activity at other 5-HT receptor minimal and makes this a relatively safe medication. It can have a bitter taste, making it more difficult to disguise for cats. Buspirone is commonly used in combination with an SSRI or TCA or used alone for anxiolytic effects, such as treating anxiety-related urine marking in cats. Some veterinary behaviorists use buspirone in combination with diazepam for treating global fear and generalized anxiety in dogs. The medication may have a modest effect of boosting social confidence.

- The degree of anxiety control is mild, making buspirone inappropriate for profound panic states.

Alpha-2 agonists

Alpha-2 adrenergic receptors are located throughout the central and peripheral nervous system. Alpha-2 agonists function as a NE receptor agonist and block NE release at the locus coeruleus in the brain.

Sedative-hypnotic effects of alpha-2 are a result of inhibition of NE release from noradrenergic receptors (autoreceptors) in the locus coeruleus section of the brainstem. Analgesic effects are principally due to spinal anti-nociception via binding to non-noradrenergic receptors (heteroreceptors) located on the dorsal horn neurons of the spinal cord. Alpha-2 agonists stimulate the alpha-2 receptors in the body at presynaptic and postsynaptic receptors. Activation of the presynaptic alpha-2 adrenoceptor inhibits the release of NE and terminates the propagation of pain signals. Activation of the postsynaptic alpha-2 adrenoceptors in the CNS inhibits sympathetic activity and can decrease blood pressure and heart rate.

Clonidine is a nonselective alpha-2 adrenergic agonist and acts on alpha-2B, alpha-1B, alpha-2A, and alpha-1A adrenergic receptors and the imidazoline receptor, whereas dexmedetomidine is a highly selective alpha-2 adrenergic agonist and it acts primarily on alpha-2A adrenergic receptors. Clonidine has a specificity of 220 : 1 (alpha-2 to alpha-1 ratio), whereas dexmedetomidine exhibits a specificity of 1620 : 1 (Giovannitti et al. 2015).

Clonidine is a centrally acting alpha-2 agonist used to control blood pressure in people but is also thought to have some analgesic and anxiolytic effects because it can decrease NE release in the brain (Schweimer et al. 2005). Clonidine can be administered as needed for fear-inducing situations up to every 12 hours. It may take up to two hours for the anxiolytic effect and is expected to have a duration of four to six hours (Ogata and Dodman 2011). Starting with a low dose and titrating up to effect is recommended. In people, it is mainly metabolized in the liver and excreted in urine. Potential side effects to monitor for include vomiting, diarrhea, hypotension, tachycardia or bradycardia, sedation, increased irritability or anxiety, or anticholinergic effects.

Dexmedetomidine oromucosal gel (Sileo®) is a FDA-approved drug for noise aversion in dogs (Sileo® for Dogs n.d.). Sileo produces calming without significant sedation within 30 to 60 minutes after administration for noise events. Sileo may be redosed every two hours up to five times per 24 hours if the dog is still experiencing anxiety. Sileo has been used off label to treat other situational anxieties including panic in dogs associated with storm phobia and increased fear, anxiety, and/or stress with veterinary visits. Oral transmucosal mean bioavailability of dexmedetomidine is 28%, due to extensive first-pass metabolism. Dexmedetomidine must be absorbed through the oral mucosa for a behavioral effect. If the preparation is swallowed, bypassing buccal mucosa, there is no effect. Sileo is well tolerated in dogs. The most common adverse effects are pale mucous membranes, and possible emesis or sedation. Reported uncommonly are gastroenteritis, periorbital edema, and inappropriate urination.

Alpha-2 agonists should be avoided in dogs with severe cardiovascular, respiratory, liver or kidney disease, or in conditions of shock, severe debilitation, or stress due to extreme heat, cold or fatigue (Sileo® n.d. Package insert).

Antidepressants

The antidepressant classes that will be discussed include TCA, SSRI, and MAOI.

Tricyclic antidepressants

TCA are structurally similar to phenothiazines (central three-ring structure) and work by inhibiting the reuptake of NE and 5-HT by the presynaptic plasma membrane transporters. Commonly used medications in this class include clomipramine (Clomicalm®), amitriptyline (Elavil®), imipramine (Tofranil®), and doxepin (Sinequan®). Certain TCA are used to treat a variety of anxiety and compulsive disorders, as well as some forms of aggression in dogs and cats. Specific diagnoses applicable to this drug class include separation anxiety, generalized anxiety, compulsive disorders, such as lick granulomas or psychogenic alopecia, and anxiety-related urine marking. Additional effects include adrenergic effects, such as sedation or syncope; anticholinergic effects, such as dry mouth, dry eye, mydriasis, urine retention, constipation, tachycardia, or other arrhythmias; and antihistaminic effects. Amitriptyline and doxepin show the most potent antihistaminic effects in this drug class. Clomipramine administration has been associated with changes in measured thyroid levels. Although it is not thought to cause clinical hypothyroidism in dogs, it can complicate monitoring maintenance levels in dogs currently being treated for hypothyroid disease (Crowell-Davis and Murray 2006).

These medications have a narrower therapeutic window than the SSRI and clinically they are associated with more side effects. An overdose of a tricyclic antidepressant near 15 mg/kg can lead to death by fatal cardiac arrhythmia within hours (Johnson 1990; Simpson and Papich 2003). Cats tend to be more sensitive to TCA than dogs. This is most likely because these drugs are metabolized by glucuronidation.

TCA may take three to four weeks for maximal effect. TCA should be weaned gradually if they are to be discontinued after three to four weeks of use. TCA are contraindicated in patients with glaucoma, keratoconjunctivitis sicca (dry eye), cardiac arrhythmias, seizures, urinary retention, or thyroid disease. They should not be used with MAOI, as this greatly increases the risk of serotonin syndrome. After discontinuing a TCA, a minimum of 14 days should elapse before starting a MAOI. Clomipramine is more specific for 5-HT than other TCA making it more likely to have anti-compulsive effects compared with other TCA. Dogs metabolize clomipramine faster than people do. The half-life in dogs is approximately 5 hours compared to 24 hours in people. The label dose for clomipramine formulated as Clomicalm is 2–4 mg/kg q 24 hours; however, many experts agree that it may be more efficacious when administered every 12 hours rather than every 24 hours in dogs (Landsburg et al. 2003; Crowell-Davis and Murray 2006).

Clomicalm is a chewable flavored tablet formulation of clomipramine that is labeled for separation anxiety in dogs. It is not recommended for use in dogs displaying aggression per the label.

Selective serotonin reuptake inhibitors

SSRI are derivatives of TCA. Their mechanism of action is by inhibiting the reuptake of 5-HT by the presynaptic plasma membrane transporters. They also desensitize the 5-HT 1A autoreceptors over time.

Commonly used medications in this class include fluoxetine (Reconcile® and Prozac®), paroxetine (Paxil®), sertraline (Zoloft®), and citalopram (Celexa®). They are used to treat various anxieties, fears, aggressions, and compulsive disorders in dogs and cats. They tend to have fewer side effects than TCA and a safer therapeutic window. Owing to the reregulation of some of the receptors, expect four to six weeks to see the full therapeutic effect. As with many of the other medications already discussed, SSRI should be weaned off gradually when dosing chronically.

Additional effects include mild lethargy or anorexia, although these are usually mild and resolve within one to two weeks. More concerning side effects include nausea, vomiting, diarrhea, constipation, insomnia, increased agitation, tremors, increased anxiety, and rarely, increased aggression. Individual variation within the spectrum of side effects can be seen.

As with TCA, SSRI should not be used in combination with MAOI because of the risk of serotonin syndrome. When changing from fluoxetine to a MAOI, it is recommended to wait five weeks after discontinuing the fluoxetine before starting the MAOI. Fourteen days should elapse after discontinuance of a MAOI and beginning a SSRI. SSRI should be used cautiously when the patient is concurrently administered with tramadol, as this synthetic opiate analgesic also has 5-HT and NE reuptake activity, and this combination can lead to serotonin syndrome. It has been documented that dogs have an increased cardiac sensitivity to citalopram (Celexa); therefore, use with caution in this species (Celexa Product Information 2013).

Fluoxetine

A common human trade name for fluoxetine is Prozac, and the veterinary trade name is Reconcile. Fluoxetine may be less likely to disinhibit aggression than other commonly used behavior modifying drugs.

The generic, tablet, and capsule form of fluoxetine is inexpensive. Transdermal formulations of fluoxetine have been used in cats to ease daily administration. Unfortunately, there is no evidence at this time that transdermal formulations result in consistent and therapeutic blood levels; therefore, rendering this formulation type ineffective and potentially harmful in cats (Ciribassi et al. 2003).

Reconcile, is a flavored chewable tablet that is FDA approved for separation anxiety in dogs when used in conjunction with a behavior modification plan. This formulation is not recommended for use with dogs displaying aggression per the label.

Paroxetine

Paroxetine (Paxil) is another commonly used SSRI. Paroxetine is used in people for disorders involving social anxiety, panic, posttraumatic stress, generalized anxiety, and obsessive compulsive behaviors. Use is similar in veterinary patients. Paroxetine may be more likely to have anticholinergic side effects, such as urine retention or constipation, than other SSRI and these side effects may be more apparent in cats. Patient monitoring is recommended. Caution should be used with prescribing paroxetine for use in a male cat. Slowly titrating the dose over the first few weeks can help to avoid or alleviate side effects. Paroxetine, in some opinions, may be less likely to cause agitation that is sometimes seen with fluoxetine. It also has a shorter half-life than fluoxetine.

Monoamine oxidase inhibitors

MAOI work by blocking oxidative deamination or breakdown of intracellular monoamine neurotransmitters (5-HT, NE, and DA) by the enzyme monoamine oxidase, found within the mitochondria. There are two types of MAO, types A and B. Type A breaks down mainly 5-HT, NE, DA, and tyramine, whereas type B preferentially destroys phenylethylamine and DA. The drugs that inhibit MAO-A are considered less selective and not routinely used in veterinary medicine. It is interesting to note that the degree of inhibition of each neurotransmitter is species specific, and individual variation can be seen within any species.

Selegiline

Selegiline, also known as L-deprenyl or Anipryl®, is the only MAOI currently used in veterinary behavior medicine. Selegiline is used primarily for Parkinson's and Alzheimer's diseases in people but used for CDS in dogs and cats. Anipryl is FDA approved for the treatment of pituitary-dependent hyperadrenocorticism in dogs and for CDS in dogs.

Selegiline has additional mechanisms of action beyond inhibiting the breakdown of neurotransmitters by monoamine in the mitochondria. It also inhibits the presynaptic reuptake of DA, NE, and 5-HT. In addition, it modulates DA levels by inhibiting some autoreceptors, preventing degradation, and increasing turnover. It decreases oxidative stress secondary to the DA degradation and may also enhance the action of superoxide dismutase and catalase, two free radical scavengers that help to increase the elimination of free radicals. It also increases levels of phenylethylamine, which is a neuromodulator of DA responses. It helps to increase the release and decrease the reuptake of DA (Campbell et al. 2001; Crowell-Davis and Murray 2006; Pfizer Inc. 1998).

The many different actions of selegiline lead to a variety of effects seen in the patient. These include elevated mood or decreased anxiety. Selegiline is used to treat a wide variety of behavioral disorders in Europe, whereas in the United States it is primarily used for CDS in dogs and cats. In Europe, anxiolysis is one of the main uses of this medication.

Selegiline has also been shown to decrease oxidative damage (Campbell et al. 2001; Crowell-Davis and Murray 2006; Pfizer Inc. 1998). This is important because oxidative damage of DA pathways is considered a significant mechanism in the pathogenesis of Parkinson's disease, and free radicals also contribute to Alzheimer's disease in people and CDS in animals.

High doses may cause stereotypic behaviors because of the increase in DA. Motor activity may be increased as a result of selegiline's metabolic products, including amphetamine and methamphetamine, as well as phenylethylamine, which also has amphetamine effects. It is therefore recommended to administer this medication in the morning so the pet does not keep the owner up at night with increased activity. In addition, vomiting, diarrhea, agitation, restlessness, or disorientation may be occasionally seen. Because of the metabolic products, this drug does have the potential for abuse by people, so monitoring and recording of prescriptions are recommended.

Before administering a MAOI, it is important to be aware of all medications, including parasiticides and herbal remedies that the pet is taking. MAOI should not be used concurrently with other TCA, SSRI, or MAOI, as there is a significant risk of developing serotonin syndrome or toxicity with these combinations.

Serotonin syndrome occurs when the concentration of 5-HT in the brain becomes too high, reaching toxic levels. Clinical signs that can be seen include nausea, confusion, agitation, muscle rigidity, tremors, salivation, and hyperthermia, and may lead to seizures, coma, and death. This is most commonly the result of a MAOI combined with another antidepressant (usually a TCA or SSRI), and the inhibition of neurotransmitter degradation from the MAOI is coupled with reuptake inhibition from the antidepressant but can occur with other combinations as well. Multiple MAOI should not be combined. Amitraz, a topical parasiticide, is also a MAOI. It is found in Mitaban®, Preventic® collars, and the spot-on flea and tick treatment, CERTIFECT™. Other combinations can potentially lead to serotonin syndrome. Diets high in tryptophan or tryptophan supplementation could also create serotonin syndrome because the amino acid tryptophan is the precursor to 5-HT. Some over-the-counter herbal supplements can have this unintended effect also. St. John's Wort can act as MAOI or broad spectrum reuptake inhibitor (Schwartz 2005), and Griffonia seed extract is comprised of 5-hydroxytryptophan, another part of the synthesis of 5-HT (Crowell-Davis and Murray 2006). Other medications commonly used to manage concurrent disease processes in older patients can also negatively interact with selegiline. The synthetic opiate analgesic, tramadol, has 5-HT and NE reuptake actions. There have been case reports of agitation, stupor, and death when selegiline was combined with other opioids. Caution should be used when these medications are combined or used concurrently (Plumb 2002). Extreme fluctuations in blood pressure may occur when selegiline is combined with phenylpropanolamine, a drug commonly used for urinary incontinence, or alpha-2 agonists. In one study of healthy dogs receiving selegiline and phenylpropanolamine, alone or in combination, no adverse effects were detected (Cohn et al. 2002).

- Before administering a MAOI, it is important to be aware of all medications, including parasiticides and herbal remedies that the pet is taking.

There is also an interaction called the *cheese effect* that occurs more commonly in people, but there have been a few cases reported in individual animals. It occurs when larger amounts of certain cheeses or wine are ingested while taking a MAOI, and the level of tyramine in the gut increases because MAOI prevent inactivation of tyramine, which leads to increased NE. This can create a phenomenon in which vasoconstriction and an increase in blood pressure occur simultaneously, leading to a hypertensive crisis. This is more likely to occur with nonselective MAOI (MAOA-I) but could potentially occur in sensitive individuals. Therefore, it may be prudent to limit the pet's cheese intake with concurrent use of selegiline (selegiline FDA professional monograph).

Mood stabilizers

Mood stabilizers are used to mediate extreme changes in mood and help treat mania and depression in people, particularly lithium. Many have historically been used to facilitate seizure control, particularly valproic acid and carbamazepine. Their behavioral effects aim to decrease impulsivity, emotional reactivity, and aggression. They are uncommonly used in veterinary behavior medicine.

Carbamazepine has a similar structure to TCA and acts on ion channels to decrease high-frequency repetitive firing. This was the mechanism implicated for seizure control, although its short half-life makes it less effective in this regard. It also has other non-specific actions on many neurotransmitters, and its psychotropic mode of action is unknown. Carbamazepine is generally used for impulsive, explosive aggression but almost always in conjunction with other behavior modifying drugs. Side effects to be aware of and to monitor for include: nausea, dizziness, elevated liver values, blood dyscrasias, and dermatologic lesions. At a minimum, a complete blood count and chemistry panel should be checked before starting therapy and again one month after treatment or after a dose increase.

Atypical antidepressants

There are several atypical antidepressants that are becoming more frequently used as adjuncts to behavior treatment plans. These include buspirone (Buspar), trazodone (Desyrel®), and mirtazapine (Remeron®, Mirataz™), but the list is expanding rapidly. Buspirone was discussed under anxiolytics.

Trazodone

Trazodone is a mixed 5-HT agonist/antagonist. It works as a weak inhibitor of 5-HT reuptake at presynaptic 5-HT receptors and as an antagonist at postsynaptic 5-HT receptors. The active metabolite *m*-chlorophenylpiperazine also has some agonistic effect at 5-HT 1 receptors, which may also increase 5-HT by mediating inhibitory effect of GABA (Simpson and Simpson 1996). Trazodone is commonly used in people as an antidepressant, anxiolytic, sleep aid, and anti-obsessional.

The synergistic effect of trazodone in combination with a SSRI or TCA can be helpful when additional anxiety control is needed but the risks or side effects of benzodiazepines are too severe (Gruen and Sherman 2008). Trazodone has also been used alone or as needed for specific events (e.g. fireworks, thunderstorms). Additionally, it has been used to facilitate postsurgical crate confinement and decrease stress associated with veterinary care.

Trazodone typically has minimal anticholinergic effects, but vomiting, diarrhea, or sedation can be noted. These are less likely if the dose is started low and titrated up and if administered with food. Uncommonly, increased anxiety, irritability, or aggression can be seen, and the pet should be monitored for these side effects. This medication has also been reported to have the lowest seizure risk of the drugs in the antidepressant class (Gruen and Sherman 2008).

Mirtazapine

Mirataz (mirtazapine transdermal ointment) is an FDA-approved transdermal for treating feline weight loss due to stress or disease. It is administered topically by applying a 1.5-inch ribbon of ointment (approximately 2 mg/cat equal to 0.1 mL) on the inner pinna of the cat's ear once daily for 14 days. Common adverse effects are application site reactions, behavioral abnormalities (vocalization and hyperactivity) and vomiting.

Mirtazapine (trade name Remeron) is also available in a generic tablet form. Traditionally, mirtazapine has been used as an antidepressant in human medicine, but it has been used as an appetite stimulant in pets. Mirtazapine is considered a second generation or tetracyclic antidepressant that works through presynaptic alpha-2 adrenergic receptor antagonist activity and increases 5-HT and NE activity (Quimby et al. 2011). Mirtazapine has sedation, anxiolytic, antiemetic, and appetite stimulant effects. In cats, mirtazapine is used for its anti-nausea, antiemetic, and appetite stimulating effects (Quimby et al. 2011). In children with a diagnosis of autistic disorder, the medication has been used to decrease inappropriate sexual behaviors (Coskun et al. 2009).

There is a potential risk for paradoxical increased anxiety or irritability whether mirtazapine is given orally in dogs, and orally or transdermally in cats. Serotonin syndrome may occur when combined with other serotonergic drugs, therefore patient monitoring should occur when combined with SSRI or TCA. Use should be avoided with MAOI because of significant risk of serotonin syndrome. Owing to the lack of glucuronidation capabilities in the cat, mirtazapine when administered orally is typically given every 72 hours rather than once to twice daily in the dog.

CNS stimulants

CNS stimulants are uncommonly used in veterinary behavior medicine and are indicated for a few behavioral disorders, mainly for narcolepsy or hyperkinesis (pathologic hyperactivity) in dogs. There are several side effects associated with this class of medication because of the stimulant nature of these drugs. They are contraindicated in patients with glaucoma, heart disease, or an animal that has taken MAOI in the last 14 days (Crowell-Davis and Murray 2006).

Dextroamphetamine is an injectable formulation, which can be used in the clinic to attempt to diagnose hyperkinesis, as its effect occurs rapidly but has short duration. It is rarely used.

Methylphenidate (Ritalin) works by enhancing DA release and inhibiting DA and NE reuptake. This leads to a paradoxical calming effect in some overactivity disorders, learning deficits, or some types of aggression in people. Methylphenidate is indicated for narcolepsy and hyperkinesis in dogs but is contraindicated in dogs showing hyperactivity from other causes, such as conditioned behaviors. True hyperkinesis is rare. Diagnosis confirmation with a drug trial using methylphenidate should only be undertaken if behavior modification treatment for the other differentials for hyperactivity has failed and the clinician has a strong suspicion for hyperkinesis as a differential diagnosis. The medication is typically started at a low dose and incrementally increased every one to two days. If at any point, the hyperactivity worsens, the drug trial is discontinued. The dose titration is important because the effect on the patient's activity level usually falls in a reverse bell curve effect. A lower dose may be ineffective, seen as no change in the degree of hyperactivity, but as the dose is incrementally increased, a point at which the activity level drops dramatically will be found. This will be considered near the therapeutic dose for that individual dog. If the dose increase is continued, the dog's activity will increase back to baseline and potentially even higher.

Anticonvulsants

Two anticonvulsants commonly used in behavioral medicine are gabapentin (Neurotin®) and pregabalin (Lyrica). These anticonvulsant medications are considered for patients with fear and anxiety-related conditions, chronic pain of neuropathic origin, and those with epilepsy. They are both in the drug family called Gabapentinoid.

Both drugs bind with high affinity to alpha 2-delta subunits of voltage activated calcium channels. They have anticonvulsant and antineuralgic effects by reduced neurotransmitter release and activity. The primary effect of gabapentin and pregabalin may be to act by reducing or inhibiting the excitatory effects of glutamate via acting as a voltage gaited calcium channel blocker. They may also act as a sodium channel blocker influencing excitatory nerve activity.

Gabapentin and pregabalin have anticonvulsant effects and do not reduce the seizure threshold like most antidepressants (TCA, SSRI, and MAOI). In humans, they are primarily used as an adjuvant to other anticonvulsants for treatment of partial seizures. In humans, they are also used to treat nerve pain (fibromyalgia, diabetic peripheral neuropathy) and restless leg syndrome. Therefore, if the veterinary patient has a history of seizures or the repetitive behavioral disorder may be a partial seizure, gabapentin or pregabalin may be the behavioral drug of choice for their antiepileptogenic and pain-relieving effects. Generally, these drugs are well tolerated, with the most common side effects being sedation and ataxia.

Gabapentin and pregabalin have been used as a sole agent for treating chronic fear, anxiety, phobia, and panic-related conditions in veterinary patients. They can be effective for generalized anxiety, social anxiety, and even some panic disorders in people, and they are used for similar conditions in veterinary patients. They can be used as adjunct medications in combination with SSRI, TCA and MAOI. Gabapentin and pregabalin can be a situational event medication for acute fear, anxiety, phobic, and panic conditions.

Gabapentin

A single dose of gabapentin in cats has been shown to reduce stress with transportation and examination within the veterinary hospital (van Haaften et al. 2017). A single dose of gabapentin in dogs has been shown to reduce lip licking behavior, a sign of stress, during veterinary visits (Stollar et al. 2022). Gabapentin is commonly used and recommended as a pre-visit pharmaceutical to reduce fear, anxiety, and stress in dogs and cats for veterinary visits and procedures. Gabapentin is more slowly and variably absorbed when compared to pregabalin. As of 2022 gabapentin is not federally recognized as a schedule V controlled substance by the Controlled Substances Act. However, some states have categorized it as a schedule V controlled substance. Therefore, additional monitoring and recording of prescriptions is necessary in those states.

Pregabalin

Pregabalin has been shown to reduce signs of anxiety in cats during transportation when given 90 minutes prior to placing the cat in the carrier and starting transportation (Lamminen et al. 2022). In dogs with Chiari-like malformation and syringomyelia, and dogs undergoing surgery for intervertebral disk disease, pregabalin has been shown to be efficacious for the treatment of neuropathic pain (Sanchis-Mora et al. 2019; Schmierer et al. 2020). Pregabalin is more readily absorbed and more potent, possibly a better anticonvulsant, has a longer half-life, and may be better tolerated in some patients than gabapentin. Pregabalin is a schedule V controlled substance under the Controlled Substances Act and carries a risk of abuse by owners; therefore, additional monitoring and recording of prescriptions is necessary.

Nutraceuticals and supplements

A nutraceutical is a nutritional supplement that has pharmaceutical properties and is used for medicinal benefits to physical or mental health. There are several nutraceuticals that are becoming more frequently used as adjuncts to behavioral medications and are used to augment behavior modification treatment plans. Behavioral effects as well as side effects of nutraceuticals are often milder than with conventional drugs.

Alpha-casozepine

Alpha-casozepine (Zylkene®) is a bioactive peptide originating from alpha S1 tryptic casein, a bovine-sourced hydrolyzed milk protein, which has been reported to have anxiolytic effects similar to benzodiazepines in dogs and cats (Beata et al. 2007a, 2007b). Alpha-casozepine has an affinity for GABA receptors in the brain and produces calming without side effects commonly associated with benzodiazepines. The oral supplement is used to help dogs and cats stay calm in challenging and unusual situations such as traveling, noise events, interactions with unfamiliar people, and separation. The product may be used solely for events or daily long term. Better effects may be observed when the supplement is started a few days up to a week before the event. Best effects may be observed if the pet is supplemented for a medium- or long-term duration (Buckley 2017). Alpha-casozepine is also available in some commercially available therapeutic diets, which may promote calming in dogs and cats (Landsberg et al. 2017).

L-Theanine

L-Theanine is an amino acid, naturally found in green, black, and white tea, which is a structural analog of glutamate. L-Theanine binds and blocks glutamate receptors, which decrease excitatory impulses and glutamate's stimulatory effects in the brain (Nathan et al. 2006). L-Theanine is thought to promote calming by increasing the neurotransmitters serotonin, dopamine, and GABA in the brain (Nathan et al. 2006). L-Theanine facilitates the generation of alpha waves in the brain that are indicative of relaxed, awake and alert states, without promoting drowsiness (Mason 2001; Dramard et al. 2018). L-theanine (Anxitane) is an oral supplement for dogs and cats, which is indicated to promote relaxation with nervousness or environmentally induced stress and anxiety. Clinical trials suggest a reduction in global anxiety scores for dogs and cats (Dramard et al. 2018; Michelazzi et al. 2010). L-Theanine has been studied for noise or storm fear and phobias in dogs (Berteselli and Michelazzi 2007; Michelazzi et al. 2010, 2015; Pike et al. 2015), travel anxiety in dogs (Berteselli and Michelazzi 2007), urine marking in cats (Dramard et al. 2018), and fear of people in dogs (Araujo et al. 2010). The oral supplement is most effective when used in conjunction with appropriate behavior modification for the specific condition.

Probiotics

Probiotics are foods or oral supplements containing live bacterial microorganisms that may provide health benefits and alter, improve, or restore normal gut flora. There is scientific evidence that certain strains of probiotics have anxiolytic effects in animals and humans (Messaoudi et al. 2011). In a blinded crossover design study of Labrador Retrievers fed Purina Pro Plan Veterinary Supplements Calming Care, anxiety-related behaviors such as spinning, pacing, jumping, and barking were reduced in 90% of dogs (McGowan 2016). Increased exploratory behavior in a novel environment was observed in the supplemented group compared to placebo (McGowan 2018). Also noted were reduced salivary cortisol concentrations, decreases in heart rate, and increases in heart rate variability, all indicative of reduced stress levels (McGowan 2018). In a study of cats with feline herpes virus (FHV-1), cats supplemented with Feline Calming Care were significantly less likely to display anxious behaviors such as pacing, had lower serum cortisol concentrations, reduced sneezing associated with FHV-1, and were more likely to have increased social activity when compared to cats supplemented with the placebo.

Omega 3

Omega 3 are nutritional supplements for dogs and cats. The best omega 3 are derived from fish oils and contain high levels of the omega 3 fatty acids, DHA (docosahexaenoic acid) and EPA (eicosapentaenoic acid).

DHA and EPA supplementation may reduce pain levels, treat inflammatory conditions in the brain and body, improve cognition and the ability to learn, reduce anxiety scores, and reduce overall levels of irritability.

Mainstay, adjunct, situational event medication and/or nutraceutical

Veterinarians should consider nutraceuticals for mild cases of fear, anxiety, and/or stress as a sole agent or as an adjunct or augmentation strategy to complement conventional behavioral medications with concurrent implementation of the behavior modification treatment plan. With conventional medication drug selection, veterinarians must consider what general category of behavior medication is most appropriate, a mainstay, an adjunct or augmentation strategy, or a situational and/or event medication.

Many chronic behavior problems are best treated with a mainstay medication on board every day while concurrently implementing an appropriate behavior modification and training plan. Mainstay medications are used long term, generally once to twice a day and fall into the class of medications called antidepressants. All antidepressants have anxiolytic effects, hence their use in veterinary behavioral medicine. Examples include the following: SSRI, TCA, or MAOI. These medications have a delayed onset of action and may take four to six weeks for evaluation of effect.

Adjunct medications are medications that are added and used in addition to the mainstay medication. They may be used routinely to augment or potentiate the mainstay medication or to further reduce fear, anxiety, and/or stress via other mechanisms. Common adjunct medications include benzodiazepines, trazodone, gabapentin, clonidine, and mirtazapine. Adjunct medications typically have a rapid onset of action with some effect within hours of administration. They may be used at the start of a mainstay medication when an anxiolytic effect is needed right away or added to the mainstay medication for further anxiety reduction. Chronic dosing of adjunct medications at a routine frequency (at least daily) may provide cumulative effects and prevent the reoccurrence of fear, anxiety and/or stress that maintains the undesirable behavior.

Acute behavior problems, like specific fears and phobias, are best treated situationally, using situational or event medications. Medication is administered just prior to the stressful event and only as needed. These medications can be used to prevent or lessen fear, anxiety, and/or stress with an event like a visit to the veterinarian. To prevent fear, anxiety, and/or stress, they work best if given prior to the onset of the undesirable behavioral reaction. This may be administering the behavioral medication well in advance of a suspected stressful situation or event. They are less effective in reducing already present fear, anxiety, and stress, but are often used in that context as well. Besides adjunct medications, common situation or event medications are benzodiazepines, trazodone, gabapentin, clonidine, and Sileo (dexmedetomidine oromucosal gel).

Conclusion

The nervous system is a complexity of neurons and neurotransmitters communicating important information at specific moments. The brain is the most intricate of all the organs in the body. The various structures in the brain work in conjunction to attain life and personality. There are over 50 neurotransmitters in the body, but the neurotransmitters most commonly associated with behavior are the monoamines and GABA. There are many different medications and drug classes that can be useful tools in the comprehensive treatment plan for behavioral disorders. Whether the main diagnosis centers around fear and anxiety, compulsive disorder, aggression, cognitive dysfunction, or hyperkinesis, the same basic plan should be followed for every patient to make an educated decision on whether behavioral medications are indicated (see Table 10.3), and if so, which is the most appropriate medication for that case. A thorough behavior and medical history should be obtained, and a working diagnosis should be made by a licensed Doctor of Veterinary Medicine after a veterinarian–client–patient relationship has been established. Potential drug interactions or concurrent illnesses should be identified prior to medication being prescribed. The client should be educated about side effects,

Table 10.3 Possible indications for drug therapy.

Behavior disorder or other considerations	
Fear and/or anxieties	Multiple stimuli
	Stimuli cannot be avoided
	Intensity of stimuli cannot be controlled
	Cannot determine a non-stressful starting point for desensitization to begin
	Self-injurious behavior
Aggression	Multiple triggers
	Triggers cannot be identified
	Triggers cannot be managed or avoided
	Threshold for aggression very low
	Little warning before aggressive response
	Non-graduated response
Compulsive disorder	Decrease frequency/intensity of behavior so behavior modification possible
	Decrease frequency/intensity of conflict behaviors that have the potential for developing into a compulsive behavior (usually from frustration)
Cognitive dysfunction	Slow progression of cognitive dysfunction
	Adjunct symptomatic therapy if new fears and anxieties, insomnia develop
Condition of the human–animal bond	Broken or severely damaged human–animal bond
	Owner is afraid of the pet
	Owner contemplating euthanasia or rehoming, seeking help as a "last resort"

contraindications, and length of time to effect for the medication prescribed for the pet. Adequate follow-up with the client and patient is imperative to monitor treatment success and to make adjustments as needed.

By obtaining a thorough understanding of neurophysiology, pharmacokinetics, and psychopharmacology, a veterinary technician can be prepared to assist and educate clients regarding the treatment of their pet's behavioral disorders, thus helping to preserve the human–animal bond.

Acknowledgement

The author acknowledges the contribution of Sara L. Bennett and Carissa D. Sparks to the first edition chapter.

References

Araujo, J.A., de Rivera, C., Ethier, J.L. et al. (2010). ANXITANE tablets reduce fear of human beings in a laboratory model of anxiety-related disorders. *Journal of Veterinary Behavior* 5 (5): 268–275.

Beata, C., Beaumont-Graff, E., Coll, V. et al. (2007a). Effect of alpha-casozepine (Zylkene) on anxiety in cats. *Journal of Veterinary Behavior* 2 (2): 40–46.

Beata, C., Beaumont-Graff, E., Diaz, C. et al. (2007b). Effects of alpha-casozepine (Zylkene) versus selegiline hydrochloride (Selgian, Anipryl) on anxiety disorders in dogs. *Journal of Veterinary Behavior* 2 (5): 175–183.

Berteselli, G.V. and Michelazzi, M. (2007). Use of L-theanine tablets (Anxitane™) and behavior modification for treatment of phobias in dogs: a preliminary study. In: *Poster. 6th IVBM, Riccione, IT.*

Bill, R.L. (2006). *Clinical Pharmacology and Therapeutics for the Veterinary Technician*, 3e. St. Louis, MO: Mosby Inc.

Blier, P. and de Montigny, C. (1998). Possible serotonergic mechanisms underlying the antidepressant and anti-obsessive–compulsive disorder responses. *Biological Psychiatry* 53: 193–203.

Buckley, L.A. (2017). Is alpha-casozepine efficacious at reducing anxiety in dogs? *Veterinary Evidence* 2 (3): https://doi.org/10.18849/ve.v2i3.67.

Campbell, S., Trettien, A., and Kozan, B. (2001). A noncomparative open-label study evaluating the effect of selegiline hydrochloride in a clinical setting. *Veterinary Therapeutics* 2 (1): 24–39.

Carlson, N.R. (2002). *Foundations of Physiological Psychology*, 5e. Boston, MA: A Pearson Education, Inc.

Celexa Product information (2013). *Forest Pharmaceuticals.* St. Louis, MO: Warner-Lambert Company.

Center, S.A., Elston, T.H., and Rowland, P.H. (1996). Fulminant hepatic failure associated with oral administration of diazepam in 11 cats. *Journal of the American Veterinary Medical Association* 209: 618–625.

Ciribassi, J., Luescher, A., and Pasloske, K.S. (2003). Comparative bioavailability of fluoxetine after transdermal and oral administration to healthy cats. *American Journal of Veterinary Research* 64 (8): 994–998.

Cohn, L., Dodam, J., and Szladovits, B. (2002). Effects of selegiline, phenylpropanolamine, or a combination of both on physiologic and behavioral variables in healthy dogs. *American Journal of Veterinary Research* 63 (6): 827–832. https://doi.org/10.2460/ajvr.2002.63.827.

Coskun, M., Karakoc, S., Kircelli, F., and Mukaddes, N.M. (2009). Effectiveness of mirtazapine in the treatment of inappropriate sexual behaviors in individuals with autistic disorder. *Journal of Child and Adolescent Psychopharmacology* 19 (2): 203–206.

Crowell-Davis, S. and Murray, T. (2006). *Veterinary Psychopharmacology*. Ames: Blackwell Publishing Company.

Cunningham, J.G. and Klein, B.G. (2007). *Textbook of Veterinary Physiology*, 4e. Philadelphia, PA: Elsevier.

Dramard, V., Kern, L., Hofmans, J. et al. (2018). Effect of l-theanine tablets in reducing stress-related emotional signs in cats: an open-label field study. *Irish Veterinary Journal* 71: 21.

Giovannitti, J.A., Thoms, S.M., and Crawford, J.J. (2015). Alpha-2 adrenergic receptor agonists: a review of current clinical applications. *Anesthesia Progress* 62 (1): 31–38.

Grilly, D.M. (2006). *Drugs and Human Behavior*, 5e. Boston, MA: Pearson Education, Inc.

Gruen, M. and Sherman, B. (2008). Use of trazodone as an adjunctive agent in the treatment of canine anxiety disorders: 56 cases (1995–2007). *Journal of the American Veterinary Medical Association* 233: 1902–1907.

van Haaften, K.A., Forsythe, L.R.E., Stelow, E.A., and Bain, M.J. (2017). Effects of a single preappointment dose of gabapentin on signs of stress in cats during transportation and veterinary examination. *Journal of the American Veterinary Medical Association* 251 (10): 1175–1181.

Hedges, D. and Burchfield, C. (2006). *Mind, Brain and Drug: An Introduction to Psychopharmacology*. Boston, MA: Pearson Education, Inc.

Horwitz, D. and Mills, D.S. (2002). *BSAVA Manual of Canine and Feline Behavioural Medicine*. Quedgeley, Gloucester: British Small Animal Veterinary Association.

Johnson, L.R. (1990). Tricyclic antidepressant toxicosis. *Veterinary Clinics of North America, Small Animal Practice* 20: 393–403.

King, A.S. (1987). *Physiological and Clinical Anatomy of the Domestic Mammals*. Oxford: Oxford University Press.

Lamminen, T., Doedée, A., Hyttilä-Hopponen, M., and Kaskinoro, J. (2022). Pharmacokinetics of single and repeated oral doses of pregabalin oral solution formulation in cats. *Journal of Veterinary Pharmacology and Therapeutics* 45 (4): 385–391.

Landsberg, G., Milgram, B., Mougeot, I. et al. (2017). Therapeutic effects of an alpha-casozepine and L-tryptophan supplemented diet on fear and anxiety in the cat. *Journal of Feline Medicine and Surgery* 19 (6): 594–602.

Landsburg, G., Hunthausen, W., and Ackerman, L. (2003). *Handbook of Behavior Problems of the Dog and Cat*, 2e. Edinburgh: Saunders.

Lindell, E.M., Erb, H.N., and Houpt, K.A. (1997). Intercat aggression: a retrospective study examining types of aggression, sexes of fighting pairs, and effectiveness of treatment. *Applied Animal Behaviour Science* 55: 153–162.

Mason, R. (2001). 200 mg of Zen: L-theanine boosts alpha waves, promotes alert relaxation. *Alternative and Complementary Therapies* 7 (2): 91–95.

McCurnin, D.M. and Bassert, J.M. (2006). *Clinical Textbook for Veterinary Technicians*, 6e. St. Louis, MO: Elsevier Saunders.

McGowan, R.T.S. (2016). "Oiling the brain" or "cultivating the gut": impact of diet on anxious behavior in dogs. In: *Proceedings of the Nestlé Purina Companion Animal Nutrition Summit, Florida*, 91–97.

McGowan, R.T.S. (2018). Tapping into those 'gut feelings': impact of BL999 (*Bifidobacterium longum*) on anxiety in dogs. In: *ACVB Symposium*.

Messaoudi, M., Lalonde, R., Violle, N. et al. (2011). Assessment of psychotropic-like properties of a probiotic formulation (lactobacillus helveticus ROO52 and Bifidobacterium longum R0175) in rats and human subjects. *British Journal of Nutrition* 105: 755–764.

Meyer, J.S. and Quenzer, L.F. (2005). *Psychopharmacology Drugs, the Brain, and Behavior*. Sunderland, MA: Sinauer Associates Inc.

Michelazzi, M., Berteselli, G., Minero, M., and Cavallone, E. (2010). Effectiveness of L-theanine and behavioral therapy in the treatment of noise phobias in dogs. *Journal of Veterinary Behavior* 5 (1): 34–35.

Michelazzi, M., Berteselli, G.V., Talamonti, Z. et al. (2015). Efficacy of L-theanine in the treatment of noise phobias in dogs: preliminary results. *Veterinária* 29 (2): 53–59.

Nathan, P.J., Lu, K., Gray, M., and Oliver, C. (2006). The neuropharmacology of L-theanine (N-ethyl-L-glutamine): a possible neuroprotective and cognitive enhancing agent. *Journal of Herbal Pharmacotherapy* 6 (2): 21–30.

Ogata, N. and Dodman, N. (2011). The use of clonidine in the treatment of fear-based behavior problems in dogs: an open trial. *Journal of Veterinary Behavior* 6: 130–137.

Overall, K. (2001). Pharmacologic treatment in behavioural medicine: the importance of neurochemistry, molecular biology and mechanistic hypotheses. *The Veterinary Journal* 162: 9–23.

Overall, K. (2004). Paradigms for pharmacologic use as a treatment component in feline behavioral medicine. *Journal of Feline Medicine and Surgery* 6: 29–42.

Pfizer Inc (1998). *Freedom of Informations Summary: Anipryl® (Selegiline Hydrochloride) Tablets for Use in Dogs*. Groton, CT: Pfizer Inc.

Pike, A.L., Horwitz, D.F., and Lobprise, H. (2015). An open-label prospective study of the use of l-theanine (Anxitane) in storm-sensitive client-owned dogs. *Journal of Veterinary Behavior* 10 (4): 324–331.

Plumb, D.C. (2002). *Veterinary Drug Handbook*, 4e. Ames: Iowa State Press.

PromAce® Package insert, Fort Dodge (2000). Fort Dodge Animal Health, Fort Dodge, IA 50501, USA (Injection); Ayerst Laboratories, Inc., Rouses Point, NY 12979, USA (Tablets) I 02300 Rev. Aug. 2000 02wc.

Quimby, J.M., Gustafson, D.L., Samber, B.J., and Lunn, K.F. (2011). Studies on the pharmacokinetics and pharmacodynamics of mirtazapine in healthy young cats. *Journal of Veterinary Pharmacology and Therapeutics* 34 (4): 388–396.

Sanchis-Mora, S., Chang, Y.M., Abeyesinghe, S.M. et al. (2019). Pregabalin for the treatment of syringomyelia-associated neuropathic pain in dogs: a randomised, placebo-controlled, double-masked clinical trial. *Veterinary Journal* 250: 55–62.

Schmierer, P.A., Tünsmeyer, J., Tipold, A. et al. (2020). Randomized controlled trial of pregabalin for analgesia after surgical treatment of intervertebral disc disease in dogs. *Veterinary Surgery* 49 (5): 905–913.

Schwartz, S. (2005). *Psychoactive Herbs in Veterinary Behavior Medicine*. Ames: Blackwell Publishing Company.

Schweimer, J., Fendt, M., and Schnitzler, H.U. (2005). Effects of clonidine injections into the bed nucleus of the striaterminalis on fear and anxiety behavior in rats. *European Journal of Pharmacology* 507: 117–124.

Sileo® for Dogs (n.d.). NADA 141-456. Approved by FDA. Revised November 2017. https://animaldrug-satfda.fda.gov/adafda/app/search/public/document/downloadFoi/942 (accessed December 2022).

Sileo® Package insert. (n.d.). Manufactured by Orion Corporation, Turku, Finland. Distributed by Zoetis Inc.

Simpson, B.S. and Papich, M.G. (2003). Pharmacologic management in veterinary behavioral medicine. *The Veterinary Clinics of North America: Small Animal Practice* **33**: 365–404.

Simpson, B. and Simpson, D. (1996). Behavioral pharmacotherapy. Part I. Antipsychotics and Antidepressants. *Compendium on Continuing Education for the Practicing Veterinarian* **18** (10): 1067–1081.

Stollar, O., Moore, G.E., Mukhopadhyay, A. et al. (2022). Effects of a single dose of oral gabapentin in dogs during a veterinary visit: a double-blinded, placebo-controlled study. *Journal of the American Veterinary Medical Association* 260 (9): 1031–1040.

Tobias, K., Marioni-Henry, K., and Wagner, R. (2006). A retrospective study on the use of acepromazine maleate in dogs with seizures. *Journal of the American Animal Hospital Association*. **42**: 283–289.

Further reading

Caspi, A., Sugden, K., and Moffitt, T.E. (2003). Influence of life stress on depression: moderation by a polymorphism in the 5-HTT gene. *Science* 301 (291–293): 386–389.

Dodman, N. and Shuster, L. (1998). *Psychopharmacology of Animal Behavior Disorders*. Malden: Blackwell Science.

Hariri, A.R., Mattay, V.S., Tessitore, A. et al. (2002). Serotonin transporter genetic variation and the response of the human amygdala. *Science* 297: 400–403.

Landsberg, G., Hunthausen, W., and Ackerman, L. (2013). *Behavior Problems of the Dog and Cat*. Saunders Elsevier: 3.

Wanamaker, B.P. and Massey, K.L. (2009). *Applied Pharmacology for Veterinary Technicians*. St. Louis, MO: Saunders Elsevier.

The PowerPoint of figures, appendices, MCQ's are available at www.wiley.com/go/martin/behavior

Appendix Section 1

Forms and Questionnaires

The appendices can be downloaded and printed at www.wiley.com/go/martin/behavior

Appendix 1
Canine behavior history form part 1

Name ______________________________ Phone ______________________________

Address ____________________ City ____________________ State ______________ Zip ________

Email: ______________________________ Alternate phone ______________________________

Household: #adults (>18 years): ______________ #children: ______________ ages: ________

#dogs (including patient): ______________ #cats: ______________ #other animals: ______________

Who is the primary caretaker of the dog?

- ❑ Husband
- ❑ Wife
- ❑ Child ______________
- ❑ Other ______________
- ❑ N/A

Name	Breed	Sex	Age (years)
Patient			
Dog 2			
Dog 3			
Dog 4			

Patient Information:

Weight (kg): _______ Body condition: Thin 1 2 3 4 5 Obese

Age neutered: _______ years __________ months ❑ Unknown

Current medical problems: ______________________________

Current medications: ______________ Dose rate (mg/kg q.): __________

______________ Dose rate (mg/kg q.): __________

Origin:

- ❑ Own breeding
- ❑ Breeder
- ❑ Private home
- ❑ Pet shop
- ❑ Humane society
- ❑ Stray
- ❑ Other ______________
- ❑ Don't know

Age removed from litter: __________ ❑ Unknown

Age obtained by owner: __________ ❑ Unknown

Canine and Feline Behavior for Veterinary Technicians and Nurses, Second Edition. Edited by Debbie Martin and Julie K. Shaw.

Companion website: www.wiley.com/go/martin/behavior

If obtained as a puppy, how was the puppy raised?

- ❑ In house
- ❑ In kennel/garage
- ❑ Loose outside
- ❑ Puppy mill
- ❑ Other
- ❑ Don't know
- ❑ N/A

If obtained as a puppy, how did you select that particular puppy from the litter?

- ❑ Breeder selected
- ❑ No choice
- ❑ Most outgoing
- ❑ Most timid
- ❑ Biggest
- ❑ Smallest
- ❑ Looks
- ❑ Other ________________
- ❑ N/A

If previously owned, for what primary purpose was the dog kept?

- ❑ Adult's pet
- ❑ Family pet
- ❑ Children's pet
- ❑ Show dog
- ❑ Breeding
- ❑ Guard dog
- ❑ Farm/outside dog
- ❑ Obedience
- ❑ Service/working dog
- ❑ Hunting dog
- ❑ Research/teaching
- ❑ Other ________________
- ❑ Don't know
- ❑ N/A

Primary purpose for which dog was obtained?

- ❑ Adult's pet
- ❑ Family pet
- ❑ Children's pet
- ❑ Show dog
- ❑ Breeding
- ❑ Watch/guard dog
- ❑ Farm/outside dog
- ❑ Obedience
- ❑ Service/working dog
- ❑ Hunting dog
- ❑ Other ________________

Average number of hours dog is left alone per week-day? ________________

Schedule on weekdays

- ❑ Is consistent
- ❑ Varies

Where is the dog when left alone?

- ❑ Cage
- ❑ Confined in a room
- ❑ Loose in living area
- ❑ Basement
- ❑ Garage
- ❑ Outside kennel
- ❑ Outside tied
- ❑ Loose in yard
- ❑ Other ________________
- ❑ N/A

Where is the dog at night?

- ❑ Cage
- ❑ Confined in a room
- ❑ Loose in living area
- ❑ Basement
- ❑ Garage
- ❑ Bedroom
- ❑ On person's bed
- ❑ Outside
- ❑ Other ________________

Exercise (walks):

- ❑ <1/week
- ❑ several/week
- ❑ once/day
- ❑ 2×/day
- ❑ 3×/day
- ❑ >3×/day

Exercise schedule

- ❑ Is consistent
- ❑ Varies during week

Average hours of walking exercise per day: ______________

Dog is walked on:

❑ Off leash
❑ Harness
❑ Flat collar
❑ Head halter
❑ Choke chain
❑ Pinch collar

Reason walked with that specific training tool:

____

Training:

❑ Dog has been trained to go into a crate readily
❑ Attended puppy classes (<four months)
❑ Dog has been trained with a clicker
❑ Dog is a trained service dog
❑ Attended classes over four months of age
❑ Dog has been shown in trials
❑ Dog is trained for other work

At what age did puppy/obedience classes start? ________ years ______ months don't know

Level of training:

❑ Basic (come, sit, down, heel on leash)
❑ Average (Basic plus: heel off leash, stay)
❑ Advanced

Performance of dog in class/training situation:

❑ Poor ❑ Fair ❑ Good ❑ Excellent ❑ Don't know/ N/A

Performance elsewhere:

❑ Poor ❑ Fair ❑ Good ❑ Excellent ❑ Don't know/ N/A

Training aids used:

❑ Off leash
❑ Head halter
❑ Choke collar
❑ Pinch collar
❑ Flat collar
❑ Harness
❑ Front clip harness
❑ Don't know/ N/A

Reason:

____

Types of discipline:

❑ None ever
❑ Response substitution
❑ Verbal reprimand
❑ Distracting
❑ Startling
❑ Physical
❑ Shock
❑ Time out
❑ "Dominance" roll
❑ Water spray
❑ Other ______________
❑ ______________

Feeding:

Diet	%	Brand
Dry		
Canned		
Table food		
Other		

Feeding schedule:

❑ once/day ❑ 2×/day ❑ >2×/day ❑ ad lib

Feeding schedule:

❑ Is regular ❑ Feeding schedule varies

Food treats type: ______________________ Contingent on behavior ❑ yes ❑ no

Temperament:

How would you generally describe your dog's temperament (check all that apply):

❑ Friendly to owner	❑ Aggressive to strangers	❑ Hyperexcitable
❑ Aloof	❑ Shy of strangers	❑ Super "submissive"
❑ Aggressive to owner	❑ Happy, outgoing	❑ Fearful (environment)
❑ Friendly to strangers	❑ Inhibited	❑ Fear of noises
❑ Aloof to strangers	❑ Anxious	❑ Don't know

Comments: ____

____

What was the temperament of the dog as a puppy:

❑ Friendly to owner	❑ Aggressive to strangers	❑ Hyperexcitable
❑ Aloof	❑ Shy of strangers	❑ Super "submissive"
❑ Aggressive to owner	❑ Happy, outgoing	❑ Fearful (environment)
❑ Friendly to strangers	❑ Inhibited	❑ Fear of noises
❑ Aloof to strangers	❑ Anxious	❑ Don't know

Comments: ____

____

Presenting problems (in order of importance to owner):

1. ____
2. ____
3. ____
4. ____

What have you tried so far to treat the problem(s)?

____

____

____

____

Comments and status of the human–animal bond?

The PowerPoint of figures, appendices, MCQ's are available at www.wiley.com/go/martin/behavior

Appendix 2
Canine behavior history form part 2

Dog's name________________________________ Owner's name ____

General behavioral profile How does your dog react to the following (if the dog has experienced the situation in the past)?								
	Neutral	**Friendly**	**Hyper**	**Fearful**	**Anxious**	**Defensive Aggression**	**Offensive Aggression**	**Don't know**
Unfamiliar people at door								
Unfamiliar people in home								
Unfamiliar people, neutral Territory, on leash								
Same, off leash								
Same approaching/ try to pet, on leash								
Children, bikes, skateboards								
Joggers (adults)								
On leash while cars, trucks go by								
Children 1–6 years								
Children 7–11								
Children 12–18								
Unfamiliar dogs on property								
Unfamiliar dogs off property on leash								
Same off leash								
Owners leaving								
Owners returning								
Nail trimming								

Canine and Feline Behavior for Veterinary Technicians and Nurses, Second Edition. Edited by Debbie Martin and Julie K. Shaw.

Companion website: www.wiley.com/go/martin/behavior

Grooming								
Bathing								
Wiping feet								
Owner reaching over head or touching on head								
Owner touching other places								
Owner lifting dog up								
Grasping collar, restraining dog								
Roughhousing								
Approach or take food dish while dog is eating								
Taking away bone/ toy/stolen object								
Approach dog on his bed								
Disturbing sleeping dog								
Stepping over lying dog								
Verbal reprimand								
Physical punishment								
Putting on/taking off collar								
Staring at dog								
Car rides								
Stranger approaching car								
Vacuum cleaner								
Broom								
Thunder								
Loud noises (other than thunder)								

Comments on behavior during consultation:

Problem history: **Problem #**

General description: What happens? Where does it happen? Who is present? What are the triggers?

How does the dog behave (including body language before and afterwards) and how do people react?

Most recent incident:

Second most recent:

____

The earliest incident:

____

Age problem started: _________ months________ years

Any changes at that time?

____

Progression:

❑ same ❑ increasing ❑ decreasing

Frequency:

❑ >10×/day ❑ 1–10×/day ❑ 1–6×/week ❑ <once/week

PRELIMINARY DIAGNOSIS:

1. ____________________ **3.** ____________________

2. ____________________ **4.** ____________________

Medication: ____________________ Dosage: ____________________

TREATMENT PLAN:

The PowerPoint of figures, appendices, MCQ's are available at www.wiley.com/go/martin/behavior

Appendix 3

Feline behavior history form part 1

Name______________________________ Phone________________

Address________________ City____________ State________ Zip______

Email:______________________________ Alternate phone________________

Household: #adults (>18 years):____________ #children:____________ ages:______

#cats (including patient):__________ #dogs:__________ #other animals:________

Who is the primary caretaker of the cat?

❑ Husband
❑ Wife
❑ Child
❑ Other ________
❑ N/A

Name	Breed	Sex	Age (years)
Patient			
Cat 2			
Cat 3			
Cat 4			

Patient information:

Weight (kg): __________ Body condition: Thin 1 2 3 4 5 Obese

Age neutered: ______ years ______ months ______ ❑ Unknown

Current medical problems: ______________________________

Current medications: ________________ Dose rate (mg/kg q..): __________

________________ Dose rate (mg/kg q..): __________

Origin:

❑ Own breeding
❑ Breeder
❑ Private home
❑ Pet shop
❑ Humane society
❑ Stray
❑ Other ________
❑ Don't know

Canine and Feline Behavior for Veterinary Technicians and Nurses, Second Edition. Edited by Debbie Martin and Julie K. Shaw.

Companion website: www.wiley.com/go/martin/behavior

Age obtained: ____________(years)____________(months)____________ ❑ Unknown

If obtained as a kitten, how was the kitten raised?

❑ In house
❑ Kennel/garage
❑ Loose outside
❑ Other
❑ Don't know
❑ N/A

If obtained as kitten, how did you select that particular kitten from the litter?

❑ Breeder selected
❑ No choice
❑ Most outgoing
❑ Most timid
❑ Biggest
❑ Smallest
❑ Prettiest
❑ Other __________
❑ N/A

Age removed from litter: ______________________________ ❑ Unknown

Age obtained by owner: ______________________________ ❑ Unknown

If previously owned, for what primary purpose was the cat kept?

❑ Adult's pet
❑ Family pet
❑ Children's pet
❑ Show
❑ Breeding
❑ Farm/outside cat
❑ Research/teaching
❑ Other__________
❑ Don't know
❑ N/A

Is the cat declawed?

❑ No
❑ Front only
❑ Front and back

Age at declawing: ____________(years)____________(months)____________ ❑ Unknown

Primary purpose for which cat was obtained:

❑ Adult's pet
❑ Family pet
❑ Children's pet
❑ Show
❑ Breeding
❑ Farm/outside cat
❑ Other __________

Average number of hours the cat is left alone per weekday: __________

Schedule on weekdays

❑ Is consistent
❑ Varies

Where is the cat when left alone?

❑ Cage
❑ Confined in a room
❑ Loose in living area
❑ Outside
❑ Basement
❑ Garage
❑ N/A

Where is the cat at night?

- ❑ Cage
- ❑ Confined in a room
- ❑ Loose in living area
- ❑ Bedroom
- ❑ On person's bed
- ❑ Outside
- ❑ Basement
- ❑ Garage

Average hours of being outside per day: ___________

Schedule

- ❑ Is consistent
- ❑ Varies

Types of discipline used:

- ❑ none ever
- ❑ response substitution
- ❑ verbal reprimand
- ❑ startling
- ❑ physical
- ❑ time-out
- ❑ water
- ❑ other __________

Feeding and litter boxes:

Diet	%	Brand
Dry		
Canned		
Table food		
Other		

Feeding schedule:

- ❑ <once/day
- ❑ 1×/day
- ❑ 2×/day
- ❑ ad lib
- ❑ Other

Feeding schedule:

- ❑ Is regular
- ❑ Feeding schedule varies

Food treats type: ______________________ Contingent on behavior ❑ yes ❑ no

Fresh water provided:

- ❑ once/day
- ❑ 2×/day
- ❑ >2×/day
- ❑ other

Watering schedule:

- ❑ Is regular
- ❑ Varies during week

Number of dishes with feed: ______________________________

Number of dishes with water: ______________________________

Number of litter boxes: ______________________________

Location of litter boxes (check all that apply):

❑ Living area	❑ Kitchen	❑ Bathroom
❑ Spare room	❑ Laundry room	❑ Closet
❑ Basement	❑ Hallway	❑ Other

Type of litter box:

❑ Open	❑ Covered	❑ Varies

Type of litter:

❑ Clumping	❑ Shavings	❑ Sand
❑ Clay	❑ Newspaper	❑ Other

Is litter

❑ Deodorized/scented	❑ No odor control	❑ Don't know

Type of litter

❑ Is consistent	❑ Varies	❑ N/A

Liners used:

❑ No	❑ Always	❑ Varies

Litter boxes scooped:

❑ <once/week	❑ several/week	❑ once/day
❑ weekly	❑ daily	❑ N/A

Litter boxes washed:

❑ <once/month	❑ weekly	❑ >daily
❑ monthly	❑ several/week	❑ N/A

Cleaner used:

❑ Strong disinfectant	❑ Bleach	❑ Other ________
❑ Pine cleaner	❑ Mild soap	❑ N/A
❑ Lemon cleaner	❑ Water only	

Temperament:

How would you generally rate the cat's temperament?

❑ Friendly	❑ Hyperexcitable	❑ Offensive aggressive
❑ Aloof	❑ Shy of people	❑ Don't know
❑ Inhibited	❑ Fearful (environment)	
❑ Anxious	❑ Fear aggressive	

Comments: ______________________________

____

What was the temperament of the cat as a kitten?

- ❑ Friendly
- ❑ Aloof
- ❑ Inhibited
- ❑ Anxious
- ❑ Hyperexcitable
- ❑ Shy of people
- ❑ Fearful (environment)
- ❑ Fear aggressive
- ❑ Offensive aggressive
- ❑ Don't know

Presenting problems (in order of importance to owner):

1. ______________________________
2. ______________________________
3. ______________________________
4. ______________________________

What have you tried so far to treat the problem(s)?

____

____

____

____

Comments and status of the human–animal bond?

____

____

____

____

____

____

____

____

The PowerPoint of figures, appendices, MCQ's are available at www.wiley.com/go/martin/behavior

Appendix 4
Feline behavior history form part 2

Cat's name ____________________ Owner's name ____________________

General behavioral profile								
How does your cat react to the following (if the cat has experienced the situation in the past):								
	Calm	**Friendly**	**Hyper**	**Neutral**	**Fearful**	**Anxious**	**Aggressive**	**Don't know**
Unfamiliar people in home								
Same approaching, wanting to pet								
Babies								
Children								
Unfamiliar cats on property								
Nail trimming								
Giving medication								
Grooming								
Petting								
Lifting cat up								
Restraining cat								
Putting cat in carrier								
Roughhousing								
Disturbing sleeping cat								
Stepping over lying cat								
Cat same household approaching								
Other cat outside								

Canine and Feline Behavior for Veterinary Technicians and Nurses, Second Edition. Edited by Debbie Martin and Julie K. Shaw.

Companion website: www.wiley.com/go/martin/behavior

Dog same household approaching								
Strange dog outside								

Comments on behavior during consultation:

Problem history: **Problem #**

General description: What happens? Where does it happen? Who is present? What are the triggers?

How does the cat behave (including body language before and afterwards) and how do people react?

Most recent incident: ______________________________

____

____

____

____

Second most recent: ______________________________

____

____

____

____

The earliest incident: ______________________________

____

____

____

____

Age problem started: ____________ months ____________ years

Any changes at that time? ______________________________

____

____

____

____

Progression:

❑ same ❑ increasing ❑ decreasing

Frequency:

❑ >10×/day ❑ 1–10×/day ❑ 1–6×/week ❑ <once/week

PRELIMINARY DIAGNOSIS:

1. ______________________ 3. ______________________

2. ______________________ 4. ______________________

Medication:______________________ Dosage:______________________

TREATMENT PLAN:

The PowerPoint of figures, appendices, MCQ's are available at www.wiley.com/go/martin/behavior

Appendix 5
Links for examples of online behavioral history forms

Feline history form:

https://veterinarybehavior.formstack.com/forms/cat_behavior_history_copy

Canine history form:

https://veterinarybehavior.formstack.com/forms/dog_behavior_history_copy

Feline follow-up history form:

https://veterinarybehavior.formstack.com/forms/cat_follow_up_copy

Canine follow-up history form:

https://veterinarybehavior.formstack.com/forms/dog_follow_up_copy

RDVM referral form example:

https://veterinarybehavior.formstack.com/forms/veterinarian_referral_copy

The PowerPoint of figures, appendices, MCQ's are available at www.wiley.com/go/martin/behavior

Canine and Feline Behavior for Veterinary Technicians and Nurses, Second Edition. Edited by Debbie Martin and Julie K. Shaw.

Companion website: www.wiley.com/go/martin/behavior

Appendix 6
Trainer assessment form

Assessment criteria	Notes	0–5 (5 is excellent)
Welcomes potential clients to observe a class prior to making a decision to enroll		
Explains a skill and gives examples of how the skill is useful in everyday life		
Demonstrates the skill		
Utilizes handouts and other instructional guides		
Circulates through the students giving assistance and guidance when needed		
Remains conscious of the emotional and motivational state of all animals in the classroom setting and acts appropriately		
Arranges the classroom to optimize the success of each handler and animal		
Does not become focused on one student		
Keeps the class moving at an appropriate pace		
Can adjust their teaching plan as needed for individual student's needs		
Is professional and respectful at all times to owners/handlers		
Is appropriate and liberal with positive reinforcement to both the owners and animals.		
Is familiar with TAGteach and utilizes it frequently and appropriately to instruct clients		

Canine and Feline Behavior for Veterinary Technicians and Nurses, Second Edition. Edited by Debbie Martin and Julie K. Shaw.

Companion website: www.wiley.com/go/martin/behavior

Uses appropriate management tools to decrease unwanted behaviors while teaching the desired behaviors		
Utilizes only humane training methods that promote and protect the human–animal bond and are not harmful to the handler or dog in any way		
Does not recommend or utilize choke collars, pinch collars, electronic shock collars, or physical or verbal punishments		
Does not coach or advocate the outdated "dominance hierarchy theory" and the subsequent confrontational training and relationship that follows from it		
Understands and addresses the emotional and motivational state of the animal.		
Recommends and utilizes training tools designed not to inflict physical pain		
Understands the value of education and attends continuing education seminars regularly		
Is a certified member of a standardized and policed credentialing program		
Because of variables in dog breeding, temperament, owner commitment, and experience, a trainer cannot and should not guarantee the results of their training, although should ensure client satisfaction		
Builds and maintains a mutually communicative, respectful, and professional relationship with veterinary professionals		
Understands their role on the veterinary behavior team and does not diagnose behavior disorders or change the prescribed treatment plan		
Total points		

The PowerPoint of figures, appendices, MCQ's are available at www.wiley.com/go/martin/behavior

Appendix 7
Determining pet owner strain

Life area	Manifestation of strain
Mental and emotional	❑ Stress and a feeling of being "used up" ❑ Worry or anxiety ❑ Anger toward your pet ❑ Fear your pet may hurt you or a loved one ❑ "Aloneness" and alienation ❑ Feelings of "hopelessness" when it comes to your pet ❑ Feelings of "not being able to go on" if your pet were to die
Health	❑ Health issues due to stress (weight loss or gain, headaches, etc.) ❑ Declined self-care ❑ Decreased energy ❑ Injury from your pet
Social	❑ Embarrassment ❑ Shame or guilt ❑ Fear of stigma/social disapproval ❑ Alienation ❑ Limit or cease having house guests ❑ Guilt when socializing outside the home ❑ Neglected relationships or giving up relationships that make you happy to tend to your pet's psychological and emotional needs ❑ Fear of being away from your pet ❑ Giving up hobbies ❑ Fear of injury to strangers
Financial	❑ Distraction during work day ❑ Financial liability/lawsuits ❑ Property damage and destruction ❑ Cost of treatment, medication, training, etc.
Family environment	❑ Fear for safety of family members ❑ Discord with significant other ❑ Strained relationship with extended family members ❑ Alienation by extended family

Source: Adapted from Mendenhall and Mount (2011), *Families in Society* 92 (2): 183–190; Anon. (2011), *Client Essays*, West Lafayette, IN: J. Shaw.

The PowerPoint of figures, appendices, MCQ's are available at www.wiley.com/go/martin/behavior

Canine and Feline Behavior for Veterinary Technicians and Nurses, Second Edition. Edited by Debbie Martin and Julie K. Shaw.

Companion website: www.wiley.com/go/martin/behavior

Appendix 8
Canine behavior plan of care

Consultation date: ____________________

Client name: ____________________ Phone: ____________________ Email: ____________________

Address: ____________________ City: ______________ State: ______________ Zip: ______________

Dogname: ____________________ Age: __________ Breed: __________ M ❑ Mx ❑ F ❑ Fx ❑

Canine Behavioral Diagnosis		
Aggression	**Target of aggression**	❑
❑ Conflict induced	❑	❑
❑ Possessive	❑	**Ingestive**
❑ Disease/pain induced	❑	❑ Coprophagia
❑ Fear/defensive induced	❑	❑ Pica
❑ Idiopathic	**Fear/Anxiety disorders**	❑ Predatory behavior
❑ IDA + motivation	❑ Generalized anxiety	**Eliminative**
❑ IDA–H + motivation	❑ Global fear	❑ Housesoiling
❑ Alliance induced	❑ Separation anxiety	❑ Urine marking
❑ Status induced	❑ Sound/thunderstorm phobia	❑ Excitement urination
❑ Learned	❑ Specific fear or phobia	❑ Extreme fear/appeasement urination
❑ Maternal/hormonal induced	❑ Acute conflict behaviors/stereotypy	**Other**
❑ Play induced	❑ Compulsive disorder	❑ Cognitive dysfunction
❑ Redirected	Specific fear(s) or phobia(s) noted:	❑ Hyperexcitability
❑ Territorial	❑	❑ Conditioned unwanted behavior
❑	❑	❑
Prescribed treatment plan (see back for details and further information)		
Management	**Training**	❑ Shape relaxation
❑ Avoid triggers	❑ Marker training	❑ Leave it/drop it
❑ Ignore attention-seeking behaviors	❑ Lure reward training	❑
❑ Ignore at specific times	❑ Other training	❑
❑ Cue→response→reward interactions	❑ Agility training	❑
❑ Environmental modifications	❑ Concept training	❑
❑	❑ K9 Nose Work® training	❑
	❑ Crate/confinement training	**Behavior modification** (see back)
❑ Crate confinement	❑	❑ Counter conditioning
❑ Other confinement	❑	❑
❑	**Training tools**	❑
❑ Umbilical cord	❑ Head halter	❑
❑ Change primary caregiver	❑ Basket muzzle	❑
❑ Increase mental stimulation	❑ Other muzzle	❑
❑ Walk off property	❑ Body harness	❑ Response Substitution
❑ Aerobic exercise	❑ Front clip harness	❑
❑ Regular schedule	❑ Anxiety clothing	❑
❑ Dietary change	❑ Calming cap	❑
❑ Meal feed twice daily	❑ Drag line	❑
❑	❑ Tether	❑
❑	❑ Interactive toys/puzzles	❑ Systematic Desensitization
Other	❑ Pheromones	❑
❑ Interruption of behavior	❑ Remote reward	❑
❑ Cease punishment	**Specific behaviors to train**	❑
❑ Remote punishment	❑ Targeting	❑
❑ Grief counseling	❑ Attention	❑
❑ Rehoming patient	❑ "Look" and "Watch"	❑ **Other**
❑	❑ Sit ❑ Down ❑ Recall	❑
❑	❑ Loose leash walking	❑
❑	❑ Go to a place	❑

Canine and Feline Behavior for Veterinary Technicians and Nurses, Second Edition. Edited by Debbie Martin and Julie K. Shaw.

Companion website: www.wiley.com/go/martin/behavior

Bite history
Has the dog bitten? yes ❑ no ❑ Does the dog redirect aggression? yes ❑ no ❑
How severe were the bites? Did not make contact ❑ Did not break skin ❑ Puncture ❑ Medical care needed ❑
Does the dog give warning before biting? yes ❑ no ❑ unknown ❑
Note known triggers and other significant bite history:

Medical conditions and medications

Comments and treatment details
Veterinarian signature: Date:

The PowerPoint of figures, appendices, MCQ's are available at www.wiley.com/go/martin/behavior

Appendix 9
Behavior problem list

Eliminative	Social	Ingestive
❑ Incontinence	❑ Barking/howling/whining	❑ Anorexia
❑ Diarrhea/vomiting	❑ Rolling in unsavory items	❑ Chewing objects
❑ House soiling	❑ Jumps up on people	❑ Coprophagia
❑ Urine marking	❑ Demands attention	❑ Compulsive eating
❑ Urination on pheromones	❑ Demands touch	❑ Compulsive drinking
❑ Other ______________	❑ Aggressive to owners	❑ Eating grass/plants
Grooming	❑ Aggressive to strangers	❑ Eating garbage
❑ Licking self	❑ Aggressive to dogs/same household	❑ Pica
❑ Sucking on self	❑ Aggressive to strange dogs	❑ Prey chasing
❑ Chewing on self	❑ Aggressive to other animals	❑ Car etc. chasing
❑ Scratching self	❑ Other ______________	❑ Light/shadow chasing
❑ Checking hind end		❑ Stealing food
❑ Other ______________		❑ Fly snapping
		❑ Air/mouth licking
		❑ Other __________

Temperament related	Reproduction	Locomotory
❑ Depressed/inappetent	❑ Cannibalism	❑ Circling/ whirling
❑ Hyperexcitable/active	❑ False pregnancy	❑ Tail biting
❑ Hyperreactive	❑ Masturbation	❑ Pacing, figure 8s
❑ Nervous/anxious	❑ Mounting people	❑ Digging
❑ Fear of thunder	❑ Mounting animals	❑ Lameness/ conditioned
❑ Fear of loud noises excl. thunder	❑ Self-nursing	❑ Roaming
❑ Fear of people	❑ Other ______________	❑ Scratching objects
❑ Fear of situations		❑ Freezing
❑ Fear of objects/animals		❑ Other ____________
❑ Other ______________		

Comments:

The PowerPoint of figures, appendices, MCQ's are available at www.wiley.com/go/martin/behavior

Canine and Feline Behavior for Veterinary Technicians and Nurses, Second Edition. Edited by Debbie Martin and Julie K. Shaw.

Companion website: www.wiley.com/go/martin/behavior

Appendix 10
Technician observation

Date: ____________ Client name: ____________ Pet name: ____________

	Start of appointment	5 min	15 min	30 min	End of appointment
Treats					
Treat proximity					
Interactions					
Trainability (1–10)					
General behavior					
Restrictions					
Significant events during appointment					

The PowerPoint of figures, appendices, MCQ's are available at www.wiley.com/go/martin/behavior

Appendix 11
Follow-up communication form

Client:					Date:		Patient name:
Problem list:							
Problem #1							
Status of problem (1 worst 1 10 best):							
	Cured		Much improved		Moderately improved		Worse
	Same		Slightly improved		No improvement		Considering euthanasia
Problem #2							
Status of problem (1 worst–10 best):							
	Cured		Much improved		Moderately improved		Worse
	Same		Slightly improved		No improvement		Considering euthanasia
Problem #3							
Status of problem (1 worst–10 best):							
	Cured		Much improved		Moderately improved		Worse
	Same		Slightly improved		No improvement		Considering euthanasia

Current medications and dose:	**Comments:**	
Current treatment plan and application:	**Comments:**	**Client compliance (poor 1–10 excellent)**

Canine and Feline Behavior for Veterinary Technicians and Nurses, Second Edition. Edited by Debbie Martin and Julie K. Shaw.

Companion website: www.wiley.com/go/martin/behavior

Specific concerns, discussion, and suggestions

Next contact scheduled for:

Signature:	Printed name:

The PowerPoint of figures, appendices, MCQ's are available at www.wiley.com/go/martin/behavior

Appendix 12
Behavior diary

Month: ____________________

Behavior																															
10 (Excellent)																															
9																															
8																															
7																															
6																															
5																															
4																															
3																															
2																															
1 (poor)																															
Day of month	**1**	**2**	**3**	**4**	**5**	**6**	**7**	**8**	**9**	**10**	**11**	**12**	**13**	**14**	**15**	**16**	**17**	**18**	**19**	**20**	**21**	**22**	**23**	**24**	**25**	**26**	**27**	**28**	**29**	**30**	**31**

Canine and Feline Behavior for Veterinary Technicians and Nurses, Second Edition. Edited by Debbie Martin and Julie K. Shaw.

Companion website: www.wiley.com/go/martin/behavior

Notes/significant events/medication

1	
2	
3	
4	
5	
6	
7	
8	
9	
10	
11	
12	
13	
14	
15	
16	
17	
18	
19	
20	
21	
22	
23	
24	
25	
26	
27	
28	
29	
30	
31	

The PowerPoint of figures, appendices, MCQ's are available at www.wiley.com/go/martin/behavior

Appendix 13
New kitten (less than 3 months) questionnaire

Owner's name: ______________________ Today's date: ______________________

Cat's name: ______________________ Cat's age (DOB): ______________________

1. Where did you obtain your kitten from (breeder, petstore, friend, shelter, rescue, humane society, etc.)?

 ____

2. How long have you had your kitten? ______________________
3. How old was your kitten when you obtained him/her? ______________________
4. How many kittens were in the litter? ______________________
5. When were the kittens taken away from the mother? ______________________
6. Where does your kitten spend most of his/her day? (inside, outside, in a room, in a kennel, with you)?

 ____

7. How would you describe your kitten's litter box training?

 ❑ Great, not having any accidents

 ❑ Good, a few accidents have occurred

 ❑ Not a clue, most elimination is happening in a location I do not prefer

 Comments: ______________________

8. How many litter boxes do you have and where are they located? ______________________

 ____

9. What is the size and type of litter box (covered, uncovered, automatic, oval, large rectangular, etc.)?

 ____

10. What type and brand of litter do you use? (scented or unscented, scoopable vs. clay)

 ____

11. Does your kitten like to play with toys? What type? ______________________
12. Does your kitten use scratching posts? What type? ______________________
13. Have your enrolled your kitten in a kitten class? If so, where? ______________________

Canine and Feline Behavior for Veterinary Technicians and Nurses, Second Edition. Edited by Debbie Martin and Julie K. Shaw.

Companion website: www.wiley.com/go/martin/behavior

14. If you have other pets in the household, describe the kitten's relationship with them ________________

____

15. Has your kitten ever shown any growling, hissing, or nipping/biting toward you or anyone else? If so, when?

____

16. Are there things your kitten is afraid of or does not like? If so, please describe

____

17. Has your kitten shown any of these signs: coughing, sneezing, itching, diarrhea, vomiting, or lack of appetite?

____

18. Any change in water or food consumption? ____

19. What type of food do you feed your kitten and how often is he/she fed? Is food available all the time or at set "mealtimes"?

____

20. Any change in frequency of urination or defecation? __________________________________

____

21. What, if any, medications (over the counter or prescription) does your kitten take or have applied routinely?____

22. What are three things you enjoy about your kitten? ___________________________________

____

____

____

23. Do you have any concerns or topics you would like to discuss? ____________________________

____

____

____

The PowerPoint of figures, appendices, MCQ's are available at www.wiley.com/go/martin/behavior

Appendix 14
New puppy (less than 4 months) questionnaire

Owner's name: ______________________ Today's date: ______________

Dog's name: ______________________ Dog's age (DOB): ______________

1. Where did you obtain your puppy from (breeder, petstore, friend, shelter, rescue, humane society, etc.)?

   ____

   ____

2. How long have you had your puppy? ______________________
3. How old was your puppy when you obtained him/her? ______________________
4. How many puppies were in the litter? ______________________
5. When were the puppies taken away from the mother? ______________________

   ____

6. Where does your puppy spend most of his/her day? (inside, outside, in a room, in a kennel, with you)?

   ____

   ____

7. How would you describe your puppy's house training?
   - ❑ Great, not having any accidents
   - ❑ Good, a few accidents when I forget to take him/her out
   - ❑ So-so, having several accidents a day
   - ❑ Not a clue, most elimination is happening in a location I do not prefer

   Comments: ____

8. Have your enrolled your puppy in a puppy socialization class? If so, where? ______________

   ____

9. If you have other pets in the household, describe the puppy's relationship with them______________

   ____

Canine and Feline Behavior for Veterinary Technicians and Nurses, Second Edition. Edited by Debbie Martin and Julie K. Shaw.

Companion website: www.wiley.com/go/martin/behavior

10. Has your puppy ever shown any growling, barking, snarling, or nipping toward you or anyone else? If so, when?

____

____

11. Are there things your puppy is afraid of or does not like? If so, please describe

____

12. Has your puppy shown any of these signs: coughing, sneezing, itching, diarrhea, vomiting, or lack of appetite?

____

____

13. What type of food do you feed your puppy and how often is he/she fed? Is food available all the time or at set "mealtimes"?

____

____

14. Any change in water or food consumption?____

15. Any change in frequency of urination or defecation?____

16. What, if any, medications (over the counter or prescription) does your puppy take or have applied routinely (at least monthly)?

____

____

____

17. What are three things you enjoy about your puppy?

____

____

____

18. Do you have any concerns or topics you would like to discuss?

____

____

____

The PowerPoint of figures, appendices, MCQ's are available at www.wiley.com/go/martin/behavior

Appendix 15

Juvenile, adolescent, or adult cat (3 months to ~12 years) questionnaire

Owner's name: ______________________ Today's date: ______________

Cat's name: ______________________ Cat's age (DOB): ______________

1. Where does your cat spend most of his/her day? (inside, outside, in a room, in a kennel, with you)?

   ____

2. How would you describe your cat's litter box training?
   - ❑ Great, not having any accidents
   - ❑ OK, a few accidents (less than once a month)
   - ❑ Could be better, several accidents a week
   - ❑ Not a clue, most elimination is happening in a location I do not prefer

   Comments: ____

   ____

3. How many litter boxes do you have and where are they located? ______________

   ____

4. What is the size and type of litter boxes (covered, uncovered, automatic, oval, large rectangular, etc.)?

   ____

5. What type of litter do you use and what brand? (scented or unscented, scoopable vs. clay)

   ____

6. Does your cat like to play with toys? What type?

   ____

7. Does your cat use scratching posts? What type? ______________

8. What is your typical routine of activities with your cat each day?

   ____

   ____

   ____

Canine and Feline Behavior for Veterinary Technicians and Nurses, Second Edition. Edited by Debbie Martin and Julie K. Shaw.

Companion website: www.wiley.com/go/martin/behavior

9. If you have other pets in the household, describe the cat's relationship with them ____________________

____

10. Has your cat ever shown any growling, hissing, or nipping/biting toward you or anyone else? If so, when?

____

____

11. Are there things your cat is afraid of or does not like? If so, please describe.

____

____

12. Has your cat shown any of these signs: coughing, sneezing, itching, diarrhea, vomiting, or lack of appetite?

____

____

13. Any changes in grooming or sleeping habits? ____________________

14. Any change in water or food consumption?

____

15. What type of food do you feed your cat and how often is he/she fed? Is food available all the time or at set "mealtimes"?

____

____

16. Any change in frequency of urination or defecation?

____

17. What, if any, medications (over the counter or prescription) does your cat take or have applied routinely?

____

____

____

18. What are three things you enjoy about your cat? ____________________

____

____

____

19. Do you have any concerns or topics you would like to discuss? ____________________

____

The PowerPoint of figures, appendices, MCQ's are available at www.wiley.com/go/martin/behavior

Appendix 16
Juvenile, adolescent, or adult dog (4 months to ~7 years) questionnaire

Owner's name: ______________________ Today's date: ____________

Dog's name: ______________________ Dog's age (DOB): ____________

1. Where does your dog spend most of his/her day? (inside, outside, in a room, in a kennel, with you)?

   ____

2. Have you taken your dog to a training class? If so, where? ______________________

   ____

3. Do you train your dog? If so, how? (with treats, clicker training, etc.) ______________________

   ____

4. Do you walk your dog? If so what type of collar does your dog wear for walks? ____________

   If not, why? ____

5. Any problems with walking your dog? ____

6. How would you describe your dog's house training?
   - ❑ Great, not having any accidents
   - ❑ Good, a few accidents when I forget to take her/him out (less than once a month)
   - ❑ Could be better, numerous accidents a week
   - ❑ Not a clue, most elimination is happening in a location I do not prefer

   Comments: ____

   ____

7. What is your typical routine of activities with your dog each day? ______________________

   ____

8. If you have other pets in the household, describe the dog's relationship with them ____________

   ____

   ____

Canine and Feline Behavior for Veterinary Technicians and Nurses, Second Edition. Edited by Debbie Martin and Julie K. Shaw.

Companion website: www.wiley.com/go/martin/behavior

9. Has your dog ever shown any growling, barking, snarling, or mouthing/biting toward you or anyone else? If so, when?

____

____

10. Are there things your dog is afraid of or does not like? If so, please describe ______________

____

11. Any coughing, sneezing, itching, diarrhea, vomiting, or lack of appetite? ______________

____

12. Any changes in grooming or sleeping habits? ______________

13. Any change in water or food consumption? ______________

____

14. What type of food do you feed your dog and how often is he/she fed? Is food available all the time or at set "mealtimes"?

____

15. Any change in frequency of urination or defecation? ______________

____

16. What, if any, medications (over the counter or prescription) does your dog take or have applied routinely?

____

____

____

17. What are three things you enjoy about your dog? ______________

____

____

____

18. Do you have any concerns or topics you would like to discuss? ______________

____

____

____

The PowerPoint of figures, appendices, MCQ's are available at www.wiley.com/go/martin/behavior

Appendix 17
Senior or geriatric cat (11+years) questionnaire

Owner's name: ______________________ Today's date: ______________________

Cat's name: ______________________ Cat's age (DOB): ______________________

1. Where does your cat spend most of his/her day? (inside, outside, in a room, in a kennel, with you)?

____

2. How would you describe your cat's litter box training?
   - ❑ Great, not having any accidents
   - ❑ OK, a few accidents (less than once a month)
   - ❑ Could be better, several accidents a week
   - ❑ Not a clue, most elimination is happening in a location I do not prefer

   Comments: ____

   ____

3. How many litter boxes do you have and where are they located?______________________

____

4. What is the size and type of litter boxes (covered, uncovered, automatic, oval, large rectangular, etc.)?

____

5. What type of litter do you use and what brand? (scented or unscented, scoopable vs. clay)

____

6. Does your cat like to play with toys? What type?

____

7. Any changes in activity, such as being more active at night, or sleeping more during the day? Any increase in vocalization?

____

8. Does your cat seem disoriented at times or unable to recognize familiar people?______________________

____

9. Does your cat seem stiff when moving, slow to rise, or less agile? ______________________

____

Canine and Feline Behavior for Veterinary Technicians and Nurses, Second Edition. Edited by Debbie Martin and Julie K. Shaw.

Companion website: www.wiley.com/go/martin/behavior

10. Does your cat use scratching posts? What kind? ______________________

11. What is your typical routine of activities with your cat each day? ______________________

____

12. If you have other pets in the household, describe your cat's relationship with them ______________________

____

13. Has your cat ever shown any growling, hissing, or mouthing/biting toward you or anyone else? If so, when?

____

14. Are there things your cat is afraid of or does not like? If so, please describe ______________________

____

15. Has your cat shown any of these signs: coughing, sneezing, itching, diarrhea, vomiting, or lack of appetite?

____

____

16. Any changes in grooming habits? ______________________

17. Any change in water or food consumption? ______________________

____

18. What type of food do you feed your cat and how often is he/she fed? Is food available all the time or at set "mealtimes"?

____

____

19. Any change in frequency of urination or defecation?______________________

____

20. What, if any, medications (over the counter or prescription) does your cat take or have applied routinely?

____

____

____

21. What are three things you enjoy about your cat?

____

____

____

22. Do you have any concerns or topics you would like to discuss?

____

____

____

The PowerPoint of figures, appendices, MCQ's are available at www.wiley.com/go/martin/behavior

Appendix 18
Senior or geriatric dog (~7+years) questionnaire

Owner's name: ______________________ Today's date: ______________

Dog's name: ______________________ Dog's age (DOB): ______________

1. Where does your dog spend most of his/her day? (inside, outside, in a room, in a kennel, with you)?

   ____

2. Have you taken your dog to a training class? If so, where? ______________

   ____

3. Do you train your dog? If so, how? (with treats, clicker training, etc.) ______________

   ____

4. Do you walk your dog? If so what type of collar does your dog wear for walks? ______________

   ____

   If not, why? ______________________________

5. Any problems with walking your dog? ______________________________

6. Have you noticed any changes in your dog's personality or activity level?
   - ❑ Less or more active
   - ❑ Difficulty rising after resting or sitting
   - ❑ Urine or stool accidents in the house
   - ❑ More needy or anxious
   - ❑ More standoffish
   - ❑ Disoriented or failure to recognize familiar people

   Comments: ______________________________

   ____

7. What is your typical routine of activities with your dog each day? ______________

Canine and Feline Behavior for Veterinary Technicians and Nurses, Second Edition. Edited by Debbie Martin and Julie K. Shaw.

Companion website: www.wiley.com/go/martin/behavior

8. If you have other pets in the household, describe the dog's relationship with them ____________________

____

9. Has your dog ever shown any growling, barking, snarling or mouthing/biting toward you or anyone else? If so, when?

____

10. Are there things your dog is afraid of or does not like? If so, please describe ____________________

11. Any coughing, sneezing, itching, diarrhea, vomiting, or lack of appetite? ____________________

12. Any changes in grooming habits? ____________________

13. Any change in water or food consumption? ____________________

____

14. What type of food do you feed your dog and how often is he/she fed? Is food available all the time or at set "mealtimes"?

____

____

____

15. Any change in frequency of urination or defecation? ____________________

____

____

16. What, if any, medications (over the counter or prescription) does your dog take or have applied routinely?

____

____

____

17. What are three things you enjoy about your dog?

____

____

____

18. Do you have any concerns or topics you would like to discuss?

____

____

____

The PowerPoint of figures, appendices, MCQ's are available at www.wiley.com/go/martin/behavior

Appendix 19
Pet selection counseling

Owner: ______________________ Email: ______________________
Address: ____
Home phone: ______________________ Alt. phone: ______________________

Pet Selection Counseling-Part 1: Lifestyle

1. Household members:

NAME	AGE	RELATIONSHIP

2. Current household pets:

NAME	AGE	SEX	SPECIES/BREED

3. Previous household pets

NAME	AGE	BREED

4. How often do adults visit?
   - ❑ Daily
   - ❑ Numerous times weekly
   - ❑ 1–4 times monthly
   - ❑ Infrequently

5. How often do children or teens visit?
   - ❑ Daily
   - ❑ Numerous times weekly
   - ❑ 1–4 times monthly
   - ❑ Infrequently

6. Would you say your current lifestyle is
   - ❑ Very hectic
   - ❑ Moderately busy/controllable
   - ❑ Calm/quiet

7. Does anyone in your family have special needs?
   ❑ Yes ❑ No
   If yes, please specify
   ____

8. Is anyone in your home allergic to animals?
   ❑ Yes ❑ No
   If yes, please specify:
   ____

9. Are there any major family changes in your near future?
   - ❑ Birth of a child
   - ❑ Household move
   - ❑ Schedule change
   - ❑ Marital change
   - ❑ Other:______________

Part 2: Care and Maintenance

10. You live
    - ❑ In a house
    - ❑ In an apartment
    - ❑ On a farm
    - ❑ Other:

11. What is your approximate yard size?
    - ❑ Large (acre or more)
    - ❑ Medium
    - ❑ Small
    - ❑ No yard to speak of

12. What type of fencing is around your yard?
    - ❑ Chain-link
    - ❑ Invisible fence
    - ❑ Privacy
    - ❑ No fence

13. Where will your pet spend most of his time?
    - ❑ Indoors
    - ❑ Outdoors
    - ❑ 50/50

14. How will a pet be managed in your back yard?
    - ❑ Fence
    - ❑ Tie-out
    - ❑ Not sure

15. What will your pet's indoor areas include?
    - ❑ Full access to rooms
    - ❑ Limited access to rooms
    - ❑ Allowed on furniture
    - ❑ Allowed on some furniture

16. Where will your pet sleep?
    - ❑ Crate
    - ❑ Their own bed
    - ❑ Family member's bed
    - ❑ Outside
    - ❑ Other

17. How long will your pet be left alone during the day?
    - ❑ <1 hour
    - ❑ 4 hours or less
    - ❑ 8 hours or less
    - ❑ >8 hours
    - ❑ Variable

18. Where will your pet be kept when you are not home?
    - ❑ Crate
    - ❑ Outside
    - ❑ Free access to house
    - ❑ Specific room

19. How much time do you plan on interacting with your dog daily?(training, playing, grooming, exercise, etc.)
    - ❑ <1 hour
    - ❑ 1–2 hours
    - ❑ >3 hours

20. Prioritize three activities you would like to do with your pet (jogging, swimming, training, etc.):
    1)

    2)

    3)

21. How often will you walk your pet off your property for mental stimulation?
    - ❑ Twice a day
    - ❑ Once daily
    - ❑ Once weekly
    - ❑ Less than once a week

22. Who will be in charge of feeding your pet?
    - ❑ Family takes turns
    - ❑ Adult
    - ❑ Child under 18 years

23. Who will be in charge of clearing up after the pet?
    - ❑ Family takes turns
    - ❑ Adult
    - ❑ Child under 18 years

Canine and Feline Behavior for Veterinary Technicians and Nurses, Second Edition. Edited by Debbie Martin and Julie K. Shaw.

Companion website: www.wiley.com/go/martin/behavior

24. How often do you plan to train your pet?
 - ❑ Multiple times a day
 - ❑ Multiple times a week
 - ❑ Occasionally
 - ❑ As little as possible

25. If acquiring a puppy will you take it to socialization classes?
 - ❑ Yes
 - ❑ No
 - ❑ Unsure, more information needed

26. Do you plan on crate training your pet?
 - ❑ Yes
 - ❑ No
 - ❑ Unsure, more information needed

27. Who will be responsible for administering your pet's medical care (medication etc.)?
 - ❑ Family takes turns
 - ❑ Adult
 - ❑ Child under 18 years

28. Would you prefer to have your pet trained:
 - ❑ Without assistance
 - ❑ With the help of a private trainer
 - ❑ Group training class
 - ❑ Leave pet at a training facility
 - ❑ Unsure, need more information

29. What will you do with your pet on occasions when you travel?
 - ❑ Take pet on trip
 - ❑ Board the pet
 - ❑ Hire a pet sitter
 - ❑ Other

Part 3: Financial Considerations

30. How much are you budgeting monthly for your pet's food?
 - ❑ $50 or less
 - ❑ $100 or less
 - ❑ more than $100

31. How much are you willing to pay for your pet?
 - ❑ Free
 - ❑ Less than $50
 - ❑ Less than $100
 - ❑ Less than $500
 - ❑ Less than $ 1000
 - ❑ $1000 or more

32. Do you plan on spaying/neutering your pet?
 - ❑ Yes
 - ❑ No
 - ❑ Unsure, need more information

33. How much are you budgeting to spend *annually* on your pet's medical care?
 - ❑ Less than $200
 - ❑ $200–$300
 - ❑ $301–$400
 - ❑ More than $400
 - ❑ Whatever is necessary

34. Which of the following pet sources are you considering?
 - ❑ Reputable breeder
 - ❑ Animal shelter/humane society
 - ❑ Breed rescue organization
 - ❑ Pet store
 - ❑ Other

Part 4: Pet Characteristics

35. What other animals (not your own) will your pet interact with?
 - ❑ Dogs
 - ❑ Cats
 - ❑ Other
 - ❑ Often
 - ❑ Rarely
 - ❑ Never

36. Primary purpose for obtaining your pet
 - ❑ Adult's pet
 - ❑ Family pet
 - ❑ Child's pet
 - ❑ Breeding
 - ❑ Show
 - ❑ Hunting
 - ❑ Protection
 - ❑ Farm/outside pet
 - ❑ Other

37. Breeds you are considering
 1)
 2)
 3)

38. Has someone in your household owned a puppy less than 6 months of age?
 - ❑ Yes
 - ❑ No

 How long ago?

39. What age would you like your pet to be when you acquire it?
 - ❑ As young as possible
 - ❑ 8 weeks
 - ❑ 6 months or older
 - ❑ Adult

40. Are you interested in training your pet?
 - ❑ Yes, I look forward to training my pet
 - ❑ No, I would like a pet that requires little training

41. House-training problems
 - ❑ Could live with problem
 - ❑ Would do whatever it takes to correct the problem
 - ❑ Problem would prompt me to part with the pet

42. Shyness with people
 - ❑ Could live with problem
 - ❑ Would do whatever it takes to to correct the problem
 - ❑ Problem would prompt me to part with the pet

43. Aloofness with family
 - ❑ Could live with problem
 - ❑ Would do whatever it takes to correct the problem
 - ❑ Problem would prompt me to part with the pet

44. Excitability
 - ❑ Could live with problem
 - ❑ Would do whatever it takes to correct the problem
 - ❑ Problem would prompt me to part with the pet

45. Demands attention
 - ❑ Could live with problem
 - ❑ Would do whatever it takes to correct the problem
 - ❑ Problem would prompt me to part with the pet

46. Jumping on people
 - ❑ Could live with problem
 - ❑ Would do whatever it takes to correct the problem
 - ❑ Problem would prompt me to part with the pet

47. Digging/yard destruction
 - ❑ Could live with problem
 - ❑ Would do whatever it takes to correct the problem
 - ❑ Problem would prompt me to part with the pet

48. Chewing/destruction
 - ❑ Could live with problem
 - ❑ Would do whatever it takes to correct the problem
 - ❑ Problem would prompt me to part with the pet

49. Excessive vocalization
 - ❑ Could live with problem
 - ❑ Would do whatever it takes to correct the problem
 - ❑ Problem would prompt me to part with the pet

50. How often do you plan to groom your pet at home?
 - ❑ Daily
 - ❑ Weekly
 - ❑ Monthly
 - ❑ As infrequently as needed

51. How important is it to you that your pet "guards your home"?
 - ❑ Very important
 - ❑ Important
 - ❑ Not important
 - ❑ Do not want a guard dog

52. What size pet do you prefer?
 - ❑ Micro (less than 5 lbs.)
 - ❑ Very small (less than 10 lbs.)
 - ❑ Small (11–25 lbs.)
 - ❑ Medium (26–50 lbs.)
 - ❑ Large (51–90 lbs.+)
 - ❑ Giant (greater than 90 lbs.)
 - ❑ No preference

53. How important is it to you that your pet wants to sit on your lap, follow you around, etc.?
 - ❑ Very important
 - ❑ Important
 - ❑ Not important
 - ❑ Would rather have an independent dog

54. Would you have your pet professionally groomed?
 - ❑ Yes
 - ❑ No
 - ❑ Occasionally

55. How much does hair on your clothing or furniture bother you?
 - ❑ Can't tolerate
 - ❑ Can tolerate somewhat
 - ❑ Does not bother me

56. Please list any questions or concerns you may have:

____

____

____

____

____

Appendix 20
Canine breeder interview questions

Canine breeder interview questions	
	What was this breed bred to do? (lap dogs, guard dogs, etc.)
	Are the dogs from a working line or a show line?
	Will we be able to meet the parents of our puppy?
	What made you choose this sire?
	What made you decide to breed this particular bitch?
	How often do you breed your bitches?
	How many litters has this bitch had?
	What has been her history with litters? (Was she a good "Mom"?)
	How many puppies are in the litter?
	At what age do you allow the puppies to go to homes?
	What type of environment are the puppies kept in? (kennel, house, etc.)
	What type of environmental enrichment do you have for the puppies?
	How much exposure do the puppies have currently with people? How often are the puppies handled by people?
	Is this bitch good with children?
	Is the sire good with children?

Canine and Feline Behavior for Veterinary Technicians and Nurses, Second Edition. Edited by Debbie Martin and Julie K. Shaw.

Companion website: www.wiley.com/go/martin/behavior

	What behavior or temperament traits do you feel are most important in this breed?
	Are there any behavior or temperament traits you try to decrease in this breed when you considered which bitch and sire to use? What are those traits?
	Are there any common breed-specific behavior problems seen in this breed?
	Do you encourage deviations from breed standards? (i.e. off colors, smaller than standard size)
	What health issues are common in this breed?
	What breed deviations, orthopedic issues, or other health problems have you seen in your particular line?
	Do you have your dogs OFA certified (or other breed-specific health screens)?
	Are your dogs bred to be working dogs? (i.e. Do you have dogs that are service dogs, herding dogs, guard dogs, etc.)
	Who is the breeder's veterinarian and would it be OK for you to speak to the veterinarian?
General considerations	
	Did the breeder "interview you" by asking you questions pertaining to your lifestyle and why you want this particular breed?
	Was the breeder open to your questions or defensive?

The PowerPoint of figures, appendices, MCQ's are available at www.wiley.com/go/martin/behavior

Appendix 21

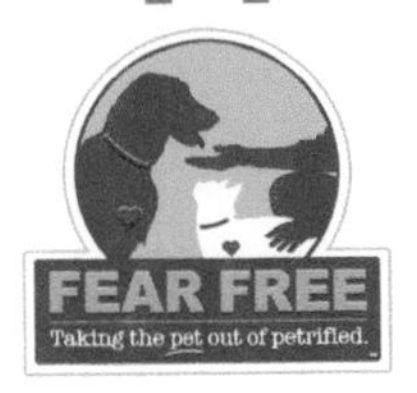

Veterinary hospital scavenger hunt **CANINE**

First and Last Name: ____________________

Date: __________ **Phone:** __________ **Email:** __________

Dog's Name: ____________________

As part of promoting Fear Free® veterinary visits, our hospital encourages you to visit us with your canine companion just for fun. We have put together a scavenger hunt of activities to help create a successful fun visit. Once you complete the card, turn it in at the hospital to be entered into our monthly drawing for a prize. To build positive memories with the veterinary hospital, we recommend frequent fun visits. You may complete a fun visit and enter the drawing as often as once a day.

As long as your dog does not already have an existing fear of the veterinary hospital, this will be a fun and appropriate game for you to play together.

> The scavenger hunt starts with at home preparation. Make sure your dog is relaxed and comfortable with travel in the car. Using a crate or dog seat belt are safe options for car travel. Acclimate your dog to the seat belt and/or crate by incorporating yummy treats with these things. A long lasting food storage toy stuffed with frozen canned dog food, may keep your dog preoccupied and relaxed during the entire car travel. During transport, a non-slip surface should be utilized to prevent your dog from sliding. Bring your dog's favorite treats, toys, and grooming brush (if your dog enjoys being brushed). Prepare the car so it promotes a calming environment; calming familiar music, calming scents, and cool or warm the car to room temperature before putting your dog in the car.

Preparing for the visit:

- ❑ Dog is hungry
- ❑ 50 to 100 very small favorite treats. Treats should be no larger than a half of a pea. You might not use all of them but you should count on using at least 40. Better to have too many than not enough.
- ❑ Favorite toys and/or grooming brush
- ❑ Your dog is acclimated to car travel and is relaxed during transport
- ❑ Your dog has an opportunity to relieve himself before getting in the car
- ❑ The car is properly prepared; calming familiar music, calming scents, appropriate temperature, non-slip surface, long lasting food storage device

Canine and Feline Behavior for Veterinary Technicians and Nurses, Second Edition. Edited by Debbie Martin and Julie K. Shaw.

Companion website: www.wiley.com/go/martin/behavior

When you arrive:

- ❑ Give your dog a small ¼-inch treat once you park
- ❑ Check with front office team members before coming into the hospital with your dog
- ❑ Verify your dog is relaxed

List 3 to 4 indicators that your dog is relaxed:

1. ______________________________
2. ______________________________
3. ______________________________
4. ______________________________

  - ❑ Give 2 or 3 small treats to your dog upon approaching the building
  - ❑ Give 2 or 3 small treats to your dog for entering the lobby. Reinforce calm behavior frequently (every 5–20 seconds) while waiting to go into an exam room.

Scale:

- ❑ Allow your dog to get on the scale by himself; keep the leash loose
- ❑ Either toss some treats on the scale or if your dog knows how to follow a hand target, cue him onto the scale and give him a treat.

In the exam room:

The goal is to make the exam room a fun and relaxing place for your dog. Engage your dog in some of his/her favorite activities. Offer your dog special treats to help create a pleasant association with the exam room. Work at your dog's pace.

- ❑ Allow your dog to explore the room at his/her own pace
- ❑ Offer treats, toys, and brushing with calm and relaxed attention from you

> Find the following Fear Free® environmental enhancements we have made in our hospital waiting area and/or exam room to create a pleasant experience for you and your dog:

- ❑ What type of music do you hear? ____________

  A slow tempo of piano music may have a calming effect on you and your dog
- ❑ We utilize calming scents in our hospital. Identify and list a calming scent and/or pheromone you see being used in our hospital.

  Scent/pheromone: ____________________

  Location: ____________________
- ❑ What type of lighting are we using to create a more relaxed and calm atmosphere?

  Lighting type: ____________________

  Location: ____________________
- ❑ We try to provide your dog with non-slip surfaces in our hospital. Identify one that you see in the exam room or lobby.

  ____

Team Member Interactions

Our team is specially trained to make our interactions with your dog as pleasant as possible. When meeting a dog, it is best to let them make the first move. Playing hard to get, will indicate to your dog that we are not threatening. Here are some things you should see us do when first interacting with animals in the hospital. Check off each interaction you see and include the team member's name or initials.

- ❑ __________ Avoid direct eye contact
- ❑ __________ Turn sideways to appear smaller and less threatening

- ❑ ____________ Allow the pet to approach rather than approaching the pet
- ❑ ____________ Move smoothly and calmly
- ❑ ____________ Talk slowly and softly (spa-like tone)
- ❑ ____________ Use treats with interactions

The PowerPoint of figures, appendices, MCQ's are available at www.wiley.com/go/martin/behavior

Appendix 22

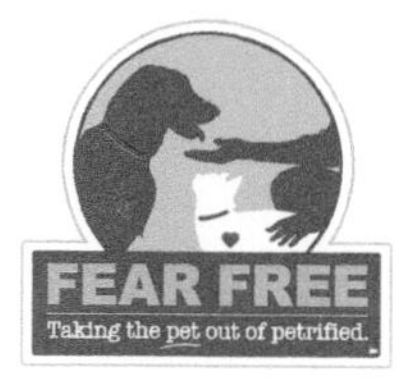

Veterinary hospital scavenger hunt **FELINE**

First and Last Name: ______________________________

Date: ____________ **Phone:** ____________ **Email:** ____________

Cat's Name: ______________________________

As part of promoting Fear Free® veterinary visits, our hospital encourages you to visit us with your feline companion just for fun. We have put together a scavenger hunt of activities to help create a successful fun visit. Once you complete the card, turn it in at the hospital to be entered into our monthly drawing for a prize. To build positive memories with the veterinary hospital, we recommend frequent fun visits. You may complete a fun visit and enter the drawing as often as once a day.

As long as your cat does not already have an existing fear of the veterinary hospital, this will be a fun and appropriate game for you to play together

The scavenger hunt starts with at home preparation. Make sure your cat is relaxed and comfortable in his/her carrier. Keep the carrier out at all times and incorporate some of these techniques to create a carrier oasis: put the cat's favorite things around the carrier, play with the cat around the carrier, place a pheromone infused towel or bed and/or an object of clothing permeated with your scent inside the carrier, place treats, catnip, and toys inside, feed the cat in or near the carrier. Let your cat enter the carrier on his/her own. You can teach your cat to enter the carrier on cue to earn a food reinforcer or toss a treat or toy into the carrier. During transport, a non-slip surface should be in the carrier and under it to prevent the cat or carrier from sliding. The floorboard behind the passenger seat is the most secure location for your cat's carrier. When carrying your cat in the carrier, be sure to minimize movement. Try to keep it still. If possible, rather than holding it by the handle, carry it from the bottom. Bring your cat's favorite treats, toys, and grooming brush (if your cat enjoys being brushed). Prepare the car so it promotes a calming environment; calming familiar music, calming scents, and cool or warm the car to room temperature before putting your cat in the car.

Preparing for the visit:

- ❑ Cat is hungry
- ❑ Favorite treats, toys, and/or grooming brush are packed
- ❑ Your cat is acclimated to a carrier and will enter on his/her own
- ❑ Carrier is properly prepared (non-slip surface, calming scents, secured in car)
- ❑ Minimize carrier movement by holding the carrier by the bottom instead of handle if possible
- ❑ Prepare the car; calming familiar music, calming scents, appropriate temperature

Canine and Feline Behavior for Veterinary Technicians and Nurses, Second Edition. Edited by Debbie Martin and Julie K. Shaw.

Companion website: www.wiley.com/go/martin/behavior

When you arrive:

- ❑ Check with front office team members before coming into the hospital with your cat
- ❑ Verify your cat is relaxed

List 3 to 4 indicators that your cat is relaxed:

1. ____
2. ____
3. ____
4. ____

In the exam room:

The goal is to make the exam room a fun place for your cat to be. Engage your cat in some of his/her favorite activities. Offer your cat special treats to help create a pleasant association with the exam room. Work at your cat's pace.

- ❑ Allow your cat to come out of the carrier on his/her own. Open the door and have a non-slip surface for the cat to step onto. If your cat prefers to stay in the carrier, that is fine. Give some treats to your cat in the carrier.
- ❑ Allow your cat to explore the room at his/her own pace
- ❑ Offer treats, toys, and brushing with calm and relaxed attention from you

> Find the following Fear Free® environmental enhancements we have made in our hospital waiting area and/or exam room to create a pleasant experience for you and your cat:

- ❑ What type of music do you hear? ________________

  A slow tempo of piano music may have a calming effect on you and your cat
- ❑ We utilize calming scents in our hospital. Identify and list a calming scent and/or pheromone you see being used in our hospital.

  Scent/pheromone: ________________________

  Location: ________________________
- ❑ What type of lighting are we using to create a more relaxed and calm atmosphere?

  Lighting type: ________________________

  Location: ________________________
- ❑ We try to provide your cat with non-slip surfaces in our hospital. Identify one that you see in the exam room.

  ____

Team Member Interactions

Our team is specially trained to make our interactions with your cat as pleasant as possible. When meeting a cat, it is best to let them make the first move. Playing hard to get, will indicate to your cat that we are not threatening. Here are some things you should see us do when interacting with animals in the hospital. Check off each interaction you see and include the team member's name or initials.

- ❑ __________ Avoid direct eye contact
- ❑ __________ Turn sideways to appear smaller and less threatening
- ❑ __________ Allow the pet to approach rather than approaching the pet
- ❑ __________ Move smoothly and calmly
- ❑ __________ Talk slowly and softly (spa-like tone)
- ❑ __________ Use treats with interactions

> The PowerPoint of figures, appendices, MCQ's are available at www.wiley.com/go/martin/behavior

Appendix Section 2
Training Exercises

The appendices can be downloaded and printed at www.wiley.com/go/martin/behavior

Appendix 23
Acclimatizing a pet to a crate

1. Crate should be located in commonly used areas of the home.
2. Always give a treat for going into the crate.
3. A food stuffed storage device will entertain a pet for a longer period of time.
4. Hide treats daily in the confinement area. When the pet explores the area he will begin to believe in the crate fairy.
5. Going into the confinement area should always be fun. Use an upbeat tone and attitude rather than a threatening or scolding manner when confining a pet.
6. Never punish a pet by sending him to his crate.
7. Supply appropriate toys in the confinement area.
8. Feed the pet's meals in the crate with the door opened or closed.
9. Minimize the length of time the pet is in his confinement area by offering scheduled breaks. Excessive confinement can result in hyperactivity.
10. When first introducing the crate, the pet should be allowed to explore it at his own pace. Reward the pet with readily consumed treats for showing interest in the crate.
11. Clicker training utilizing shaping can be an easy and fun way to teach a pet to enter a kennel on cue.

    Video 7.3 on the companion website illustrates introducing a puppy to a crate.

The PowerPoint of figures, appendices, MCQ's are available at www.wiley.com/go/martin/behavior

Canine and Feline Behavior for Veterinary Technicians and Nurses, Second Edition. Edited by Debbie Martin and Julie K. Shaw.

Companion website: www.wiley.com/go/martin/behavior

Appendix 24
Elimination training log

Time	Walking outside on leash in backyard, record urine/stool	Feed	Walk around the block	Train using small food treats
6 am				
7 am				
8 am				
9 am				
10 am				
11 am				
12 pm				
1 pm				
2 pm				
3 pm				
4 pm				
5 pm				
6 pm				
7 pm				
8 pm				
9 pm				
10 pm				

Walk outside every hour when home during the day, feed twice a day, walk around the block twice a day, train twice a day.

The PowerPoint of figures, appendices, MCQ's are available at www.wiley.com/go/martin/behavior

Canine and Feline Behavior for Veterinary Technicians and Nurses, Second Edition. Edited by Debbie Martin and Julie K. Shaw.

Companion website: www.wiley.com/go/martin/behavior

Appendix 25

Shaping plan for teaching a dog to ring a bell to go outside to eliminate

Shaping plan for teaching a dog to ring a bell to go outside to eliminate	
Hold a bell on a string directly in front of the dog's nose	C/T head turn toward bell
	C/T nose or paw touching bell
Dog may begin using paw to move bell	
Before taking dog outside to eliminate (may need to keep on a leash to prevent wandering) hold the bell directly in front of him	Dog touches bell, door opens as reward, outside to eliminate
Hang bell at door, before taking dog outside (may need to keep on leash at door) wait for dog to orient to bell	Any orientation to bell and door opens as reward, outside to eliminate
	Continue raising criteria gradually for more movement of the bell before going outside
Dog may begin ringing the bell any time he would like to go out to play	Initially, take the dog out every time he rings the bell, then begin only taking him out when you suspect he may have to eliminate, and ignore other times. Make sure the dog is provided adequate social and exploratory activities.

C/T: click then treat.

The PowerPoint of figures, appendices, MCQ's are available at www.wiley.com/go/martin/behavior

Canine and Feline Behavior for Veterinary Technicians and Nurses, Second Edition. Edited by Debbie Martin and Julie K. Shaw.

Companion website: www.wiley.com/go/martin/behavior

Appendix 26

Preventive handling and restraint exercises

Handling

1. The dog should be calm and relaxed before starting the exercise. Attend to changes in body language at all times.
2. The dog should have previous clicker training experience and understand the association between the click and treat delivery.
3. Use small easily consumed treats and have your clicker ready.
4. Keep sessions short; 1–3 minutes.
5. Go slow and make it fun and positive (a negative experience could have a long-lasting negative consequence).
6. Desensitization and counter conditioning will be utilized to facilitate relaxation with handling.
7. Begin by touching the dog gently in a neutral location for 1 second. Click while touching him. Remove your hand. Give the dog a treat. Always start with your hand touching the dog in a neutral location, such as the shoulder or neck. Glide your hand to other body parts while assessing response.

   Body parts to touch and pair with food include

head	mouth
ears	neck
nose	shoulders
back	flank
tail	elbows
chest	legs
belly	feet

8. After the dog is relaxed and comfortable with you gently touching him for 1 second on the various body parts, then increase to 2, 3, 4 seconds, and so on. Vary the length so it does not always get longer and longer.
9. Gradually increase the pressure of the touch and decrease the duration of contact. Reset duration to 1 second. Click while you are touching, then remove your hand, and offer a treat. Gradually increase the level of pressure.
10. Use one hand to touch and the other hand for the clicker. Avoid clicking near the dog's ears.

Canine and Feline Behavior for Veterinary Technicians and Nurses, Second Edition. Edited by Debbie Martin and Julie K. Shaw.

Companion website: www.wiley.com/go/martin/behavior

Restraint

1. The dog should be calm and relaxed before starting this exercise. Consider starting on the floor or you may use a table for a small dog. Use a non-slip surface. Attend to changes in body language at all times.

2. Use special, readily consumed treats such as canned cheese. Have your clicker ready.

3. The dog should have previous clicker training experience and understand the association between the click and treat delivery.

4. Keep sessions short; 1–3 minutes.

5. Go slow and make it fun and positive (a negative experience could have long-lasting negative consequences).

6. Gently place an arm around your dog and click. Release and offer a treat. Arm goes over his back and under the belly/chest.

7. Progress to cradling with one arm over his back and under his belly/chest and the other arm under his neck.

8. With each consecutive repetition, gradually increase the pressure and/or duration.

9. If while performing these exercises, your dog *mildly* struggles (1 or 2 seconds) to get down:

   - Continue to hold him. (Note if the dog is panicking then it is best to release him rather than waiting.)
   - Say nothing.
   - Wait until he calms down.
   - Give him a treat.
   - Put him down.

   Next time progress slower to avoid stress and struggling.

If struggling for more than 3 seconds, release rather than waiting for your dog to calm down. If your dog has shown aggression or extreme fear with restraint, do not attempt these exercises.

Video 7.5 on the companion website illuminates the process of acclimating a dog to restraint.

The PowerPoint of figures, appendices, MCQ's are available at www.wiley.com/go/martin/behavior

Appendix 27
Preventive food bowl exercises

1. Other pets in the household should be out of sight or confined before implementing the exercise.

2. Place a few kibbles in the bowl and place the bowl on the ground. Allow the dog to eat *all* the food. Pick up the empty bowl and place a few more kibbles in the bowl. Repeat until the entire meal is fed. If the dog knows a "sit" cue you may ask him to sit prior to lowering the bowl.

3. Another variation: Start with a few kibbles in the bowl and as the dog is eating add a few more kibbles to the bowl until the entire meal is fed.

4. Toss a special treat into the bowl from a distance as you enter the room in which the dog is eating. This teaches the dog that human presence means something better will fall from the sky. It is a positive association with your presence.

   If a dog has shown aggression toward people over food in the past, do not attempt this prevention exercise.

   Video 7.6 on the companion website details playing the food bowl game with a young puppy.

The PowerPoint of figures, appendices, MCQ's are available at www.wiley.com/go/martin/behavior

Canine and Feline Behavior for Veterinary Technicians and Nurses, Second Edition. Edited by Debbie Martin and Julie K. Shaw.

Companion website: www.wiley.com/go/martin/behavior

Appendix 28
Teaching tug

1. The game should be initiated by bringing out a specific tug toy that is not always available to the dog. Using a 3–4 ft tug toy or a toy with a rope attached to it, allows the toy to be further from the person and helps prevent the dog accidently making contact with the person's hand while learning the game.

2. Give the verbal cue "take it" and present the tug toy. Move the tug toy slightly back and forth to foster interest or chase.

3. When the dog has the toy in his mouth, engage him in a gentle game of tug. Verbally reward his interest in the tug. Move the tug gently back and forth rather than up and down.

4. Freeze (stop tugging and any toy movement). Give the verbal cue "drop it" and prompt the release with a treat directly under the dog's nose. Reward with the treat for dropping the toy. Pick up the toy. If the dog is over aroused and unable to release the toy, calm down the level of tugging or verbal encouragement initially. Also consider a less exciting toy.

5. Add the cue, "sit" or "down," and reward the behavior with "take it" and presentation of the tug toy. This helps to control the dog's arousal.

6. Repeat the above steps. Eventually, you will delay your presentation of the treat after giving the "drop it" cue so that the treat does not need to prompt the behavior. Still reward dropping the item with a treat or the "take it" cue.

7. When the game is over, give the dog several treats and place the tug toy out of sight.

The PowerPoint of figures, appendices, MCQ's are available at www.wiley.com/go/martin/behavior

Canine and Feline Behavior for Veterinary Technicians and Nurses, Second Edition. Edited by Debbie Martin and Julie K. Shaw.

Companion website: www.wiley.com/go/martin/behavior

Appendix Section 3
Samples and Letters

The appendices can be downloaded and printed at www.wiley.com/go/martin/behavior

Appendix 29

Canine behavior plan of care sample

Consultation Date: 1-1-14

Client's Name: Mary and Betty　Phone: 555-1212　Email: maryandbetty@happy.com

Address: 555 Happy Drive　City: Happy town　State: Oregon　Zip: 55555

Dog's Name: Roo　Age: 3 years　Breed: Redtick　M ☐ Mx ☐ F ☐ Fx■

Canine Behavioral Diagnosis		
Aggression	**Target of aggression**	☐
☐ Conflict induced	☐	☐
☐ Possessive	☐	**Ingestive**
☐ Disease/pain induced	☐	☐ Coprophagia
■ Fear/defensive induced	☐	☐ Pica
☐ Idiopathic	**Fear/Anxiety disorders**	☐ Predatory behavior
■ IDA + motivation	■ Generalized anxiety	**Eliminative**
☐ IDA-H + motivation	☐ Global fear	☐ Housesoiling
☐ Alliance induced	☐ Separation anxiety	☐ Urine marking
☐ Status induced	☐ Sound/thunderstorm phobia	☐ Excitement urination
☐ Learned	☐ Specific fear or phobia	☐ Extreme fear/appeasement urination
☐ Maternal/hormonal induced	☐ Acute conflict behaviors/stereotypy	**Other**
☐ Play induced	☐ Compulsive disorder	☐ Cognitive dysfunction
☐ Redirected	Specific fear(s) or phobia (s) noted:	☐ Hyperexcitability
☐ Territorial	■ strangers	☐ Conditioned unwanted behavior
☐	■ unknown dogs	☐

Prescribed treatment plan (see back for details and further information)		
Management	**Training**	☐ Shape relaxation
■ Avoid triggers	■ Marker training	☐ Leave it/ drop it
■ Ignore attention-seeking behaviors	☐ Lure reward training	☐
☐ Ignore at specific times	☐ Other training	☐
■ Cue→response→reward interactions	☐ Agility training	☐
☐ Environmental modifications	☐ Concept training	☐
☐	☐ K9 Nose Work® training	☐
	☐ Crate/confinement training	**Behavior modification** (see back)
☐ Crate confinement	☐	■ Counter conditioning
☐ Other confinement	☐	▣ On walks if needed
☐	**Training tools**	▣ When other dogs are present
☐ Umbilical cord	■ Head halter	☐
■ Change primary caregiver	☐ Basket muzzle	☐
☐ Increase mental stimulation	☐ Other muzzle	☐
■ Walk off property	☐ Body harness	■ Response substitution
☐ Aerobic exercise	☐ Front clip harness	▣ On walks if needed
☐ Regular schedule	☐ Anxiety clothing	☐
☐ Dietary change	☐ Calming cap	☐
☐ Meal feed twice daily	☐ Drag line	☐
☐	☐ Tether	☐
☐	☐ Interactive toys/puzzles	☐ Systematic desensitization

Canine and Feline Behavior for Veterinary Technicians and Nurses, Second Edition. Edited by Debbie Martin and Julie K. Shaw.

Companion website: www.wiley.com/go/martin/behavior

Other	☐ Pheromones	☐
☐ Interruption of behavior	☐ Remote reward	☐
☐ Cease punishment	**Specific behaviors to train**	☐
☐ Remote punishment	■ Targeting	☐
☐ Grief counseling	■ Attention	☐
☐ Rehoming patient	☐ "Look" and "Watch"	☐ Other
☐	■ Sit ■ Down ☐ Recall	☐
☐	■ Loose leash walking	☐
☐	■ Go to a place	☐

Bite history

Has the dog bitten? ■ yes ☐ no Does the dog redirect aggression? ☐ yes ☐ no

How severe were the bites? Did not make contact ■ Did not break skin ☐ Puncture ☐ Medical care needed ☐

Does the dog give warning before biting? ☐ yes ☐ no ☐ unknown

Note known triggers and other significant bite history:
Very defensive warning, would prefer to run

Medical conditions and medications

No known medical issues, normal blood chemistry profile and thyroid profile. We have started Roo on Fluoxetine 1 mg/kg q 24 hr (once daily). There may be a decrease in appetite short term. Please report back to me routinely with changes in behavior.

Comments and treatment details

Helix,
Thank you so much for assessing Roo for us. We agree with your assessment and feel very lucky to have your on our behavior team.
My name is Nancy and I am Dr. Happy's technician. I will be working to help coordinate communication and treatment.
From your astute observations and what history we were able to obtain we agree Roo seems to have poor social skills that are aggravated by her generalized anxiety. She will become aggressive but it certainly isn't her first choice for getting out of a situation.

1) Avoid triggers – this will be almost impossible to do until the medication begins to take effect
2) Marker training to build confidence (we are thrilled she is not afraid of the clicker)
3) We are going to ask Mary and Betty to ignore all three dogs unless they are interacting with them in a cue→response→reward format (please reinforce that behavior in Mary and Betty!) until their next appointment. There is tension between the dogs and we'd like to decrease any potential alliance that may be developing while Roo's medication takes effect.
4) They can train Roo and tether Cocoa and Misty in the room. Cocoa and Misty get tossed treats just for being in the room with Roo. (CC) Either have Roo on leash or the other dog's on the other side of a barrier to prevent Roo from running after a tossed treat intended for the other dogs.
5) On walks when another dog approaches use foundations skills and CC to turn away from the approaching dog. A head halter may be required. That is your choice.

We are intentionally keeping the treatment plan short at this time. We'd like to recheck Roo in one month to reassess how she is doing on the medication and then add further aspects to the treatment plan.

Please call anytime and we look forward to working with you on this and other behavior cases.
Dr. Happy and Nancy Happyday, RVT

Dr. Happy 1-1-14

Veterinarian signature: Date:

The PowerPoint of figures, appendices, MCQ's are available at www.wiley.com/go/martin/behavior

Appendix 30
Sample field assessment

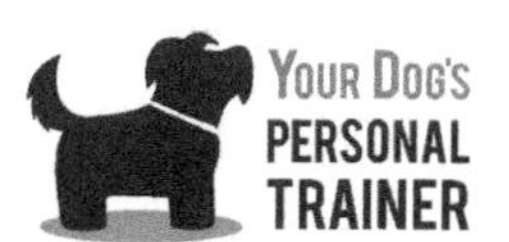

Mary – Owner, 60 years old. Female
Betty – Owner, 55 years old. Female, pending shoulder surgery

Owner concerns

1. Aggression toward unknown dogs
2. Relationship with other dogs in the household
3. Aggression toward unknown people.

Signalment and history: Roo (patient)

Roo is a three-year-old spayed female Redtick Coonhound adopted from a shelter at approximately five months of age. In her time following adoption, she experienced a number of aversive experiences regarding other dogs and people:

- approx. six months of age – attacked by two Poodles
- approx. seven months of age – attacked by a dog being fostered by the household
- approx. nine months of age – attacked by a Pit Bull
- approx. two years of age – attacked by a Boston Terrier who latched onto an ear
- whipped and beaten off in two separate incidents following Roo's charging at strangers
- almost two years of shock collar training regarding her triggers (bikers, joggers, skateboarders, other dogs, other people). Betty and Mary subsequently learned this made things worse for Roo and have stopped using the shock collar.

***Despite the above history, Roo has no bite history with humans or dogs.

History: Misty (housemate)

Misty is a four-year-old spayed female (probably) Springer Spaniel/Pointer mix. She was adopted from a shelter at approximately one year of age. Betty and Mary have worked hard to rehabilitate her and have had huge success in that endeavor.

History: Cocoa (housemate)

Cocoa is a two-year-old neutered male Lab–Border Collie mix who was adopted from a shelter 11 months ago.

None of the dogs have been to formal training classes. Betty and Mary are seeking help at this time due to having to keep Roo away from people and other dogs, the possibility of serious altercations if they don't keep her away and the increasing difficulties with interactions among the dogs in the home. They feel there is a growing tension between the dogs within the household.

Canine and Feline Behavior for Veterinary Technicians and Nurses, Second Edition. Edited by Debbie Martin and Julie K. Shaw.

Companion website: www.wiley.com/go/martin/behavior

Medical information

It is reported that none of the dogs have any ongoing medical issues at this time.

Assessment – Meeting observations

We met for the assessment at their home. Betty and Mary have developed many routines for taking care of their dogs' physical needs, such as runs in a nearby field, leash walks, hide-it games, and household "cuddle times".

Roo

Roo was reported to be the dog whose issues are a priority for them. Roo charged into the room to greet me with, at first, no barking. She was eagerly taking treats although she exhibited intense wrinkling of the forehead and a tightly pulled forward commissure. One of my movements startled her and she jumped back, weight shifted over her rear, barking with an almost closed mouth.

In subsequent barking at me, her body weight was shifted well forward with mouth puckered and wrinkled forehead. It was understandable that members of the public would feel threatened upon being rushed in this manner. Roo has been beaten in two incidents when she was off leash in public and charged at people barking in this manner.

As I worked with Roo doing some clicker training, I observed her easily startle with flicks of my hand to toss a treat. Each time she startled she would jump back with the above described body language and barking. Throughout my two-hour assessment with her, she responded in this "never relaxed" fashion the entire time. She jumped at slight hand movements, my moving my head back (very small movement), to my lanyard dangling on the clicker, to my turning my body. She was NEVER relaxed. Betty and Mary report that Roo responds in this manner to many ordinary events that happen suddenly in her environment. In other words, there are multiple triggers for Roo's intense reactions and these are often events that cannot be controlled, prevented or managed.

I attempted a bit of impromptu counter conditioning to the sight of my lanyard. With a dog who has a mild fear response to an item, one can expect to see forward progress in a trial session such as this. In the case of Roo, I observed signs that counter conditioning to hanging straps would be possible. I believe she was reacting more to the quick movements than to the lanyard itself.

Throughout the two-hour assessment, Roo had moments of relaxed body features and facial features. She appeared to be a completely different dog at those times. However, those times did not last very long as another triggering event would occur.

I consider Roo to be exhibiting conflict-related responses. Because there are so many triggers, it's possible she is in a frequent state of anxiety and conflict (she wants to interact but her fear takes over).

In the course of my visit, we sat on living room furniture discussing the dogs while the dogs carried on their normal interactions. In observing Roo's interactions with her housemates, I observed that she does not give appropriate communication to the young dog, Cocoa. By observing Cocoa, I conclude he's not getting the information he needs from Roo as he persists in unacceptable behaviors until Roo suddenly has had enough and then attacks.

In my experience, I have observed other dog pairs with this type of interaction. Owners presume the issue is "dominance" or "bullying." I suspect that Roo's underlying anxiety and poor social skills lead to a much greater than necessary "correction," which then leads to an actual fight between the dogs.

Misty

My observations of Misty were of a relaxed dog, eager to greet, eager to work with a stranger. She has certainly come a long way from her described fear issues of the past. Betty and Mary are doing "happy visits" to the veterinarian's office to help Misty learn to be more comfortable there. Clicker training will give them a big boost forward in that process. I observed ordinary self-control issues with Misty such as grabbing treats roughly and jumping on me excitedly. These can easily be smoothed out in training sessions focused on teaching her what TO do in given situations.

Cocoa

Cocoa is just approaching the age of social maturity. Because none of the household dogs are effective communicators, there are no peace-keepers in the group. Cocoa, being the youngest, appears to me a bit adrift as a result. He continues to badger the other dogs to play with him. Misty can communicate to him with subtle head or body turns that she isn't interested and he does respond to those – IF the entire context is one of low stimulus. When there's too much arousal and activity, he loses the ability to pay attention to the subtleties of communication.

I am concerned about his being described as biting the throats of the other dogs. I did not observe an example of this at this time.

Assessment of responses to another dog when on leash

Roo was assessed on leash, starting at about a distance of 80 feet, with both a lifelike, stuffed dog on leash and a live Bearded Collie on leash. In both cases, Roo alerted to the other dog and gave off moderate excited barking indicating, to me, curiosity. We closed distance in both cases significantly without evoking her typical reactive response. Her typical response was not observed. However, using Betty and Mary's observations of Roo's responses to me in their home, I have a good sense of her reaction to certain dogs when spotted in public. I have enough information to know that she does have a threshold distance we can work with and that there are low-level dogs we can use for establishing a baseline of acceptable responses.

Current problems to be addressed

1. Roo's responses to triggers are frequent and they involve triggers that cannot be easily controlled. Addressing this underlying anxiety would be the first step.***See **Specific concerns**
2. Roo's responses to her two major triggers – humans and dogs – when on leash and in public.
3. Building inter-dog communication skills.

Current training and management plan

- **CLICKER TRAINING** (marker-based training) as a fast, efficient communication tool ("that's it, what you are doing right now is what I want")
- **FOUNDATION SKILLS**
  These are tools that will be used in the introductions to other people and to other dogs. These will also be used for teaching a household relaxation mode that will not only help Roo's anxiety and the other dogs' over-arousal, but will aid Betty in her recuperation from surgery. These will likely be a review for the dogs in some cases. Nevertheless, it's important to have a very large reinforcement history for these skills so that Betty and Mary can count on the dog being able to respond in real-life, arousal-packed situations. These foundation skills are:
  - **Relaxation on a mat** to be used as a safety zone and a signal that now it's time to bring down the arousal level and become calm again.
  - **Attention to the handler** under ever-increasing challenges, volunteered by each dog, until it becomes habit.
  - **Leave it** – the ability to break off from that which the dog is about to do. This is very helpful in interrupting a reactive response before it even starts.
  - **Instant name response, sit, down, target to hand.**

- **PUBLIC SKILLS**
  These are skills that will be used in behavior modification exercises involving other dogs. They are also the skills needed for navigating leash walks in the neighborhood. These skills are:
  - **Fast and fun about turn with loose leash walking**
  - **Learning to read the precursor signs** that predict a reactive response is not far behind.

Interactions with Betty and Mary and current status of the human–animal bond

All three dogs are well cared for and interacted with. It's obvious how much Betty and Mary care for their dogs and the time they put into giving them a good life. With Betty's increasing shoulder difficulties, culminating in surgery in December, there needs to be a more relaxed, calm nature to the household and that can be taught to the dogs rather than continual attempts to impose it by Betty and Mary. It is obvious Betty and Mary are deeply bonded to Roo.

Betty and Mary use food treats in training and the dogs respond to two or three trained cues when no triggering events are occurring. They are committed to improving the dog–dog interactions in their household.

***Specific concerns

After observing Roo in her home environment, it is my profesional opinion that Roo's general anxiety is inhibiting her learning process and causing conflict and significant anxiety between her and the other dogs in the household. I am concerned that the stress could potentially lead to serious relationship issues down the road between the housemates. I am recommending Betty and Mary take Roo to their veterinarian for an examination, behavioral diagnosis and treatment plan that may or may not include anxiolytic medications.

I would very much like to assist with helping Betty and Mary in the application of the prescribed treatment plan and look forward to working with the hospitals behavior team in Roo's follow-up care.

Source: Printed with permission:
Helix Fairweather, Karen Pryor Academy Certified Training Partner
Your Dog's Personal Trainer
helixfairweather@gmail.com

The PowerPoint of figures, appendices, MCQ's are available at www.wiley.com/go/martin/behavior

Appendix 31
Sample of a pet selection report

The husband of a family consisting of wife, 38 years old, husband, 49 years old, and two daughters, 8 and 11 years old, sought assistance with obtaining a dog for the family. This will be their first dog. The client was sent a pet selection questionnaire to be completed by the entire family.

Questionnaire results

The financial consideration part of the questionnaire revealed that the client was willing to spend $1000 or more on the purchase of a dog. They wanted to obtain a puppy from a reputable breeder. They were also willing to pay "whatever is necessary" on annual medical costs and would budget $100 or less monthly for food. They would like more information on neutering.

The questions pertaining to pet characteristics revealed that they were interested in a dog for the children, one that requires little training, and they would like to obtain the dog as young as possible. They would be willing to do "whatever it takes to correct the problem" should the dog develop house soiling issues, shyness with people, aloofness with family members, attention-demanding behavior, jumping on people, digging, destructive chewing, or excessive vocalization. They could live with a dog that is excitable. It was not important to them that the dog guard the house. They were planning to devote time to grooming the dog at home weekly and also have it professionally groomed routinely. They wanted a small dog less than 10 lbs. It was important to them that the dog would want to sit on their lap. They would not tolerate hair on clothing or furniture. Three breeds of dogs that they were considering: Maltese, Cavalier King Charles Spaniel, and Mini-Havanese.

Consultation

A two-hour in-home appointment was performed and the following information was provided in writing and discussed with the entire family:

Recommendations:

❑ Suggested breed options:
- Miniature Poodle:
  - Pros: Small, lively, playful, bright, attentive, usually (should be) good with people and other animals, variety of colors, does not shed
  - Cons: Barking, joint or eye problems, grooming, may be difficult to find a good breeder
- Maltese:
  - Pros: Very small, bright, playful, usually (should be) good with people and other animals, does not shed
  - Cons: FRAGILE, difficult to house train, barking, grooming, medical concerns (orthopedic, liver)
- Havanese:
  - Pros: Small but sturdy, playful, entertaining, does not shed
  - Cons: Difficult to house train, barking, grooming, very expensive ($2500), not a large breeding stock (potential for genetic problems)

Canine and Feline Behavior for Veterinary Technicians and Nurses, Second Edition. Edited by Debbie Martin and Julie K. Shaw.

Companion website: www.wiley.com/go/martin/behavior

- Bichon Frise:
  - Pros: Small but sturdy, does not shed, does not require much exercise, usually (should be) good with people and other animals
  - Cons: Difficult to house train, barking, grooming, skin problems
- Yorkie:
  - Pros: Small, lively, curious, does not need extensive exercise
  - Cons: FRAGILE, excitable (terrier), barking, difficult to house train, grooming

❑ Male versus female

❑ Choosing a breeder:
- NEVER buy a puppy from a pet store! No reputable breeder will sell his/her puppies to a pet store.
- Poor breeders:
  - Not interested in improving the breed and does not care about breed standards
  - AKC registration does not guarantee quality
  - Breeds 3+ different breeds
  - Dogs are kept or managed in kennels or in separate building
- Good breeders:
  - Know and follow breed standards
  - Know health issue of the breed
  - They want to tell you everything about their dogs
  - Understand puppy development and puppies are properly socialized
  - Will not sell the puppy until it is at least eight weeks old
  - Choose prospective owners carefully
  - Encourage you to meet the puppy's parents
  - Willing to give references
  - Have done medical testing and provide written proof that the sire and dam are free of potential genetic medical problems associated with the breed
- Breeder quiz:
  - What are the breed standards?
  - What are the common health issues for the breed?
  - What testing has the breeder done with the Sire and Dam prior to breeding?
  - How old are the puppies' parents?
  - What made the breeder decide to breed these two dogs?
  - What is the history of the breed?
  - What environment are the puppies kept in?
  - What is their socialization/enrichment/handling program for the puppies?
  - At what age are the puppies allowed to go to their new home?
  - Ask for references from the breeder's veterinarian and owners of dogs previously bred by the breeder

❑ Things to do before bringing the puppy home:
- Set a routine or schedule for feeding and walking. A chart can be very helpful especially if multiple people will be sharing the responsibility.
- Small breed dogs may need to be fed three times a day until four months old to avoid hypoglycemia
- Purchase a crate and maybe also an exercise pen
- Purchase food (breeder should send some home with you)
- Purchase food and water bowls
- Purchase a collar and leash
- Purchase two or more Kong toys or other food storage toys
- *Puppy Start Right: Foundation Training for the Companion Dog* by Kenneth and Debbie Martin
- Decide and write down "Rules of the House"
- Have Karo syrup on hand in case of a hypoglycemic event
- Schedule an appointment with a veterinarian within a few days of obtaining the dog
- Consider using the Adaptil® diffuser (dog-appeasing pheromone) near the kennel

- ❑ Things to look for in a puppy
  - Should be excited to meet new people
  - Should eagerly approach you, tail wagging, and curious
  - A shy or fearful puppy will become worse as it gets older
  - Hair coat should be shiny and clean
  - Eyes and nose should be clean and clear (no discharge)
- ❑ Problem prevention:
  - Socialization!!!!
  - House training
  - Crate training
  - Play biting
  - Food bowl safety
  - Prevent fear of the veterinary hospital/groomer

Resources

Books

Culture Clash by Jean Donaldson

Living with Kids and Dogs. . .Without Losing Your Mind by Colleen Pelar, CPDT

Puppy Start Right: Foundation Training for the Companion Dog by Kenneth and Debbie Martin

Puppy Training for Kids by Sarah Whitehead

On Talking Terms with Dogs: Calming Signals by Turid Rugaas

Websites

Some websites for potential breeders in the geographical area of the client were provided.

Follow-up

After the consultation, the client decided they would look for a female Maltese puppy. They were interested in obtaining a puppy in the next two to three months. It was stressed during the consultation that Malteses can be difficult to house train due to their size. The owners understood this and were interested in pursuing the breed.

The clients hired me to help them find a reputable breeder. I contacted a breeder who was within 1.5 hours of the client and engaged in actively showing their dogs in conformation. The owner of the kennel spoke with me for over 40 minutes. He was eager to discuss his dogs. He stated that in the past 15 years of breeding Malteses, they had had one dog with a liver shunt and 10 patent ductus arteriosis. They screen for patella luxation. He gave me several veterinary references.

The breeder stated that they do not let their puppies leave until they are at least 12 weeks old. He felt they were able to provide better socialization than most pet owners and was also attempting to prevent separation anxiety. He allows the bitch to wean the puppies. Puppies and the bitch stay in the house and have exposure to people and household sounds. They are also taken outside in exercise pens on grass for short periods of time each day. They currently had four litters about two to three weeks apart. They would be ready to be adopted in about two months. The breeder was open to a visit from me or the family.

After talking with my client about the breeder, I recommended that I visit the breeder's home and meet some of their dogs. An hour visit in the breeder's home was performed. The puppies and bitches were very clean. The adult dogs were friendly and eagerly jumped into my lap. The breeder gave me a tour through the kennel area adjoining the home to allow me to meet the male dogs. Although they barked, they appeared friendly and outgoing. The facility was clean and the dogs were taken care of appropriately. They owned a total of 18 dogs. Some were old (16–18 years old) retired show dogs that were living as pets in the home. I was pleased with the visit and recommended the owners contact the breeder to obtain a puppy. The cost of the dog was more than the owner had anticipated, but the client was willing to pay the price.

The clients visited the breeder about two weeks later and were shown a four-month-old female that had been at a friend's house. I advised the client that I would be concerned about the socialization history, house training and why it was returned to the breeder. I contacted the breeder and determined the dog had been sold as the pick of the litter and was being co-owned by the breeder. However, she was "low in the legs." Her patellas were good but she was not going to be the correct proportion for conformation. She had been managed in the kitchen at the previous home and was trained to pee pads.

The breeder would have another 12-week-old female available in the middle of May. I discussed the pros and cons of obtaining a four-month-old puppy. Although I encouraged the owner to wait for the younger puppy, I left the decision to the client. The client decided to obtain the four-month-old puppy.

Five training appointments were performed over a 1.5-month period. The entire family attended each appointment. The parents and girls were taught how to teach "Riley" to sit, down, come, leave it, drop it, place (go to bed), stay, and walk on a loose leash using lure reward and clicker training. The biggest challenge for the owner was the house training. Management and prevention options were discussed at each appointment. Two months after obtaining (the dog was now six months of age) "Riley," she was only having occasional urine accidents in the house (~3 times a week). Stool was always outside in the designated elimination area.

A follow-up email from the owner nearly two years after obtaining the dog, revealed that the dog was completely house trained and a terrific companion for the family. The husband reported, "My two biggest concerns were sleeping through the night and pottying outside. She does great at both of these. She does seem to bark a lot but we were forewarned by you about this."

Discussion

Although a four-month-old Maltese would not have been my first pick for this family, they were educated on the pros and cons of a variety of small-breed dogs that would fit their desires. Consequently, they were able to make an informed decision and set realistic expectations for their canine companion.

Provided courtesy of Debbie Martin, LVT, VTS (Behavior)

The PowerPoint of figures, appendices, MCQ's are available at www.wiley.com/go/martin/behavior

Appendix 32

Dr. Andrew Luescher's letter regarding puppy socialization

To Whom It May Concern:

This letter's purpose is to define Purdue University's recommendations for Puppy Class protocols.

The main objectives of puppy classes are exposure and desensitization to potentially frightening stimuli, socialization, and the teaching of appropriate dog–owner interaction. Although simple commands are trained as well, obedience training is not a main objective of puppy classes.

Puppies go through well-defined developmental stages. Puppy classes are designed to utilize the sociability of young puppies. **However, the socialization period of dogs ends at around 12–14 weeks of age.** Up to that age, puppies can readily learn not to fear new things, and to develop appropriate social behavior. If this opportunity to shape puppy behavior is missed, the puppies are likely to show behavior disturbances later in life. **Therefore, in order to maximize the benefits of puppy classes, puppies should be enrolled at 7–10 weeks of age if possible, the sooner the better.**

The puppy classes at Purdue University's Animal Behavior Clinic start any time between 7 and 14 weeks of age *and* at least 10 days after initial vaccination for the Distemper/Parvo combination and Bordatella. We encourage the use of an intranasal Bordatella/Parainfluenza (+/− Adeno) combination and the use of a high-titer, low-passage Parvo vaccination. These should be vaccinations administered after a thorough veterinary exam. Several vaccines are currently on the market, which meet these requirements.

Trainers and veterinarians have had concerns about placing puppies at risk in an environment where they may pick up an infectious disease. As with anything, one must always weigh the risks and benefits. "Puppy cuteness" only lasts so long and many more puppies currently lose their homes due to behavior reasons than die of viral diseases.

We are aware of only one Parvo problem in a puppy preschool class in Minnesota in the early 90s and none since high titer Parvo vaccines gained mainstream use in 1995. There have been no Puppy Class participants infected with Parvo virus in any puppy classes offered at Ohio State or Purdue University. These are both facilities that treat high humane society caseloads and numerous Parvo cases annually.

Preliminary investigations underway at the University of Pennsylvania suggest that low-level exposure to pathogens, like what might occur in a clean although not completely sterile environment, may actually promote a "stronger" or more responsive immune system (verbal communication with Dr. Karen Overall, dipl ACVB 1998).

Canine and Feline Behavior for Veterinary Technicians and Nurses, Second Edition. Edited by Debbie Martin and Julie K. Shaw.

Companion website: www.wiley.com/go/martin/behavior

Let's welcome new puppies into our society by showing them what we expect, not dispose of them because we failed to communicate our expectations at a time when the puppies are most impressionable.

Sincerely,

Andrew Luescher, DVM, PhD, Diplomate ACVB
Director, Animal Behavior Clinic, Purdue University

Steve Thompson, DVM, Diplomate ABVP,
Certified in Canine/Feline Practice
Director, The Pet Wellness Clinic, Purdue University

The PowerPoint of figures, appendices, MCQ's are available at www.wiley.com/go/martin/behavior

Appendix 33
Dr. R.K. Anderson's letter regarding puppy socialization

TO: My Colleagues in Veterinary Medicine:

Common questions I receive from puppy owners, dog trainers, and veterinarians concern:

1. What is the most favorable age or period of time when puppies learn best?
2. What are the health implications of my advice that veterinarians and trainers should offer socialization programs for puppies starting at 8 to 9 weeks of age?

Puppies begin learning at birth and their brains appear to be particularly responsive to learning and retaining experiences that are encountered during the first 13 to 16 weeks after birth [Dr. Anderson is saying that the prime time for puppy socialization stops somewhere between 13 and 16 weeks, although more socialization occurs after that time]. This means that breeders, new puppy owners, veterinarians, trainers and behaviorists have a responsibility to assist in providing these learning/socialization experiences with other puppies/dogs, with children/adults and with various environmental situations during this optimal period from birth to 16 weeks.

Many veterinarians are making this early socialization and learning program part of a total wellness plan for breeders and new owners of puppies during the first 16 weeks of a puppy's life – the first 7–8 weeks with the breeder and the next 8 weeks with the new owners. This socialization program should enroll puppies from 8 to 12 weeks of age as a key part of any preventive medicine program to improve the bond between pets and their people and keep dogs as valued members of the family for 12–18 years.

To take full advantage of this early special learning period, many veterinarians recommend that new owners take their puppies to puppy socialization classes, beginning at 8 to 9 weeks of age. At this age they should have (and can be required to have) received a minimum of their first series of vaccines for protection against infectious diseases. This provides the basis for increasing immunity by further repeated exposure to these antigens either through natural exposure in small doses or artificial exposure with vaccines during the next 8–12 weeks. In addition the owner and people offering puppy socialization should take precautions to have the environment and the participating puppies as free of natural exposure as possible by good hygiene and caring by careful instructors and owners.

Experience and epidemiologic data support the relative safety and lack of transmission of disease in these puppy socialization classes over the past 10 years in many parts of the United States. In fact, the risk of a dog dying because of infection with distemper or parvo disease is far less than the much higher risk of a dog dying

Canine and Feline Behavior for Veterinary Technicians and Nurses, Second Edition. Edited by Debbie Martin and Julie K. Shaw.

Companion website: www.wiley.com/go/martin/behavior

(euthanasia) because of a behavior problem. Many veterinarians are now offering new puppy owners puppy socialization classes in their hospitals or nearby training facilities in conjunction with trainers and behaviorists because they want socialization and training to be very important parts of a wellness plan for every puppy. We need to recognize that this special sensitive period for learning is the best opportunity we have to influence behavior for dogs and the most important and longest lasting part of a total wellness plan.

Are there risks? Yes. But 10 years of good experience and data, with few exceptions, offers veterinarians the opportunity to generally recommend early socialization and training classes, beginning when puppies are 8 to 9 weeks of age. However, we always follow a veterinarian's professional judgment, in individual cases or situations, where special circumstances warrant further immunization for a special puppy before starting such classes. During any period of delay for puppy classes, owners should begin a program of socialization with children and adults, outside their family, to take advantage of this special period in a puppy's life.

The PowerPoint of figures, appendices, MCQ's are available at www.wiley.com/go/martin/behavior

Appendix 34
Sample puppy socialization class curriculum[1]

[1] With permission from Kenneth and Debbie Martin from Puppy Start Right for Instructors online course via www.karenpryoracademy.com

All classes are approximately one hour in length and meet once a week. After completing orientation, owners then complete four classes with their puppy.

Orientation presentation

Orientation allows for the human participates to learn about what to expect in puppy class and is a prerequisite to attending class with a puppy. Ideally orientation should be offered weekly in order to enroll new puppies immediately.

Orientation covers

- class format and what to expect
- socialization defined
- introduction to clicker training
  - begin to teach attention and targeting at home
- positive proactive socialization
- body language and signs of fear
- what to do if my puppy is afraid
- successful canine parenting
- positive behavior solutions
- what to bring to class.

Health and handling class

- Health and handling class includes the following topics:
- Training topic: Sit
- Problem prevention and behavior solutions topics
  - Crate/confinement training
  - Handling and restraint
  - Muzzle training
  - Elimination training.

Canine and Feline Behavior for Veterinary Technicians and Nurses, Second Edition. Edited by Debbie Martin and Julie K. Shaw.

Companion website: www.wiley.com/go/martin/behavior

Wheels and children's toys class

Wheels and children's toys class includes the following topics:

- Training topic: Loose leash walking
- Problem prevention and behavior solutions topics
  - Counter surfing and stealing objects
  - Digging
  - Independence training
  - Hide and seek or Find it game.

Obstacles and sounds class

Obstacles and sounds class includes the following topics:

- Training topic: Leave it and drop it
- Problem prevention and behavior solutions topics
  - Play biting/mouthing
  - Gotcha game (collar grab)
  - Food bowl exercise.

Costumes and appearances class

Costumes and appearances class includes the following topics:

- Training topic: Recall/come
- Problem prevention and behavior solutions topics
  - Chewing
  - Jumping
  - Spay and neuter.

The PowerPoint of figures, appendices, MCQ's are available at www.wiley.com/go/martin/behavior

Appendix 35
Sample kitten class curriculum

Each class is approximately 1 hour in length. Kittens should be less than 14 weeks of age when starting class.

Week 1 Topics

Feline communication and body language

Appropriate owner–kitten play with toys

Litter box preferences and recommendations

Environmental enrichment

Handling for routine at home medical care

Teaching a come when called

Week 2 Topics

Importance of daily routine

Acclimating a kitten to a harness and leash

Scratching

Multi-cat household recommendations

Reintroduction of cats after a vet visit

Handling for routine at home medical care AGAIN!

Teaching sit and high five

The PowerPoint of figures, appendices, MCQ's are available at www.wiley.com/go/martin/behavior

Canine and Feline Behavior for Veterinary Technicians and Nurses, Second Edition. Edited by Debbie Martin and Julie K. Shaw.

Companion website: www.wiley.com/go/martin/behavior

Index

Canine and Feline Behavior for Veterinary Technicians and Nurses, Second Edition. Edited by Debbie Martin and Julie K. Shaw.

Companion website: www.wiley.com/go/martin/behavior

W

Z